SLEEP AND ITS DISORDERS.

Volume 14 in the Series

Major Problems in Neurology
SIR JOHN WALTON, TD, MD, DSc, FRCP
Consulting Editor

OTHER MONOGRAPHS IN THE SERIES

SLEEP
AND ITS DISORDERS

J.D. PARKES
MD FRCP

Reader in Neurology
University Department of Neurology
King's College Hospital and Institute of
Psychiatry, London
and
Honorary Consultant Neurologist
King's College Hospital and Maudsley
Hospital, London
ENGLAND

1985
W. B. Saunders Company   London   ·   Philadelphia   ·   Toronto
Mexico City   ·   Rio de Janeiro   ·   Sydney   ·   Tokyo   ·   Hong Kong

W. B. Saunders Company 1 St Anne's Road
Eastbourne, East Sussex, BN21 3UN, England

West Washington Square
Philadelphia, PA 19105, USA

1 Goldthorne Avenue
Toronto, Ontario M8Z 5T9, Canada

Apartado 26370—Cedro 512
Mexico 4, D.F. Mexico

Rua Evaristo da Veiga 55, 20° andar
Rio de Janeiro – RJ, Brazil

9 Waltham Street
Artarmon, N.S.W. 2064, Australia

Ichibancho Central Building, 22–1 Ichibancho
Chiyoda-ku, Tokyo 102, Japan

10/fl, Inter-Continental Plaza, 94 Granville Road
Tsim Sha Tsui East, Kowloon, Hong Kong

First published 1985

Typeset by Phoenix Photosetting, Chatham
Printed in Great Britain by Mackays of Chatham Ltd

British Library Cataloguing in Publication Data

Parkes, J.D.
  Sleep and its disorders.—(Major problems
in neurology; v. 14)
  1. Sleep disorders
  I. Title   II. Series
  616.8'49   RC547

  ISBN 0-7216-1858-8

CONTENTS

Colour plates appear between pages 40 and 41

Foreword

'Sleep that knits up the ravell'd sleave of care', as Lady Macbeth put it, has long been something of a medical mystery. Mechanisms which induce and control it and determine its length, nature and content have long exercised the interest of physiologists, philosophers and practising doctors as well as psychologists, poets and writers of prose. The remarkable advances resulting from new knowledge of physiological processes acquired through electrophysiological studies in man and animals, as well as through greater understanding of endocrine and biochemical processes and their influence upon the brain, have solved many mysteries though there are still a great many more yet to be elucidated. As new knowledge has emerged, it has thrown new light upon those clinical disorders of the sleep mechanisms which have long been recognized, such as narcolepsy, sleep paralysis and various forms of hypersomnia to name but three, and slowly we are beginning to learn more about processes such as dreaming and circadian rhythms along with disorders such as the familiar jet lag which result when these are disturbed.

Thus I would regard the publication of a monograph dealing with sleep and its disorders as being timely, and I believe that Dr. David Parkes has produced a volume which will stand as the authoritative work of reference for many years to come. Readers of former volumes published in this series will at once recognize that this book is longer than any we have previously included, but this has been the result of a deliberate decision since this work is not only exceptionally comprehensive and detailed, with abundant references to the relevant literature, but it is remarkably up-to-date, thoughtful and scholarly. Nuggets of fascinating historical information abound throughout its lively text and are invariably brought into context by reference to modern scientific thinking, research and experiment. Despite its scope and the remarkable amount of detail that it contains about anatomy, physiology, psychology, biochemistry and pharmacology, as well as clinical neurology, I have found it to be splendidly, clearly and logically organized and immensely readable and entertaining. I am in no doubt that scientists in many fields and doctors working in a wide range of specialties will find it exciting and illuminating, as I have done, and will feel the need to turn to its pages often in the future for reference purposes. Dr. Parkes has done his profession an outstanding service by writing it.

SIR JOHN WALTON
Oxford
February, 1985

Preface

This book is in three sections. The first describes the biology of normal sleep; the second, diseases of sleep in man; and the third, the treatment of these diseases. The first two sections aim to be a comprehensive guide for physicians interested in sleep, whilst the third section contains exact details about the treatment of sleep–wake disorders.

Most of what we know about sleep has been learned since 1953, when REM sleep was first recognized. Major developments in the last quarter century have included the discovery of sleep apnoea, the development of benzodiazepines, the recognition of the extraordinary association between human leucocyte antigens and narcolepsy, and the expansion of sleep laboratory medicine, particularly in the USA. The classification of sleep disorders in 1979 was a major milestone.[1]

The new and rapidly expanding field of sleep disorder medicine stems directly from the pioneering research work of sleep laboratories, and the establishment of definitive recording techniques.[2] However, these facilities are scarce and expensive, and we have nothing in the UK to match California, Texas or New York. The problem is therefore to know best how these scarce resources should be used. The general physician is capable of diagnosing and treating the vast majority of patients with sleep disorders without over-relying on sleep laboratory diagnostic studies. Of course patients with special problems may be referred to appropriate specialists. From the clinical viewpoint, the indications for sleep laboratory investigations are minute. Only sleep apnoea and sleep myoclonus, as elicited by the history, warrant further sleep laboratory diagnostic studies.[3]

The psychiatric aspects of sleep disorders have sometimes received too little attention. Every sleep disorder centre needs a psychiatrist far more than an EEG machine. We are indeed fortunate at King's College Hospital in having Brian Toone, Hilary Nissenbaum, and their colleagues, to whom I owe an enormous debt of gratitude.

Despite the advances in sleep research of the last quarter century, a great deal was known about sleep even in Old Testament times. Much of this historical knowledge is still valuable today, despite the absence of detailed EEG studies at the start of the encephalitis lethargica epidemic in 1917–1927, or for example in one of the first patients with akinetic mutism described by Cairns in 1952, a girl of 14 with a cyst in the third ventricle. It is surely as important to know that encephalitis lethargica may have been responsible for the rise of National Socialism in Germany as that rapid eye movements are not continuous throughout the rapid eye movement phase of sleep. The terms often used by patients to describe their sleep, such as 'good' and 'bad', 'deep' and 'light', are less easy to define than the electrophysiological terminology of sleep, but both types of information have to be considered in any book about sleep.

A note on the illustrations. These mainly concern the biological function of sleep and the reality of sleep disorders rather than the pattern of electrical discharge from the brain during sleep and wakefulness. A few pictures are included which highlight popular conceptions as well as fallacies about sleep, from Rip van Winkle to Charlie Brown.

I would like to dedicate this book to the memory of two great physicians, Bob Schwab from Boston, and Pierre Passouant from Montpellier. I owe my first interest in sleep research to Bob Schwab. During a visit to Boston to learn of the secrets of Parkinson's disease, Bob gave me a very large sealed tin to take home, containing, he said, enough material to treat all the post-encephalitic parkinsonians in Britain. In retrospect, I suspect that the activities of the FDA had limited his use of the contents. I later found that I had taken, unknowingly and undeclared, several kilograms of levamphetamine through both the USA and UK customs. Our last meeting, just before his death, was enjoyable as any, and we shared instead of the usual lettuce sandwich a gigantic meal of reindeer steak. This may have been unwise, since Bob was a bad diabetic. His illness gave him a special concern for patients with long-term diseases, both narcolepsy and parkinsonism. Pierre Passouant, the Director of the Laboratory of Experimental Medicine at Montpellier, was more cautious than Bob Schwab, although the two men were great friends. Pierre Passouant's approach was highly scientific, and he produced over a quarter of a century a series of outstanding reviews of sleep problems. I remember with gratitude the enthusiastic teaching and personal kindness of both these physicians.

I am deeply grateful to many friends and colleagues who helped to write this book. Foremost amongst these are Nicola Langdon, who critically reviewed each chapter over countless cups of coffee, and Peter Rose, who traced nearly all the references about sleep anatomy. Many readers and referees, known and unknown, made helpful suggestions about individual chapters, EEG technology and the sleep of their children. These included William Gardner, Peter Robson, Alan Bennett, Martin Rossor, Robin Manser, Graham Kennedy, Maureen Woolley, Peter and Pam Asselman, and John Rothwell. Many colleagues unhesitatingly allowed me to use their illustrations. My thanks are also due to the library staff at King's College Hospital Medical School, and to Jean Kilshaw for cheerful and unremitting help in tracing obscure and old references, and to Mrs. Elizabeth Nash and Mrs. Lesley Gibson for numerous typings of the manuscript.

This book would not have been written without the continuous help and encouragement, as well as the editorial skills, of Nicholas Dunton and David Cross of W. B. Saunders, and Sir John Walton, to all of whom I am most grateful.

REFERENCES

1. Association of Sleep Disorder Centres. Diagnostic classification of sleep and arousal disorders, *Sleep* (1979) **2**, 1–137.
2. Guilleminault, C. (ed.) *Sleeping and Waking Disorders, Indications and Techniques*, Menlo Park, California: Addison-Wesley (1982) 435 pp.
3. Kales, A., Kales, J.D. & Soldatos, C.R. Insomnia and other sleep disorders, *Med. Clin. North. Am.* (1982) **66**, 971–991.

PART I

NORMAL SLEEP

CHAPTER 1

NORMAL SLEEP, ITS VARIANTS AND RELATED STATES

INTRODUCTION

Waking, not sleeping, is considered to be the normal state for mankind, but this is not so in all animals. Regular cycles of rest and activity occur during fetal development, even perhaps in the human fertilized ovum. Newborn babies spend more than half their lives asleep, mostly in the rapid eye movement (REM) state, but as we get older we sleep less and much of our deep sleep is lost by three score years and ten. Young adults spend about a third of their lives asleep and a tenth dreaming. Like human infants, young animals of many species sleep a lot more than do the old, but the sleep habits and patterns of animals, irrespective of age, are very different from those of humans. A well fed domesticated cat, but not a wild cat, spends only a quarter of its entire life awake, and both the gorilla and the opossum possibly less than a fifth. At the other extreme are many birds such as the albatross, which, unless they sleep whilst flying, may spend 99% of their lives awake. As well as the time spent sleeping, the ways in which animals sleep vary widely. Rapid eye movement sleep occurs in most of the mammals and birds that have been investigated, although this sleep phase has not been recognized in either the spiny anteater, considered to be a very primitive animal, or the dolphin, one of the most advanced. Indeed, the dolphin has unihemisphere sleep, slow activity localized to one or other hemisphere alone. Environment and life style largely determine these different patterns, and the winter torpor of hibernating animals commences with slow-wave sleep. So various are the patterns of sleep throughout the animal kingdom, that it is disturbing to consider this from the viewpoint of man alone.

No-one knows what sleep is for. One record for going without any sleep at all and without any serious consequence is held by a man from San Diego who achieved this for 11 days. Some psychologists have believed that the bounds of consciousness extend vaguely in sleep to cover not only the whole past life of the sleeper, but the whole consciousness of the species, and even its predecessors. Hall thus accounted for the fact that the best and most honest of men sometimes execute in their dreams the most dishonest and cruel deeds.[8] This theory appears unlikely. However, there is no doubt that our waking performance, vigilance and vigour, our health and happiness, the whole quality of our waking lives are profoundly affected by the way we sleep. Some of these features can be measured, but others, such as peace of mind,[9] cannot. Sleep has many functions. As well as providing restoration for the mind, good sleep seems essential for our bodies. One of the most important functions of sleep, as shown by the high prevalence of sleep in the young of all species, may be the promotion of learning and brain development. Perhaps even the achievement of waking consciousness, the 'knowledge of what passes within our own minds' is dependent on sleep.

The exact anatomical basis of sleep, waking and the sleep–wake cycle as well as the neurotransmitters involved are not known. Pharmacologists have hunted with little success for sleep 'juices'. Despite much attention to 5-hydroxytryptamine (5-HT) and catecholamines, other neurotransmitters may be of more importance for sleep control and over 20 different peptides and other neurotransmitters occur in a single cubic centimetre of brain stem. Recently, the calcium antagonist nifedipine and benzodiazepine antagonists have been shown to possess intrinsic alerting activity. Vasoactive intestinal peptide (VIP) has been located in the major contender for the role of central body clock, the suprachiasmatic nucleus, and melatonin is being given to jet pilots in an attempt to reset body rhythms after transmeridian flights.[1]

Poor sleep is sometimes viewed as the root of many different human ailments whilst waking, these ailments being as diverse as dementia and fibrositis.[17] Much of the normal physiology of sleep remains unexplained, and the reason for many of the parasomnias, which occur in children more often than adults, is unknown. Although these are not psychiatric disorders, the Church still attempts to banish incubi, terrors-by-night, with prayer; there is no doubt that behavioural therapy is sometimes effective in preventing night terrors. Notable achievements in sleep research in the last decade include recognition of the importance of breathing disorders during sleep, and the practical application of knowledge of man's circadian rhythms, obtained from experiments in caves and cellars, to everyday work schedules, including those of doctors as well as of nuclear submarine crews. During the same period, there has been a steady increase in knowledge of many sleep disorders.

This introduction describes basic facts about behaviour and electrophysiology during sleep and dreaming in animals and man, and explores some theories about the nature of sleep.

NATURE OF SLEEP

All known animals and plants, even unicellular amoebae, have regular cycles of activity and rest. These are determined by *external* factors, day and night, and other changes in the environment, but also by *internal* pacemakers or biochemical clocks. Only higher animals, mammals and man, have regular sleep–wake cycles as opposed to rest–activity cycles. The old idea that sleep is simply a time of rest for the organ of wakefulness[25] is clearly incorrect.

Von Economo, working in a Viennese psychiatric clinic, observed two opposite syndromes in patients seen at the start of the 1917–1927 encephalitis lethargica epidemic. One group of patients slept too much. At autopsy they had lesions mainly in the mesencephalic tegmentum and posterior hypothalamus. A second group, insomniac patients, had lesions mainly in the forebrain. These observations led von Economo to the concept of a *wakefulness centre* in the posterior hypothalamus, and a *hypnogenic centre* in the basal forebrain.[27, 28] At the time these ideas were not widely accepted, not least because of the diffuse rather than focal nature of pathology in encephalitis lethargica. Nevertheless, later studies have confirmed von Economo's ideas (see Chapter 2).

At the time of Pavlov, sleep was thought to be the final result of an internal irradiation of inhibition to both hemispheres and possibly the midbrain. During this period, nothing was known of the physiology of inhibition, later recognized to be an active, not a passive, process.[23, 24] Evarts' microelectrode studies[7] on single cortical neurones in free-moving, unanaesthetized animals demonstrated beyond criticism that a general inhibition of the cerebral cortex did not occur during sleep, and finally abolished the ancient idea that sleep is a passive, not an active, process.

SLEEP STAGES

Last century, Macnish[16] suggested that there were two forms of sleep, *complete sleep* with total suppression of movement, sensation, and all mental activity, and *incomplete sleep* with retention of some mental activity, as in dreaming. However, the different stages of sleep were not clearly recognized until the development of the electroencephalogram (EEG). Bremer was the first to show striking changes in the electrical activity of the brain during sleep.[3–5] Subsequently, Loomis and his colleagues delineated five different patterns of EEG activity connected with different states or levels of sleep. This system formed the basis for all subsequent classifications of sleep stages.[12–15] The next major advance came in 1953 when Aserinsky and Kleitman reported that, during sleep, periodic rapid eye movements occurred, different from the slow rolling eye movements that had long been known to accompany the onset of sleep (Fig. 1.1).[2] These periodic eye movements were associated with dreaming by Dement and Kleitman.[6] The bursts of eye movement are now commonly called rapid eye movements (REMs), and the state of sleep REM sleep.

During the same period, evidence emerged from many laboratories, notably those of Moruzzi and Jouvet, that sleep was an active physiological process with clearly defined electrocorticographic and behavioural changes, dependent on specific neurochemical mechanisms and the activity of brain stem nuclei and areas extending from the medulla to the posterior diencephalon.[10, 18–22] 'The maintenance of wakefulness was revealed as the responsibility of a postulated ascending reticular activating system including part of the posterior hypothalamus, whilst the promotion of sleep was the pleasant task assigned to the lower brain stem and basal forebrain areas.'[26]

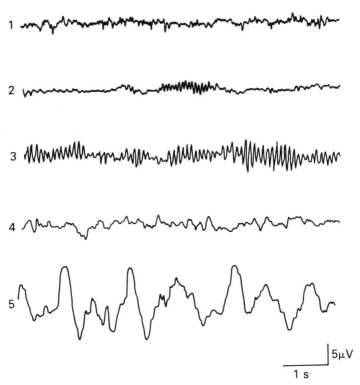

Figure 1.1   *Samples of the main EEG frequencies of interest in the different states of alertness. 1: beta activity; 2: spindle; 3: alpha rhythm; 4: theta activity; 5: delta activity. Reprinted with permission from Gaillard.*[78]

BEHAVIOUR BEFORE AND DURING SLEEP

PRE-SLEEP BEHAVIOUR IN ANIMALS

In all species, sleep is preceded by learned and instinctive behaviour designed to find a safe environment and a natural sleep posture that allows for good thermoregulation. As an example of this, both natural and electrically induced sleep in the cat are heralded by a stereotyped behaviour pattern, the animal searching for a quiet, restful and safe environment before finally curling up in a corner and going to sleep.[64] Ritual behaviour at this stage is not uncommon. The orang utan builds a sleeping platform every night before sleep commences,[68] whilst many birds, whose daily activities may be dozens of miles from their sleeping places, congregate in their hundreds to fly to a traditional sleeping tree.[45] Some animals paw the ground before lying down, and elephants prepare a genuine pillow out of soft material. Animals with bushy tails can adopt a sleep posture with the tail over the eyes, and bears sometimes hold one paw over their eyes.[41, 43–45]

SLEEP ONSET IN MAN

As in animals, both learned and unconditioned mechanisms are of great importance in determining sleep onset in man. Sleep requires the absence of sudden external stimuli, a suitable environment, the daily regular stereotypy of bedtime, and relaxation of antigravity muscles with a comfortable bed.[55] Spontaneous conditioning may explain several habits which are regarded as necessary or convenient procedures in order to fall asleep — daytime exercise more than 2 h before bedtime and sexual activity both promote sleep.

MONOTONY AND SLEEP

Rhythmic, monotonous, sensory stimulation promotes sleep.[39] Thus, a mother rocks her baby, rhythmic womb sounds may help newborn infants to rest, and Balinese masseurs tickle the soles of their clients' feet to induce sleep. However, a background of relaxed wakefulness or light drowsiness is usually required. In cats, *electrical stimulation* of group 2 afferent fibres, related to touch, hair and pressure receptors, in trains of repetitive volleys, will produce EEG synchronization and induce sleep, although stimulation of group 1 muscle afferent fibres from muscle spindles does not affect the EEG or cause drowsiness.[65, 66] *Photic stimulation* will very occasionally produce EEG and behavioural signs of sleep in man,[39] and strong afferent volleys from arterial baroceptors will cause sleep-like behaviour and EEG synchronization in animals.[53] *Skin pressure* produces behavioural sleep and EEG signs of deactivation in rabbits.[75] However, the final outcome of some of these manoeuvres is not sleep, but animal hypnosis.[34, 40, 74]

CHARACTERISTICS OF SLEEP

Piéron[63] characterized behaviour during sleep by the presence of quiescence and the absence of wakefulness, but also by an increased threshold of arousal to external sensory stimuli, and the ability to become aroused spontaneously. Sleep and waking occur at about the same time every day, and an important characteristic of sleep is this strong circadian rhythmicity. In addition, mammals have the ability to make up for lost sleep.

SLEEP POSTURE

Adler's 'Problems of Neurosis'

When we see a person sleeping upon the back, stretched out like a soldier at attention, it is a sign that he wishes to appear as great as possible. One who lies curled up like a hedgehog with a sheet drawn over his head is not likely to be a striving or courageous person, but is probably cowardly.

. . . A person who sleeps on his stomach betrays stubbornness and negativity.

(see Bates, J. *Lancet* (1942) 1, 186)

The waking posture of most infants is supine. Good sleep is dependent on a comfortable posture and both infants and adults sleep more often supine than prone.[36] Jovanovič in his book *Der Schlaf* (Barth, Munich, 1969, p. 223) reported that adult sleeping positions, in order of preference, were supine, on the right side, on the left side and on the stomach. (The combination of a heavy meal, alcohol and sleeping face upwards will predispose to obstructive apnoea in adults – see Chapter 7.)

Parmeggiani and Rabini[62] suggested that sleep posture is influenced by the need for thermoregulation, and that decreased postural muscle activity resulted from changes in the regulation of muscle innervation rather than from a generalized tendency to hypotonia. The resulting posture reduces energy expenditure to a minimum. However, frequent changes in posture during sleep do occur, and are probably necessary to prevent pressure necrosis. Postural shifts are accompanied or preceded by changes in autonomic activity.[29]

MUSCLE TONE DURING SLEEP

In man, the phasic stretch reflexes are depressed during sleep[56] as well as the H reflex,[48, 49] although there is tonic contraction of the orbicularis oculi[47] and Bell's phenomenon occurs[54] with contraction of the extrinsic muscles of the eye. Oswald[59] recalls the observation that Chinamen sleep with the eyes half closed owing to the peculiar development of the facial musculature in this race. An extensor Babinsky response sometimes occurs during both REM and NREM sleep.[31, 38] Sleep atonia, persisting into partial wakefulness, accounts for the phenomenon of sleep paralysis (see p. 202).

During REM sleep, *muscle activity* is markedly reduced, and *postural activity* in neck and intercostal muscles is absent,[50] although there is random myoclonic twitching as a result of phasic excitation of brain stem structures,[67] as well as rapid eye movements and phasic contractions of middle ear muscles.[32] Diaphragm electromyograms remain as in wakefulness.

AUTONOMIC ACTIVITY DURING NREM AND REM SLEEP

Very marked changes in parasympathetic and sympathetic activity occur during sleep, with a marked difference in behaviour of both respiration and blood pressure during REM and NREM sleep. These changes are summarized below.

NREM sleep
During NREM sleep, there is intense *myosis*,[47] *reduction in sweating* and *loss of skin galvanic responses*.[42] *Thermoregulatory* mechanisms remain intact, although set at lower levels than in wakefulness. *Core temperature* falls slightly. *Gastrointestinal mobility* and *secretion* may separately or together increase, decrease or remain unaltered.[33, 73]

Loss of sympathetic activity during NREM sleep is reflected by a *slight reduction in heart rate*, 1–2 beats/min, accompanied by a *fall in blood pressure*[30, 69] and a *fall in cardiac output*. In man, arterial pressure usually falls 10–20% during sleep, with a minimum reached 1.5–2.5 h after sleep onset, and a gradual rise to waking values towards the morning. The lowest blood pressure coincides with NREM stage 3–4 sleep, but may depend more on the time of night and sleep posture than sleep stage.[71, 72] In hypertensive subjects, blood pressure changes during sleep are usually similar to those found in normal subjects.[52]

REM sleep

Different changes occur during REM sleep. Brain temperature rises during REM sleep in animals, with a simultaneous increase in cerebral blood flow and cerebral metabolism. Despite rise in temperature, temperature regulation is impaired during REM sleep,[61] and both shivering and thermal sweating may be lost or decreased more than in NREM sleep.[46] Parmeggiani[60] has related loss of temperature control during REM sleep to changes in hypothalamic unit activity.

In the few subjects in whom cerebral blood flow has been measured during sleep, there is an increase in cortical blood flow of around 40% during REM sleep. Mangold *et al.*[57] using the Kety–Schmidt rebreathing method found that five of six subjects had a mean reduction of cerebral oxygen consumption of 11% during sleep, whereas the remaining subject had an increase of 34%. Using [133]Xenon inhalation, Sakai *et al.*[70] found that cerebral blood flow was lower in all cortical regions during NREM sleep compared with wakefulness (10–15% reduction in stages 1 and 2, 25–30% in stages 3 and 4).

Cerebral metabolism in man during REM sleep has not yet been reported using radioactive deoxyglucose and positron-emission tomographic (PET) scanning, although Kennedy *et al.*[51] studied local cerebral glucose utilization during NREM sleep in monkeys. All areas of the brain studied had an equal or lower metabolic rate in NREM sleep than in wakefulness. Also, the metabolism of cortical layers was much more homogeneous during sleep than wakefulness. The experimenters searched for a hypnogenic centre, controlling sleep onset, and with increased metabolic activity at this time in the brain of monkeys, but no such centre has yet been found.[58]

During REM sleep, heart rate and systemic arterial blood pressure generally increase with respect to NREM sleep.[35] However, both heart rate and blood pressure during REM sleep in humans are very variable, with sudden increases of systolic pressure to higher values than are recorded during wakefulness.[35] Sudden large falls, as well as increases in blood pressure, may occur, and in animals these falls are greatly enhanced after baroceptor denervation.

Fisher *et al.*[37] first demonstrated that *penile erections* occur during REM sleep.

Respiratory changes during sleep are discussed in Chapter 7.

The result of sympathetic and parasympathetic changes during REM sleep, at least in animals, is a generalized decrease in vasoconstrictor outflow involving skin, mesenteric and renal vessels.[60] All these variables show phasic, as well as tonic, changes.

ELECTROPHYSIOLOGY DURING SLEEP

NOMENCLATURE

EEG changes observed in awakening from sleep have been referred to variously as activation, desynchronization, EEG arousal or the blocking reaction. *Activation* and *deactivation*, 'facilitation' and 'withdrawal' of tone, imply historical concepts held in the 1930s, but are still terms used to describe the change from quiet sleep to relaxed or alert wakefulness and the reverse. *Synchronization* and *desynchronization* apply to EEG patterns. Overall the degree of synchronization increases with the amount of slow activity present and the degree of drowsiness. Desynchronization accompanies arousal. The slow-wave phase of sleep is interrupted by low-voltage fast activity, muscle relaxation and phasic events with rapid eye movements. The EEG resembles that of wakefulness, but the animal is asleep, hence *paradoxical sleep* as alternative terminology for fast, *desynchronized* or *REM sleep* (Table 1.1).

The concept of different levels of brain activity and the term *vigilance* were introduced by Head[79] to indicate the degree of physiological efficiency of an animal or experimental preparation. 'Vigilance' was used initially in such a broad way as to be meaningless, but was revived with concepts of an ascending reticular formation and other cortical projection systems, and used to indicate the level of arousal.[87] According to Moruzzi, the level of alertness and general

Table 1.1 *Nomenclature of sleep stages*

Non-REM sleep (NREM)	
Quiet sleep	Sometimes applied to NREM sleep in infants
Synchronized sleep	Similar EEG waveforms occur at the same time over all areas in scalp recordings
Deep sleep	Applied to NREM stages 3 and 4, since the threshold for arousal is greater than in NREM stages 1 and 2
Delta sleep	Applied to NREM stages 3 and 4, where delta activity (1–3 Hz) is very prominent, or dominates the recording
Slow-wave sleep	Similar to delta sleep
REM sleep	
Active sleep	The opposite of quiet sleep, with prominent and frequent limb, body and eye movements
Desynchronized sleep	D sleep: absence of EEG synchronization
Paradoxical sleep	Although the subject is behaviourally asleep, the EEG tracing is of low voltage and desynchronized, resembling that of wakefulness

The different terms for NREM sleep (and also for REM sleep) are sometimes used in a reciprocal manner, although this is not always strictly correct. The different phases of sleep do not have similar characteristics in all mammalian species. The REM sleep phase can be difficult to identify in humans when eye movements themselves are deficient (due to either brain stem or neuromuscular disease). And how should we classify REM sleep in an animal that lacks the ability to move its eyes?

In this book the terms *NREM* and *REM* sleep are used to characterize the two main human sleep stages when these have been identified.

Light, deep, good and *bad* sleep are terms that cannot be quantified in the same way as EEG sleep stages and are purely subjective. However, since these terms are used often by patients they are used in this book. No association with any specific sleep stage or pattern is implied by this usage (see p. 23).

aspects of drive are related to the activity of the reticular activating system, coma being regarded as a unique zero level, with absent or very low rates of reticular discharge, whereas hyperactivity, mania and rage represent the opposite extreme.

Sleeping infants born at term spend approximately 50% of sleep time in one of two states, *quiet* and *active* sleep. These occur alternately, with a cycle time of about 45 min. *Quiet* sleep in infants is characterized by regular heart rate and respiration, no eye or limb movements, and an alternating EEG pattern (*tracé alternant*) between discrete bursts of generalized delta activity and faster components lasting a few seconds. This state corresponds to NREM sleep of adults. *Active* sleep in infants is characterized by irregular heart and respiration rates, many eye and limb movements, and a more constant EEG pattern. This phase is analogous to the REM sleep of adults.

SLEEP STAGES

Three basic parameters are needed to define the stage of sleep, *EEG* (electroencephalogram), *EOG* (electro-oculogram, recording eye movement) and *EMG* (electromyogram, recording muscle activity). The classification of sleep stages mostly used today distinguishes two main phases of sleep, *NREM* or *slow sleep* according to the French terminology, and *REM* or *paradoxical sleep*. In man, sleep stages are generally more differentiated than in animals, but the possibility of subcortical recording in animals permits the identification of additional phenomena such as hippocampal theta activity and ponto-geniculo-occipital spikes.[78]

Electroencephalographically, sleep is composed of four NREM stages and one REM stage. The two very different kinds of sleep alternate in regular cycles throughout the night. In addition to characteristic variation in *spontaneous* activity of the brain during alertness and sleep, there are also changes in *evoked activity* with sensory stimulation.

During both wakefulness and sleep, the different types of spontaneous EEG activity can be divided into four frequency bands: *beta* (above 12 Hz), *alpha* (8–12 Hz), *theta* (4–8 Hz) and *delta* (1–3 Hz). The amplitude of these waves is generally greater for slow than for fast frequencies, partly because of a low-pass filter effect of scalp and skull tissue (Fig. 1.1).

At sleep onset, the 8–12 Hz occipital and posterior part of the head alpha rhythm of relaxed wakefulness begins to disappear. Initially the alpha rhythm becomes more diffuse on the scalp, more abundant, and slower in frequency. The alpha rhythm may wax and wane, giving way to a low-voltage irregular pattern with the relatively flat EEG tracing that marks *stage 1 NREM sleep*. In this stage, the EEG consists mainly of low-to-moderate voltage mixed theta frequencies (4–6 and 5–7 Hz). Slow rolling or horizontal eye movements replace the rapid eye movements of wakefulness. Stage 1 NREM sleep lasts from about 30 s to 7 min. If aroused, subjects usually describe being half awake rather than asleep.

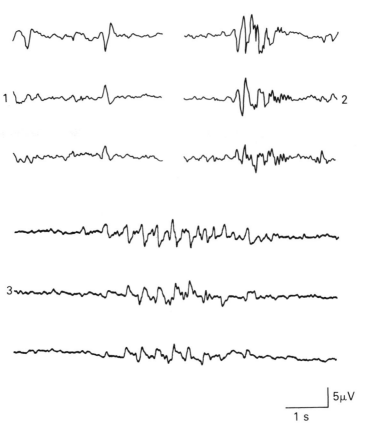

Figure 1.2   *Three waveforms characteristic of sleep stages. 1: vertex sharp wave in stage 2; 2: K potential immediately followed by a spindle also in stage 2; 3: sawtooth waves in paradoxical sleep. Each sample consists of three bipolar leads from the anterior (top), middle (middle) and posterior (bottom) part of the scalp. Reprinted with permission from Gaillard.*[78]

In stage 2 NREM sleep, unequivocal sleep occurs. Stage 2 is characterized by three different patterns: sleep spindles, vertex sharp waves and K potentials (Fig. 1.2). *Sleep spindles,* so called because the waves at the start and end of each brief burst of 12–15 Hz activity are smaller than the waves in the middle, occur throughout stages 2–4 NREM sleep. Since they are superimposed on large amplitude slow waves in stages 3–4, spindles are difficult to see with the naked eye, although they can be detected with electronic analysis. About five spindles occur each minute in normal stage 2 sleep. Spindles are often associated with *K complexes*. These complexes, an initial negative wave followed 0.75 s later by a positive wave, appear simultaneously over all areas of the head. Most appear to be spontaneous, but some occur in response to external sensory stimuli, and also possibly to changes in internal autonomic system activity, gut and bladder contractions.[83] Meaningful auditory stimuli, e.g. the subject's name given forwards rather than backwards, are said to

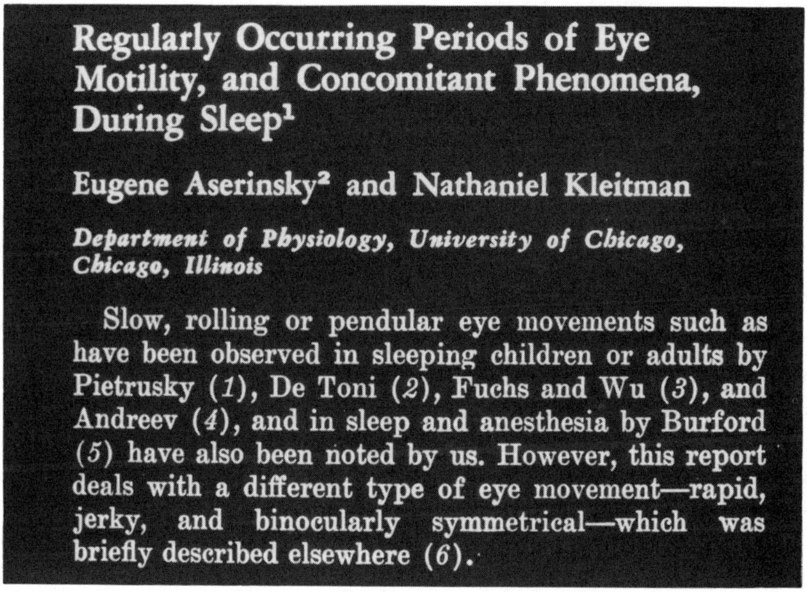

Regularly Occurring Periods of Eye Motility, and Concomitant Phenomena, During Sleep[1]

Eugene Aserinsky[2] and Nathaniel Kleitman

Department of Physiology, University of Chicago, Chicago, Illinois

Slow, rolling or pendular eye movements such as have been observed in sleeping children or adults by Pietrusky (*1*), De Toni (*2*), Fuchs and Wu (*3*), and Andreev (*4*), and in sleep and anesthesia by Burford (*5*) have also been noted by us. However, this report deals with a different type of eye movement—rapid, jerky, and binocularly symmetrical—which was briefly described elsewhere (*6*).

Figure 1.3   *The recognition of REM sleep. From* Science, *(1955)* **118**, *273, with kind permission.*

provoke K complexes more readily than meaningless stimuli.[88] Between two and three K complexes occur each minute. K complexes appear to be non-specific evoked potentials characteristic of NREM sleep, and which combine a frontal slow wave, a central spindle, and a *vertex sharp wave*.

Stage 3 NREM sleep is marked by a continuous increase in EEG voltage, and a decrease in frequency. With the increase in voltage, the EEG pattern becomes more and more synchronized. Stage 3 sleep is defined by the occurrence of at least 20% of waveforms with a frequency of 0.5–3 Hz (mainly 1–2 Hz), and amplitude greater than 75 μV. (Stage 3 sleep is very stable across different age groups, but alters with many pathological conditions.)

The domination of the EEG record by delta waves indicates the presence of *stage 4 NREM sleep*. A high abundance of slow waves is typical of sleep in young adults, and this stage rapidly declines with age.

There is a progressive increase in the *stimulus threshold necessary to produce arousal* between stages 1 and 2, and stages 3 and 4 NREM sleep. During stages 3 and 4, noise stimuli that are sub-threshold for arousal may not cause any alteration in the EEG pattern.

Upon falling asleep, and after the alpha rhythm disappears, stages 1 and 2 NREM sleep occur within a few minutes, and stages 3 and 4 NREM sleep within 30–45 min in normal healthy young adults. NREM stage 3–4 sleep may last from a few minutes to an hour, and is usually followed by a brief episode of stage 2 NREM sleep before the first appearance of REM sleep. The first REM period of the night usually commences 75–90 min after sleep onset, and lasts for 5–10 min. This first episode is the least intense REM period of the night, both in physiological manifestations, frequency of eye movements and respiratory irregularity, and in the intensity of dreams.

There are usually between 4 and 5 NREM–REM cycles during a normal night's sleep. The duration and intensity of each REM period increases with each cycle, and the final REM periods last 20–60 min. In contrast, NREM stage 3–4 sleep is progressively lost, with less NREM stage 3–4 sleep in the second than in the first NREM–REM cycle, and often no NREM stage 3–4 sleep at all in late cycles. Final night sleep is composed therefore mainly of stage 2 NREM, and REM sleep.

Hippocampal theta activity, remarkably regular high-amplitude waves recorded from the hippocampus of animals and of a few humans during subcortical recording for the investigation of epilepsy, occurs during REM sleep and wakefulness, but becomes desynchronized during NREM sleep.

Ponto-geniculo-occipital waves (PGO waves) are sleep-related sharp waves recorded in some but not all animal species. They have been most studied in the cat, where they are the most conspicuous EEG pattern of REM sleep. Waves with somewhat similar characteristics have been described in man,[89] but are much less visible than in other species. In the cat, PGO waves appear shortly before the onset of REM sleep, and occur throughout the episode in association with rapid eye movements, although this is not the case in the monkey.[76]

Evoked potentials to sensory stimuli show little change in latency or waveform with sleep. In general, short latency components of evoked potentials are not affected by drowsiness or sleep and long latency components show only minor changes. *Auditory* and *visual* potentials show prolonged latencies associated with focal deficits in their respective pathways, but only minor alterations with changes in alertness. Habituation to sensory stimuli with repeated monotonous signals during wakefulness is, however, accompanied by a progressive decline in voltage of evoked brain potentials, and during sleep there is an overall reduction in the amplitude of evoked responses. With *auditory evoked responses*, potentials are of greatest amplitude during wakefulness, reduced during all stages of NREM sleep, and of lowest amplitude during REM sleep. The various components of evoked responses are altered by sleep in different ways. Sleep, coma due to brain disease, metabolic disturbance, drugs or alcohol, cause non-specific changes in the early components of somatosensory evoked potentials, unless these are blocked by lateral pontine lesions. Some authors have shown that late responses can be enhanced in sleep with an increase in late negative components in the auditory evoked response with drowsiness.[77] In contrast, Larson *et al.*[84] found no relationship between evoked potential waveform and the clinical level of responsiveness in adults following head injury. Lille *et al.* [85,86] concluded that evoked potentials of all modalities become simpler, broader, flatter and of more prolonged latency with a progressive decline in awareness in children.

REM periods alternate with NREM periods at about 90 min intervals. The rapid eye movements that give this stage its name are jerky, horizontal, vertical and oblique, binocularly symmetrical, and may be accompanied by phasic muscle twitches (Fig. 1.3). Eye movements and muscle twitches, particularly of the hands, legs and face, may be grouped in bursts or isolated, and slow rolling as well as rapid eye movements occur. Otherwise, skeletal muscle tone (with the exception of the diaphragm) is low or abolished. Muscle tone in jaw and neck muscles is particularly low, and the deep tendon reflexes are very reduced or abolished. Muscle atonia, interrupted by phasic events, is associated with a low-voltage fast (15–20 Hz) electroencephalogram intermixed with theta waves, similar to that of alertness (Fig. 1.4).

In a few subjects during REM sleep, 8–12 Hz activity (with the same spatial distribution as alpha activity during wakefulness) is present, and sawtooth waves (theta activity with rapid rise and slow decline) can be distinguished, usually in association with rapid eye movements.

The proportions of total sleep time occupied by NREM and REM sleep are shown in Table 1.2.

REM sleep is characterized by the occurrence of rapid eye movements, but these are not continuous, in contrast to the EEG pattern and (with the exception of muscle twitches) loss of muscle tone during REM sleep.

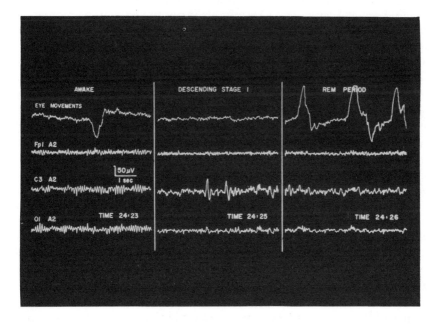

Figure 1.4 *Under normal conditions in adults, sleep commences with non-REM activity. However, REM sleep occurs within a few minutes of sleep onset in narcolepsy (from Rechtschaffen, A. et al., Electroenceph. Clin. Neurophysiol. (1963)* **15,** *599–609), with permission of the author and editor.*

Table 1.2   *Average percentage of total sleep time occupied by NREM and REM sleep in healthy young (aged 20–30) adults*

	Men	Women
NREM sleep		
Stage 1	4	4
2	45	50
3	6	5
4	15	12
REM sleep	28	25

DEPTH OF SLEEP

Depth of sleep can be determined by the EEG as well as by the strength of stimulus necessary to cause arousal. EEG slowing and synchronization, viewed as a result of withdrawal of the reticular influence on the thalamocortical system, gives some indication of the level of drowsiness, whilst absence of rhythmic features in the EEG is generally regarded as evidence of arousal. This change in the EEG is often very obvious in hepatic encephalopathy, where the EEG dominant frequency usually correlates well with the degree of drowsiness as well as with the severity of liver damage (but see p. 78).

In man, the stimulus required to produce arousal from REM sleep is similar to that necessary in stage 2 NREM sleep, but in many laboratory animals, especially the cat, REM sleep is very deep, and arousal requires a large stimulus similar to that necessary in NREM stage 3–4 sleep.[94] The concept of *depth of sleep*, based purely on the threshold for arousal stimulus, is however somewhat artificial. Despite high thresholds for both auditory and direct electrical stimulation of the mesencephalic reticular formation during REM sleep in cats,[80,81] there is a greater spontaneous activity in the reticular formation during REM than NREM sleep.[82]

LEVEL OF ALERTNESS

The assessment of level of alertness during wakefulness depends on the nature of the specific stimulus, as well as on the general sensory background. Physiological, objective and subjective methods have been developed to measure levels of momentary or sustained alertness, but these often depend on the motivation, cooperation and interest of the subject. *Physiological measures* include the determination of pupillary diameter under infra-red illumination (pupillography), which is very sensitive to rapid changes in alertness level,[90, 95] and the *contingent negative variation*, which is of highest voltage over the frontal cortex when attention is concentrated on an unexpected signal and the need to make a decision or take action. This correlates well with other objective or subjective measures of attention. Many different auditory and visual *vigilance tasks*, reaction time tests, flicker fusion studies and letter sorting problems have been developed to study attention levels over short or long periods.[91-93]

Some level of attention is preserved during sleep, as suggested by the son of Pavlov, reading a lecture to the Physiology Society in Scotland in 1923. 'The miller is awoken if his mill stops grinding in the night, and a mother is awoken by the crying of her child.'

Whatever the reason, only a very small proportion of external events that stimulate the sense organs are noticed, and awareness is usually a highly selective phenomenon, determined not so much by the intensity or sensory modality of signals, as by their context, significance and information content. The state of alert awareness and responsiveness during wakefulness, in contrast to the lack of awareness and unresponsiveness during sleep, implies some level of *conscious* appreciation. *Consciousness* (defined by John Locke in 1690 as the perception of what passes in a man's own mind), as opposed to alertness, is a philosophical, as well as psychological concept. Studies of sleep deprivation, and of the action of central stimulant and hypnotic drugs, often investigate the effects on alertness and memory, but not on consciousness. However, changes in consciousness may be more important consequences of sleep disruption than changes in attention.

NORMAL SLEEP

The average time spent asleep falls from about 16 h in every 24 in neonates, to 8 h at the age of 12, 7 h in adults and 6 in extreme old age[129] (Fig. 1.5).

BABIES AND INFANTS

At 30–32 weeks of gestation, a regular sleep–wake cycle is established in the human fetus with, in premature infants, a REM sleep time percentage of around 80% at 30 weeks and 60% at 36 weeks, falling to 50% at full term. In young babies the EEG phase shifts much more often (every 20–35 min) than in adults and the sleep cycle commences with REM, not NREM, activity.[121]

By four months of age the onset of sleep shifts from the newborn mode of entry through REM sleep to the adult mode of entry through NREM sleep. The proportion of total sleep time that is 'active' sleep steadily decreases, and the proportion that is 'quiet' sleep increases (see p. 12). Babies and young children show a clear distinction between the two sleep phases, with conspicuous fast and slow eye movements, muscle twitching, facial smiles, grimaces and frowns, lip sucking, small amplitude limb and finger movements, brief vocalizations and transient eye openings during active sleep. All these movements become less obvious with growth.

Effects of feeding on sleep in young infants have been claimed for a long time. Specific rhythms of sleeping and waking can be imposed by feeding at fixed times and Mills[113] considered that meal timing was critical for the

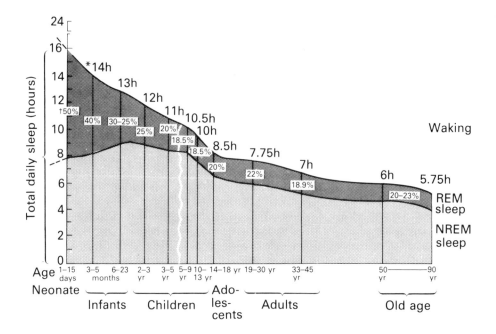

Figure 1.5   *Changes with age in total amounts of daily sleep and daily REM sleep.*
* Total daily amount of sleep (hours).
† REM sleep as percentage of total sleep.
(Redrawn with permission and modification from the original publication by Roffwarg et al.[122])

development of normal sleep–wake cycles as well as total sleep time, REM latency and REM length in young children. However, rhythmic sleep does develop in infants who are not subject to regular feeding habits, with normal maturation of sleep rhythms despite continuous intravenous feeding.[122]

CHILDREN

At the age of one, children spend 12–13 h of each 24 asleep, 30% of which is REM sleep; and by adolescence a little over 8 h, 20% of which is REM sleep.

ADULTS AND THE ELDERLY

As life progresses sleep becomes poor. There is an increase in the number of nocturnal awakenings, and the amount of NREM stage 1 sleep increases from about 5% in childhood to 15% of sleep in old age. This lengthening of the period spent entering sleep has been attributed to loss of neurones in the brain and a general 'weakening' of the sleep processes.[99, 133] Whilst stage 1 NREM sleep slightly increases, stage 3–4 NREM sleep gradually decreases from the age of 20 onwards, and usually little or none is left by the age of 60. In contrast, REM sleep (as a percentage of total sleep time) remains remarkably constant from the age of puberty onwards.

SLEEP AND LIFESTYLE

Sleep depends on sex, environment, occupation, social class, personality and even pre-sleep diet, as well as age.[109, 125, 126, 128] In pre-school age children, there are national differences, dependent on climate, habit, learning, clothing, daylight, season and, most important, maternal expectation. Swiss, American and Scandinavian children go to bed at slightly different times, and country boys and girls sleep differently from town children. In adults, some of the main variations in sleep pattern observed depend on the day of the week and occupation.

Healthy Oxford villagers on average go to bed at 2300, fall asleep in 12 min, wake not at dawn but at 0700, and spend another 12 min in bed. On week days this adds up to 7½ h sleep each night, longer at weekends. A 30–45 min day nap is common, often as compensation for short sleep at night. Such a nap may improve subsequent alertness.[124] Retired, unemployed or ill men all sleep longer at night and have more extensive naps by day than fit subjects.[118] University *students*,[105, 119, 130] *hospital patients*[97, 106] and even people who regard themselves as chronically *poor sleepers*[108, 110] show only slight variations from this normal pattern. However, any change in lifestyle will upset sleep habit or sleep need. Most patients feel they have a greater need of sleep at times of stress, depression, change in occupation, or with increased mental, physical or emotional work,[102] although they may not sleep for longer. Acute stress – as before sky diving or deep sea diving – may prevent prior sleep altogether, and excessive intellectual labour is a recognized cause of insomnia: Solberg described in 1871 the case of a boy of eight who developed insomnia as a result of anxiety about his approaching examinations. In contrast, when things go well, work is enjoyable and life is good, sleep is usually excellent, although the need for sleep may be reduced.[102]

MICROSLEEPS

With tiredness, or after sleep deprivation, short *microsleeps* occur during periods of wakefulness. These are short, 1–10 s bursts of stage 1 sleep, with loss of alpha activity, synchronized 4–7 Hz activity, or stage 2 NREM sleep.[96, 98, 114, 116, 117, 132] Microsleeps are associated with brief lapses of awareness during periods of normal alertness, and are especially common in narcoleptics.[100, 132] Microsleeps probably represent a low level of vigilance, and do not account for prolonged periods of impaired attention or for episodes of automatic behaviour.[101, 127]

Some early observations on sleep habits from de Manacéine *(1897)* are reproduced overleaf.[97a]

Börner tried the experiment of placing a heavy cover-
let over the faces of persons in deep sleep; without
awaking, the sleepers always removed the impediment
which hindered their free respiration. Occasionally
persons arise from bed and empty a distended
bladder without awaking. Certain birds always sleep
on one leg, and those which sleep on the water in this
way, as Headley points out, have a habit of gently
paddling with the foot, thus slowly revolving in a
circle; so that a group of voluntary muscles continues
to act uninterruptedly during sleep. In the old days
before railways, postillions and others often slept on
the journey. Hammond has frequently seen soldiers
asleep on horseback during a night march, and has
so slept himself. Infantry often fall asleep during
forced marches; in such cases they continue to
make all the necessary movements, walk at a regulated pace, hold their guns, etc., without awaking.
Cuming knew a punkah-wallah who could work
the punkah with his foot fairly well while sound
asleep.

LONG AND SHORT SLEEPERS

Chou en Lai and Napoleon regularly slept for less than 5 h each night,
although the French Emperor, after his defeat at the battle of Aspern in 1809,
the first battle he had lost after 17 victories, reportedly slept for 36 h, with
invincible somnolence, so that his suite feared for his life. In contrast, Albert
Einstein was said to sleep a great deal.[112] Although most adults sleep for 7½ h a
night, some sleep for much less or more. Natural long and natural short
sleepers have equal amounts of delta sleep, but long sleepers have much more
REM sleep.[103, 104, 131] The mental development, achievement and personality of
natural long sleepers (over 9½ h a night) do not greatly differ from short
sleepers (under 5½ h a night),[130, 131] although Hartmann[102] suggested that long
sleepers tended to be worriers, and short sleepers non-worriers. Hartmann *et
al.*[103] thought that short sleepers (under 6 h) might be more efficient, hard
working and conformist, but less creative than long sleepers.

A number of extremely short sleepers have been described, although these
are very uncommon. Meddis *et al.*[111] reported a 70-year-old lady who claimed to
have slept for only an hour each night for many years. On investigation she
slept for an average of 67 min every 24 h, with no indication of tiredness. Jones
and Oswald[107] studied two unusually short sleepers, men who had slept about
2½ h per night for many years without ill effects. These short sleepers all had a

high proportion of slow-wave sleep. Very long sleepers have attracted less notice. Natural long sleepers obtain much more REM sleep than average, since REM sleep is concentrated at the end of the night, not at the beginning.

'GOOD' AND 'POOR' SLEEPERS

Some people habitually sleep well, others badly, independent of the length of sleep. 'Poor' sleepers are mainly light sleepers, easily aroused, whilst 'good' sleepers sleep heavily.[115] Light sleepers find it difficult to get off to sleep, and may need absolute quiet. Zimmerman[134] showed that light sleepers also have a higher heart rate and body temperature, a faster respiratory rate, more spontaneous awakenings, and more body movements during sleep than deep sleepers. The expectation of either 'good' or 'poor' sleep may influence subsequent sleep patterns. 'Good' sleepers adapt more rapidly to changes of sleep environment than do 'poor' sleepers. Robinson[120] showed that 'good' sleepers slept even better after two hours of bedtime study, whilst 'poor' sleepers had even worse nights. However, it is a well known paradox that some 'poor' sleepers who constantly complain about their sleep go to sleep rapidly in sleep laboratories, and then sleep deeply for the expected time, and with normal sleep patterns.

DREAMS

Much of the Koran was revealed to Mahomet in dreams, but no dreams dreamt by Christ are recorded in the New Testament.[176] The earliest dream poem in the English language is a lyric by an unknown poet, *The Dream of the Rood* (crucifix), known originally from an eighth century runic inscription on the Rothwell Cross, Dumfriesshire.

Adults wake spontaneously with dream recall about once every 3–4 nights. The most vivid and the best remembered dreams occur at the end of the night. Some form of mentation occurs throughout the night and in all phases of sleep, although there are clear and consistent differences in the nature of dream reports and the frequency of dreams from the different stages of sleep in laboratory subjects. Overall, egocentric, vivid, hallucinatory images are reported in between 60 and 80% of awakenings from REM sleep, whilst vague, fragmentary and poorly described thoughts are noted in between 30 and 50% of awakenings from NREM sleep.

The *sensory errors* and *hypnagogic hallucinations* of sleep onset differ in many ways from dreams. Awareness of the environment drops rapidly on going to sleep, but the level of cortical arousal remains sufficiently high to allow some appreciation of external stimuli. Hypnagogic hallucinations normally include a reworking of scenes from the previous few hours, and, despite fantasy, lack an essential dream-like quality. These sensory errors are often accompanied by feelings of weightlessness, loss of balance or support, falling or floating, perhaps due to partial sensory deafferentation from vestibular and muscle sensor inputs, and imagery may be interrupted by a hypnic jerk. End-of-dream-sleep dreams, *hypnopompic hallucinations,* are qualitatively different from hypnagogic hallucinations, intense dreaming being accompanied by perceptual release.

REM SLEEP DREAMS

Dreams from REM sleep are more visual than auditory, although some auditory component is often present. The dreamer may feel odd or strange as compared with waking reality, although the dream content is usually sequenced, occurring in a familiar setting with the dreamer as the central actor on the stage. When emotional overtones do occur, the dream is more often unpleasant than not. Characteristically, sudden scene shifts occur whilst dreaming. Experiments reported by Berger[138] suggest that most people dream in colour most of the time, although Hall[158] at the Institute of Dream Research, Santa Cruz, California, concluded that whether a dream is coloured or not has little if any significance.

Dreams are mostly short, but appreciation of the real-time content may be absent or distorted. Psychologists and psychiatrists have mainly studied the dream content of healthy young subjects in laboratories, which may be different from dream accounts with spontaneous waking under normal conditions. In healthy young subjects, the frequent finding of dreams with a high sexual content or prominent emotional overtones is perhaps not surprising, and, in any case, these dreams may be better remembered than others. Webb[181] pointed out that morning dream reports are usually more rich and complex than those collected early at night.

There have been many attempts to link dream content with REM physiology, although most of these have proved fruitless. Major respiratory abnormalities during REM sleep are sometimes linked to a current dream experience of laughing, talking or choking,[160] and when sleep–talking takes place in REM sleep it may relate to the dream situation.[172] The nature of dream content has been associated with the appearance and disappearance of penile erections during REM sleep, which, since these occupy 100–200 min each night, are, not surprisingly, often reported to be accompanied by dreams of sexual activity.[149, 178]

Wolpert[185] found an association between dreamed movements of the arms and action potentials in the wrist muscles. Others have connected limb movement and small muscle jerking with dream activity[155] and the deaf and dumb, for example, are said to make appropriate sign language with their hands during REM sleep. Roffwarg *et al.*[175] have tried to relate dream content to middle ear EMG activity; and several attempts have been made to connect the direction and amount of eye movements during REM sleep with visual scanning of dream material.[137] Dement and Wolpert[146] found that REMs were in abundance at times of frequent alteration of gaze in dreams, whereas total absence or few REMs correlated with staring at immobile objects or with breaks in pictorial imagery. Roffwarg et al.[174] attempted to show that the number and direction of REMs could be predicted with reasonable accuracy by treating the dream scene as a visual event that the dreamer scanned as he would if awake; and, more recently, Herman et al.[159] have reinvestigated the evidence for a directional correspondence between eye movements and dream imagery in REM sleep, and suggested that there may be some pairing of dream narratives with EOG recordings in the same axis of gaze. Interruption of the motor pathways for eye movements does not interfere with visual imagery in REM sleep, and REMs do not necessarily need the presence of an intact frontal or visual cortex. REMs occur in sleep in congenitally blind people as well as in functionally decorticate humans.[135, 162]

NREM SLEEP DREAMS

There are clear differences in the reported character of dreams in NREM and REM sleep. After awakenings from NREM sleep stages early in the night, brief thoughts rather than dreams are reported; whilst awakenings from NREM sleep late in the night, during which sleep is lighter than in early NREM stages, yield more dream reports than from earlier wakings.[151] However, light sleepers, who are aroused easily and who say that they sleep poorly, report dreams from NREM awakenings almost as often as they do from REM awakenings;[186] and dream reports are known from awakenings before the occurrence of the first REM phase of the night.[166, 179, 180] It has been suggested that failure to confine dreaming to REM sleep is a pathological state of affairs, and Foulkes[152] found that the capacity for spillover of dream-like fantasy into NREM sleep was greatest in individuals who score highly on schizophrenia scales of the MMPI. However, it looks as if some kind of dream-like mentation continues throughout sleep,[151, 182] and basic dream characteristics are not due solely to REM sleep-specific mechanisms.[168]

Dream recall depends on both the duration and degree of EEG arousal which follows the arrival of the information as well as the degree of familiarity of the information.[164, 167] Thus everyone dreams, but not everyone has good dream recall. Recall depends on the amount of arousal,[156, 182] and according to Foulkes[150] is more likely after awakenings which occur during or after the REM stage of sleep, with higher, nearer waking, EEG wave frequency than during slow-wave sleep.

NIGHTMARES AND NIGHT TERRORS

Nightmares, bad dreams during REM sleep with a powerful emotional content, severe anxiety, terror or dread, are mainly confined to children. Fear is rapidly controlled, and there is not the intense autonomic activity of a night terror. *Night terrors,* in contrast, are arousals from NREM, not REM sleep, and usually occur at the end of the first sleep NREM cycle.[141, 148] Dream recall is poor, but autonomic activity is extreme. The child awakes but is only partially aroused, with intense fear, screaming, widely dilated pupils, tachycardia and sweating, lasting up to 30 min (see *Parasomnias*) (Fig. 1.6).

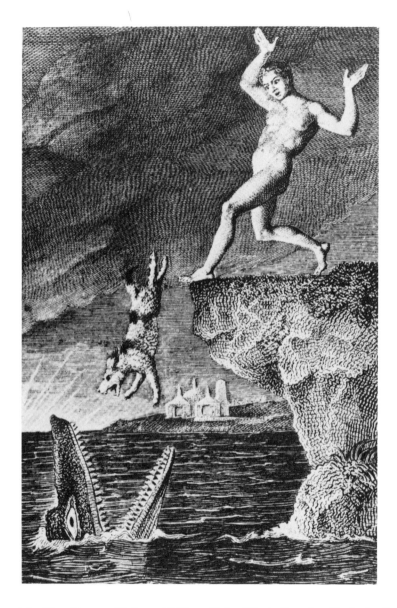

Figure 1.6 The Dream Vision, *William Blake (illustration for* Hayley's Ballads: *Frontispiece:* The Dog, 1805).

HEMISPHERE LATERALITY AND DREAMING

After Charcot's first description[142] there are many reports indicating that cerebral lesions may cause the loss of dream recall. Murri et al.[169] examined 53 patients with acute unilateral brain lesions. Patients with posterior but not anterior lesions had a frequent loss of dream recall. The dominant visual character of REM dreams has led some investigators to consider that dreaming is constructed more from visual memory stored in the right hemisphere than from verbal memory stored in the left hemisphere. In three patients with posterior right hemisphere damage, Humphrey and Zangwill[161] reported cessation of dream recall. However, Jus et al.[163] reported that damage to the frontal lobes was associated with loss of REM dream reports, and Epstein and Simmons[147] mentioned a partial aphasiac with reported lack of dreaming. Some split brain subjects show a decrease in dreaming after surgery.[140] If the EEG is used as an index of hemisphere function, and it is assumed that the hemisphere with less power is the one more actively involved in on-going mentation,[173] then right hemisphere power may be less than left during dreaming.[136]

MALE AND FEMALE DIFFERENCES IN DREAMS

Individual differences (e.g. young v. old, well v. ill, male v. female) in dream content are discussed by Cohen.[144] There are remarkably few differences between the dreams of men and women, although female dreams are said to take place more often indoors[184] and there is slight evidence that male homosexuals also tend to set their dreams indoors.[183] Cohen[143] stressed that males have slightly more aggressive dreams than females, and differentiated between masculine and feminine types of male personality. Cohen suggested that these personality differences were more important than sex distinctions for the nature of dreaming, and gave obvious examples of 'feminine' and 'masculine' male dreams.[144]

> I see G and L in Herman Park in Houston. I want G to go to the Winnipeg Royal Ballet with me that night. She already has tickets to go to some other club. I blow it off and am somewhat disappointed.

> I dreamed that I was some kind of merchant dealing with both sides in the American Civil War. I took my payments in sex with Northern and Southern women.

CHILDREN'S DREAMS

Children's reports of dreams should be considered with some circumspection. According to Foulkes[153] young three-year-old children report short dreams from both REM and NREM sleep: the younger the child, the smaller the difference between mentation during sleep and during wakefulness. Neubauer,[170] a child psychiatrist and analyst, says that very young children tend to dream of being bitten or chased; children of four tend to dream of animals and of good or bad people who either protect or attack them; whilst children of five or six dream of being killed or injured or seeing ghosts.

DREAMS OF THE BLIND

Blind people who have been sighted can see in their dreams for over a decade after losing their sight. Blind people who have never been sighted dream, but the dream lacks visual imagery. Berger et al.[139] described three men who had been blind for 3, 10 and 15 years respectively. All reported that they still saw things in their dreams, but two others who had been blind for 30 and 40 years reported that they no longer did.

PSYCHIC DREAMS

Ella Sharpe[177] quotes an impressive dream dreamt by an 81-year-old woman three days before her death: 'I saw all my sicknesses gathered together, and as I looked there was no longer sickness but roses and I knew that the roses would be planted and that they would grow'.

PSYCHIATRIC ILLNESS AND DREAMS

Freud[154] stated that the dreams of neurotics do not differ in any important way from the dreams of normal people. This is largely untrue: anxious people have anxious dreams; phobic people dream of being in dangerous or safe places; depressive people dream of violence and failure to repair damage; schizoid people dream of remote places, catastrophe and devastation.[176] Oddly enough, dreams of schizophrenics may be less bizarre, less affective and relatively more often about family members than dreams of normal subjects.[171]

FUNCTION OF DREAMS

From Minerva to the present-day gypsy fortune teller, dreams have been used as a source of prophecy, and they are still used today as a guide to conduct by children of the Malaysian peninsula, who are taught by their parents to act out their sleeping experiences. The German chemist Kekule allegedly discovered the structure of the benzene ring following a dream of snakes with their tails in their mouths,[145] and Elias Howe, inventor of the sewing machine, was led to this discovery by dreaming of a spear with a hole in the tip.[165] These problems must have occupied much of the waking thoughts of both men, and there is no scientific evidence that dreaming has any creative value in solving problems, or in literary and artistic efforts. However, Rycroft[176] considered that the conception of ideas, from the poetry of Kubla Khan to the children's stories of Enid Blyton, was independent of the will, but perhaps dependent on dreaming.

The dream theory that continues to attract the widest following is based in total or in part on Freud's original theory of sleep and dreams, that dreams are mechanisms for reducing psychic tensions that occur whilst awake, and allow the fulfilment of our unconscious wishes. According to the psychoanalytical view of dreams, these may reflect need, as well as immediate and remote past experience. There is surprisingly little evidence for these ideas, or that dreams are a royal road to the unconscious. It is difficult to influence dream content by suggestion during wakefulness, and stimulation subthreshold for arousal during REM sleep rarely produces appropriate dreams. The Freudian analyst was supposed to determine what the dream represented, and find the latent meaning by a process of free association. An up-to-date view is that of Greenberg[157] who concludes that 'dreams . . . are important for psychological function, not as a vehicle for satisfying unfulfilled or forbidden wishes, but because they provide a mechanism for maintaining a continuity and meaningfulness in our life experience' (Table 1.3).

Table 1.3   *Mechanisms of visual imagery during sleep*

Visual hallucinations with psychosis
Focal epilepsy (fronto-temporal or occipital in origin)
Hypnagogic hallucinations at sleep onset
Hypnagogic hallucinations at sleep termination
Dreams and nightmares (mainly REM sleep)
Night terrors (stage 3–4 NREM sleep)

ANIMAL SLEEP

Sleep, as we know it in man, is the monopoly of vertebrates. Among animals, many different sorts of sleep, such as deep sleep, half sleep (dozing), paradoxical sleep and winter sleep (hibernation) can be distinguished. There are solitary sleepers and group sleepers, animals who sleep at home and animals who sleep abroad. Home and sleeping place are often, but not always, the same. The hedgehog and squirrel sleep all winter in order to live, the woodchuck in Finland is asleep for 87–88% of his life, the newborn baby pays for one hour of wakefulness with two hours of sleep, whilst adult humans are asleep for only one third of their lives.[204] Amongst the birds, woodpeckers, sparrows, tits and swallows live and sleep partly in their nests, but many birds have different home and sleeping places. The three great apes, gorilla, chimpanzee and orang utan build a new sleeping nest every evening: cocks and several other birds keep to the same sleeping place, not only for years, but for several generations.[198]

It is difficult to determine reliably the sleep habits of many species. Much of the data has been obtained under zoo or circus conditions, and only a very small percentage of the world's 5000 mammalian species have been studied. Although the heroic study of Zeppelin and Rechtschaffen[225] catalogued the sleep habits of 50 different mammalian species, and Allison and Cichetti[189] evaluated REM sleep in 39 animal species, it is notoriously difficult to study the sleep of wild animals. Thus, in the Brazilian tapir, sleep has been characterized by observing two animals for one day, with twitching taken as evidence of paradoxical sleep, and giraffes with their heads resting on the ground or on their body are considered to have neck atonia and be in REM sleep. Gorillas are often said to sleep constantly except in daylight, but few have watched gorillas sleep at night.[192]

Invertebrates do not sleep, if we use criteria necessary for the definition of animal sleep, such as physical quiescence, increased threshold for arousal, reversibility and stereotyped posture. However, many invertebrates spend part of the day immobile or show striking changes in behaviour. The sea hare, *Aplysia california*, comes to rest at dusk at a specific location, takes up a stereotyped resting posture in its tank, and indulges in periodic tentacle waving likened by Sturmwasser[219] to rapid eye movements. Many insects appear to have typical 'sleep' postures, and the activity of the cockroach is reduced by previous 'rest' deprivation.

Sleep in *non-mammalian vertebrates* is widely different from that in man. Amphibians, toads and frogs do not really sleep, although the EEG of bullfrogs has high-amplitude waves when the frogs are most alert, and the stimulus threshold necessary to cause obvious change in the EEG is different during rest and activity in the tree toad *Hyla*.[200, 201] These animals tend to be nocturnal and rest in a relaxed, unresponsive posture by day. Reptiles, lizards, crocodiles and tortoises have regular cycles of rest and activity. In most reptilian species neither typical NREM nor REM sleep occurs, although the diurnal lizard *Otenosaura pectinata* may have short bursts of REM activity, and behavioural sleep in the crocodile is correlated with slow-wave EEG changes.[194]

In birds, the familiar sleep patterns of man can be identified with NREM–REM cycles, although paradoxical sleep is not prevalent – brief episodes of REM sleep last about 10 s in pigeons.[222] Tymicz *et al*.[221] showed that REM sleep varied with the season in starlings, with more REM sleep during the winter resting period of February (2.3%) than in spring and autumn migration (0.7%). During migration, rest may be impossible for long periods. It is not known whether birds such as swifts and albatrosses can sleep on long ocean voyages. In birds, EEG changes of REM sleep may not be accompanied by eye movements or limb atonia, although birds of prey, hawks and falcons, which have excellent visual acuity, spend 10% of sleep time in paradoxical sleep, with myoclonus, atonia and eye movements.[213] The pigeon relies on head movements rather than saccades to fix a visual image, but paradoxical sleep, which occupies 7% of total sleep time, is accompanied by bursts of rapid eye movement. The owl, whose eyes cannot move, sleeps with claws holding fast to a tree branch: its EEG exhibits short paradoxical periods, but without loss of tone in the body muscles, and with no rapid eye movements.[203, 220] To make up for lack of eye movement, the burrowing owl can rotate the head through more than 180°. Bruce Durie[192] records that, in the woods of New England, the way to catch an owl is to walk very slowly around the branch where the bird perches.

Unable to see clearly, the owl will follow carefully by turning its head. When the hunter has walked around three times, the owl has throttled itself.

Special adaptations are needed for sleep in *aquatic animals*. A shark is said to sleep rarely, if ever, due to the need to swim constantly or drown, but this is not true of most fish, some of whom have circadian rest–activity cycles. The EEG in fish is not an adequate measure of sleep, but that of tench has been studied for several days. Many fish neither appear to sleep nor have the anatomical substrate of sleep, raphe nuclei or locus coeruleus, although they may possess structures with similar functions. Big aquatic mammals, which cannot breathe in water, are forced to lie sleeping on the surface, with the breathing aperture at the top of the head just above the water. The blind Indian river dolphin has the shortest sleeping period yet to be shown in mammals, 1–8 s, when the sonar clicks (normally continually emitted for orientation) cease.[209, 212] However, the animal, which lives in flowing water, has to swim incessantly all its life.

Most species of *mammals* so far studied, including the mouse and the elephant, the monkey and man, have rhythmically alternating periods of NREM and REM activity, sleep spindles almost identical in frequency, and similar patterns of sleep behaviour.

Rodents, hedgehogs, cats and lower *primates* sleep about two thirds of their lives, with a high proportion of NREM sleep. Man and dog sleep less, at the expense of NREM sleep. In primates, the succession from wakefulness to slow-wave sleep occurs in definite stages, but in many animals the transition is more abrupt.

Sleep occupies as much as 60% of the life of some adult carnivores, whilst the opossum, considered to be a primitive animal, and possibly the gorilla, stay awake for only 20% of their lives.[205, 217] Examples of long and short animal sleepers are the cat and the guinea pig respectively, which are awake for 30 and 70% of their lives.[211] Careful observation and EEG studies have disposed of the old idea that some mammals, particularly ruminants, do not sleep.

The ratio of NREM to REM sleep varies widely, and sleep cycle length differs between animal species. The NREM–REM cycle of the rat lasts about 10 min, that of cats and dogs about 20 min and that of adult man 90 min.

The rat has twice the REM sleep percentage of the mouse, whilst the cat and the guinea pig respectively spend 20% and 4% of their total sleep time in REM sleep.[211] However, in general, the percentage of REM sleep of many adult animals is remarkably similar to that of man, around 20–25%, as in cats and dogs. In all animal species, the proportion of REM sleep is greatly affected by age. Newborn mammals may spend more than three-quarters of their lives in REM sleep, and gradually assume the adult pattern.[223] Some animals have monocyclic sleep, with a single sleep period every 24 h, whilst others have several sleep–wake cycles.[205]

Early in history, two types of mammals developed, the viviparous mammals with live-born young, and the egg-laying mammals of which only the platypus and the spiny anteater survive today. The spiny anteater resembles reptiles in its hibernating and fasting habits, and has been considered to be an unsuccessful and primitive animal. The sleep of the spiny anteater but not other *Echidna* has been studied in detail. Allison and Van Twyver[191] found that *Echidna* sleep for 8.6 h per 24 h, but unlike other mammals have no REM sleep. This finding has been challenged by Meddis,[207] but Allison and Van Twyver[190] considered that REM sleep arose in evolution 130 million years ago with the separation of viviparous and egg-laying mammals. However, the primitive dentate armadillo does have paradoxical sleep.[188] Mammals and birds derived independently from ancient reptiles; the presence of REM sleep in birds suggests that this was present also in ancient reptilian groups and disappeared in *Echidna*, or that it evolved independently in birds and therian mammals. The anteater has very large and convoluted frontal lobes, not present in other groups of animals that do have paradoxical sleep. Perhaps the frontal lobes of the anteater perform the same function as taken over by paradoxical sleep in other mammals[193, 197, 224] – or maybe they merely help in catching ants.

The sleep of the Black Sea dolphin is the most curious of all animals studied. Dolphins lay asleep near the water surface and thrust the head with the breathing hole out of the water at intervals of about half a minute, keeping their eyes closed. This can be done both sleeping and waking. Kovalzon[206] in Moscow found that one hemisphere of the dolphin can be synchronized, with slow waves and spindles, at a time when the other is desynchronized, the animal swimming slowly or floating, immobile. The slow-wave hemisphere side may stay the same for long periods, 2–24 h, but then the hemispheres change. Unihemispheric slow-wave sleep is the main type of sleep in the dolphin brain but has not yet been observed in any other animal. This is not only a cortical, but also a subcortical phenomenon, and records from thalamic nuclei demonstrate that the thalamus can also generate slow-wave activity unilaterally and concurrently with the neocortex. The total time percentage of right-side and left-side sleep is usually unequal. In some specimens of bottlenose dolphin and porpoise the right hemisphere sleeps more than the left, and in others vice versa. As in the spiny anteater, REM sleep has not been detected in the dolphin.

Dolphins provide an opportunity of sleep-depriving only one half of the brain. Unihemispheric sleep deprivation results in a rebound of delta sleep in this hemisphere only: each hemisphere independently shows the need for sleep. Perhaps dolphins need one hemisphere to remain active to ensure respiratory activity and muscular tone whilst the other hemisphere sleeps.[209]

BEHAVIOUR DURING ANIMAL SLEEP

Sleep postures in various animals are very diverse. The flamingo sleeps upright, standing on one leg, but bats sleep head down. Long-legged birds may take an abdominal lying position, whilst the ostrich stretches its long neck on the ground in sleep. Most mammals and man sleep on their sides, but this posture is very rare in other vertebrates.[198] Preparation for sleep is often complex. When an elephant lies down, it is already sleeping. Adult elephants sleep for about 4 h, interrupted by standing to excrete faeces and urine.

Phasic twitches of REM sleep are more violent and frequent in some species than others, and cats and dogs have marked extraocular muscle twitches, with various facial and limb movements most obvious in the distal portions of the limbs, especially the digits. Dogs, more than cats, paddle with all four limbs, and this behaviour with vocalization may suggest to dog owners that their dog is dreaming.[199] The vocalization of dogs during REM sleep is a caricature of normal barks, howls and yelps, probably due to changes in upper airway diameter induced during this sleep phase.

Attempts have been made to relate animal sleep to environment, behavioural patterns, size of brain or body, metabolic rate, longevity, energy metabolism and external temperature. Environment and life style are amongst the most important of these. The *environment* of farm animals greatly affects sleep, and wild animals with secure sleeping places and a safe den sleep more than species sleeping in the open.[189] Ponies have about an hour more total sleep time when in their stalls than when outdoors, and although the horse has been celebrated for its ability to sleep whilst standing, it is said to have to lie down to enter REM sleep.[216] Horses spend much less time, approximately 3% of sleep time, in REM sleep than man. In ruminants, drowsiness is closely associated with feeding, and the munching cow is often in slow-wave sleep. A change in diet from long hay to pelleted grass markedly reduces the percentage of the day spent in drowsiness and rumination, but REM sleep is not altered.[214, 215]

In their study of animal sleep, Zeppelin and Rechtschaffen[225] showed there was no correlation between REM sleep and any other parameter, except possibly security. Allison and Cicchotti[189] considered that the amount of REM sleep for any species related to its *life style*, the amount of danger from predators and the degree of exposure of the sleeping place. Predators spend a greater percentage of a 24 h period sleeping than do prey species and, overall, have more REM sleep.

There is some correlation between slow-wave sleep time and basal metabolic rate in animals. The higher the basal metabolic rate, the more the sleep an animal requires, although in shorter episodes and over a shorter life span. However, there are many exceptions. One function of sleep – or at least hibernation in animals – must be energy conservation, although there is no evidence for this view in man.[210, 218]

Animals sleep in a much more variable and less regimented way than we care to recognize, and the nature and function of sleep may differ depending on the conditions in which the animal lives.[192]. Sleep as we know it, with two distinct states, occurs only in animals with well developed cerebral hemispheres, with a neocortex, and with great ability to learn from experience.[187, 202] REM sleep may be particularly important for the young, perhaps essential for normal brain development and learning, although it is not found in either the spiny anteater or the dolphin. The first of these, with most terrestrial homeothermic animals, shares with the Spaniard a regular midday siesta of 1–2 h.[198]

An account of the sleep of the spiny anteater from *Cassel's Natural History* published in 1897 is given overleaf:

THE GREAT ANT-EATER. †

A DESCRIPTION of this animal—often called the Great Ant-Bear—might have been met with in Zoological works; but in October, 1853, the visitors to the Gardens in the Regent's Park had an opportunity of seeing the first living specimen brought into Europe, from the interior of Brazil, at a cost of £200.

Proceeding to its apartment, if the creature were taking its siesta, they would be reminded, as they saw it on its heap of clean straw, in one corner, of a large gray or grizzled Newfoundland dog. On looking more closely, the body appeared to be covered with long, flowing hair, proceeding from the reverted tail—a good defence from the sunbeams, nor less so from a heavy rain.

If, however, it had shaken off its slumbers, it would have been seen that, if the Ant-Eater were as tall as a Newfoundland dog, it was much longer in the proportion of the body to that of its height.

SLEEP DISORDERS IN ANIMALS

Narcolepsy occurs in spaniels, Dobermans and Labradors,[195, 208] and the genetic patterns in some canine species may be similar to man. Narcolepsy has also been recognized by clinical presentation, as well as EEG recordings and pharmacological tests, in horses and a Shetland Welsh pony.[196] *Obstructive sleep apnoea* occurs in Persian cats and bulldogs, and some grossly obese animals cannot sleep supine at all.[199] Persian cats and bulldogs with upper respiratory obstructive problems prefer to sleep with their head elevated, presumably to straighten the airway. *Parasomnias* occur in cats and dogs. Brief periods of violent limb movements, tossing the animal around the cage, confined to REM sleep and followed by arousal, may occur in domestic cats,[199] and there is a rare enuretic syndrome in dogs when well trained and otherwise continent pets persistently leave pools of urine when they sleep. This occurs in dogs of all ages, and is unrelated to any established anatomical abnormality. When observed in the act, the dogs are seen to begin to urinate whilst sleeping, with subsequent arousal.

SLEEP DEPRIVATION

The length of time a person can go without sleep is the same as that during which he can survive without food. There are some accounts of very long periods of wakefulness, but a careful examination would doubtless dispose of most of these. David Jones, a citizen of Anderson, Arizona, attracted the entire American medical profession in 1893 by a sleepless spell of 93 days, attributed to his use of tobacco whilst young.[247]

Sleep deprivation experiments in man have not revealed the hidden function of sleep. The longest period for which subjects have been kept awake is between 100 and 200 h, and more prolonged deprivation has proved impossible to achieve. After a certain time it becomes impossible to prevent sleep, or to awaken the subject, or to tell whether he or she is waking or sleeping. Frequent microsleeps (see p. 21) occur, and interrupt the performance of tasks designed to keep subjects awake.

Selective sleep stage deprivation, the attempt to study the function of REM or NREM sleep by preventing it, was first studied by Dement.[239] By awakening subjects at the start of each REM period, he effectively reduced the amount of REM sleep. Similarly, NREM sleep deprivation can be achieved by waking the subject each time the polygraph indicates that this sleep stage is present. In animals, REM sleep deprivation methods mostly rely on REM sleep atonia to wake the animal, which is balanced on a flower pot or raft, and surrounded by water. *Partial sleep deprivation*, waking the subject after the first half of sleep, achieves some degree of selective REM deprivation, since REM sleep is most preponderant in the second half of sleep.

The effects of total sleep deprivation, REM and NREM sleep deprivation are considered below.

TOTAL SLEEP DEPRIVATION

There have been numerous investigations dating back to the turn of the century into the effects of total sleep deprivation in man. These are reviewed in detail by Wilkinson,[309] Naitoh[278] and Horne.[253] The main conclusion of all these studies has been that, although total sleep deprivation for short periods undoubtedly impairs psychological performance, initial changes in most other body functions are only slight. *The main initial effect of total sleep deprivation in man is not any striking alteration in mood, performance or behaviour, but sleepiness.*[253, 254] However, in the long term, sleep deprivation may be far more serious, and prolonged periods without any sleep may ultimately result in death (see below).

There are many problems in the interpretation of the results of sleep deprivation experiments. Many of the studies of total sleep deprivation in man have depended on unnatural regimes, have been of short duration, and have involved mostly fit, intelligent and young males. Many of the reported changes of statistical significance have no physiological meaning,[253] and at least some of the results of sleep deprivation experiments are non-specific, the result of mental of physical stress. These include loss of adrenal weight in animals, elevation of blood corticosteroid levels, and stomach (duodenal) ulceration in animals and man.[277]

The major effects of total sleep deprivation are considered below.

Sleep deprivation in young subjects

Sleep, and in particular REM sleep, appears to be especially important early in development, and may be vital for brain development in the fetus as well as in the growing child. Sleep deprivation in early development affects both adult brain development and behaviour of animals.[273] Mirmiran *et al.*[272] have shown that pharmacological suppression of REM sleep before weaning in rats adversely affects subsequent cortical growth, and conditioned reflex development in the animal may fail after sleep deprivation.[265] There have been few studies of the effects of sleep deprivation in very young human subjects, and none in infancy.

Psychological effects of sleep deprivation

Many of the most obvious effects of sleep deprivation lie in the psychological sphere. A variety of aviation and naval mishaps have been attributed to lack of sleep,[231] as have mistakes made by doctors after being up all night.[228] Perhaps sleepy men are unable to give important activities the special attention that they require.[251] The many and extensive studies on the effects of sleep deprivation on psychological performance were carefully reviewed by Naitoh.[278] After loss of sleep for a single night, the effect is generally greater in the next afternoon and evening rather than morning, and is slightly greater in old than in young people.[304, 307] Vigilance is lowered, and the ability to direct attention to specific and in particular visual stimuli is reduced. Sanders and Reitsma[294, 295] have shown that the main effects of short periods of total sleep deprivation are greater on reactions to peripheral than to central visual field stimuli, and on wider than on closer visual displays. Also, there are minor changes in long latency evoked response components following sleep deprivation.[285]

In addition to reduction in vigilance, occasionally periodic lapses of short-term memory can be demonstrated after 24–48 h without sleep.[284] Subjective assessments show that vigour is decreased, mood is depressed, and fatigue, aggression and sleepiness are increased.[250, 292] Webb and Agnew[306] showed that rest alone could not compensate for sleep lack, and whether the subject rested (but did not sleep) or took active exercise through two nights of sleep deprivation made little overall difference to performance the next day.

Severe fatigue, irritability, episodes of misrepresentation, and sometimes feelings of persecution develop after 72–98 h without sleep, with in some instances minor disturbances in perception and orientation. These changes are coloured by the subject's previous personality.[255, 276] However, there are few if any long-term psychological effects in most subjects who have been sleep deprived for less than 100 h.[255] In only a very small proportion of cases (2–3%) do gross psychotic changes follow total sleep deprivation for long periods.[248, 281] Tyler[301] found psychotic features in only seven of 350 subjects kept awake for 112 h.

The longer the period of sleep deprivation, the greater are the subsequent changes in circadian rhythmicity of sleep and other sleep-related variables.[266]

In contrast to the laboratory situation, chronic sleep deprivation over months or years, as for example in chronic prostatism or sleep apnoea, can have many and severe deleterious effects, even resulting in apparent dementia. The effects of frequent nocturnal arousals and sleep fragmentation can sometimes be reversed by treatment of the cause of the sleep disturbance.[259]

Metabolic effects of sleep deprivation

Short periods of sleep deprivation cause minor changes in biochemical, physiological and metabolic activity whilst prolonged sleep deprivation may result in severe pathology and death. *Hormonal changes* are minor and result from non-specific mental and physical stress, as well as changes in circadian rhythmicity.[230] Overall, there is little change in plasma or urinary 17-hydroxycorticosteroid levels, at least for the first three days of total sleep deprivation.[253] Circadian and stress factors probably account for loss of sleep-onset growth hormone release, attenuation of the gastrin response to meals, and reduction in circulating androgen levels in healthy men.[237] *Urinary catecholamine output* shows little alteration,[267] and the effects of sleep lack on general *body metabolism* and physical work ability are very minor,[253] although there are slight alterations in body temperature, thermoregulatory function, cardiovascular activity, respiratory activity, skin conductance and EMG activity.[254] Short-term sleep loss will alter the *breathing pattern* and respiratory responses to inhaled gases.[236]

Serotonin receptor activation,[308] *MAO activity* in platelets, *dopamine metabolism* and receptor sensitivity[300] and *plasma circadian rhythms* for heavy metals[266] are all altered by short periods of sleep deprivation. Palmblad *et al.*,[279, 280] in two studies of 2–3 nights' sleep deprivation, showed that this was followed by increased *interferon production* and decreased *lymphocyte reactivity*, but the effect of sleep deprivation on *immune function* is probably not biologically significant.

Neurological effects of sleep deprivation
The neurological effects of total sleep deprivation are few. Most relate to stereoscopic vision, which has a high degree of cerebral control. Apart from visual problems, Ross[291] could find no neurological abnormality in a single subject after prolonged sleep deprivation, although Sassin[296] reported weakness of neck flexion, hand tremors, unsteadiness and horizontal nystagmus after 60 h without sleep. Gunderson *et al.*[249] reported seizures in non-epileptic soldiers who had been continuously awake for at least 24 h whilst travelling, but this report is unusual, for although lack of sleep may lower the seizure threshold in certain types of epilepsy, it is rarely if ever responsible for a seizure disorder in otherwise normal subjects.

Miles and Laslett[271] found that total sleep deprivation was followed by impairment of saccadic eye movements, whilst Clark and Warren[233] reported myopia and a decrease in accommodation, with a reduction in binocular convergence. Similar results were obtained by Horne[252] who showed that sleep deprivation resulted in a progressive loss of accommodation with exophoria.

Sleep deprivation and mood
The insomnia of endogenous depression is discussed on p. 253 and changes in the circadian rhythm of sleep and wakefulness with depressive illness on p. 132. Although depression causes insomnia, loss of sleep sometimes has an antidepressant effect.

Experimental sleep deprivation in normal young subjects usually causes a slight depression in mood. However, total night sleep deprivation is said to produce a transient antidepressant effect in between 40 and 75% of depressed subjects studied.[246, 261, 264, 303] The effect, which is not important in the practical treatment of depression, is not entirely due to suggestion or other psychological factors, although it is independent of the degree of sleep deprivation produced.[264] An antidepressant effect of sleep deprivation is seen most often, but not always, in patients with endogenous depression.[283] Sometimes the response may be spectacular, as in a 50-year-old Klinefelter patient with a psychotic depression, described by King et al.[263] Here, sleep deprivation for 24 h caused a change from melancholia to outgoing, jovial, singing and dancing behaviour. The patient said he had never before felt so good. However, the usual response is much more modest and short-lived. According to King et al.,[262] the antidepressant effect of sleep deprivation is mainly confined to depressed patients who have an abnormal dexamethasone suppression test. Such abnormality is sometimes considered to be a sensitive and highly specific marker of endogenous depression or melancholia,[232] although the results probably depend entirely on the severity of previous circadian disturbance of cortisol rhythms (see p. 138).

Sleep deprivation and death

Prolonged sleep deprivation may cause death. This finding, from many old animal studies, has often been neglected or discounted, since the stress or the constant fatigue of the stimulus necessary to prevent sleep, and not sleep loss itself, was considered to account for the animal's death.[229, 238, 268, 269, 305] However, Rechtschaffen et al.[290] in a careful study showed that sleep deprivation, not stress, caused the death of rats as early as 5 days to as long as 33 days after starting the experiment. Severely sleep-deprived rats became debilitated, yellow and ungroomed, with severe motor weakness and ataxia before death. The EEG amplitude fell to less than half of normal waking values, and, at autopsy, loss of body weight, intestinal haemorrhages, stomach ulcers, testicular atrophy, and collapsed lungs were found. Whether sleep deprivation eventually leads to death in man remains unknown.

SELECTIVE REM SLEEP DEPRIVATION

REM sleep deprivation in animals causes a number of changes in behaviour.[241, 256] These include persistent tachycardia,[256] increased cortical excitability,[235] occasionally stimulus-provoked aggression[275] and hypersexuality in sleep-deprived cats.[241] The most important of these findings is the demonstration that short-term REM deprivation in animals *impairs memory* for past events and for the acquisition of new data.[282, 299] In addition, suppression of REM sleep in animals by experimental destruction of the nucleus pontis caudalis or bilateral locus coeruleus lesions causes hyperirritability and hallucinatory-like behaviour.[256] Animals who do not recover any capacity for REM sleep progress to a stage of insomnia, agitation and eventually die; and also show increased mortality from electric shock.

REM sleep deprivation in man has proved extremely difficult to produce for long periods. After a week or two of selective arousal it becomes impossible to awaken subjects promptly at each REM sleep onset, and so prolonged deprivation can not be achieved.[234, 302] Overall, a few nights' REM deprivation has surprisingly little effect on human behaviour or memory.[243, 245, 270] The behavioural effects of REM sleep deprivation in man are not grossly different from those of total sleep deprivation, and may be due mainly to procedural stress, perhaps associated with multiple awakenings and loss of sleep resulting in subsequent tiredness, irritability and mild motor incoordination, rather than to REM sleep loss itself.

The most obvious specific effect of REM sleep deprivation is a subsequent dramatic rise in REM sleep, and reduction in REM latency. Many experiments in animals and man have confirmed this tendency to compensate for lost REM sleep.[240, 242, 244, 256, 260] The central nervous system mechanisms that support REM sleep recovery after REM suppression, although of unknown function, must be important. REM rebound may be abolished by disease or drugs. In *narcolepsy*, normal REM rebound does not occur.[298] *Clonidine, amphetamine, bromocriptine* and other dopamine and noradrenaline agonists, as well as alpha-receptor antagonists, alter or abolish REM rebound.[286-289] REM sleep rebound is also reduced by the 5-HT receptor stimulant quipazine.[312] During REM sleep rebound in the rat, brain dopamine metabolism is increased.[311] Many of the drugs listed above, in addition to their effects on REM sleep rebound, cause major alterations in REM sleep latency or prevalence. Benzodiazepines, alcohol, amphetamine and tricyclic antidepressants will halve REM sleep in acute studies, whilst tetrabenazine, reserpine, lysergic acid, diethylamide and butyrolactone increase REM sleep. Gammahydroxybutyrate is one of the few drugs known that will induce sleep-onset REM activity. However, the study of the action of these different drugs on REM sleep has given little or no information about the behavioural consequences of an increase, decrease or change in latency of REM sleep.

In the early 1960s, it was thought that total deprivation of REM sleep for a few nights might lead to psychosis. Dement and Fisher[242] described a study in which 21 subjects were REM deprived for 2–7 nights. Both they and Sampson[293] described psychological difficulties that developed in these subjects, and subsequently Dement[240] described dramatic psychological disturbances in two subjects who were sleep deprived for up to two weeks by a combination of amphetamines and awakenings. However, most subsequent studies have not confirmed these findings,[257, 297] and it seems unlikely that REM sleep deprivation produces severe psychological problems.

SELECTIVE NREM SLEEP DEPRIVATION

NREM stage 3–4 sleep deprivation has different effects from deprivation of REM sleep.[226] Loss of NREM stage 3–4 sleep produces physical rather than mental symptoms. Agnew et al.[227] reported that stage 3–4 NREM sleep deprivation resulted in physical discomfort, withdrawal and manifest concern about vague physical complaints and changes in bodily feelings. After NREM stage 3–4 sleep deprivation, muscles may become more sensitive to pressure, and volunteers can withstand less musculoskeletal pain.[247a] However, it is of course difficult to produce NREM deprivation without affecting REM sleep, and these results have not been confirmed in all studies.

RECOVERY FOLLOWING SLEEP DEPRIVATION

Not all sleep seems necessary. Following the loss of three nights' sleep, only one is made up, and loss of sleep for a week may be compensated for by only 20 h of sleep. Even after ten days of total sleep deprivation, a person rarely sleeps for more than 14–20 h at any one stretch.[258, 310] After 24–28 h without sleep, the sleep latency is short. There is an increase in NREM stage 3–4 sleep, and often a decrease in REM sleep on the first recovery night. Most of the NREM stage 3–4 sleep, but only about half of REM sleep, is regained. Increased NREM stage 3–4 sleep occurs in both young and old subjects.[304] Thus, under normal circumstances, the first half of sleep, with its high concentration of NREM stage 3–4 sleep, may be more necessary than the second half.

FUNCTION OF SLEEP

> Sleep is a natural, repeated unconsciousness that we do not even know the reason for. (Popper and Eccles[379])

> Sleep that may me more vigorous make
> To serve my God when I awake. (Bishop T. Ken, 1637–1711)

> Qui dort, dîne. (He who sleeps, dines – French proverb)

Although the statement of Popper and Eccles is as true today as it was in 1977, there has been intense speculation about the function of sleep. The main problems and lines of investigation are discussed below under the following headings:

1.   evolutionary theories of sleep;
2.   humoral theories of sleep;
3.   body restitution theories of sleep;
4.   sleep and the motor system;
5.   sleep, memory and learning;
6.   sleep and unlearning.

The first two theories are of historical interest only, and can be quickly discarded. There is considerable interest at present in the next two theories, but the narrow view that sleep restores the body, not the brain – or vice versa – is too selective.

In view of present research about sleep and learning, the last two sections are given prominence here. The old French view, that sleep is food for the mind as well as the body may be near to the truth, and it is now apparent that sleep has an important memory function.

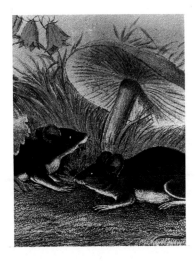

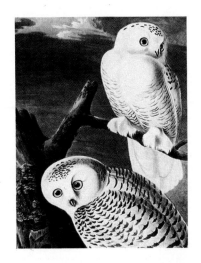

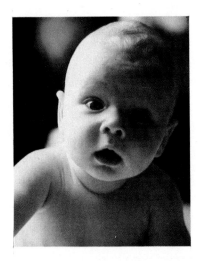

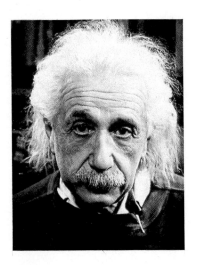

Plate 1
Different species have different ways of sleeping. Winter hibernation starts with NREM sleep. Many birds have brief periods of paradoxical sleep, although some species cannot move their eyes. Human infants spend half their lives in REM sleep. Adults sleep for 30% of their lives, and dream for 6%. Photograph of Einstein by Philippe Halsman (Magnum Photos).

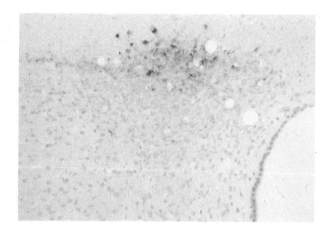

Plate 2a

Sagittal section through the suprachiasmatic nucleus (SCN) of rat, immunohistochemically stained for vaso-active intestinal peptide (VIP). VIP neurones and fibres in the SCN are stained. VIP neurones are located in the ventral part of the nucleus. Third ventricle in lower right corner. By kind courtesy of A. Weindl, Neurologischklinik, Munich.

Plate 2b

The awakening of Kumbhakarna. *The giant demon Kumbhakarna, who spends most of his life asleep, is woken up in order to defend his brother Rāvana from the attack of Rāma and his monkey allies. A miniature painting by the artist Sahib Din from an illustrated manuscript of the Sanskrit epic* Rāmāyana, *prepared between 1649 and 1653 for Maharana Jagat Singh of Udaipur. Udaipur (Western India), AD 1652. © 1977, The British Library Board.*

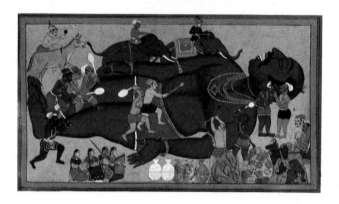

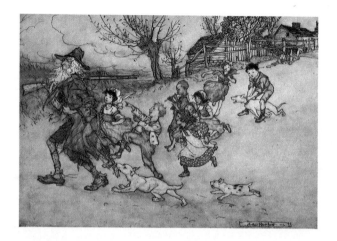

Plate 3a

Washington Irving's Rip van Winkle *was an alcoholic who slept for 20 years. Illustration by Arthur Rackham from* Fairy Tales, *reprinted by permission of the publishers, William Heinemann Ltd and Viking Penguin Inc.*

Plate 3b

A 'modern Rip van Winkle'. News of the World *11 October 1970.*

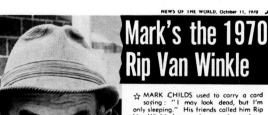

Mark's the 1970 Rip Van Winkle

☆ MARK CHILDS used to carry a card saying: "I may look dead, but I'm only sleeping." His friends called him Rip Van Winkle because he was always dropping off over his pint in his local at Chiddingly, Sussex.

But it wasn't a joke to 56-year-old Mark, an engineer, who couldn't keep a job because of sleeping sickness, a rare disease called Narcolepsy, he'd had since a child. He has passed out and woken up in railway sidings, ambulances and hospitals.

Once he found a priest administering the last rites over him—and decided to carry his warning card from then on.

His fame spread to top Russian doctors who prescribed a cure which included a daily injection of Epsom salts.

It worked, and now Mark can hardly manage a yawn.

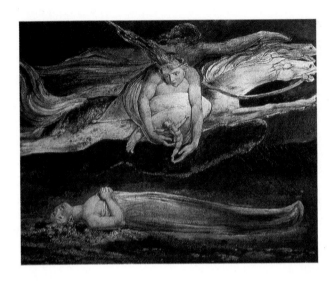

Plate 4a
The artist's view of sleep. William Blake: Pity, *ca. 1795.*

Plate 4b
Antoine Wiertz: Buried alive. *Musée Wiertz, Royal Museums of Fine Arts of Belgium, Brussels. By kind permission of the Director.*

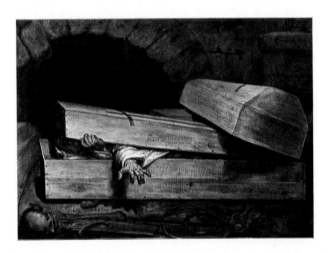

EVOLUTIONARY THEORIES OF SLEEP

Kleitman[353] (pp. 363–370) and Berlucchi[318] have reviewed the evolutionary theories of sleep and wakefulness. It has been suggested often that the development of sleep in the animal kingdom from insects, fish, reptiles, birds to primates, is also seen in the changes in sleep which occur as the human infant grows to the adult man. However, as we have seen (p. 29), animals sleep in many different ways. In the animal kingdom, sleep is often more determined by environment and life style than by evolutionary status, and the idea that the ontogeny of sleep in man repeats the phylogeny of sleep in animals is probably false. A general feature of *mammalian sleep* (see p. 9) is the capacity for sleep regulation with marked rebound of REM sleep and enhancement of slow-wave sleep following sleep deprivation in many species – the cat, dog and rabbit as well as man. Despite intensive investigation, REM sleep has not been found in the dolphin, and there is still insufficient data to justify the conclusion of Allison and van Twyver[315] that paradoxical sleep arose 130 millions years ago with the divergence of *Echidna* ancestors from the main line of mammalian evolution (see p. 32). *Many invertebrates* show characteristic behaviour similar to that of the sleep of vertebrates, and a knowledge of sleep-like states throughout the animal kingdom is necessary to understand the meaning of sleep.

Moruzzi[370] viewed the adult human sleep–wake cycle as the result of both inborn factors, basically the development and maturation of the cerebral cortex from infancy[353] and its relationship with the brain stem, and learnt factors under the influence of day and night and social influences.

HUMORAL THEORIES OF SLEEP

The hypnotoxin theory of sleep, in one form or other, dies hard. Kleitman[353] reviewed some 16 possible hypnotoxins, although all have now been discarded. Hypnotoxin theories propose that the production and accumulation of some sleep toxin results in sleep, which in turn modifies this state with subsequent awakening. Sleep-promoting substances have been claimed to be released as a consequence of both sleep deprivation[356] and sleep induction by electrical thalamic stimulation.[354] It is puzzling that these substances may appear in the brain, blood or cerebrospinal fluid both as a consequence of prolonged wakefulness and also of induced sleep.[370]

If sleep were due to a hypnotoxin, Siamese twins should sleep and wake at the same times. Kleitman[353] discussed the sleep of Siamese twins observed by Geoffrey Saint-Hilaire in 1836, and others exhibited by Barnum and Bailey. In these infants, sleeping and waking were independent. Later reports by Alekseyeva[316] and Webb[394] have demonstrated convincingly that thoracopagus as well as craniopagus conjoined twins sleep at different times, have a different duration and depth of sleep, and have independent NREM and REM sleep. There is no evidence that sleep is caused by any hypnotoxin, or that one function of sleep is to remove toxic waste.

BODY RESTITUTION THEORIES OF SLEEP

Sleep was considered by Sherington[385] to be a state of enhanced *tissue growth and repair* following the wear and tear of wakefulness. Four lines of evidence support this idea. (1) Sleep length increases with body mass, both in human subjects[313] and across species.[396] (2) Boyar et al.[320] suggested there was an increased release of anabolic hormones during sleep. (3) Occasionally, a graduated increase of stage 3 and 4 NREM sleep follows graded increases in exercise[343] (but see p. 50). (4) Increased mitosis during sleep and faster bone growth during sleep were reported by Valk and van der Bosch.[391] Also, the release of growth hormone from the pituitary at sleep onset with peak levels during NREM stage 3–4 sleep[382] is often considered to indicate that NREM sleep is a time for body repair. However, sleep-related growth hormone release is rare in mammals, and, in man, somatomedin growth hormone factors show highest levels waking, not sleeping.[366] If the function of growth hormone in adults is to permit protein synthesis, it is surprising that insulin does not show sleep-related release.

Peak rates of cell division occur during sleep, but are not due to sleep itself. Scheving[383] found that the peak mitosis rate over 24 h was influenced by feeding, with an inverse relationship to cortisol output.[336] Increased cell division at night still occurs without sleep, and the stimulus to body tissue repair is probably feeding, not sleep. The fasting state of sleep may be associated with tissue breakdown, and not repair, in which case growth hormone release, with a protein-sparing effect during sleep, possibly may be beneficial.[338, 339]

SLEEP AND THE MOTOR SYSTEM

Is sleep necessary for the normal function of the motor system? Horne[349] has shown that the mechanical efficiency at different work loads of the body is not reduced by three days without sleep. On the other hand, poor sleep, alpha–delta sleep, sleep deprivation and NREM sleep deprivation may result in subsequent muscle aching.[367] A recent 120 h sleep deprivation investigation of the activity of skeletal muscle enzymes, sampled by biopsy at the end of deprivation, reported changes in enzyme activity, as well as increased serum lactate.[393]

Any abnormality of sleep, hypersomnia, insomnia or fragmented sleep may be followed by impaired motor control on waking. Minor degrees of morning weakness, usually involving distal muscles, skilled hand function and cortical movements are found for brief periods in some normal subjects immediately after waking. Although sleep deprivation does not affect work ability, there is a definite circadian rhythm to physical performance, which is maximal between 1200 and 2100.[372]

Sleep has profound effects on waking motor control. In *parkinsonism*, irrespective of drug treatment, between a third and a half of all subjects show considerable sleep benefit, and, in the late illness, early morning foot dystonia is a characteristic feature on waking.[362] In *hereditary progressive dystonia*, with marked diurnal fluctuation, sleep, but not rest in the afternoon, will abolish dystonia.[384] This variation may be due to sleep-related rhythms in 5-HT, noradrenaline and dopamine in the brain. Regional monoamine oxidase and brain dopamine concentrations, and also dopamine receptor sensitivity, are different sleeping and waking, or altered by sleep deprivation;[390] and Stern and Morgane[389] suggested that sleep may be a time of maintenance of catecholamine systems involved in motor control. However, all the functions of the brain and body are influenced by the alternation of sleep and wakefulness, and it is easy to show that the aim of sleep is not to give a period of rest to the skeletal muscles, nor to permit the recovery of the spinal cord or autonomic nervous system.[368, 369] The body and muscles, but perhaps not the brain, can rest to a similar extent in quiet wakefulness as in sleep. Horne[349] has suggested therefore that the major function of sleep is to maintain not the body but the brain. However, in the final analysis, many if not all aspects of mammalian life depend on sleep.

SLEEP, MEMORY AND LEARNING

Descartes, Liebnitz and Kant taught that we think and dream continuously during sleep, although we frequently forget that we have done so. 'In sleep, the mind is not engaged with thoughts but with molecular processes, and these processes are the great factor in the aetiology of dreams.' These philosophical ideas are supported by recent evidence that sleeping and dreaming are necessary for memory. Learning, the consolidation of memory, the mutual interaction between innate and acquired information and programming – perhaps specially important for genetic functions – all depend on sleep, particularly on REM sleep.[325, 346, 352, 378] However, it is of course unrealistic to separate functionally NREM from REM sleep, since the two processes are closely related and may have complementary memory functions.

The idea that sleep is necessary for memory has a greater experimental basis than any other theory. Just over half a century ago, psychologists showed the beneficial effects of sleep upon the retention of memories acquired during wakefulness.[351, 392] The special significance of REM sleep for memory has been established in four main ways: (1) by REM sleep deprivation experiments in animals and man; (2) by a study of the characteristics of REM sleep following new learning or environmental changes; (3) by examination of the effects of lesions of REM sleep-generating mechanisms in animals and of REM sleep disorders in man; and (4) by observation of the effects on memory of drugs that alter REM sleep.

Most reports linking REM sleep with learning come from animal studies. The main evidence is the finding of high levels of REM sleep after learning tasks; and interference with learning following REM sleep deprivation.[335, 364, 377] REM sleep at specific times following training is necessary for many learning tasks.[387]

However, the outcome of these studies has been very mixed, with negative as well as positive results. The exact experimental design is critical, and the slightest variation in animal weight, age, previous activity or sleep may upset the experiment. It is generally assumed that the critical period for sleep is within a few hours of the task in polycyclic animals, but long latency REM sleep responses, up to 12 h after learning, may occur.[387] The acquisition of many simple learning tasks in animals is followed by an augmentation of REM sleep,[319, 360] without any modification of NREM sleep; augmentation of REM sleep after learning has even been described in human babies.[376]

Memory consolidation is enhanced by drugs with stimulant properties (e.g. amphetamine, picrotoxin and strychnine), before or after learning, although these drugs may interfere with sleep.[363] Drug effects on attention, sleep and memory are thus very complex and findings such as that the combination of imipramine with physostigmine will prevent the deleterious effect of REM sleep deprivation on learning in rodents[346] are difficult to interpret.

Lesions that interfere with REM sleep mechanisms in animals interfere with learning. Fishbein and Gutwein[335] showed that lesions of the catecholamine-containing cells of the locus coeruleus, sufficient to cause up to 50% reduction of phasic PGO waves and eye movements in REM sleep, resulted in an increase in the period during which new memory traces may be disrupted by electroconvulsive shock. The most recent memories are the most susceptible to disruption.[397] Bilateral but not unilateral locus coeruleus lesions are necessary to interfere with REM sleep, but unilateral lesions will extend the labile period of a memory trace.

Sleep may be particularly important for RNA and DNA synthesis linked to memory processes. The effect of sleep on the synthesis of brain nucleic acids (RNA and DNA) has been investigated after injection of radioactive precursors, and the RNA content of neurones and glia determined. There is some evidence that during sleep RNA is more actively synthesized, less rapidly degraded or more slowly transported into the cytoplasm. This has been attributed to more active involvement of nuclear RNA and slowing down of ribosomal RNA activity in large nuclei of astrocytes or neurones during slow-wave sleep.[340] This molecular approach to sleep function has not yet determined whether new molecules are synthesized during sleep as the result of learning during wakefulness.

In human adults, as in animals, there is some evidence that REM sleep may increase following learning. Hartmann[347] and Greenberg[341] indicated that an increase of REM sleep time occurs after days of increased learning, mental stress and especially demanding events, although these results are very inconsistent, and Lester et al.,[358] who studied the effect of real life stress associated with final medical examinations upon sleep in the laboratory, found no increase in REM sleep, although there was a decrease in NREM sleep. Other stressful situations, such as Skylab with zero gravity, do not produce any immediate increase in REM sleep,[337] although this may occur several days after return to earth. Sitaram et al.[386] showed that increased vigilance whilst awake may be followed by an increase in REM sleep. During an intensive language course, the best learners were found to have an increase in REM sleep, whilst those who did not improve language scores also showed no change in REM sleep time.[324]

Absent or markedly reduced REM sleep has been documented in many human diseases, for example in progressive supranuclear palsy,[332, 344, 359, 361, 373, 388] but in none of these disorders in which REM sleep is reduced has any major change in memory or personality been clearly attributed to lack of REM sleep. The pattern of memory impairment in subcortical dementia[365] with marked forgetfulness and lack of motivation[314] has been linked to loss of REM sleep. However, patients with progressive supranuclear palsy can and do continue to learn until late in the disease, although they are apathetic and disinterested, with poor motivation. Awareness, personality, motivation and behaviour may be entirely normal in patients with spinocerebellar ataxia despite marked reduction in REM sleep. Dementia in Huntington's chorea or progressive supranuclear palsy is not dependent upon sleep disruption or lack of REM sleep, although the present data is scanty. However, Castuldo and Krynicki showed that REM sleep measurements vary with the degree of intelligence in mentally retarded patients, and that the degree of correlation that exists is independent of neurological impairment.[321]

Many attempts have been made to relate REM reduction after brain trauma with loss of memory in man.[327] Also, linkage of recovery of REM sleep with recovery of intellectual function has been suggested after head injury, but the evidence is inconclusive.[330, 331] Following up a group of nine patients with severe traumatic brain damage, Ron et al.[381] found a correlation between cognition and REM sleep improvement in seven patients, but not in two. If massive learning does cause an increase in REM sleep, brain-damaged patients who are improving should have a higher proportion of REM sleep than patients showing no improvement. Greenberg and Dewan compared the percentage of REM sleep in improving and non-improving aphasic patients and found that the latter group did in fact have lower levels.[342] In 32 patients with Down's syndrome, phenylketonuria and other forms of brain damage, Feinberg[329] found a positive relation between the amount of eye movement during REM sleep and estimates of intellectual function, whilst in a comparison of 38 normal individuals and 15 brain-damaged subjects, Feinberg[328] showed that the mentally retarded patients had less REM sleep. It is obvious that none of these observations establishes a role for REM sleep in human learning or memory, and convincing evidence for this idea has still to be obtained in brain-damaged subjects.

In normal, not brain-damaged, humans there is considerable evidence that those subjects who sleep following learning remember slightly more than those subjects who are awake for the same length of time. Sleep appears to be most beneficial to human learning when it follows immediately after. However, results are very variable and the benefit of sleep when compared with wakefulness following learning is neither great nor long-lasting.[345] High arousal at the time of learning, although not improving immediate recall, results in better long-term retention than low arousal. It is possible that memory for neutral material such as nonsense syllables and word pairs is consolidated during NREM sleep, whilst REM sleep may play a more active role in consolidation of more vivid and emotive material.

Can learning occur during sleep? The best case that can be made comes from the study of physiological responses to external stimuli during sleep. Pressing a switch in response to noise may occur in light stage 1–2 NREM sleep, but rarely in deep NREM or REM sleep.[395] The meaningfulness of stimulus during sleep affects the response. Thus the nature of the stimulus (personal name versus electric shock) will affect the complexity of physiological response, change in heart rate, stimulus-evoked K complex, or galvanic skin response.[317, 375] If the stimulus is repeated, habituation of the EEG arousal response, galvanic skin and other physiological responses occurs during sleep.[333, 374]

Reliable, prolonged or useful sleep-learning has not been demonstrated. Short-term memory for very simple stimuli such as a single figure may be possible if presented in stage 1–2 NREM sleep, but the stimulus presentation is often followed by arousal. Learning of complex information does not occur if presented in uninterrupted (alpha-free) sleep, and is not followed by arousal.[322] Although there may be no difficulty in the storage of simple learned responses during sleep, later waking recall is impossible.[326, 355, 357]

SLEEP AND 'UNLEARNING'

Hughlings Jackson[350] attributed to sleep the function of sleeping away unnecessary memories as well as consolidation and reprogramming of more vital material. Newman and Evans[371] assigned a specific 'unlearning' function to REM sleep and Crick and Mitchison[323] suggested that REM sleep may have a 'cleaning-up' function, to remove unwanted memory traces from information nets in the brain. Any 'unlearning' system might remove weak memories, but reinforce strong ones, and might conceivably prevent fantasy, obsessions and hallucinations. Relative isolation of the cortex from environmental stimuli during sleep may be a necessary requisite for a system which delivers a non-specific noise signal, e.g. the series of electric discharges or spike potentials of PGO waves. Electrical discharges may reduce the storage of all information, but totally abolish only weak memories. If PGO waves reached the limbs, sleep would be disturbed by muscle jerking, and hence possibly a need for motor as well as sensory disconnection.

Is there any evidence that REM sleep does have an 'unlearning' function? As long ago as 1917, Pötzl showed that dream material was sometimes derived from unimportant or unnoticed details, in keeping with the idea that these might be swept away by REM sleep.[380] He showed subjects brief exposures of complicated pictures, and observed which items were missed. These items were found to appear in distorted form in drawings from memory, and also appeared in dreams. More recently, studies of mathematical models of nerve nets in the brain have shown that random input, as occurs during REM sleep, will reduce spurious memories, but also enhance access to real ones.[348] Also, in animals, procedures (e.g. reserpine administration) that should enhance the amount of REM sleep after a learning exercise sometimes result in poorer, not better, retention.[334] None of this evidence is conclusive, and much of what we remember, as well as much of what we forget, must be determined by waking rather than sleeping processes.

THE ENVIRONMENT OF SLEEP

Good sleep is widely accepted as a component of good health, but what constitutes or is considered to be 'good' sleep varies widely. The proverb 'early to bed and early to rise makes a man healthy, wealthy and wise' is possibly true. However, there is little scientific support for the British public school view of the requirements for good sleep (a freezing dormitory with wide open windows); what is needed are quiet surroundings, freedom from light and noise and a comfortable bed. A strange situation, even in comfortable surroundings, will disturb sleep. First-night recordings in sleep laboratories are notoriously unreliable and often show very disturbed sleep, even in otherwise good sleepers.[398] Even bed position can be important. Charles Dickens claimed that he could detect the Earth's magnetic field and required correct north–south bed orientation for good sleep.

NOISE

Noise sensitivity during sleep varies markedly from one person to another, from an awakening threshold of 15 dB for one sleeper to over 100 dB for another, but everyone has a noise level which will disturb sleep. The level of tolerated noise tends to be lowest latest in the night[407] and the sound of the early morning delivery of milk may be particularly disturbing, since this also corresponds with the period at which the bladder becomes distended.[406]

Women are awoken more easily by a sudden noise than men,[400] perhaps owing to the inherent need for maternal awakening, and old people's sleep is more disturbed by noise than that of young people. A noise level sufficient to awaken a 70-year-old causes only a temporary shift to stage 1 NREM sleep at the age of 25, and sonic booms cause arousal much more often in old than in young people.[404, 409]

The awakening threshold varies with the stage of sleep. This is lowest in stage 1, greatest in delta sleep and variable in REM sleep.[407] The threshold for arousal to a meaningful stimulus, personal name or baby's whimper, is said to be less than for non-meaningful stimuli; and the sound level required to produce disturbance can be high if the sound is such that it is incorporated into the dream content but low if it conflicts with the dream.

Traffic and airport noise markedly disturb sleep, even in people who do not awaken from it and may not remember the noise in the morning. In a comparison of residents living close to the Los Angeles International Airport and others in quieter areas, Globus et al.[401] found that people living near to the Airport had 45 min less delta, stage 2 and REM sleep than the other subjects each night. Under these circumstances earplugs will promote sleep.

THE BED

Some people sleep most comfortably on a hard bed, others on one which is soft and yielding, although, as would be expected, hard surfaces and wooden floors cause more body movements, more awakenings and more stage 1 sleep than do softer surfaces.[403] However, exotic beds, water beds, bean beds and the like have little effect on sleep in normal subjects.[399, 402, 408, 410]

SLEEPING PARTNER

In a double bed with a partner, a change in sides on which they lie may be the answer to poor sleep. Monroe[405] investigated good sleeper couples who habitually slept in the same bed. When the couples slept together in a sleep laboratory, they had less delta sleep and more REM sleep than when they slept apart. Sleeping in separate beds may prevent arousals due to changes in the posture of the sleeping partner and improve the depth and quality of sleep.

SLEEP AND FOOD

Food assists sleeping. Early this century Pavlov[421, 422] showed that a carbohydrate meal induced sleep in dogs, and more recently Fara et al.[416] have shown that the introduction of milk or fat directly into the duodenum of cats improves sleep. There is a loose association between feeding, sleeping and thyroid function, hyperthyroidism being associated with weight loss and short but intensive sleep, whereas hypothyroidism results in weight gain and long sleep times with a relative loss of delta sleep.[418] It has been suggested that sleep-promoting factors are present in bacteria taken in with food.

Weight gain, when food intake is more than body need, leads to quiet and long sleep periods; and weight loss, as a result of low food intake, can lead to more fragmented and shortened sleep. Crisp and McGuiness[413] found that fatter people sleep longer and judge themselves happier than thin people, and Adam[411] found a significant correlation between being above or below ideal weight and the duration of sleep. Regularity of evening food intake seems to be good for sleep,[412] although it is counterproductive to indulge in heavy eating or drinking before bedtime. In babies, alteration in 5-hydroxytryptophan (5-HTP) in the diet may alter sleep patterns, but the effect is slight.[423] The amount of 5-HTP in even high-protein foods is low and unlikely to alter adult sleep.

Most people normally stop eating between 2200 and 0800 and sleep is usually a time of fasting. This fast results in a reduction in protein turnover during sleep; this is determined by the night-time fast, not by sleep itself.[417] However, severe and prolonged fasting may cause insomnia. Patients with anorexia nervosa tend to have disturbed sleep, particularly in the middle of the night, and wake early. This is not related to mood changes but depends probably on the severity of the nutritional disturbance. In patients with both depression and poor appetite, weight loss is frequently associated with complaints of poor sleep and weight increase with long and sound sleep.[414, 415] In 364 attenders at a psychiatric outpatient clinic, Crisp and Stonehill[414] found that early morning waking and broken sleep in the latter part of the night were associated with recent weight loss independent of mood.

In *depression*, most patients lose weight and become insomniacs, although a minority show the reverse pattern, put on weight and sleep for excessively long times.[420] In *anorexia nervosa*, sleep often improves when these patients are fed.[419] However, near-starvation can cause sleepiness, not increased alertness. Observations in prison camps during the Second World War on prisoners with rations of about 1000 calories a day, with a bare minimum of vitamins to prevent clinical manifestations of deficiency, showed that the inmates were very sleepy as well as hungry and weak.

SLEEP AND WEATHER

The season of the year, the weather, temperature, barometric pressure and hours of daylight all affect sleep. The onset of sleep in aviation personnel showed some relationship with barometric pressure when investigated by Raboutet *et al.*[433] The higher the barometric pressure was during a routine EEG, the fewer people fell asleep. Webb and Ades suggested that both very high and very low barometric pressures were associated with increasing sleepiness during EEGs.[436]

Many people living in Norway north of the Arctic circle complain about insomnia during the dark season during the midwinter when the sun does not rise above the horizon. This complaint can affect up to one-third of school children and adolescents[425, 427] and also adults. This type of insomnia is usually characterized by difficulty in going to sleep in the evening, and is sometimes very severe. Those suffering from winter insomnia feel ill at ease and tired in the morning and sometimes for most of the day.[428]

Sleep varies with the environmental temperature, but there is no ideal temperature for everyone. It has been shown that sleeping in a hot climate with room temperatures above 24 °C (75 °F) does reduce the quality of sleep, with a decrease in both REM and delta sleep, more awakenings and more movements,[434] and sometimes a greater recall of dreams. Gradually reducing the room temperature to 12 °C, however, may increase the unpleasant and emotional aspects of dreams.

Some animals seem to have an ideal external sleep temperature, 30–32 °C in the rat, 22 °C in the cat,[431, 437] but no consistent differences in sleep in human psychiatric patients sleeping at 18 °C, 23 °C and 29 °C have been shown.[432]

Euler and Söderburg[426] reported that gentle local heating of the hypothalamus had a damping effect on the reticular formation and promoted EEG changes of sleep in the cat and the rabbit, whilst excessive heating caused arousal. In man, body core temperature has been reported to be higher throughout the night in poor than in good sleepers,[429] and in a study of Adam and Tomeny reported by Oswald[430] poor sleepers were also hotter throughout the day than good sleepers.

During REM sleep, temperature regulation is impaired in animals, as well as humans.[424, 435]

SLEEP AND EXERCISE

Oswald[452] and Adam[438] have suggested that slow-wave sleep is necessary for physical restoration. If this is so, one might expect people who take little exercise, who are lazy, or who spend much of the day in bed resting but not asleep, to have little NREM sleep at night, whilst athletes and Olympic runners might have long periods of NREM sleep. However, the evidence that exercise influences subsequent sleep in any way, or that good sleep is followed the next day by an increased capacity for exercise, is very slight (Table 1.4). Indeed, Hobson[448] showed that exercise taken too near to bedtime will prevent sleep, and Ryback et al.[453] showed that prolonged bed rest during the day, without exercise, over a five-week period, actually increased, not decreased, the amount of delta sleep during the night. Despite these findings, there have been many studies of the effect on sleep of mild (gentle jogging), moderate (3–4 mile fast walking) or severe (marathon running) exercise, taken by either normal

Table 1.4 *Sleep and exercise – reported effects in various studies*

Horne[449]	No effect on sleep
Torsvall[457]	No effect on sleep
Baekeland and Lasky[439] Shapiro et al.[455] Shapiro et al.[454] Malotnev et al.[451] Griffin and Trinder[444] Shapiro and Verschoor[456]	Enhanced at night All physically well trained subjects
Walker et al.[460] Buguet et al.[441] Bonnet[440] Trinder et al.[459] Horne and Staff[450]	No NREM stage 3–4 sleep increase
Browman[442]	Effect on first sleep cycle only
Bonnet[440] Buguet et al.[441]	Increase or decrease of different stages of NREM sleep
Torsvall et al.[458]	Reduced REM sleep No change in slow-wave sleep

sedentary young men or trained athletes; and at periods between 1 and 10 h before sleep onset. Hauri[445-447] found that intensive exercise for 6 h on one evening, and complete relaxation for 6 h on another evening, did not greatly alter the subsequent sleep of non-athletic students. With athletes, the position is somewhat different, and those in good training may have a greater proportion of deep sleep (NREM stages 3 and 4) than others.[439, 461] In contrast to these findings, Torsvall *et al.*[458] have shown that athletic races may cause a delay or decrease in REM sleep, but little change in NREM sleep. In view of these conflicting results, there is considerable scepticism as to whether exercise has any effect on sleep.

DEATH AT NIGHT

Statistics from Berlin,[468] Glasgow[466] and San Diego[469] fix the highest peak of mortality at night, between 0400 and 0700. The commonest time of sudden death in many conditions is at night.[462]

Hammond,[463] in a study of over 1 million individuals for the American Cancer Society, found that during a 2-year follow-up period of mortality, men who said that they slept about 7 h per night had lower death rates than those who reported sleeping either less or more. In a separate study, Kripke *et al.*[465] analysed recent cause-specific mortality in relation to sleep length and health status over a 6-year follow-up period. Men sleeping 4 h or less had a 2.8-fold mortality risk compared with those sleeping 7–7.9 h. For those sleeping 10 h or more, the mortality risk was 1.8. This was true for coronary heart disease, stroke and cancer, as well as for suicide.

Death from heart disease is especially common during sleep. Partinen *et al.*[467] examined the effect of sleep length on heart disease. Short (less than 6 h) or long (more than 10 h) sleepers had more complaints relating to coronary heart disease than those who slept for 7–8 h per night. Short sleep was especially related to angina pectoris, and pain of possible infarction. On the other hand, long sleepers had the highest diagnosed incidence of myocardial infarction. This may be due to the excess in long sleepers of REM sleep, which has been associated with nocturnal coronary attacks.

As well as heart disease, excess nocturnal deaths have been related to sleeping pill and tranquilliser use, and possibly sleep apnoea. In data from the barbiturate era, Kripke and Garfinkel[464] gave evidence that more people who took sleeping pills died at night. In 661 subjects, the hour of death was as shown in Table 1.5. There is a significant difference in the temporal distribution

Table 1.5   *Hour of death and sleeping pill use.*

Hour of death	No sleeping pills	Frequent sleeping pills
2300–0600	81	125
0700–1400	112	118
1500–2200	121	104
Total	314	347

of these deaths, but illnesses which cause an excess of deaths during sleep may of course lead to an increased intake of sleeping pills.

HYPNOSIS

Hypnosis is a very different state from sleep, and sleep induced by hypnotic drugs is different from the condition known as hypnosis, although there are behavioural similarities between hypnosis, automatic behaviour and sleep walking.[470, 472] Mesmer, who considered that the stars and planets had an effect on man, exerted by a force comparable to magnetism, was the discoverer of the phenomenon now called hypnosis, a state of altered awareness induced by suggestion and associated with abnormal suggestibility (Fig. 1.7). Animals, including crabs, rabbits and hens, as well as man, may be hypnotized. Approximately 10% of Western Europeans will enter deep hypnosis, and 90% light hypnosis.

In addition to heightened suggestibility, with highly focussed attention and obliteration of peripheral distractions induced by the hypnotist, the state of hypnosis is characterized by confabulation, loss of critical judgement, amnesia, and sometimes sensory obliteration, time regression and the ability to sustain fixed postures. Critical judgement may be entirely lost and the idea that hypnosis can somehow reactivate original memory traces is largely false. Memory is a shifty thing and easily altered by suggestion, and confabulation during hypnosis may result in failure of self-monitoring, disturbed time sense, and convincing descriptions of abduction by flying saucer or life as a slave in ancient Greece. Despite this, the forensic use of hypnotism is on the increase in the USA.

Amnesia, unlike that of head injury not retrograde, only occurs with deep hypnosis. Suggestibility and post-hypnotic suggestion is well documented, and distortion of perception, 'flashbacks' and false perception correspond somewhat to the dreaming state with visual imagery.

Under hypnosis, atonia comparable to that of sleep may be induced, or alternatively either segmental or generalized catalepsy. The alpha rhythm of relaxed wakefulness is abolished during deep hypnosis, and replaced by diffuse low to moderate voltage 4–7 Hz components, but sleep spindles or other sleep-specific changes do not occur.

The production of hypnosis is dependent upon directed, rather than neglected, attention to a repetitive, monotonous and sometimes conditioned stimulus. This stimulus is usually mundane, although autohypnosis may be conditioned by a variety of strange and monotonous stimuli. The Hesychasts of Mount Athos remained motionless for several days with the gaze fixed on the navel; the Taskodrugites remained statuesque for long periods with the finger applied to the nose; and the Jogins could apparently hibernate at will. The Dandus of India become cataleptoid by 12 000 repetitions of the sacred word 'Om'. In the appropriate setting, repeated stimuli may provoke either hypnosis or sleep. St. Simon Stylites, perched on his lofty pillar, preserved an attitude of saintly withdrawal from worldly things for days, and likewise Socrates would stand for hours motionless and wordless.[471]

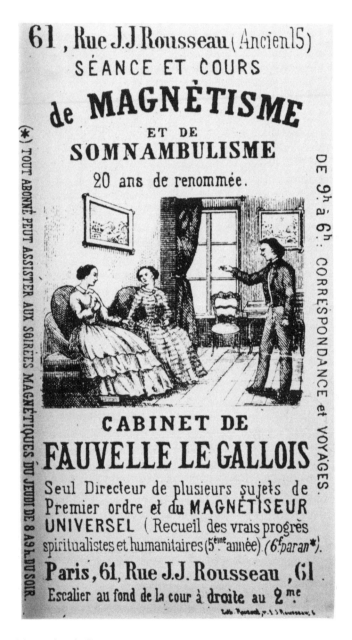

Figure 1.7 *Mesmerism in France.*

REFERENCES

INTRODUCTION

1. Arendt, J. & Marks, V. Can melatonin alleviate jet-lag? *Brit. Med. J. (Clin. Res.)* (1983) **287**, 426.
2. Aserinsky, E. & Kleitman, N. Regularly occurring periods of eye motility and concomitant phenomena during sleep, *Science* (1953) **118**, 273–274.
3. Bremer, F. Cerveau 'isolé' et physiologie du sommeil, *C. R. Soc. Biol.* (1935) **118**, 1235–1241.
4. Bremer, F. L'activité cérébrale au cours du sommeil et de la narcose. Contribution à l'étude du mécanisme du sommeil, *Bull. Acad. Roy. Méd. Belg.* (1937) **4**, 68–86.
5. Bremer, F. L'activité électrique de l'écorce cérébrale et le problème physiologique du sommeil, *Bull. Soc. Ital. Biol.* (1938) **13**, 271–290.
6. Dement, W.C. & Kleitman, N. The relation of eye movements during sleep to dream activity: an objective method for the study of dreaming, *J. Exp. Psychol.* (1957) **53**, 339–346.
7. Evarts, E.V. Activity of individual cerebral neurons during sleep and arousal, *Res. Publ. Ass. Nerv. Ment. Dis.* (1967) **45**, 319–337.
8. Hall, S. A study of fears, *Am. J. Psychol.* (1897) 244.
9. Horne, J.A. Human sleep and tissue restitution; some qualifications and doubts, *Clin. Sci.* (1983) **65**, 569–578.
10. Jouvet, M. Neurophysiology of the states of sleep, *Physiol. Rev.* (1967) **47**, 117–177.
11. Lombard, W.P. The variations of the normal knee-jerk and their relation to the activity of the central nervous system, *Am. J. Psychol.* (1887) **1**, 1.
12. Loomis, A.L., Harvey, E.N. & Hobart, G.A. Potential rhythms of the cerebral cortex during sleep, *Science* (1935) **81**, 597–598.
13. Loomis, A.L., Harvey, E.N. & Hobart, G.A. Further observations on the potential rhythms of the cerebral cortex during sleep, *Science* (1935) **82**, 199–200.
14. Loomis, A.L., Harvey, E.N. & Hobart, G.A. Cerebral states during sleep as studied by human brain potentials, *J. Exp. Psychol.* (1937) **21**, 127–144.
15. Loomis, A.L., Harvey, E.N. & Hobart, G.A. Distribution of disturbance-patterns in the human electroencephalogram, with special reference to sleep, *J. Neurophysiol.* (1938) **1**, 413–430.
16. Macnish, R. *The Philosophy of Sleep,* Glasgow: E. McPhun (1830).
17. Moldofsky, H. & Scarisbrick, P. Induction of neurasthenic musculoskeletal pain syndrome by selective sleep stage deprivation, *Psychosom. Med.* (1976) **38**, 35–44.
18. Moruzzi, G. The physiology of sleep, *Endeavour* (1963) **22**, 31–36.
19. Moruzzi, G. Active processes in the brain stem during sleep, *Harvey Lect.* (1963) **58**, 233–297.
20. Moruzzi, G. The historical development of the deafferentation hypothesis of sleep, *Proc. Am. Phil. Soc.* (1964) **108**, 19–28.
21. Moruzzi, G. Sleep and instinctive behaviour, *Arch. Ital. Biol.* (1969) **107**, 175–216.
22. Moruzzi, G. & Magoun, H.W. Brain stem reticular formation and activation of the EEG, *Electroenceph. Clin. Neurophysiol.* (1949) **1**, 455–473.
23. Pavlov, I.P. 'Innere Hemmung' der bedingten Reflexe und der Schlaf—ein und derselbe Prozess, *Skand. Arch. Physiol.* (1923) **44**, 42–58.
24. Pavlov, I.P. *Conditioned Reflexes. An Investigation of the Physiological Activity of the Cerebral Cortex.* Anpep. G.V. (ed.) Oxford: Oxford University Press (1927) 430.
25. Purkinje, J.E. Wachen Schlaf Traum und verwändte Zustände. In: Wagner, R. (ed.) *Handwörterbuch der Physiologie,* (9 Bande). Braunschweig: Friedr Vieweg & Sohn (1846) Bd 3 (Abt 2), S 412–480.
26. Salamy, J.G. Sleep: some concepts and constructs. In: Williams, R.L. & Karacan, I. (eds.) *Pharmacology of Sleep,* New York: Wiley (1976) 53–82.
27. von Economo, C. Die Pathologie des Schlafes. In: Bethe, A. von, Bergman, G.V., Embden, G. & Ellinger, A. (eds.) *Handbuch der normalen und pathologischen Physiologie.* Berlin: Springer (1926) Vol. 17 S 591–610.
28. von Economo, C. Schlaftheorie, *Ergebn. Physiol.* (1929) **28**, 312–339.

BEHAVIOUR BEFORE AND DURING SLEEP

29. Alihanka, J. Sleep movements and associated autonomic nervous activities in young male adults, *Acta Physiol. Scan. (Suppl.)* (1982) **511**, 1–85.
30. Aserinsky, E. & Kleitman, N. Two types of ocular motility occurring during sleep, *J. Appl. Physiol.* (1955) **8**, 1–10.
31. Batini, C., Fressy, J. & Gastaut, H. A study of the plantar cutaneous reflex during the different phases of sleep, *Electroenceph. Clin. Neurophysiol.* (1964) **16**, 412–413.
32. Baust, W., Berlucchi, G. & Moruzzi, G. Changes in the auditory input during arousal in cats with tenotomized middle ear muscles, *Arch. Ital. Biol.* (1964) **102**, 657–674.
33. Baust, W. & Rohrwasser, W. Das Verhalten von pH und Motilität des Magens in natürlichen Schlaf des Menschen, *Pflüeger Arch. Ges. Physiol.* (1969) **305**, 229–241.
34. Carli, G. Dissociation of electrocortical activity and somatic reflexes during rabbit hypnosis, *Arch. Ital. Biol.* (1969) **107**, 219–234.
35. Coccagna, G., Mantovani, M., Brignani, F., Manzini, A. & Lugaresi, E. Arterial pressure changes during spontaneous sleep in man, *Electroenceph. Clin. Neurophysiol.* (1971) **31**, 277–281.
36. De Koninck, J., Gagnon, P. & Lallier, S. Sleep positions in the young adult and their relationship with the subjective quality of sleep, *Sleep* (1983) **6**, 52–59.
37. Fisher, G. Gross, J. & Zuch, J. Cycle of penile erection synchronous with dreaming (REM) sleep – preliminary report, *Arch. Gen. Psychiat.* (1965) **12**, 29–45.
38. Fujiki, A., Shimizu, A., Yamada, Y., Yamamoto, J. & Kaneko, Z. The Babinski reflex during sleep and wakefulness, *Electroenceph. Clin. Neurophysiol.* (1971) **31**, 610–613.
39. Gastaut, H. & Bert, B. Electroencephalographic detection of sleep induced by repetitive sensory stimuli. In: Wolstenholme, G.E.W. & O'Connor, M. (eds.) *On the Nature of Sleep*, London: Churchill (1961) 260–283.
40. Gilman. T.T. & Marcuse, F.L. Animal hypnosis, *Psychol. Bull.* (1949) **46**, 151–165.
41. Hassenberg, L. *Ruhe und Schlaf bei Säugetieren*, Wittenberg-Lutherstadt: A. Ziemsen (1965) 160.
42. Hawkins, D., Puryear, H., Wallace, C., Deal, W. & Thomas, E. Basal skin resistance during sleep and 'dreaming', *Science* (1962) **136**, 321–322.
43. Hediger, H. *The Psychology of Animals in Zoos and Circuses*, New York: Dover Publications (1968) 166.
44. Hediger, H. Comparative observations on sleep, *Proc. Roy. Soc. Med.* (1969) **62**, 153–156.
45. Hediger, H. The biology of natural sleep in animals, *Experientia* (1980) **36**, 13–18.
46. Henane, R., Buguet, A., Roussel, B. & Bittel, J. Variations in evaporation and body temperatures during sleep in man, *J. Appl. Physiol.* (1977) **42**, 50–55.
47. Hess, W.R. Das Schlafsyndrom als Folge dienzephal Reizung, *Helv. Physiol. Pharmacol. Acta* (1944) **2**, 305–344.
48. Hishikawa, Y., Sumitsuji, K., Matsumoto, K. & Kaneko, Z. H reflex and EMG of the mental and hyoid muscles with special reference to narcolepsy, *Electroenceph. Clin. Neurophysiol.* (1965) **18**, 487–492.
49. Hodes, R. & Dement, W.C. Depression of electrically induced reflexes (H-reflexes) in man during low voltage EEG 'sleep', *Electroenceph. Clin. Neurophysiol.* (1964) **17**, 617–629.
50. Jouvet, M. Recherches sur les structures nerveuses et les mécanismes responsables des différentes phases du sommeil physiologique, *Arch. Ital. Biol.* (1962) **100**, 125–206.
51. Kennedy, C., Gillin, J.C., Mendelson, W., Suda, S., Miyaoka, M., Ito, M., Nakamura, R.K., Storch, F.I., Petigrew, K., Mishkin, M. & Sokoloff, L. Local cerebral glucose utilization in non-rapid eye movement sleep, *Nature* (1982) **297**, 325–327.
52. Khatri, I.M. & Freis, E.D. Hemodynamic changes during sleep in hypertensive patients, *Circulation* (1969) **39**, 785–790.
53. Koch, E. Die Irradiation der pressor-receptorischen Kreislaufreflexe, *Klin. Wschr.* (1932) **11**, 225–227.
54. Koella, W.P. *Sleep: its Nature and Physiological Organization*, Springfield, Illinois: Charles C. Thomas (1967)
55. Konorski, J. *Integrative Action of the Brain*, Chicago/London: Chicago University Press (1967) 531.
56. Lee, M.A.M. & Kleitman, N. Studies on the physiology of sleep: attempts to demonstrate functional changes in the nervous system during experimental insomnia, *Am. J. Physiol.* (1923) **67**, 141–152.

57. Mangold, R., Sokoloff, L., Connor, E., Kleinerman, J., Therman, P.G. & Kety, S.S. The effect of sleep and lack of sleep on the cerebral circulation and metabolism in normal young men, *J. Clin. Invest.* (1955) **34**, 1092–1100.
58. Nakamura, R.K., Kennedy, C., Gillin, J.C., Suda, S., Ito, M., Storch, F.I., Mendelson, W., Sokoloff, L. & Mishkin, M. Hypnogenic centre theory of sleep: no support from metabolic mapping in monkeys, *Brain Res.* (1983) **268**, 372–376.
59. Oswald, I. *Sleeping and Waking: Physiology and Psychology* Amsterdam: Elsevier (1962).
60. Parmeggiani, P.L. Behavioural phenomenology of sleep (somatic and vegetative), *Experientia* (1980) **36**, 6–11.
61. Parmeggiani, P.L., Agnati, L.F., Zamboni, G. & Cianci, T. Hypothalamic temperature during the sleep cycle at different ambient temperatures, *Electroenceph. Clin. Neurophysiol.* (1975) **38**, 589–596.
62. Parmeggiani, P.L. & Rabini, C. Sleep and environmental temperature, *Arch. Ital. Biol.* (1970) **108**, 369–388.
63. Piéron, H. *Le Problème Physiologique du Sommeil*, Paris: Masson (1913) 520.
64. Ploog, D. Über den Schlaf und seine Beziehungen zu endogenen Psychosen, *Münch. Med. Wschr.* (1953) **95**, 897–900.
65. Pompeiano, O. Ascending and descending influences on somatic afferent volleys in unrestrained cats: supraspinal control of spinal reflexes during natural and reflexly induced sleep. In: Jouvet, M. (ed.) *Aspects Anatomo-Fonctionnels de la Physiologie du Sommeil*, Paris: CNRS (1965) 309–395.
66. Pompeiano, O. Muscular afferents and motor control during sleep. In: Granit, R. (ed.) *Muscular Afferents and Motor Control* (First Nobel Symposium), Stockholm: Almqvist & Wiksell (1966) 415–436.
67. Pompeiano, O. & Morrison, A.R. Vestibular influences during sleep. 1. Abolition of the rapid eye movements of desynchronized sleep following vestibular lesions, *Arch. Ital. Biol.* (1965) **103**, 569–595.
68. Portielje, A.F.J. Triebleben bzw. intelligente Äusserungen beim Orang-utan *(Pongo pigmaeus Hoppius), Bijdr. Dierk.* (1939) **27**, 61–114.
69. Richardson, D.W., Honour, A.J., Fenton, G.W., Stott, F.H. & Pickering, G.W. Variation in arterial pressure throughout the day and night, *Clin. Sci.* (1964) **26**, 445–460.
70. Sakai, F., Meyer, J.S., Karacan, I., Derman, S. & Yamamoto. M. Normal human sleep: regional cerebral hemodynamics, *Ann. Neurol.* (1979) **7**, 471–478.
71. Snyder, F. Autonomic nervous system manifestations during sleep and dreaming, *Res. Publ. Assoc. Res. Nerv. Ment. Dis.* (1967) **45**, 469.
72. Snyder, F., Hobson, J.A., Morrison, D.F. & Goldfrank, F. Changes in respiration, heart rate and systolic blood pressure in human sleep, *J. Appl. Physiol.* (1964) **19**, 417–422.
73. Stacher, G., Presslich, B. & Stärker, H. Gastric acid and secretion and sleep stages during natural night sleep. *Gastroenterology* (1975) **68**, 1449–1455.
74. Steiniger, F. Die Biologie der sog. 'tierischen Hypnose', *Ergebn. Biol.* (1936) **13**, 348–451.
75. Takagi, K. Über den Einfluss des mechanischen Hautdruckes auf die vegetativen Funktionen, *Acta Neuroveg. (Wien)* (1957) **16**, 439–446.

ELECTROPHYSIOLOGY DURING SLEEP

76. Bert, J. Caractères génériques et caractères spécifiques de l'activité de pointes 'ponto-géniculo-occipitales' (PGO) chez deux babuins, *Papio hamadryas* et *Papio papio, Brain Res.* (1975) **88**, 362–366.
77. Callaway, E. *Brain Electrical Potentials and Individual Psychological Differences*, New York: Grune and Stratton (1975).
78. Gaillard, J.M. Electrophysiological semeiology of sleep, *Experientia* (1980) **36**, 3–7.
79. Head, H. The conception of nervous and mental energy II. ('Vigilance'; a physiological state of the nervous system), *Brit. J. Psychol.* (1923) **14**, 126–147.
80. Hodes, R. & Suzuki, J.I. Comparative thresholds of cortex, vestibular system and reticular formation in wakefulness, sleep, and rapid eye movement periods, *Electroenceph. Clin. Neurophysiol.* (1965) **18**, 239–248.
81. Huttenlocher, P.R. Effects of state of arousal on click responses in the mesencephalic reticular formation, *Electroenceph. Clin. Neurophysiol.* (1960) **12**, 819–827.
82. Huttenlocher, P.R. Evoked and spontaneous activity in single units of medial brain stem

during natural sleep and waking. *J. Neurophysiol.* (1961) **24**, 451–468.

83. Johnson, L.C. & Karpan, W. Autonomic correlates of the spontaneous K-complex, *Psychophysiology* (1968) **4**, 444–452.

84. Larson, S.J., Sances, A.Jr., Ackmann, J.J. & Reigel, D.H. Non-invasive evaluation of head trauma patients, *Surgery* (1973) **74**, 34–40.

85. Lille, F., Borlone, M., Lérique, A., Scherrer, J. & Thieffry, S. Evaluation de la profondeur du coma chez l'enfant par la technique des potentials évoqués, *Rev. Neurol.* (1967) **117**, 216–217.

86. Lille, F., Lerique, A., Pottier, M., Scherrer, J. & Thieffry, S. Evoked cortical responses during coma in childhood, *Presse. Med.* (1968) **76**, 1411–1414.

87. Moruzzi, G. The sleep–waking cycle, *Ergebn. Physiol.* (1972) **64**, 1–165.

88. Oswald, I. *Sleeping and Waking*, Amsterdam: Elsevier (1962).

89. Salzarulo, P., Lairy, G.C., Bancaud, J. & Munari, C. Direct depth recording of the striate cortex during REM sleep in man: are there PGO potentials? *Electroenceph. Clin. Neurophysiol.* (1975) **38**, 199–202.

90. Schmidt, H.S. & Fortin, L.D. Electronic pupillography in disorders of arousal. In: Guilleminault, C. (ed.) *Sleeping and Waking Disorders. Indications and Techniques*, Menlo Park, California: Addison-Wesley (1982) 127–143.

91. Valley, V. & Broughton, R. The physiological (EEG) nature of drowsiness and its relation to performance deficits in narcoleptics, *Electroenceph. Clin. Neurophysiol.* (1983) **55**, 243–251.

92. Wilkinson, R.T. & Ashby, S.M. Selective attention, contingent negative variation, and the evoked potential, *Biol. Psychol.* (1974) **1**, 167–179.

93. Wilkinson, R.T. & Haines, E. Evoked response correlates of expectancy during vigilance, *Acta Psychol. (Amst.)* (1970) **33**, 402–413.

94. Williams, H.L., Hammack, J.T., Daly, R.C., Dement, W.C., & Lubin, A. Responses to auditory stimulation, sleep loss and the EEG stage of sleep, *Electroenceph. Clin. Neurophysiol.* (1964) **16**, 269–279.

95. Yoss, R.E., Moyer, N.J. & Ogle, K.N. The pupillogram and narcolepsy, *Neurology* (1969) **19**, 921–928.

NORMAL SLEEP

96. Bjerner, B. Alpha depression and lowered pulse rate during delayed reactions in a serial reaction task, *Acta. Physiol. Scand.* (1949) **19**, 1–93.

97. Costello, G.C. & Smith, C.M. The relationship between personality, sleep and the effects of sedatives, *Brit. J. Psychiat.* (1963) **109**, 568–571.

97a. de Manacéine, M. *Sleep: Its Physiology, Pathology, Hygiene and Psychology*, London: Scott (1897).

98. Dement, W.C. & Mitler, M. An introduction to sleep. In: Petre-Quadens, O. & Schlag, J. (eds.) *Basic Sleep Mechanisms*, New York: Academic Press (1974) 271–296.

99. Feinberg, I. Effects of age on human sleep patterns. In: Kales, A. (ed.) *Sleep, Physiology and Pathology: a Symposium*, Philadelphia, Pennsylvania: Lipincott (1969) 39–52.

100. Guilleminault, C., Billiard, M., Montplaisir, J. & Dement, W.C. Altered states of consciousness in disorders of daytime sleepiness, *J. Neurol. Sci.* (1975) **26**, 377–393.

101. Guilleminault, C. & Dement, W.C. 235 cases of excessive daytime sleepiness. Diagnosis and tentative classification, *J. Neurol. Sci.* (1977) **31**, 13–27.

102. Hartmann, E. *The Functions of Sleep*, New Haven, Connecticut: Yale University Press (1973).

103. Hartmann, E., Baekeland, F. & Zwilling, G.R. Psychological differences between long and short sleepers, *Arch. Gen. Psychiat.* (1972) **26**, 463–468.

104. Hartmann, E., Chung, R. & Chien, C.P. L-tryptophan and sleep, *Psychopharmacologia* (1971) **19**, 114–127.

105. Johns, M.W. Methods for assessing human sleep, *Arch. Int. Med.* (1971) **127**, 484–492.

106. Johns, M.W., Egan, P., Gay, T.J.A. & Masterton, J.P. Sleep habits and symptoms in male medical and surgical patients, *Brit. Med. J.* (1970) **2**, 509–512.

107. Jones, H.S. & Oswald, I. Two cases of healthy insomnia, *Electroenceph. Clin. Neurophysiol.* (1968) **24**, 378–380.

108. Kales, A., Caldwell, A.B., Preston, T.A., Healey, S. & Kales, J.D. Personality patterns in insomnia, *Arch. Gen. Psychiat.* (1976) **33**, 1128–1134.

109. McGhie, A. & Russell, S.M. The subjective assessment of normal sleep patterns, *J. Ment. Sci.* (1962) **108**, 642–654.

110. Marks. P.A. & Munroe, L.J. Correlates of adolescent poor sleepers, *J. Abnorm. Psychol.* (1976) **83**, 243–246.
111. Meddis, R., Pearson, A. & Langford, G. An extreme case of healthy insomnia, *Electroenceph. Clin. Neurophysiol.* (1973) **35**, 213–214.
112. Mendelson, W.B., Gillin, J.C. & Wyatt, R.J. *Human Sleep and its Disorders,* New York: Plenum Press (1977) 14.
113. Mills, J.N. Development of circadian rhythms in infancy. In: Davis, J.A. & Dobbing, J. (eds.) *Scientific Foundations of Paediatrics,* London: Heinemann (1974) 758–772.
114. Mirsky, A.F. & Cardon, P.V. A comparison of the behavioural and physiological changes accompanying sleep deprivation and chlorpromazine administration in man, *Electroenceph. Clin. Neurophysiol.* (1962) **14**, 110.
115. Monroe, L.J. Transient changes in EEG sleep patterns of married good sleepers: the effects of altering sleeping arrangements, *Psychophysiology* (1969) **6**, 330–337.
116. Naitoh, P. & Townsend, R.E. The role of sleep deprivation research in human factors, *Hum. Fact.* (1970) **12**, 253–257.
117. Oswald, I. *Sleeping and Waking: Physiology and Psychology,* New York: Elsevier (1962).
118. Palmer, C.D., Harrison, G.A. & Hiorns, R.W. Sleep patterns and life style in Oxfordshire villages, *J. Biosoc. Sci.* (1980) **12**, 437–467.
119. Price, V.A., Coates, T.J., Thoresen, C.E. & Grinstead, O.A. Prevalance and correlates of poor sleep among adolescents, *Am. J. Dis. Child.* (1978) **132**, 583.
120. Robinson, T.M. *Presleep Activity and Sleep Quality of Good and Poor Sleepers,* University of Chicago, unpublished doctoral dissertation, June 1969 (cited by Hauri, P., in *The Sleep Disorders,* Kalamazoo, Michigan: Upjohn (1977) 75.
121. Roffwarg, H.P., Muzio, J.N. & Dement, W.C. Ontogenetic development of the human sleep–dream cycle, *Science* (1966) **152**, 604–619.
122. Salzarulo, P., Fagioli, L., Salomon, F., Ricour, C., Raimbault, G., Ambrosi, S., Cicchi, O., Duhamel, J.F. & Rigoard, M.T. Sleep patterns in infants under continuous feeding from birth, *Electroenceph. Clin. Neurophysiol.* (1980) **49**, 330–336.
123. Solberg, G. *Allgemeìne Zeitschrift für Psychiatrie.* Cited in: Gould, G.M. & Pyle, W.L. *Anomalies and Curiosities of Medicine,* London: Rebman (1898).
124. Taub, J.M. Effects of scheduled afternoon naps and bedrest on daytime alertness, *Int. J. Neurosci.* (1982) **16**, 107–127.
125. Tune, G.S. Sleep and wakefulness in normal human adults, *Brit. Med. J.* (1968) **2**, 269.
126. Tune, G.S. Sleep and wakefulness in 509 normal human adults, *Brit. J. Med. Psychol.* (1969) **42**, 75–80.
127. Valley, V. & Broughton, R. The physiological (EEG) nature of drowsiness and its relation to performance deficits in narcoleptics, *Electroenceph. Clin. Neurophysiol.* (1983) **55**, 243–251.
128. Vitiello, M.V., Prinz, N.P. & Halter, J.B. Sodium-restricted diet increases nighttime plasma norepinephrine and impairs sleep patterns in man, *J. Clin. Endocrinol. Metab.* (1983) **56**, 553–556.
129. Webb, W.B. The measurement and characteristics of sleep in older persons, *Neurobiol. Aging* (1982) **3**, 311–319.
130. Webb, W.B. & Agnew, H.W. Sleep stage characteristics of long and short sleepers, *Science (NY)* (1970) **168**, 146–147.
131. Webb, W.B. & Friel, J. Sleep stage and personality characteristics of 'natural' long and short sleepers, *Science* (1971) **171**, 587–588.
132. Williams, H.L., Granda, L., Jones, R.C., Lubin, A. & Armington, J.C. EEG frequency and finger pulse volume as predictors of reaction time during sleep loss, *Electroenceph. Clin. Neurophysiol.* (1962) **14**, 64–70.
133. Williams, R.L., Karacan, I. & Hursch, C.J. *Electroencephalography (EEG) of Human Sleep: Clinical Applications,* New York: Wiley (1974).
134. Zimmerman, W.B. Sleep mentation and auditory awakening thresholds, *Psychophysiology* (1970) **6**, 540–549.

DREAMS

135. Antrobus, J.S., Dement, W.C. & Fisher, C. Patterns of dreaming and dream recall: An EEG study, *J. Abnorm. Soc. Psychol.* (1964) **69**, 341–344.
136. Antrobus, J.S. & Ehrlichman, H. The 'dream' report: attention, memory, functional

hemispheric asymmetry, and memory organization. In: Fishbein, W. (ed.) *Sleep, Dreams and Memory*, New York: Spectrum (1981) 135–145.

137. Aserinsky, E. The maximal capacity for sleep: rapid eye movement density as an index of sleep satiety, *Biol. Psychiat.* (1969) **1**, 147–154.

138. Berger, R.J. Experimental modification of dream content by meaningful verbal stimuli, *Brit. J. Psychiat.* (1963) **109**, 722–740.

139. Berger, O.J., Olley, P. & Oswald, I. The EEG, eye movements and dreams of the blind, *Am. J. Exp. Physiol.* (1966) **14**, 183–186.

140. Bogen, J.E. The other side of the brain. II: an appositional mind, *Bull. Los Angeles Neurol. Soc.* (1969) **34**, 73–105.

141. Broughton, R. Sleep disorders – disorders of arousal? *Science* (1968) **159**, 1070–1078.

142. Charcot, J.M. Un cas de suppression brusque et isolée de la vision mentale des signes et des objets (formes et couleurs), *Prog. Med.* (1883) **2**, 568–571.

143. Cohen, D.B. Sex role orientation and dream recall, *J. Abnorm. Psychol.* (1973) **82**, 246–252.

144. Cohen, D.B. *Sleep and Dreaming*, Oxford: Pergamon Press (1979) 246.

145. Dement, W.C. *Some Must Watch Whilst Some Must Sleep*, San Francisco: W.H. Freeman (1972) 101.

146. Dement, W.C. & Wolpert, E.A. The relation of eye movements, body motility, and external stimuli to dream content, *J. Exp. Psychol.* (1958) **55**, 543–553.

147. Epstein, A.W. & Simmons, N.N. Aphasia with reported loss of dreaming, *Am. J. Psychiat.* (1983) **140**, 108–109.

148. Fisher, C.J., Byrne, J., Edwards, R. & Kahn, E. A psychophysiological study of nightmares, *J. Am. Med. Assoc.* (1970) **18**, 747–782.

149. Fisher, C., Gross, J. & Zuch, J. Cycle of penile erections synchronous with dreaming (REM) sleep, *Arch. Gen. Psychiat.* (1965) **12**, 29–45.

150. Foulkes, D. Dream reports from different stages of sleep, *J. Abnorm. Soc. Psychol.* (1962) **65**, 14–25.

151. Foulkes, D. *The Psychology of Sleep*, New York: Scribner (1966).

152. Foulkes, D. Non-rapid eye movement mentation, *Exper. Neurol.* (1967) Suppl **4**, 28–38.

153. Foulkes, D. *Children's Dreams: Longitudinal Studies*, New York: Wiley (1982).

154. Freud, S. *Introductory Lectures on Psycho-analysis*. London: Hogarth Press (1953–1974) 456–457.

155. Gardner, R., Grossman, W.I., Roffwarg, H.P. & Weiner, H. The relationship of small limb movements during REM sleep to dreamed limb action, *Psychosom. Med.* (1975) **37**, 147–159.

156. Goodenough, D.R. Dream recall. In: Arkin, A.M., Antrobus, J.S. & Ellman, S.J. (eds.) *The Mind in Sleep*, Hillsdale, New Jersey: Lawrence Erlbaum (1978).

157. Greenberg, R. Dreams and REM sleep – An integrative approach. In: Fishbein, W. (ed.) *Sleep, Dreams and Memory*, Lancaster: MTP (1981) 125–134.

158. Hall, C.S. *The Meaning of Dreams*, New York: McGraw-Hill (1966).

159. Herman, J.H., Erman, M., Boys, R., Peiser, L., Taylor, M.E. & Roffwarg, H.P. Evidence for a directional correspondence between eye movements and dream imagery in REM sleep, *Sleep* (1984) **7**, 52–63.

160. Hobson, J.A., Goldfrank, F. & Snyder, F. Respiration and mental activity in sleep, *J. Psychiat. Res.* (1965) **3**, 79–90.

161. Humphrey, M.E. & Zangwill, O.L. Cessation of dreaming after brain injury, *J. Neurol. Neurosurg. Psychiat.* (1951) **14**, 322–325.

162. Jouvet, M., Pellin, B. & Mounier, D. Polygraphic study of the different phases of sleep during chronic consciousness disorders (prolonged comas), *Rev. Neurol.* (1961) **105**, 181–186.

163. Jus. A., Jus, K., Villeneuve, A., Pires, A., Lachance, R., Fortier, J. & Villeneuve, R. Studies on dream recall in chronic schizophrenic patients after prefrontal lobotomy, *Biol. Psychiat.* (1973) **6**, 275–293.

164. Koukkou, M. & Lehmann, D. Dreaming: the functional state-shift hypothesis. A neuropsychophysiological model, *Brit. J. Psychiat.* (1983) **142**, 221–231.

165. Krippner, S. & Hughes, W. Dreams and human potential, *J. Humanist Psychol.* (1970) **10**, 1–20.

166. Kuhlo, W. & Lehmann, D. Das Einschlaferleben und seine neurophysiologischen Korrelate, *Arch. Psychia. Nervenkrankheiten* (1964) **205**, 687–716.

167. Lehmann, D. & Koukkou, M. Computer analysis of EEG wakefulness – sleep patterns during learning of novel and familiar sentences, *Electroenceph. Clin. Neurophysiol.* (1974) **37**, 73–84.

168. McCarley, R.W. & Hobson, J.A. The neurobiological origins of psychoanalytic dream theory, *Am. J. Psychiat.* (1977) **134**, 1211–1221.
169. Murri, L., Arena, R., Siciliano, G., Mazzotta, R. & Muratorio, A. Dream recall in patients with focal cerebral lesions, *Arch. Neurol.* (1984) **41**, 183–185.
170. Neubauer, P. Children's dreams. In: Freedman, A.M. & Kaplan, H.I. (eds.) *The Child: His Psychological and Cultural Development*, Vol. 1, New York: Atheneum (1972).
171. Okuma, T., Sunami, Y., Fukuma, E., Takeo, S. & Motoike, M. Dream content study on chronic schizophrenics and normals by REMP-awakening technique, *Fol. Psychiat. Neurol. Jap.* (1970) **24**, 151–162.
172. Rechtschaffen, A., Goodenough, D.R. & Shapiro, A. Patterns of sleep talking, *Arch. Gen. Psychiat.* (1962) **7**, 418–426.
173. Robins, K.E. & McAdam, D.W. Interhemispheric alpha asymmetry and imagery mode, *Brain Lang.* (1974) **1**, 189–193.
174. Roffwarg, H.P., Dement, W.C., Muzio, J.N. & Fisher, C. Dream imagery: relationship to rapid eye movements of sleep, *Arch. Gen. Psychiat.* (1962) **7**, 235–238.
175. Roffwarg, H., Herman, J. & Lamstein, S. The middle ear muscles: predictability of their phasic activity in REM sleep from dream material, *Sleep Res.* (1975) **4**, 165.
176. Rycroft, C. *The Innocence of Dreams*, London: Hogarth Press (1979) 148, 163.
177. Sharpe, E.F. *Dream Analysis*, New York: Brunner Mazel (1978).
178. Snyder, F. In: Greenfield, N.S. & Lewis, W.C. (eds.) *Psychoanalysis and Current Biological Thought*, Madison, Wisconsin: University of Wisconsin (1965) 275.
179. Vogel, G.W. Sleep-onset mentation. In: Askin, A.M., Antrobus, J.S. & Ellman, S.J. (eds.) *The Mind in Sleep*, Hillsdale, New Jersey: Lawrence Erlbaum (1978).
180. Vogel, G.W., Barrowclough, B. & Giesler, D.D. Limited discriminality of REM and sleep onset reports and its psychiatric implications, *Arch. Gen. Psychiat.* (1972) **26**, 449–455.
181. Webb, W.B. In: *The Encyclopaedia Brittanica*, Vol. 5, Chicago: Encyclopaedia Brittanica Inc. (1982) 1011.
182. Webb, W.B. & Cartwright, R.D. Sleep and dreams, *Ann. Rev. Psychol.* (1978) **29**, 223–252.
183. Winget, C. & Farrell, R.A. A comparison of the dreams of homosexual and non-homosexual males. Paper presented at the annual meeting of the Association for the Psychophysiological Study of Sleep, Bruges, Belgium, June 1971.
184. Winget, C., Kramer, M. & Whitman, R.M. Dreams and demography, *Can. Psychiat. Assoc. J.* (1972) **17**, 203–208.
185. Wolpert, E.A. Studies in psychophysiology of dreams. II. An electromyographic study of dreaming, *Arch. Gen. Psychiat.* (1960) **2**, 231–241.
186. Zimmerman, W.B. Sleep mentation and auditory awakening thresholds, *Psychophysiology* (1970) **6**, 540–549.

ANIMAL SLEEP

187. Adey, W.R., Kado, R.T. & Rhodes, J.M. Sleep: cortical and subcortical recordings in the chimpanzee, *Science* (1963) **141**, 932–933.
188. Affani, J. Observations on the sleep of some South American marsupials and edentates. In: Chase, M.H. (ed.) *The Sleeping Brain*, Los Angeles: BIS (1972) 21–23.
189. Allison, T. & Cicchetti, D.V. Sleep in mammals: ecological and constitutional correlates, *Science* (1976) 194, 732–734.
190. Allison, T. & Van Twyver, H. The evolution of sleep, *Nat. Hist.* (1970) **79**, 56–65.
191. Allison, T. & Van Twyver, H. Electrophysiological studies of the echidna, *Arch. Ital. Biol.* (1972) **110**, 145–184.
192. Bruce Durie, D.J. Sleep in animals. In: Wheatley, D. (ed.) *Psychopharmacology of Sleep*, New York: Raven Press (1981) 1–18.
193. Crick, F. & Mitchison, G. The function of dream sleep, *Nature* (1983) **304**, 111–114.
194. Flanigan, W.F., Jr. Sleep and wakefulness in inguanid lizards, *Ctenosaura pectinata* and *Iguana iguana*, *Brain Behav. Evol.* (1973) **8**, 401–436.
195. Foutz, A.S., Mitler, M.M., Cavalli-Sforza, L.L. & Dement, W.C. Genetic factors in canine narcolepsy, *Sleep* (1979) **1**, 413–421.
196. Foutz, A.S., Mitler, M.M. & Dement, W.C. Narcolepsy, *Ven. Clin. North Am. (Small Anim. Pract.)* (1980) **10**, 65–80.
197. Hartmann, E. The functions of sleep and memory processing. In: Fishbein, W. (ed.) *Sleep, Dreams and Memory*, Lancaster: MTP (1981) 111–124.

198. Hediger, H. The biology of natural sleep in animals, *Experientia* (1980) **36**, 13–16.
199. Hendricks, J.C. & Morrison, A.R. Normal and abnormal sleep in mammals, *J. Am. Vet. Med. Assoc.* (1981) **178**, 121–126.
200. Hobson, J.A. Electrographic correlates of behaviour in the frog, with special reference to sleep, *Electroenceph. Clin. Neurophysiol.* (1967) **22**, 113–121.
201. Hobson, J.A., Goin, O. & Goin, C. Electrographic correlates of behaviour in tree frogs, *Nature* (1968) **220**, 386–387.
202. Jouvet, M., Michel, F. & Mounier, D. Comparative electroencephalographic analysis of physiological sleep in the cat and in man, *Rev. Neurol. (Paris)* (1960) **103**, 189–205.
203. Karadzic, V., Kovacevic, R. & Momirov, D. In: Koella, W.P. & Levin, P. (eds.) *Proceedings of the 1st European Congress on Sleep Research*, Basel: S. Karger (1973).
204. Kleitman, N. Discussion. In: Wolstenholme, G.E.W. & O'Connor, M. (eds.) *Ciba Foundation Symposium on the Nature of Sleep*, London: Churchill (1961) 388.
205. Kleitman, N. *Sleep and Wakefulness*, 2nd ed., Chicago: Chicago University Press (1963).
206. Kovalzon, V.M. Brain temperature variations and ECoG in free-swimming bottle-nose dolphins, *Sleep* (1976) Basel: S. Karger 239–241.
207. Meddis, R. On the function of sleep, *Anim. Behav.* (1975) **23**, 676–691.
208. Mitler, M., Boyson, B., Campbell, L. & Dement, W.C. Narcolepsy–cataplexy in a female dog, *Exp. Neurol.* (1974) **45**, 332–340.
209. Mukhametov, L.M. Sleep in marine mammals. In: Borbély, A. & Valtax, J.-L. (eds.) *Sleep Mechanisms*, Berlin: Springer Verlag (1984) 227–238.
210. Parmeggiani, P.L. Regulation of physiological functions during sleep in mammals, *Experientia* (1982) **38**, 1405–1408.
211. Pellet, J. & Beraud, G. Organisation nychtémérale de la veille et du sommeil chez la cobaye *(Cavia porcellus)*, *Physiol. Behav.* (1967) **2**, 131–137.
212. Pilleri, G. *Die Geheimnisse der blinden Delphine*, Berne: Hallweg (1975).
213. Rojas-Ramirez, J.A. & Tauber, E.S. Paradoxical sleep in two species of avian predator *(Falconi formes)*, *Science* (1970) **167**, 1754–1755.
214. Ruckebusch, Y. Comparative effects of sleep and wakefulness in farm animals. In: Chase, M.H. (ed.) *The Sleeping Brain*, Los Angeles: UCLA Brain Information Service (1972) 23–28.
215. Ruckebusch, Y. The relevance of drowsiness in the circadian cycle of farm animals, *Anim. Behav.* (1972) **20**, 637–643.
216. Ruckebusch, Y., Barbey, P. & Guillemot, P. Les états de sommeil chez le cheval *(Equus caballus)*, *C.R. Soc. Biol.* (1970) **164**, 658–665.
217. Schaller, G.B. The year of the gorilla, Chicago: Chicago University Press (1964) (quoted by Kleitman, N. *Sleep and Wakefulness*, Chicago: Chicago University Press (1967) 552.
218. Shapiro, C.M. Energy expenditure and restorative sleep, *Biol. Psychol.* (1982) **15**, 229–239.
219. Sturmwasser, F. The cellular basis of behaviour in *Aplysia, J. Psychiat. Res.* (1971) **8**, 237–257.
220. Susic, V.T. & Kovatcevic, R.M. Sleep patterns in the owl *(Strix aluce), Physiol. Behav.* (1973) **11**, 313–317.
221. Tymicz, J., Narebski, J. & Jurkowlaniec, E. Circadian sleep–wakefulness rhythm of the starling, *Sleep Res.* (1975) **4**, 146.
222. Walker, J.M. & Berger, R.J. Sleep in the domestic pigeon *(Columbia livea), Behav. Biol.* (1972) **7**, 195–203.
223. Webb, W.B. *Sleep: The Gentle Tyrant*, Englewood Cliffs, New Jersey: Prentice-Hall (1975) 180.
224. Winson, J. In: Hartmann[197] p. 112.
225. Zeppelin, H. & Rechtschaffen, A. Mammalian sleep, longevity and energy metabolism, *Brain Behav. Evol.* (1974) **10**, 425–470.

SLEEP DEPRIVATION

226. Agnew, H.W., Webb, W.B. Comparison of stage four and 1-REM sleep deprivation, *Percept. Mot. Skills* (1967) **24**, 851–858.
227. Agnew, H.W., Webb, W.B., & Williams, R.L. The effects of stage four sleep deprivation, *Electroenceph. Clin. Neurophysiol.* (1964) **27**, 68–70.
228. Asken, M.J. & Raham, D.C. Resident performance and sleep deprivation: a review, *J. Med. Educ.* (1983) **58**, 382–388.
229. Bast, T.H. & Bloemendal, W.B. Studies in experimental exhaustion due to lack of sleep: effects on nerve cells in medulla, *Am. J. Physiol.* (1927) **82**, 140–146.

230. Bast, T.H., Supernaw, J.S., Lieberman, B. & Munro, J. Studies in exhaustion due to lack of sleep: effect on thyroid and adrenal glands with special reference to mitochondria, *Am. J. Physiol.* (1928) **85**, 135–140.
231. Borowsky, M.S. & Wall, R. Naval aviation mishaps and fatigue, *Aviat. Space Environ. Med.* (1983) **54**, 535–538.
232. Carroll. B.J., Feinberg, M., Greden, J.F., Tarka, J., Albala, A.A., Hasket, R.F., James, N.McL., Kronfol, Z., Lohr, N., Steiner, M., de Vigne, J.P. & Young, E. A specific laboratory test for the diagnosis of melancholia. Standardization, validation and clinical utility. *Arch. Gen. Psychiat.* (1981) **38**, 15–23.
233. Clark, B. & Warren, N. The effect of loss of sleep on visual tests, *Am. J. Optometry* (1939) **16**, 80–95.
234. Cohen, D.B. The cognitive activity of sleep, *Prog. Brain Res.* (1980) **53**, 307–324.
235. Cohen, H., Thomas, J. & Dement, W.C. Sleep styles, REM deprivation and electroconvulsive thresholds in the cat, *Brain Res.* (1970) **19**, 317–321.
236. Cooper, K.R. & Phillips, B.A. Effect of short-term sleep loss on breathing, *J. Appl. Physiol.* (1982) **53**, 855–858.
237. Cortés-Gallegos, V., Casteneda, G., Alonso, R., Sojo, I., Carranco, A., Cervantes, C. & Parra, A. Sleep deprivation reduces circulatory androgens in healthy man, *Arch. Androl.* (1983) **10**, 33–37.
238. Crile, G.W. In: Rowland, A.F. (ed.) *A Physical Interpretation of Shock, Exhaustion and Restoration: An Extension of the Kinetic Theory*, London: H. Frowde/Hodder and Stoughton (1921) 232.
239. Dement, W. The effect of dream deprivation, *Science* (1960) **131**, 1705–1707.
240. Dement, W.C. Experimental dream studies. In: *Academy of Psychoanalysis: Science and Psychoanalysis* Vol. 7, New York: Grune and Stratton (1964) 129–184.
241. Dement, W.C. Recent studies on the biological role of REM sleep *Am. J. Psychiat.* (1965) **122**, 404–408.
242. Dement, W.C. & Fisher, C. Experimental interference with the sleep cycle, *Can. Psychiat. Assoc. J.* (1963) **8**, 400–405.
243. Ellman, S.J., Spielman, A.J., Luck, D., Steiner, S.S. & Halperin, R. REM deprivation: a review. In: Arkin, A.M., Antrobus, J.S. & Ellman, S.J. (eds.) *The Mind in Sleep: Psychology and Psychophysiology*, Hillside, New Jersey: Lawrence Erlbaum (1978) 419–457.
244. Ferguson, J. & Dement, W.C. Paper presented to the Association for the Psychophysiological Study of Sleep, Washington DC, March 1965.
245. Fishbein, W. & Gutwein, B.M. Paradoxical sleep and memory storage processes, *Behav. Biol.* (1977) **19**, 425–464.
246. Gillin, J.C. The sleep therapies of depression, *Prog. Neuropsychopharmacol. Biol. Psychiat.* (1983) **7**, 351–364.
247. Gould, G.M. & Pyle, W.L. *Anomalies and Curiosities of Medicine*, London: Rebman (1898) 863.
248. Gulevich, G., Dement, W. & Johnson, L. Psychiatric and EEG observations on a case of prolonged (264 hours) wakefulness, *Arch. Gen. Psychiat.* (1966) **15**, 29–35.
249. Gunderson, C.H., Dunne, P.B. & Feher, T.L. Sleep deprivation seizures, *Neurology (Minneap.)* (1973) **23**, 678–686.
250. Hartmann, E., Orzack, M.H. & Branconnier, R. Deficits produced by sleep deprivation: Reversal by d- and l-amphetamine, *Sleep Res.* (1974) **3**, 151.
251. Hockey, G.R.J. Stress and the cognitive component of skilled performance. In: Hamilton, V. & Warbarton, D.M. (eds.) *Human Stress and Cognition*, New York: Wiley (1979).
252. Horne, J.A. Binocular convergence during total sleep deprivation in man, *Biol. Psychol.* (1975) **3**, 309–319.
253. Horne, J.A. A review of the biological effects of total sleep deprivation in man, *Biol. Psychol.* (1978) **7**, 55–102.
254. Horne, J.A. Human sleep and tissue restitution: some qualifications and doubts, *Clin. Sci.* (1983) **65**, 569–578.
255. Johnson, L.C. Psychological and physiological changes following total sleep deprivation. In: Kales, A. (ed.) *Sleep, Physiology and Pathology*, Philadelphia: Lipincott (1969) 206–220.
256. Jouvet, D., Vimont, P., Delorme, F. & Jouvet, M. Étude de la privation sélective de la phase paradoxale de sommeil chez le chat, *C. R. Soc. Biol.* (1964) **158**, 756–759.
257. Kales, A., Hoedamaker, F.S., Jacobson, A. & Lichtenstein, E.L. Dream deprivation: an experimental reappraisal, *Nature* (1964) **204**, 1337–1338.
258. Kales, A., Tan, T.L. & Kollar, E.J. Sleep patterns following 205 hours of sleep deprivation,

Psychosom. Med. (1970) **32**, 189–200.

259. Kelly, J. & Feigenbaum, L.Z. Another cause of reversible dementia: sleep deprivation due to prostatism, *J. Am. Geriatr. Soc.* (1982) **30**, 645–646.

260. Khazan, N. & Sawyer, C.H. 'Rebound' recovery from deprivation of paradoxical sleep in the rabbit, *Proc. Soc. Exp. Biol. Med.* (1963) **114**, 536–539.

261. King, D. Pathological and therapeutic consequences of sleep loss. A review, *Dis. Nerv. Syst.* (1977) **38**, 873.

262. King, D., Dowdy, S., Jack, R., Gardner, R. & Edwards, P. The dexamethasone suppression test as a predictor of sleep deprivation antidepressant effect, *Psychiat. Res.* (1982) **7**, 93–99.

263. King, D., Russell, M. & Smith, D. Response to dexamethasone suppression and total night sleep deprivation in an affectively disordered Klinefelter patient, *J. Nerv. Ment. Dis.* (1983) **171**, 59–61.

264. Knowles, J.B., Southmayd, S.E., Delva, N., Prowse, A., MacLean, A.W., Cairns, J., Letemendia, F.J. & Waldron, J. Sleep deprivation: outcome of controlled single case studies of depressed patients, *Can. J. Psychiat.* (1981) **26**, 330–333.

265. Koridze, M.G. & Nemsadze, N.D. Effect of deprivation of paradoxical sleep on the formation and differentiation of food conditioned reflexes, *Neurosci. Behav. Physiol.* (1982) **12**, 369–373.

266. Kuhn, E. & Brodan, V. Changes in the circadian rhythm of serum iron induced by a 5-day sleep deprivation, *Eur. J. Appl. Physiol.* (1982) **49**, 215–222.

267. Kuhn, E., Rysanek, K., Kujalova, V., Brodan, V., Valek, J. & Rotreki, J. Diurnal rhythms of excretion of catecholamine metabolites during sleep deprivation, *Activitas Nerv. Sup.* (1973) **15**, 129–131.

268. Licklider, J.C.R. & Bunch, M.E. Effects of enforced wakefulness upon growth and maze-learning behaviour of white rats, *J. Comp. Physiol.* (1946) **39**, 339–350.

269. Manacéine, M. de, *Arch. Ital. Biol.* (1894) **21**, 322 (quoted in: *Sleep: its Physiology, Pathology, Hygiene and Psychology*, London: W. Scott (1897) 355).

270. McGrath, M.J. & Cohen, D.B. REM sleep facilitation of adaptive waking behaviour: a review of the literature, *Psychol. Bull.* (1978) **85**, 24–57.

271. Miles, W.R. & Laslett, H.R. Eye movement and visual fixation during profound sleepiness, *Psychol. Rev.* (1931) **38**, 1–13.

272. Mirmiran, M., Scholtens, J., van de Poll, N.E., Uylings, H.B., van der Gugten, J. & Boer, G.J. Effects of experimental suppression of active (REM) sleep during early development upon adult brain and behaviour in the rat, *Brain Res.* (1983) **283**, 277–286.

273. Mirmiran, M., Uylings, H.B. & Corner, M.A. Pharmacological suppression of REM sleep prior to weaning counteracts the effectiveness of subsequent environmental enrichment on cortical growth in rats, *Brain Res.* (1983) **283**, 102–105.

274. Moldofsky, H. & Scarisbrick, P. Induction of neurasthenic musculoskeletal pain syndrome by selective sleep stage deprivation, *Psychosom. Med.* (1976) **38**, 35–44.

274a. Moldofsky, H., Scarisbrick, P. & England, H. Musculoskeletal symptoms and non-REM sleep disturbance in patients with 'fibrositis syndrome' and healthy subjects, *Psychosom. Med.* (1975) **37**, 341–351.

275. Morden, B., Conner, R., Mitchell, G., Dement, W. & Levine, S. Effects of rapid-eye-movement (REM) sleep deprivation on shock-induced fighting, *Physiol. Behav.* (1968) **3**, 425–432.

276. Morris, G. & Singer, M.T. Sleep deprivation: transactional and subjective observations, *Arch. Gen. Psychiat.* (1961) **5**, 453–465.

277. Murison, R., Usin, R., Coover, G.D., Lien, W. & Ursin, H. Sleep deprivation procedure produces stomach lesions in rats, *Physiol. Behav.* (1982) **29**, 693–694.

278. Naitoh, P. Sleep deprivation in human subjects: a reappraisal, *Waking Sleeping* (1976) **1**, 53–60.

279. Palmblad, J., Cantell, K., Strander, H., Froberg, J., Karlsson, C.-G., Levi, L., Granstrom, M. & Unger, P. Stessor exposure and immunological responses in man: interferon-producing capacity and phagocytosis, *J. Psychosom. Res.* (1976) **20**, 193–199.

280. Palmblad, J., Petrini, B., Wasserman, J. & Akerstedt, T. Lymphocyte and granulocyte reactions during sleep deprivation, *Psychosom. Med.* (1979) **41**, 273–278.

281. Pasnau, R.O., Naitoh, P., Stier, S. & Kollar, E.J. The psychological effects of 205 hours of sleep deprivation, *Arch. Gen. Psychiat.* (1968) **18**, 496–505.

282. Pearlman, C.A. Rat models of the adaptive function of REM sleep. In: Fishbein, W. (ed.) *Sleep, Dreams and Memory*, Lancaster: MTP (1981) 37–46.

283. Pflug, B. The effect of sleep deprivation on depressed patients, *Acta Psychiat. Scand.* (1976) **53**, 148.
284. Polzella, D.J. Effects of sleep deprivation on short-term recognition memory, *J. Exp. Psychol.* (1975) **104**, 194–200.
285. Pressman, M.R., Spielman, A.J., Pollak, C.P. & Weitzman, E.D. Long-latency auditory evoked responses during sleep deprivation and in narcolepsy, *Sleep* (1982) **5**, Suppl 2, S147–156.
286. Radulovacki, M., Wojcik, W.J. & Fornal, C. Effects of bromocriptine and α-flupenthixol on sleep in REM sleep-deprived rats, *Life Sci.* (1979) **24**, 1705–1712.
287. Radulovacki, M., Wojcik, W.J., Fornal, C. & Miletich, R. Elimination of REM sleep rebound in rats by α adrenoceptor blockers, phentolamine and phenoxybenzamine, *Pharmacol. Biochem. Behav.* (1980) **13**, 51–55.
288. Radulovacki, M., Wojcik, W.J., Walovitch, R. & Brodie, M. Phenoxybenzamine and bromocriptine attenuate need for REM sleep in rats, *Pharmacol. Biochem. Behav.* (1981) **14**, 371–375.
289. Radulovacki, M. & Zak, R. Amphetamine abolishes REM sleep rebound in rats: effect of a single injection, *Brain Res.* (1981) **217**, 420–424.
290. Rechtschaffen, A., Gilliland, M.A., Bergman, B.M. & Winter, J.B. Physiological correlates of prolonged sleep deprivation in rats, *Science* (1983) **221**, 182–184.
291. Ross, J.J. Neurological findings after prolonged sleep deprivation, *Arch. Neurol.* (1965) **12**, 399–403.
292. Roth, T., Kramer, M., Leston, W. & Lutz, T. The effect of sleep deprivation on mood, *Sleep Res.* (1974) **3**, 154.
293. Sampson, H. Deprivation of dreaming sleep by two methods. I. Compensatory REM time, *Arch. Gen. Psychiat.* (1965) **13**, 79–86.
294. Sanders, A.F. & Reitsma, W.D. Lack of sleep and covert orienting of attention, *Acta Psychol. (Amst.)* (1982) **52**, 137–145.
295. Sanders, A.F. & Reitsma, W.D. The effects of sleep loss on processing visual information in the functional visual field, *Acta Psychol. (Amst.)* (1982) **51**, 149–162.
296. Sassin, J.F. Neurological findings following short-term sleep deprivation, *Arch. Neurol.* (1970) **22**, 54–56.
297. Snyder, F. The new biology of dreaming, *Arch. Gen. Psychiat.* (1963) **8**, 381–391.
298. Spielman, A.J., Pressman, M., Pollak, C.P., Rubinstein, M., Lanstein, S., Roffwarg, H.P. & Weitzman, E.D. REM deprivation of narcoleptics, *Sleep Res.* (1979) **8**, 216.
299. Stern, W.C. The relationship between REM sleep and learning. Animal studies. In: Hartmann, E. (ed.) *Sleep and Dreaming*, Boston: Little Brown and Co (1970) 249–257.
300. Tufik, S., Lindsey, C.J. & Carlini, E.A. Does REM sleep deprivation induce a supersensitivity of dopaminergic receptors in the rat brain? *Pharmacology* (1978) **16**, 98–105.
301. Tyler, D.B. Psychological change during experimental sleep deprivation, *Dis. Nerv. Syst.* (1955) **16**, 239–299.
302. Vogel, G.W. A review of REM sleep deprivation, *Arch. Gen. Psychiat.* (1975) **32**, 749–761.
303. Vovin, R.Y., Aksenova, I.O. & Sverdlov, L.S. Sleep deprivation in the treatment of chronic depressive states, *Neurosci. Behav. Physiol.* (1982) **12**, 92–96.
304. Webb, W.B. Sleep stage responses of older and younger subjects after sleep deprivation, *Electroenceph. Clin. Neurophysiol.* (1981) **52**, 368–371.
305. Webb, W.B. & Agnew, H.W. Jr. Sleep deprivation, age, and exhaustion time in the rat, *Science* (1962) **136**, 1122.
306. Webb, W.B. & Agnew, H.W. Effects on performance of high and low energy-expenditure during sleep deprivation, *Percept. Mot. Skills* (1973) **37**, 511–514.
307. Webb, W.B. & Levy, C.M. Age sleep deprivation and performance, *Psychophysiology* (1982) **19**, 272–276.
308. Wesemann, W., Weiner, N., Rotsch, M. & Schulz, E. Serotonin binding in rat brain: circadian rhythm and effect of sleep deprivation, *J. Neural Transm. (Suppl.)* (1983) **18**, 287–294.
309. Wilkinson, R.T. Sleep deprivation. In: Edholm, O.G. & Bacharach, A.L. (eds.) *Physiology of Survival*, London: Academic Press (1965) 399–430.
310. Williams, H.L., Hammack, J.T., Daly, R.L., Dement, W.C. & Lubin, A. Responses to auditory stimulation, sleep loss and the EEG stages of sleep, *Electroenceph. Clin. Neurophysiol.* (1964) **16**, 269–279.

311. Wojcik, W.J. & Radulovacki, M. Selective increase in brain dopamine metabolism during REM sleep rebound in the rat, *Physiol. Behav.* (1981) **27**, 305–312.
312. Zak, R. & Radulovacki, M. Quipazine has a biphasic effect on slow wave sleep and reduces REM sleep rebound in REM sleep deprived rats, *Brain Res. Bull.* (1982) **8**, 329–331.

FUNCTION OF SLEEP

313. Adam, K. Body weight correlates with REM sleep, *Brit. Med. J.* (1977) **1**, 813–814.
314. Albert, M.L., Feldman, M.G. & Willis, A.L. The subcortical dementia of progressive supranuclear palsy, *J. Neurol. Neurosurg. Psychiat.* (1974) **37**, 121–130.
315. Allison, T. & Van Twyver, H. The evolution of sleep, *Nat. Hist.* (1970) **79**, 56–65.
316. Alekseyeva, T.T. Correlation of nervous and humoral factors in the development of sleep in non-disjointed twins, *Zh. Vyssh. Nerv. Deyat. Pavlova* (1958) **8**, 835–844.
317. Beh, H.C. & Barratt, P.E.H. Discrimination and conditioning during sleep as indicated by the electroencephalogram, *Science* (1965) **147**, 1470–1471.
318. Berlucchi, G. Mechanismen von Schlafen und Wachen. In: Baurt, W. (ed.) *Ermüdung, Schlaf und Traum*, S 145–203, Stuttgart: Wissenschaftliche Verlags (1970) 314.
319. Block, V., Hennevin, E. & Leconte, P. The phenomenon of paradoxical sleep augmentation after learning: experimental studies of its characteristics and significance. In: Fishbein, W. (ed.) *Sleep, Dreams and Memory*, Lancaster: MTP (1981) 18.
320. Boyar, R.M., Rosenfeld, R.S., Kapen, S., Finkelstein, V.W., Roffwarg, H.P., Weitzman, E.D. & Hellman, L. Simultaneous augmented secretion of luteinizing hormone and testosterone during sleep, *J. Clin. Invest.* (1974) **54**, 609–618.
321. Castuldo, V. & Krynicki, U. Sleep patterns and intelligence in functional mental retardation, *J. Ment. Defic. Res.* (1973) **17**, 231–235.
322. Cohen, D.B. The cognitive activity of sleep, *Prog. Brain Res.* (1980) **53**, 307–324.
323. Crick, F. & Mitchison, G. The function of dream sleep, *Nature* (1983) **304**, 111–114.
324. de Koninck, J., Proulx, G., Healey, T., Arsenault, R. & Prevost, F. Intensive language learning and REM sleep, *Sleep Res.* (1975) **4**, 150.
325. Dewan, E.M. *The Programming (P) Hypothesis for REM Sleep*, Physical Sciences Research Paper No. 368, Bedford, Massachusetts: Air Force Cambridge Research Laboratories (1969).
326. Emmons, W.H. & Simon, C.W. The non-recall of material presented during sleep, *Psychology* (1956) **20**, 76–81.
327. Fanjaud, G., Calvet, U., Rous de Feneyrois, A., Barrere, M., Besset, L. & Arbus, A. The role of paradoxical sleep in learning in man, *Rev. EEG Neurophysiol.* (1982) **12**, 337–343.
328. Feinberg, I. Eye movement activity during sleep and intellectual function in mental retardation, *Science* (1968) **159**, 1256.
329. Feinberg, I. The ontogenesis of human sleep and the relationship of sleep variables to intellectual function in the aged, *Compr. Psychiat.* (1968) **9**, 138–147.
330. Feinberg, I., Braum, M. & Schulman, E. EEG sleep patterns in mental retardation, *Electroenceph. Clin. Neurophysiol.* (1969) **27**, 128–141.
331. Feinberg, I., Koresko, R.L. & Heller, N. Sleep: electroencephalographic and eye movement patterns in patients with chronic brain syndrome, *J. Psychiat. Res.* (1967) **5**, 107–144.
332. Feldman, M.H. Physiological observations in a chronic case of 'locked-in' syndrome, *Neurology (Minneap.)* (1971) **21**, 459–478.
333. Firth, H. Habituation during sleep, *Psychophysiology* (1973) **10**, 43–51.
334. Fishbein, W. Interference with conversion of memory from short-term to long-term storage by partial sleep deprivation, *Commun. Behav. Biol.* (1970) **5**, 171–175.
335. Fishbein, W. & Gutwein, B.M. Paradoxical sleep and memory storage processes, *Behav. Biol.* (1977) **19**, 425–464.
336. Fisher, L.B. The diurnal mitotic rhythm in the human epidermis, *Brit. J. Dermatol.* (1968) **80**, 75–80.
337. Frost, J.D., Shumate, W.H., Salamy, J.G. & Booher, C.R. Skylab sleep monitoring experiment (M133). *Proceedings of the Skylab Life Sciences Symposium*, Vol. 1, Houston, 27–29 August 1974, 239–285.
338. Garlick, P.J., Glugston, G.A., Swick, R.W. & Waterlow, J.C. Diurnal pattern of protein and energy metabolism in man, *Am. J. Clin. Nut.* (1980) **33**, 1983–1986.
339. Garlick, P.J., Glugston, G.A., Waterlow, J.C. & Swick, R.W. Diurnal pattern of protein and energy metabolism in man: a defence, *Am. J. Clin. Nut.* (1981) **34**, 1626–1628.

340. Giuditta, A., Neugebauer-Vitale, A., Grassi-Zucconi, G., Ambrosini, M.V. & Scaroni, R. Synthesis of brain RNA and DNA during sleep. In: Borbély, A. & Valtax, J.-L. (eds.) *Sleep Mechanisms*, Berlin: Springer Verlag (1984) 146–154.
341. Greenberg, R. Dreams and REM sleep – an integrative approach. In: Fishbein, W. (ed.) *Sleep, Dreams and Memory*, Lancaster: MTP (1981) 125–135.
342. Greenberg, R. & Dewan, E.M. Aphasia and rapid eye movement sleep, *Nature* (1969) **223**, 183–184.
343. Griffin, S.J. & Trinder, J. Physical fitness, exercise and human sleep, *Psychophysiology* (1978) **15**, 447–450.
344. Gross, R.A., Spehlmann, R. & Daniels, J.C. Sleep disturbances in progressive supranuclear palsy, *Electroenceph. Clin. Neurophysiol.* (1978) **45**, 16–25.
345. Grosvenor, A. & Lack, L.C. The effect of sleep before or after learning on memory, *Sleep* (1984) **7**, 155–167.
346. Harris, P.F., Overstreet, D.H. & Orbach, J. Disruption of passive avoidance memory by REM sleep deprivation: methodological and pharmacological considerations, *Pharmacol. Biochem. Behav.* (1982) **17**, 119–122.
347. Hartmann, E. *The Functions of Sleep*, New Haven, Connecticut: Yale University Press (1976).
348. Hopfield, J.J., Feinstein, D.I. & Palmer, R.G. 'Unlearning' has a stabilizing effect in collective memories, *Nature* (1983) **304**, 158–159.
349. Horne, J.A. Human sleep and tissue restitution: some qualifications and doubts, *Clin. Sci.* (1983) **65**, 569–578.
350. Jackson, J.H. *Selected Writings of John Hughlings-Jackson*, Taylor, J. (ed.) London: Hodder and Stoughton (1932).
351. Jenkins, J. & Dallenbach, K. Oblivescence during sleep and waking, *Am. J. Psychol.* (1924) **35**, 605.
352. Jouvet, M. The role of monoamines and acetylcholine containing neurons in the regulation of the sleep–waking cycle, *Ergebn. Physiol.* (1972) **64**, 166–307.
353. Kleitman, N. *Sleep and Wakefulness*, Chicago: University of Chicago Press (1963) 552.
354. Kornmüller, A.E., Lux, H.D., Winkel, K. & Klee, M. Neurohumoral ausgelöste Schlafzustände an Tieren mit gekreuztem Kreislauf unter der Kontrolle von EEG-Ableitungen, *Naturwissenschaften* (1961) **48**, 503–505.
355. Koulack, D. & Goodenough, D.R. Dream recall and dream recall failure: an arousal-retrieval model, *Psychol. Bull.* (1976) **83**, 975–984.
356. Legendre, R. & Pieron, H. Recherches sur le besoin de sommeil consécutif à une vielle prolongée, *Z. Allg. Physiol.* (1913) **14**, 235–262.
357. Lehmann, D. & Koukkou, M. Learning and EEG during sleep in humans. In: Koella, W.P. & Levin, P. (eds.) *Sleep* (1973); *Physiology, Biochemistry, Psychology, Pharmacology, Clinical Implications*, Basel: S. Karger (1974).
358. Lester, B.K., Burch, N.R. & Dossett, R.C. Nocturnal EEG-GSR profiles: The influence of pre-sleep states, *Psychophysiology* (1967) **3**, 238–248.
359. Leygonie, F., Thomas, J., Degos, J.D., Bouchareine, A. & Babizet, J. Troubles du sommeil dans la maladie de Steele–Richardson. Étude polygraphique de trois cas, *Rev. Neurol.* (1976) **132**, 125–136.
360. Lucero, M. Lengthening of REM sleep duration consecutive to learning in the rat, *Brain Res.* (1970) **20**, 319–322.
361. Markland, O.N. & Dyken, M.L. Sleep abnormalities in patients with brain-stem lesions, *Neurology (Minneap.)* (1976) **26**, 769–776.
362. Marsden, C.D. 'On-off' phenomenon in Parkinson's disease. In: Rinne, U.K., Klinger, M. & Stamm, G. (eds.) *Parkinson's Disease – Current Progress, Problems and Mangement*, Amsterdam: Elsevier/North-Holland (1980) 241–254.
363. McGaugh, J.L. & Herz, M. *Memory Consolidation* San Francisco: Albion, p. 204, cited in Block et al.[319]
364. McGrath, M.J. & Cohen, D.B. REM sleep facilitation of adaptive waking behaviour: a review of the literature, *Psychol. Bull.* (1978) **85**, 24–57.
365. McHugh, P.R. & Folstein, M.F. *Subcortical Dementia*. Address to the American Academy of Neurology, Boston, April 1973 (unpublished).
366. Minuto, F., Underwood, L.E., Grimaldi, P., Furlanetto, R.W., van Wyk, J.J. & Giordano, G. Decreased serum somatomedin C concentration during sleep: temporal relationship to the nocturnal surges of growth hormone and prolactin, *J. Clin. Endocrin. Metab.* (1981) **52**, 399–403.

367. Moldofsky, H. & Scarisbrick, P. Induction of neurasthenic musculoskeletal pain syndrome by selective sleep stage deprivation, *Psychosom. Med.* (1976) **38**, 35–44.
368. Moruzzi, G. Summary statement, *Prog. Brain Res.* (1965) **18**, 241–243.
369. Moruzzi, G. The functional significance of sleep with particular regard to the brain mechanisms underlying consciousness. In: Eccle, J.C. (ed.) *Brain and Conscious Experience*, Berlin/Heidelberg/New York: Springer (1966) 345–388.
370. Moruzzi, G. The sleep–waking cycle, *Ergebn. Physiol.* (1972) **64**, 1–165.
371. Newman, E.A. & Evans, C.R. Human dream processes as analogous to computer programme clearance, *Nature* (1965) **206**, 534.
372. Nicholson, A.N. & Marks, J. *Insomnia*, Lancaster: MTP (1983) 22.
373. Osorio, I. & Daroff, R.B. Absence of REM and altered NREM sleep in patients with spinocerebellar degeneration and slow saccades, *Ann. Neurol.* (1980) **7**, 277–280.
374. Oswald, I. *Sleeping and Waking*, Amsterdam: Elsevier (1962).
375. Oswald, O., Taylor, A.M. & Treisman, M. Discrimination responses to stimulation during human sleep, *Brain* (1960) **83**, 440–453.
376. Paul, K. & Dittrichova, J. Sleep patterns following learning in infants. In: Levin, P. & Koella, U. (eds.) *Sleep 1974*, Basel: S. Karger (1975) 388–390.
377. Pearlman, C.A. REM sleep and information processing. Evidence from animal studies, *Neurosci. Biobehav. Rev.* (1979) **3**, 57–68.
378. Pearlman, C.A. & Greenberg, R. Post trial REM sleep: a critical period for consolidation of shuttlebox avoidance, *Anim. Learn. Behav.* (1973) **1**, 49–51.
379. Popper, K.R. & Eccles, J.C. *The Self and its Brain*, Berlin: Springer Verlag (1977) 496.
380. Pötzl, O. Experimentell erregte Traumbilder in ihren Beziehungen zum indirekten Sehen. *Z. Gesamte Neurol. Psychiat.* (1917) **37**, 278–349.
381. Ron, S., Algom, D., Hary, D. & Cohen, M. Time-related changes in the distribution of sleep stages in brain injured patients, *Electroenceph. Clin. Neurophysiol.* (1980) **48**, 432–441.
382. Sassin, J.F., Parker, D.C., Mace, J.W., Gotlin, R.W., Johnson, L.C. & Rossman, L.G. Human growth hormone release relation to slow-wave sleep and sleep–waking cycles, *Science* (1969) **165**, 513–515.
383. Scheving, L.E. Mitotic rhythm in the human epidermis, *Anat. Rec.* (1959) **135**, 7–20.
384. Segawa, M., Hosaka, A., Miyagawa, F., Nomura, Y. & Imai, H. Hereditary progressive dystonia with marked diurnal fluctuation. In: Eldridge, R. & Fahn, S. (eds.) *Adv. Neurol.*, Vol. 14, New York: Raven Press (1976) 215–243.
385. Sherington, C.S. *Man on his Nature*, Cambridge: Cambridge University Press (1946) 413.
386. Sitaram, N., Wyatt, R.J., Dawson, S. & Gillin, J.C. REM sleep induction by physostigmine infusion during sleep, *Science* (1976) **191**, 1281–1283.
387. Smith, C. & Butler, S. Paradoxical sleep at selective times following training is necessary for learning, *Physiol. Behav.* (1982) **29**, 469–473.
388. Steele, J.C., Richardson, J.C. & Olszewski, J. Progressive supranuclear palsy, *Arch. Neurol. (Chic.)* (1964) **10**, 333–359.
389. Stern, W.C. & Morgane, P.J. Theoretical view of REM sleep function: maintenance of catecholamine systems in the central nervous system, *Behav. Biol.* (1974) **11**, 1–32.
390. Tufik, S., Lindsey, C.J. & Carlini, E.A. Does REM sleep deprivation induce a supersensitivity of dopaminergic receptors in the rat brain? *Pharmacology* (1978) **16**, 98–105.
391. Valk, I.M. & van der Bosch, J.S.G. Intra daily variation of the human ulnar length and short term growth – a longitudinal study in eleven boys, *Growth* (1974) **42**, 107–111.
392. Van Ormer, E.G. Retention after intervals of sleep and waking, *Arch. Psychol.* (1932) **137**, 5–49.
393. Vondra, K., Brodan, V., Bass, A., Kuhn, E., Teisinger, J., Anděl, M. & Veselková, A. Effects of sleep deprivation on the activity of selected metabolic enzymes in skeletal muscle, *Eur. J. Appl. Physiol.* (1981) **47**, 41–46.
394. Webb, W.B. The sleep of conjoined twins, *Sleep* (1978) **1**, 205–211.
395. Williams, H.L., Morlock, H.C. & Morlock, J.V. Instrumental behaviour during sleep, *Psychophysiology* (1966) **2**, 208–216.
396. Zeppelin, H. & Rechtschaffen, A. Mammalian sleep, longevity and energy metabolism, *Brain Behav. Evol.* (1974) **10**, 425–470.
397. Zornetzer, S.F. The locus coeruleus and memory. In: Fishbein, W. (ed.) *Sleep, Dreams and Memory*, Lancaster: MTP (1981) 47–72.

THE ENVIRONMENT OF SLEEP

398. Agnew, H.W., Jr., Webb, W.B. & Williams, R.L. The first night effect: An EEG study of sleep, *Psychophysiology* (1966) **2** 263–266.
399. Dement, W.C., Kales, A. & Zarcone, V. Effect of the fluidized bed on the sleep pattern of normal subjects. Paper presented at the first International Congress of the Association for the Psychophysiological study of sleep, Bruges, Belgium 19–23 June 1971.
400. Dobbs, M.E. Behavioural responses during sleep of men and women to aircraft noises. Paper presented at the 12th Annual Meeting of the Association for the Psychological Study of Sleep, Lake Minnewaska, New York, 4–7 May 1972.
401. Globus, G., Friedmann, J. & Cohen, H. The effects of aircraft noise on sleep electrophysiology as recorded in the home. In: Ward, W.D. (ed.) *Proceedings of the International Congress on Noise as a Public Health Problem*, Washington DC: US Environmental Protection Agency (1974) 587–591.
402. Hauri, P. *The Sleep Disorders*, Kalamazoo, Michigan: Upjohn (1977) 1–76.
403. Kinkel, H.J. & Maxion, H. Schlafphysiologische Untersuchungen zur Beurteilung verschiedener Matratzen, *Int. Z. Angewand. Physiol.* (1970) **28**, 247–262.
404. Lucas, J.S. & Kryter, K.D. Awakening effects of simulated sonic booms and subsonic aircraft noise on six subjects 7 to 72 years of age, NASA CR-1599 Stanford Research Institute (1970) 1–56.
405. Monroe, L.J. Transient changes in EEG sleep patterns of married good sleepers: The effects of altering sleeping arrangement, *Psychophysiology* (1969) **6**, 330–337.
406. Nicholson, A. & Marks, J. *Insomnia. A Guide for Medical Practitioners*, Lancaster: MTP (1983) 57.
407. Rechtschaffen, A., Hauri, P. & Zeitlin, M. Auditory awakening thresholds in REM and NREM sleep stage, *Percept. Mot. Skills* (1966) **22**, 927–942.
408. Rosekind, M., Phillips, P. & Rappaport, J. Effects of waterbed surface on sleep: A pilot study. In: Chase, M.H., Mitler, M.M. & Walter, W.P. (eds.) *Sleep Research*, Vol. 5, Los Angeles: BRIS UCLA (1976) 132.
409. Roth, T., Kramer, M. & Trinder, J. The effect of noise during sleep on the sleep patterns of different age groups, *Can. Psychiat. Assoc. J.* (1972) 197–201.
410. Shurley, J.T. Effect of the air-fluidized bed on sleep patterns in healthy human subjects. In: Artz, C.P. & Haigert, T.S. (eds.) *Air-Fluidized Bed Clinical and Research Symposium*, Charleston: Medical University of South Carolina (1971) 38–49.

SLEEP AND FOOD

411. Adam, K. Brain rhythm that correlates with obesity, *Brit. Med. J.* (1977) **2**, 234.
412. Adam, K. Dietary habits and sleep after bedtime food drinks, *Sleep* (1980) **3**, 47–58.
413. Crisp, A.H. & McGuiness, B. Jolly fat: relation between obesity and psychoneurosis in the general population, *Brit. Med. J.* (1976) **1**, 7–9.
414. Crisp, A.H. & Stonehill, E. Aspects of the relationship between sleep and nutrition: A study of 375 psychiatric outpatients, *Brit. J. Psychiat.* (1973) **122**, 379–394.
415. Crisp, A.H., Stonehill, E., Fenton, G.W. & Fenwick, P.B.C. Sleep patterns in obese patients during weight reduction, *Psychother. Psychosom.* (1973) **22**, 159–165.
416. Fara, J.W., Rubinstein, E.H. & Sonnenschein, R.R. Visceral and behavioural responses to intraduodenal fat, *Science* (1969) **166**, 110–111.
417. Horne, J.A. Human sleep and tissue restitution: some qualifications and doubts, *Clin. Sci.* (1983) **65**, 569–578.
418. Kales, A. & Kales, J.D. Sleep disorders. Recent findings in the diagnosis and treatment of disturbed sleep, *New Engl. J. Med.* (1974) **290**, 487–499.
419. Lacey, J.H., Crisp, A.H., Kalucy, R.S., Hartmann, M.K. & Chen, C.N. Weight gain and the sleeping electroencephalogram: study of ten patients with anorexia nervosa, *Brit. Med. J.* (1975) **4**, 556–558.
420. Michaelis, R. & Hoffman, E. Zur Phenomenologie und Atiopathogenese der Hypersomnie bei endogen-phasisischen Depressionen. In: Jovanović, U.J. (ed.), *The Nature of Sleep*, Stuttgart: Gustav Fischer (1973) 190–193.
421. Pavlov, I.P. Conditioned reflexes; an investigation of the physiological activity of the

cerebral cortex, *Trans Anrep G.V.*, New York: Oxford University Press (1927).
422.   Pavlov, I.P. *Lectures on Conditioned Reflexes. II. Conditioned Reflexes and Psychiatry*, Gantt, W.H. (ed./trans.) New York: International Publishing Co. (Review by Kudie, L.S., *Psychoanal. Quart.* (1942) **11**, 565–570.)
423.   Yogman, M.W. & Zeisel, S.H. Diet and sleep patterns in newborn infants, *New Engl. J. Med.* (1893) **309**, 1147–1149.

SLEEP AND WEATHER

424.   Baker, M.A. & Hayward, J.N. Autonomic basis for the rise in brain temperature during paradoxical sleep, *Science* (1967) **157**, 1586–1588.
425.   Devold, O., Barlindhaug, E. & Backer, J.E. Søvnforstyrreiser i mørketiden, *T. Norske Laegeforen* (1957) **77**, 836–837.
426.   Euler, C., Von, & Söderberg, M.K. The influence of hypothalamic thermoceptive structures on the electroencephalogram and gamma motor activity, *Electroenceph. Clin. Neurophysiol.* (1957) **9**, 391–408.
427.   Kjos, K. Søvnforstyrreiser som skolehygienisk problem i Nord-Norge, *T. Norske Laegeforen* (1959) **79**, 1241–1245.
428.   Lingjaerde, O. & Bratlid, T. Triazolam (Halcion) versus flunitrazepam (Rohypnol) against midwinter insomnia in Northern Norway, *Acta Psychiat. Scand.* (1981) **64**, 260–269.
429.   Monroe, I.J. Psychological and physiological differences between good and poor sleepers, *J. Abnorm. Psychol.* (1965) **72**, 255–265.
430.   Oswald, I. Symptoms that depress the doctor: Insomnia, *Brit. J. Hosp. Med.* (1983) **31**, 219–224.
431.   Parmeggiani, P.L. & Rabini, C. Sleep and environmental temperature, *Arch. Ital. Biol.* (1970) **108**, 369–387.
432.   Presley, J.M., Ellen, P. & Foshee, D.P. Environmental temperature and sleep in psychiatric patients, *Newslett. Res. Ment. Health Behav. Sci.* (1973) **15**, 17–19.
433.   Raboutet, J., Lesèvre, N. & Remond, A. Involuntary sleeping during EEG, research on promoting factors, *Rev. Neurol.* (1959) **101**, 404–408.
434.   Schmidt-Kessen, W. & Kendel, K. Einfluss der Raumtemperatur auf den Nachtschlaf, *Res. Exp. Med. (Berlin)* (1973) **160**, 220–233.
435.   Shapiro, C.M., Moore, A.T. & Mitchell, D. How well does man thermoregulate during sleep? *Experientia* (1974) **30**, 1279–1280.
436.   Webb, W.B. & Ades, H. Sleep tendencies: Effects of barometric pressure, *Science* (1964) **143**, 263–264.
437.   Valatx, J.L., Roussell, B. & Cure, M. Sommeil et température cérébrale du rat au cours de l'exposition chronique en ambiance chaude, *Brain Res.* (1973) **55**, 107–122.

SLEEP AND EXERCISE

438.   Adam, K. Sleep as a restorative process and a theory to explain why, *Prog. Brain Res.* (1980) **53**, 289–306.
439.   Baekeland, F. & Lasky, R. Exercise and sleep patterns in college athletes, *Percept. Mot. Skills* (1966) **23**, 1203–1207.
440.   Bonnet, M.H. Sleep, performance and mood after the energy expenditure equivalent of 40 hours of sleep deprivation, *Psychophysiology* (1980) **17**, 56–63.
441.   Buguet, A., Roussel, B., Angus, R., Sabiston, B. & Radomski, M. Human sleep and adrenal individual reactions to exercise, *Electroenceph. Clin. Neurophysiol.* (1980) **49**, 515–523.
442.   Browman, C.P. Sleep following sustained exercise, *Psychophysiology* (1980) **17**, 577–580.
443.   Bunnell, D.E., Bevier, W. & Horvath, S.M. Effects of exhaustive exercise on the sleep of men and women, *Psychophysiology* (1983) **20**, 50–58.
444.   Griffin, S.J. & Trinder, J. Physical fitness, exercise, and human sleep, *Psychophysiology* (1978) **15**, 447–450.
445.   Hauri, P. Effects of evening activity on early night sleep, *Psychophysiology* (1968) **4**, 267–277.
446.   Hauri, P. The influence of evening activity on the onset of sleep, *Psychophysiology* (1969) **5**, 426–430.

447. Hauri, P. Evening activity, sleep mentation and subjective sleep quality, *J. Abnorm. Psychol.* (1970) **76**, 270–275.
448. Hobson, J.A. Sleep after exercise, *Science* (1968) **162**, 1503–1505.
449. Horne, J.A. The effects of exercise upon sleep: a critical review, *Biol. Psychol.* (1981) **12**, 241–290.
450. Horne, J.A. & Staff, L.H.E. Exercise and sleep: body-heating effects, *Sleep* (1983) **6**, 36–46.
451. Malotnev, V.I., Telia, Z.A. & Chachanashvili, M.G. Changes in the structure of night sleep in man after intensive muscular work, *Sechenov Physiol. J. USSR* (1977) **63**, 11–20. (in Russian).
452. Oswald, I. Human brain protein, drugs and dreams, *Nature (Lond.)* (1969) **223**, 893–897.
453. Ryback, R.S., Lewis, O.F. & Lessard, C.S. Psychobiologic effects of prolonged bed rest (weightlessness) in young healthy volunteers (Study 11), *Aerospace Med.* (1971) **42**, 529–535.
454. Shapiro, C.M., Bortz, R., Mitchel, D., Bartel, P. & Jooste, P. Slow-wave sleep: a recovery period after exercise, *Science* (1981) **214**, 1253–1254.
455. Shapiro, C.M., Griesel, R.D., Bartel, P.R. & Jooste, P.L. Sleep patterns after graded exercise, *J. Appl. Physiol.* (1975) **39**, 187–190.
456. Shapiro, C.M. & Verschoor, G.J. Sleep patterns after a marathon, *S. Afr. J. Med. Sci.* (1979) **75**, 415–416.
457. Torsvall, L. Sleep after exercise: a literature review, *J. Sport Med.* (1981) **21**, 218–225.
458. Torsvall, L., Åkerstedt, T. & Lindeck, G. Effect on sleep stages and EEG power density of different degrees of exercise in fit subjects, *Electroenceph. Clin. Neurophysiol.* (1984) **57**, 347–353.
459. Trinder, J., Buck, D., Paxton, S.J., Montgomery, I. & Bowling, A. Physical fitness, exercise, age and human sleep, *Aust. J. Psychiat.* (1982) **34**, 131–138.
460. Walker, J.M., Floyd, T.C., Fein, G., Cavness, C., Lualhati, R. & Feinberg, I. Effects of exercise on sleep, *J. Appl. Physiol.* (1978) **44**, 945–951.
461. Zloty, R.B., Burdick, J.A. & Adamson, J.D. Sleep of distance runners, *Activitas Nervosa Superior (Praha)* (1973) **15**, 217–221.

DEATH AT NIGHT

462. Baron, R.C. & Kirschner, R.H. Sudden night-time death among South-East Asians too (letter), *Lancet* (1983) **1**, 764.
463. Hammond, E.C. Some preliminary findings of physical complaints from a prospective study of 1 064 004 men and women, *Am. J. Publ. Health* (1964) **54**, 11–23.
464. Kripke, D.F. & Garfinkel, L. Excess nocturnal deaths related to sleeping pill and tranquillizer use, *Lancet* (1984) **1**, 99.
465. Kripke, D.F., Simons, R.N., Garfinkel, L. & Hammond, E.C. Short and long sleep: sleep and pills, *Arch. Gen. Psychiat.* (1979) **36**, 103.
466. MacWilliam, J.A. Blood pressure and heart action in sleep and dreams: their relation to haemorrhages, angina and sudden death, *Brit. Med. J.* (1923) **2**, 1196–1200.
467. Partinen, M., Putkonen, P.T., Kaprio, J., Koskenvuo, M. & Hilakivi, I. Sleep duration in relation to coronary heart disease, *Acta Med. Scand. (Suppl.)* (1982) **660**, 69–83.
468. Schneider, C.F. Ein Beitrag zur Ermittelung der Sterblichkeits-Verhältnisse in Berlin nach den Todeszeiten, *Arch. Pathol. Anat. Physiol. Klin. Med.* (1859) **16**, 95.
469. Wingard, D.L. & Berkman, L.F. Mortality risk associated with sleeping pattern among adults, *Sleep* (1983) **6**, 102–107.

HYPNOSIS

470. Gerebtzoff, M.A. État fonctionnel de l'écorce cérébrale au cours de l'hypnose animale, *Arch. Int. Physiol.* (1941) **51**, 365–378.
471. Gould, G.M. & Pyle, W.L. *Anomalies and Curiosities of Medicine*, London: Rebman (1898).
472. Klemm, W.R. Electroencephalographic-behavioural dissociations during animal hypnosis, *Electroenceph. Clin. Neurophysiol.* (1941) **51**, 365–378.

CHAPTER 2

THE ANATOMICAL AND PHYSIOLOGICAL BASIS OF THE SLEEP–WAKE CYCLE

WAKING, SLEEP AND COMA

WAKING AND SLEEP

Alertness and sleep are dependent on the activity of the brain as a whole, although the different levels of consciousness are determined primarily by areas of the brain stem. These areas are discussed in detail in this chapter. In summary, the systems involved are as follows.

Wakefulness
Wakefulness depends on the activity of the brain stem diencephalic ascending reticular activating system. This system is extremely complex, and is a physiological rather than an anatomical entity (see p. 88). Reduction in the activity of this system is accompanied by sleep.[19, 21]

Sleep onset
Sleep onset depends on (1) reduction or absence of normal waking sensory stimuli, (2) reduction of the activity of the ascending reticular activating system, and (3) the activity of a postulated 'hypnogenic' centre (see p. 11).

   Many have sought for such a hypnogenic centre. In patients with encephalitis lethargica, von Economo observed that subjects who were insomniac often had anterior hypothalamic lesions (see p. 81). He therefore attributed to this area a hypnogenic function. Much more recently, however, metabolic studies of cerebral glucose oxidative metabolism in primates have failed to show any single area of the brain with an increased metabolic rate at sleep onset (see. p. 11). There is no biochemical evidence that any sleep-onset centre exists, although the marker of a postulated hypnogenic centre may be a change in protein, not carbohydrate, metabolism.

   The mechanisms that determine sleep onset are of particular importance in anxiety and other causes of difficulty in first falling asleep.

Sleep maintenance
Sleep maintenance and NREM sleep are probably determined by feedback mechanisms between the hemispheres and the brain stem, as well as by the absence of arousal stimuli. However, neither the anatomical nor the biochemical basis for sleep maintenance is fully understood.

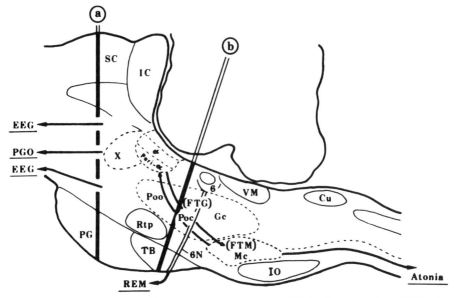

Figure 2.1 *Representation of brain stem structures responsible for the generation of REM sleep in a sagittal plain.* Abbreviations – 6, 6N: abducens nucleus and nerve, respectively; α: locus coeruleus α; Cu: cuneate nucleus; FTG: gigantocellular tegmental field, comprising the nuclei reticularis pontis oralis (Poo), caudalis (Poc) and gigantocellularis (Gc); FTM: magnocellular tegmental field corresponding to the nucleus reticularis magnocellularis (Mc); IC: inferior colliculus; PG: pontine gray; Rtp: nucleus reticularis tegmenti pontis; SC: superior colliculus; TB: trapezoid body; VM: medial vestibular nucleus; X: area X. *Reprinted with permission from Sakai.*[32]

Long-acting neurohormones or even exogenous sleep peptides such as the muramyl peptide isolated by Pappenheimer, considered to be involved in sleep onset and discussed in Chapter 8, may be more involved in sleep maintenance than the classic short-acting neurotransmitters.

Sleep maintenance rather than sleep onset is disturbed in endogenous depression.

REM sleep
REM sleep is dependent on the activity of executive neurones (REM sleep 'on' neurones) which have been localized (in cats) to magnocellular–gigantocellular areas of the pontine tegmentum (Fig. 2.1). These neurones, or contiguous neurones, also play a part in the generation of saccadic eye movements during wakefulness (see p. 102).[33, 35, 37] Focal injury to this area in man has been associated with the near-total absence of REM sleep.[15]

All EEG signs and behavioural signs of REM sleep are related to, and partially produced by, neuronal discharges arising in the pons. Jouvet[14] considered that the mediodorsal pontine tegmentum, and in particular the locus coeruleus complex, was responsible for the generation of REM sleep, since large lesions in this area almost completely abolished REM sleep. However, Jones and her colleagues[11] showed that small discrete bilateral lesions including the locus coeruleus had little effect on REM sleep, although kainic acid lesions of this area, which destroy neuronal cell bodies but not fibres of passage, are followed by about 50% reduction in paradoxical sleep and complete suppression of sleep atonia.[32]

Sakai[32] suggested that each subsystem of REM sleep (cortical desynchronization, PGO waves, sleep atonia, dreaming) was under the control of both tonic excitatory 'on' neurones and inhibitory 'off' neurones. An integrated state of neuronal activity of all the 'on' neurones and the inhibition of all the 'off' neurones seems to be essential for the generation of REM sleep. It is not known if excitation of REM sleep 'on' neurones leads to inhibition of 'off' neurones, or whether some humoral factor can act simultaneously on these two neuronal populations.

In man, sleep is always accompanied by *eye movements*. Minor movements of the eyes occur at sleep onset and both slow pursuit and rapid saccadic eye movements are characteristic of sleep. Blind men, although unable to see, move their eyes whilst sleeping. Tiredness, sleep deprivation and narcolepsy all produce impaired ocular fixation and defective eye movements, and, when eye movements are affected by brain stem disease, sleep itself is usually abnormal. Eye movements, as well as sleep, are disturbed in many diseases, encephalitis lethargica being an example of a mesencephalitis with impaired oculomotor control accompanied by a sleep disturbance. Pupillary as well as oculomotor changes are conspicuous during sleep. Rossi[31] observed that the mydriasis of a blind man (due to loss of the tonic pupilloconstrictor neuronal activity with loss of the light reflex) was replaced by meiosis during sleep. Osorio and Daroff[24] considered that the same pontine neuronal system which generates fast saccadic eye movements whilst waking may also generate the REMs of sleep, and an early indicator of chronic brain stem degenerative disease is sometimes impairment of phasic eye movements during sleep.[22] As well as saccadic eye movements, dreaming may be lost.

The regular NREM–REM sleep cycle

The anatomical and biochemical basis of the regular NREM–REM sleep cycle, which occurs 5–6 times each night in human adults, is not known. Hypothalamic lesions in man, which may damage the suprachiasmatic nucleus, disrupt the rhythmicity and entrainment of the normal 24 h sleep–wake cycle, but may not cause any major alteration in the normal rhythmicity of NREM–REM cycles within sleep itself.

Arousal

Arousal is dependent primarily on the duration of the previous sleep period as well as on the usual morning external zeitgebers – dawn, alarm clocks, a full bladder, the milkman, and so on (see Chapter 3) – rather than upon the activity of a specific arousal centre.

The systems which control the structure of sleep itself are linked to, although they have a measure of independence from, the central circadian clock timer (or timers) which organize the onset of NREM and REM sleep periods. In addition, the anatomical mechanisms of sleep and thermal regulation are linked.

Thermal regulation is closely associated with sleep, although desynchronization of the sleep–wake and temperature rhythms occurs under conditions of temporal isolation, and all homeothermic animals exhibit 24 h cycles of body temperature that are independent of sleep. If a person stays awake at night, his body temperature continues to drop, as normally would occur during NREM sleep. However, there is some overlap between the hypothalamic, thermoregulatory and sleep-inducing structures;[25] warmth induces sleep;[26] and, in many pathological disorders, hypersomnia may be accompanied by hyperpyrexia. Cairns[5] showed that acute injuries to the hypothalamus, as well as producing hypersomnia, stupor or coma, sometimes caused the temperature to rise by 1–2 °C.

Contiguity of, and connections between, sleep systems and *sensory pathways* may account for the occasional sensory features that occur at the onset of sleep. These include a sudden sensory flash, feelings of weightlessness, and limb paraesthesiae. The medial lemniscus is located at the boundary between the pontine tegmentum and the basis pontis, and sensory symptoms are prominent features of pontine lesions causing sleep disturbance. A careful sensory examination of patients with pontine lesions causing sleep disturbance often reveals evidence of dorsal brain stem involvement which may accompany disruption of sleep-related medial tegmental structures.[8]

THE STUDY OF THE ANATOMY OF SLEEP AND COMA

Early this century, surgeons discovered that handling or electrical stimulation of the human medulla oblongata and pons could cause immediate loss of consciousness, although this may have been due sometimes to vaso-vagal episodes rather than to direct interference with the caudal extremity of the reticular formation. Foerster and Spielmeyer[9] showed that digital compression of the medulla produced unconsciousness as well as stertorous breathing, bradycardia and tonic fits. Similarly, Reichardt[29] found that puncture of the medulla oblongata in the course of cisternal tapping was often but not invariably followed by loss of consciousness. Although REM sleep was not recognized at the time, Cairns[5] showed that high spinal lesions producing complete tetraplegia did not impair awareness (although Adey *et al.*[1] subsequently showed that some quadriplegic patients with cervical lesions did have reduced amounts of NREM sleep). In contrast, Cairns showed that lesions in the pons often disturbed consciousness. With *low pontine* lesions, most of which also involved the medulla, loss of awareness was often a late event, and usually accompanied by respiratory and cardiac collapse, voluntary muscle hypertonus and rapid death; whilst with *high pontine* and *diencephalic* lesions, the usual variety of loss of awareness sometimes resembled sleep more than coma, and this was accompanied by ocular and not by respiratory abnormalities.[5]

The first major landmark in the study of the anatomical localization of the mechanisms of coma, sleep and waking followed the outbreak of encephalitis lethargica in 1917–1927. Because of the importance of this topic, the occurrence of sporadic cases of encephalitis lethargica today, and the possibility of a future epidemic, encephalitis lethargica is discussed in some detail on p. 81, although EEG studies were not available in 1917. At that time, the work of von Economo firmly established that focal diencephalic and brain stem lesions affect sleep and wakefulness in man. More recently, a major distinction has been made between the effects on sleep and wakefulness of *ventral pontine lesions* (which affect the classic ascending and descending pathways but not the reticular formation); and *dorsal pontine tegmental lesions* which interrupt the ascending reticular activating system and may involve the mechanisms of REM sleep. The effects of such brain stem lesions on human sleep are described on p. 98.

During the same era, animal physiologists confirmed and greatly extended knowledge of the anatomical basis of sleep learned from studies in man. Although animals sleep in many different ways from man, the anatomical basis of the sleep–wake cycle appears to be very similar in most of the mammalian species that have been investigated. Thus the behavioural as well as the electrophysiological consequences of a midbrain transection just behind the third nerve (cerveau isolé) and cervical-medullary junction transection (encéphale isolé), in cats, bear more than a superficial resemblance to the consequences of pontine and low medullary lesions, respectively, in man.

Table 2.1 *Major behavioural and electrophysiological characteristics of wakefulness, sleep and coma in man*

	Wakefulness	Locked-in syndrome	Sleep	Coma	Akinetic mutism
Clinical characteristics	Regular 24 h rhythm. State of alert attention. Consciousness of self and environment	As in wakefulness. Voluntary motor response limited to eye movements. Minor abnormalities of sleep are present	Regular 24 h rhythm. Arousal always possible. Sleep-related events, e.g. hypnic jerks, sleep atonia	Continuous unresponsiveness. Arousal not possible. No spontaneous behavioural changes. Eyes closed	Minor self-sustained changes in activity. Arousal not possible. Eyes half closed
Electrophysiological accompaniments	Desynchronized EEG. Alpha activity with relaxed wakefulness	Overall as in wakefulness. Minor changes in sleep (see text)	NREM–REM cycles. Minor changes in somatosensory potentials	Usually monotonous sequence of slow activity. Somatosensory potentials blocked depending on lesions in specific pathway (absence of criteria for brain death)	Some evidence of EEG cyclical activity. Alpha activity may be present
Pathological changes	–	Ventral pontine lesion	–	Dorsal pontine tegmental lesion or generalized metabolic cause	Chronic coma with brain stem lesion

SLEEP AND COMA

Wakefulness, sleep and the different levels of coma are distinguished by clinical, electrophysiological and pathological criteria (Table 2.1). There is usually little or no difficulty in distinguishing between these different states, the rare instances of brain stem damage with preservation of alpha activity (alpha coma), and states of psychogenic unresponsiveness.

> Coma lacks many of the basic elements of sleep. State transitions between wakefulness, slow-wave sleep and REM sleep do not occur. Also, the phasic events of REM sleep, twitches of the limbs and facial musculature, REMs, PGO waves and cardiorespiratory irregularities, do not occur in coma. The variations in behaviour and physiology seen in normal sleep are often replaced by a monotonous sequence of slow activity in the EEG, the threshold for arousal is not achieved, and there is a reduction in cerebral oxygen uptake.[20, 28] Many patients in coma have a primary brain stem lesion, and the signs of this are obvious. Visual evoked potentials, which depend on a specific pathway via the lateral geniculate body to the visual cortex, may not be disturbed in coma due to a brain stem lesion,[6] but other somatosensory evoked potentials that depend upon the integrity of brain stem pathways are abolished, unlike the situation in sleep.

Despite these obvious differences, there are a number of similarities between coma and NREM sleep. At the start of this century, coma and sleep were thought to be similar conditions. Moruzzi[21] considered that there was a continuum of alertness between states of coma, sleep, waking and high arousal. The borderland between sleep and coma is considered below.

Sleep, hibernation and coma
Stupor and coma in man have some similarity to hibernation in animals, with decreased metabolism and body temperature. Alpine ground squirrels exposed to near-freezing temperature enter hibernation during periods of sleep, accompanied by an initial 1–2 °C drop in body temperature. Initially, both slow-wave and REM sleep occur, but as hibernation continues the temperature falls further and REM sleep occurs less frequently, only to disappear at temperatures below 75 °F.[39] This accords well with one suggested function of REM sleep; coma prevention by an increase in the ascending reticular barrage whenever a dangerous level of reticular deactivation is attained.

Electroencephalographic characteristics of sleep and coma
The criterion of EEG synchronization does not necessarily correspond to sleep. The electrical pattern of cortical desynchronization during REM sleep is very similar to that of wakefulness, although the level of consciousness is not. Loeb and Poggio[18] and Chatrian et al.[7] gave examples of pontine lesions in man which produced coma, although with preserved alpha, not slow-wave, EEG activity. On rare occasions, signs of consciousness may persist despite complete destruction of the pontine reticular core.[23] Also, Lindsley et al.[17] showed that the behavioural and electrocorticographic changes of arousal can be separated in the cat by destruction of the subthalamic reticular core, with preservation of more rostral structures.

Although data from metabolic and drug studies are difficult to interpret, the prevalence of slow activity in the electroencephalogram in hepatic encephalopathy, which is usually a good index of the degree of stupor, does not always correlate with this, and fairly marked slowing can occur without obvious reduction in awareness. This is also seen after toxic doses of anticholinergic drugs.[36]

Dissociation between REM sleep and sleep atonia
REM sleep, but without the normal atonia of this sleep stage, is observed in animals with small bilateral pontine tegmental lesions. In man, atonia equivalent to that of sleep may appear in the waking state during attacks of sleep paralysis and cataplexy, and REM sleep without atonia has been reported in a child with a brain stem tumour (see p. 97).[2]

PGO waves of REM sleep during wakefulness
PGO waves do not unequivocally occur during human sleep, although PGO-like waves from the graphic point of view have been recorded in patients with periaqueductal grey matter implants. PGO wave-like activity and trains of theta waves herald the occurrence of rapid eye movement, and have been found during sleep in patients with implanted electrodes and epilepsy, or severe pain problems.[40] These waveforms are the most conspicuous EEG pattern of REM sleep in the cat. 5-HT synthesis inhibition in the cat causes insomnia, and, after a short latency, characteristic PGO waveforms of REM sleep occur during wakefulness.

Arousal from sleep and coma
The threshold for arousal increases with the depth of NREM sleep. When NREM sleep is facilitated (as after sleep deprivation, in some forms of hypersomnia, and in children with NREM parasomnias), arousal from sleep may be difficult. In light (but not deep) coma, spindles similar to those of NREM sleep occur in reaction to external stimuli. Spindles are always a sign of favourable prognosis in coma, whilst the absence of any reactivity to external stimuli indicates a very unfavourable outcome.[27]

Different effects of acute and chronic lesions on sleep and coma
Sudden pontine vascular lesions or head injury cause immediate coma rather than stupor or sleep, whilst slowly progressive brain stem tumours may not cause hypersomnia, followed by stupor or coma, until a late stage in their development. Thus severe head injury, haemorrhage into the diencephalon or pons, or thrombosis of the posterior inferior cerebellar artery, is usually followed by immediate loss of awareness.[3, 10] Immediate regaining of consciousness from the state of akinetic mutism may follow puncture of an intraventricular cyst, whilst the transition between different levels of consciousness during recovery from coma is usually very gradual.

Recovery of sleep–wake cycles after coma
Following coma due to severe head injury, encephalitis and vascular lesions in humans, and in the cerveau isolé preparation in the cat, sleep–wake cycles gradually recover. This takes weeks or months to achieve; the normal cycles are sometimes never regained.[30]. However, after severe head injury, different EEG sleep stages can often be identified, even in chronically unresponsive patients.[4]

In the cat with a chronic cerveau isolé preparation with a low pontine–medullary junction level section, spontaneous periods of EEG desynchronization, perhaps corresponding to wakefulness, occur after 7–15 days, or may be produced in response to cortical stimulation, olfactory stimulation, or by cooling the animal. As well as EEG changes, recovery of normal pupillary behaviour occurs. Recovery is similar but faster following small midbrain lesions. Although periodic synchronization–desynchronization in the cerveau isolé preparation does not represent normal sleep cycles, and other components of REM sleep may be lacking,[13, 38] these results show that a genuine state of wakefulness can be maintained by the isolated cerebrum. The cerebral activating centres responsible for wakefulness were localized by Moruzzi[21] to the upper pathways of the reticular formation, coinciding with or related to the hypothalamic centres where stimulation causes outbursts of sham rage and defence aggression behaviour in animals after decortication. Destruction of these areas by encephalitis lethargica in man leads to hypersomnia.

Akinetic mutism and alpha coma
Akinetic mutism (see p. 104) is a state characteristic of partial recovery from deep coma or occurring with chronic states of reduced consciousness. The subject is immobile, with no spontaneous motor activity, unresponsive and with half-open eyes. Usually, some electrophysiological as well as behavioural evidence of self-sustained sleep–wake cycles is present. Cairns originally described this state in a 14-year-old girl with a craniopharyngiomatous cyst compressing the walls of the third ventricle, but many different lesions affecting different brain areas, including large bilateral frontal lobe lesions, will cause a similar picture.

The state of alpha coma may be related to that of akinetic mutism. Although in a state of coma, a few patients with brain stem infarcts maintain normal alpha activity. In these patients, the EEG pattern may be indistinguishable or closely similar to that of wakefulness, although the alpha rhythm is usually less responsive to loud noises, photic stimulation, eye opening and other stimuli.

REM sleep rebound after coma
Under normal circumstances, in human adults, REM sleep is dependent on previous NREM sleep. When this falls below a certain critical level with brain stem lesions, REM sleep is reduced or absent, as also occurs in experimental insomnia in animals. However, REM sleep is not always dependent on previous NREM sleep. Under normal conditions, there is a system within the brain which records REM sleep time and determines REM rebound following deprivation. One distinction between coma and sleep lies in suppression of this mechanism which measures REM sleep during coma. However, the majority of detailed studies in comatose humans have involved subjects with destruction of the pontine tegmentum rather than metabolic lesions which might be expected to have less specific effects on the mechanisms of REM sleep. In many instances, recovery from alcoholic coma or hepatic encephalopathy is accompanied by a rebound of REM sleep.

ENCEPHALITIS LETHARGICA AND SLEEP

Encephalitis lethargica appeared mysteriously in France and Vienna in 1917, and may have been transported to Europe from the Chinese province of Yunnanfou by returning French soldiers. The disease spread rapidly through Western Europe and England, where 126 cases, a fifth of which were fatal, were reported during the first six months of 1918. Between then and 1927, when the disease disappeared, more than 65 000 cases were seen. Nothing like encephalitis lethargica in extent, nature or severity had appeared before, apart from the sleeping sickness called nona and in which Gayet had identified lesions in the mesencephalon and hypothalamus in 1875.[43]

The cause of encephalitis lethargica was never definitely established. It occurred in the same years as an influenza pandemic, but the two conditions had a different prevalence, different clinical features and different after-effects, and were separate, unrelated disorders. Pathological features were typical of a virus infection, with microscopic foci of inflammation mainly in the grey matter of the midbrain and basal ganglia. No definite causative organism was ever identified, but the disease was thought to be due to an airborne virus, and was transmitted to monkeys by injection of brain tissue from infected patients. In 1890, Mauthner took part in a discussion of a case of nona – probably encephalitis lethargica – and foretold that the lesions causing sleep in the disease would be found in the grey matter around the aqueduct of Sylvius.[46] He had never seen a case of nona, but based his prediction on his knowledge of pathological conditions in which ocular palsies and excessive sleep are cardinal conditions, a combination seen, for example, in Wernicke's encephalopathy, and with tumours and other morbid processes that damage the walls of the third ventricle and adjacent parts. This region became known as *Mauthner's area*.

The presentation of encephalitis lethargica was variable in different years and in different localities. Von Economo saw his first patient in a Viennese psychiatric clinic, and psychiatric disturbances and compulsive behaviour were common. These took many bizarre forms; for example, one patient experienced episodic paranoia confined to one side of the body, and accompanied by oculogyric crises. Children could develop cruel, psychotic or criminal behaviour. Several young children committed murder; a boy of 10 tried to knife his mother, cut up his brother, and kill his sister with a hatchet. According to Stolk,[49] the rise of national socialism in Germany and the violence, aggression and gesticulation of Hitler may have resulted, at least in part, from encephalitis lethargica.

During the acute illness, or after apparent recovery for as long as 3–4 years, and in a fashion reminiscent of syphilis, unexpected features could first appear; parkinsonism, oculogyric crises and, the strangest of all, bizarre sleep disturbances. *Parkinsonism* was usually something more than the idiopathic disease, with dystonic postures, fits, hiccough, chorea, myoclonus, tics and respiratory abnormalities. Once established, the severity of parkinsonian features did not increase greatly over the following decades.

Oculogyric crises, with forced adversive eye movements, sometimes accompanied by compulsive thoughts, were a characteristic feature but tended to die out over the years. *Sleep disturbances* could take any form in both the acute and chronic stages of disease. Total insomnia, hypersomnia, sleep reversal, narcolepsy and cataplexy were all reported. Sleep disturbances, like the oculogyric crises, but unlike parkinsonism, tended slowly to recover.

Von Economo[53-55] described three major patterns of sleep disturbance in encephalitis lethargica; excessive sleepiness, sleeplessness and reversal of the sleep rhythm. From a study of the lesions of the disease, he recognized the definite importance of involvement of the grey matter of the midbrain and caudal part of the third ventricle. The most important lesions accounting for sleep disturbances were located in the posterior wall of the third ventricle and the adjoining grey matter of the interpeduncular region, the aqueduct and the tegmentum. Initial pathological changes in encephalitis lethargica were mostly widespread, but affected particularly the midbrain and subthalamic region, with marked involvement of the locus coeruleus. The cortex, caudate, putamen and globus pallidus with thalamus were normal in all cases, with minor changes in the corpora Luysii and substantia innominata, the greatest destruction occurring in the midbrain and pons.[42, 47]

Von Economo separated lesions causing *insomnia,* which were mainly situated in the basal forebrain, from those causing *hypersomnia,* situated in the mesencephalic tegmentum and posterior hypothalamus. Because of the widespread nature of the lesions causing encephalitis, this work was largely disbelieved at the time, but by the end of the encephalitis lethargica era had been often confirmed.[45]

Other attempts to localize sleep in the brain at the start of the 20th century were less successful than that of Von Economo. Trömner, in his book *Das Problem der Schlaf* (1912) reviewed the existing theories of sleep, only to condemn them, and replaced these with the hypothesis that sleep is regulated from a centre in the optic thalamus. He argued that sleep resulted from a sudden complete interruption of sensory impressions on their way to the cortex, and that an organ must exist that was capable of producing this sudden blockade. By virtue of its known connections with all the senses in all parts of the cortex, the thalamus has this power: 'sleep is initiated and controlled by one organ, the optic thalamus'. Unfortunately for this argument, isolated lesions of the thalamus never cause sleep disturbances, although in a case reported by Hirsch,[44] a thalamic abscess as big as a hen's egg was found in a patient who slept excessively in the last days of his illness.[41]

The acute form of encephalitis lethargica was usually accompanied by fever, somnolence and ophthalmoplegia, whilst in a second form of the disease, hyperkinesis, tics, myoclonus and chorea were accompanied by sleep inversion. When acute parkinsonism occurred, this was sometimes associated with a catatonic-like stupor.[55] Typically, narcolepsy–cataplexy was a late development following the acute attack. Initially, coma might last a week or two, followed by stupor, from which the patient could be aroused only by deep painful stimuli, progressing to a quiet, awake and sometimes akinetic state, lying with the eyes open but not initiating any activity. EEGs recorded during recent sporadic cases of probable encephalitis lethargica in this stage of the illness have shown diffuse, high-voltage delta and theta activity.[48] Recovery of normal awareness with clear sleep–wake cycles was often delayed for several months.

Narcolepsy and cataplexy seem to have occurred more frequently as late sequelae in cases presenting insomnia or sleep reversal, than following coma, stupor or hypersomnolence. Both narcolepsy and cataplexy gradually improved over the following decade.

Adie[41] described a boy of 14 who in 1923 developed sleeplessness, fever, delirium and jerking of the limbs, followed by restlessness at night and excessive sleep during the day, with double vision. He recovered from this state in about three months, sufficient to get about, but by this time his features were expressionless, his movements were slow, and he became very stout, bad-tempered and argumentative. He was still apt to drop off to sleep during the day. Attacks of overwhelming drowsiness occurred with any monotonous task. He then had attacks in which, if he laughed, his knees gave way and he fell to the ground. He said 'at the Scout camp the boys used to amuse themselves by making me laugh and then run away, leaving me helpless on the ground'. 'I cannot go to the pictures now, because if I am amused my head flops about and people look at me instead of the pictures.' By 1926 the attacks were becoming less frequent and he was beginning to lose weight, but was still much fatter than he used to be.

Symonds[50, 51] described an Icelander who developed typical narcolepsy following encephalitis lethargica and acute parkinsonism in 1918. Although he was slow to move and had bilateral ptosis and a blinking tic, his chief initial complaint was of insomnia at night, although on getting up at about 0900 he became so sleepy that he had to go to bed again. He was at his best in the evening, seldom getting off to sleep until well on in the early morning hours. In the Summer of 1919, this sleep pattern changed, and the patient first complained of excessive sleepiness followed by a period of delirium and visual hallucinosis. After this he noticed that whenever he laughed or was excited, he fell down. He began to improve spontaneously in 1922, but remained liable to falling attacks. Symonds witnessed one of these: 'a little twitching of the facial muscle, short interval of silence, he talked vaguely in Icelandic; then said "I can't move my arms".'

Many cases of post-encephalitic parkinsonism are still seen today, but there must be few if any remaining cases of narcolepsy–cataplexy as a sequel to the 1917–1927 pandemic of this illness.

The status of *secondary* narcolepsy–cataplexy following encephalitis lethargica remains in doubt. As in the above examples, persistent daytime drowsiness and sub-alertness, rather than brief attacks of true narcolepsy, characterize the illness. *Primary* narcolepsy–cataplexy depends on environmental as well as genetic factors for its development. Encephalitis lethargica may be one environmental factor that will precipitate primary narcolepsy in susceptible (possibly DR2 positive) subjects.

ANATOMY OF SLEEP AND WAKING

THE CEREBRAL CORTEX AND SLEEP

Studies by Goltz[106] on chronic decorticate dogs first showed that sleep and wakefulness may be observed even after complete ablation of the cerebral cortex.[60, 137, 171, 173] In chronic decerebrate animals, and also in anencephalic children, cyclical changes of behaviour occur, closely similar to the normal physiological alteration of sleep and wakefulness.[103, 133] The evidence from human anencephalic and hydrocephalic infants who survive long enough suggests that even with a totally absent cerebral cortex, sleep and waking occur. In addition, the child also responds to hunger, loud sounds and visual stimuli, and may even possibly see and hear, taste and smell, cry and smile, utter crude sounds and make crude movements of the limbs.[169, 183]

Although sleep–wake cycles occur in the absence of the cortex, this is essential for the normal regulation and maintenance of NREM sleep, as well as playing an active role in the maintenance of wakefulness. Proof that the regulation of sleep–wake cycles is influenced by the cortex came with the demonstration of Kleitman and Camille[138] that decortication in adult dogs produced the sleep pattern and behaviour of young puppies; and also by the finding of Bremer and Terzuolo[73] that the cortex can activate the reticular formation, resulting in turn in activation of the cortex and a general arousal response. This physiological finding has implications for the study of memory, behaviour and awareness in human cortical and subcortical disease, where in some instances it is difficult or impossible to separate clearly aspects of dementia from reduction in awareness.

Do localized cortical and subcortical lesions alter sleep in man? Considerable areas of cortex can be removed from any part of the cerebral hemispheres in man without gross alterations of sleep–wake patterns. However, sleep is often very abnormal in patients with generalized cortical disease. Generalized demyelination and sclerosis of the white matter of the cerebrum and cerebellum, although with relative preservation of brain stem structures in *Pelizaeus–Merzbacher disease,* as well as causing profound mental deterioration, oculomotor abnormalities and intermittent involuntary movements, result in a highly abnormal pattern of sleep. Wilkus and Farrell[225] described a 20-year-old severely disabled man with Pelizaeus–Merzbacher disease who had highly abnormal NREM sleep, but well preserved REM sleep. There were no identifiable spindles, vertex sharp waves or K complexes during NREM sleep, whilst REM sleep was almost normal, occurring cyclically five times throughout the night for 18% of total sleep time. Similar but less marked changes, with preservation of some vertex sharp waves and sleep spindles, were described in three less severely affected patients with Pelizaeus–Merzbacher disease by Niakan *et al.*[168] Even more dramatic sleep changes occur in *GM₂ gangliosidosis* (Tay–Sachs disease). The EEG becomes abnormal in the early stages of the illness, with paroxysmal slow waves and multiple spikes, and in young children in the late stage of illness there may be a lack of any recognizable stage of sleep.[134]

CEREBELLUM

Neurologists have been led to regard the cerebellum as a structure mainly concerned with the control of movements and posture, not with sleep. However, major behavioural manifestations of sleep include postural adjustments, autonomic control of respiratory movements, and movements of the eyes and limbs, as well as alteration in muscle tone, and the cerebellum must be involved in motor control during sleep as well as during wakefulness. Both EEG activating and synchronizing impulses arise in the fastigial nuclei, at least in the encéphale isolé cat with a low brain stem section.[97]

Cerebellar lesions affect the mechanism of muscle atonia during REM sleep,[107] although Jouvet[127] in his EEG studies of the antigravity tonus of the cat during desynchronized sleep, and Hobson[115] showed that, following ablation of the anterior lobe of the cerebellum, neither sleep atonia of the normal cat nor cataplectic-like episodes seen in decerebrate cats were greatly altered. However, there is some cerebellar component in sleep atonia. Marchesi and Strata[153] showed that the firing rate of cerebellar climbing fibre complexes increases at the onset of REM sleep atonia, and may contribute to the development of this.

Cerebellectomy does not greatly modify the sleep–wakefulness cycle itself, although cortical and subcortical cerebellar lesions favour a slight increase in REM sleep and sleepiness. Changes in sleep have been found after fastigial nuclei lesions, middle cerebellar peduncle lesions and stimulation, and after superior cerebellar peduncle and cerebellar cortex lesions.[90] The main conclusions to emerge are the existence of a functional antagonism between cerebellar cortex and deep cerebellar nuclei in regulating sleep and wakefulness. One main effect of vermis or hemisphere cerebellar lesions on sleep in man is the production of numerous sleep spindles.[152]

BASAL GANGLIA

Are the basal ganglia involved in sleep control? Neurones from the substantia nigra innervate the striatum, which is intimately involved in the control of movement. Each dopamine neurone gives rise to approximately 500 000 synaptic contacts in the striatum, and virtually every neurone in the striatum apparently receives a dopaminergic input.[59] The spontaneous activity in nigral units in cats shows little alteration between quiet waking and sleep, and there is no relationship between phasic events during sleep and unit discharge.[215] These are rare examples of neurones that show no change in activity during REM sleep. In parkinsonism, spontaneous movement is reduced in sleeping as well as waking, but REM sleep loss in this disease is unlikely to be the result of the basal ganglia lesion.

THALAMUS AND SLEEP SPINDLES

In 1927, Hess presented at the Frankfurt meeting of the German Physiological Society a film on sleep produced by electrical thalamic stimulation of a freely moving, unanaesthetized cat.[113] Low-frequency stimulation of midline thalamic nuclei caused pre-sleep behaviour followed by sleep. The area from which sleep was obtained was very limited; lateral to the massa intermedia and limited caudally by the habenulo-interpeduncular tract and rostrally by the mamillo-thalamic bundle. Stimulation of anterior thalamic nuclei also sometimes gave good results. Many physiologists at first were reluctant to accept these results, since the low rate of stimulation, and often the need for the stimulus to be repeated, as well as the delayed response in a naturally sleepy animal, were all very different from the classic results of high-frequency stimulation of the autonomic and motor system. Additionally, the cat often remained asleep for prolonged periods.[162] However, these findings have been often repeated and confirmed: the problem is their interpretation. It must be remembered that in Montreal, having obtained evidence that minor epilepsy with loss of consciousness may arise in or near the thalamus, Penfield and his colleagues claimed that the seat of consciousness is situated in the diencephalon.[176] Hess produced by electrical stimulation what may be regarded as a form of pre-sleep behaviour. The cat looked around for a sleeping place, searched for a quiet corner, and finally curled up in a quiet position, perhaps accompanied by a genuine feeling of drowsiness. According to Koella,[139] Hess's thalamic sleep centre would be the head ganglion of sleep.

In man, the thalamus does not appear to be essential for sleep, although it is essential for sleep spindle production. Sleep may occur in the absence of a thalamus,[164, 165] but lesions of the thalamus abolish EEG sleep spindles,[74] which fits the classic idea of a thalamic pacemaker driving cortical neurones and cortical synchronization during NREM sleep.[186]

There is good evidence that the periodic bursts or trains of high-amplitude cortical waves or spindles which occur more frequently as the animal sinks deeper through light and moderate sleep are generated by non-specific thalamic nuclei and their diffuse thalamocortical projections. Spindles can be driven from a medial thalamic recruiting zone. This corresponds very closely in area to that from which sleep can be promoted by low-frequency electrical stimulation.[96] Quite what the function of sleep spindles is remains unknown. They are never found in decerebrate animals, but are constantly present in normal individuals. Presumably they have an important function in the regulation of slow-wave sleep,[224] and their prevalence is greatly affected by hypnotic drugs.[114] Sleep spindles and K complexes occur with spontaneous phasic arousal in sleeping human subjects, but they are never seen during normal wakefulness.[163]

HYPOTHALAMUS

The posterior, lateral and medial hypothalamus is a continuation of the ascending activating reticular system and is closely related to it.[174] The observations made by von Economo[221–223] on cases of sleeping sickness were the first to draw the attention of clinicians as well as sleep physiologists to this area. Removal of the posterior hypothalamus abolishes wakefulness in the encéphale isolé preparation,[189] and the eventual recovery of wakefulness in the chronic cerveau isolé preparation as well as following brain stem injury in man may be attributed to the action of the posterior hypothalamus.[218, 219] In many species, posterior hypothalamic lesions cause lethargy and hypersomnolence. In 1939, Ranson showed that bilateral damage to posterolateral hypothalamic areas caused somnolence with decrease or abolition of emotional reactions, whilst hypothalamic stimulation caused the reverse.[187] These changes are not, however, invariable. Small localized posterior hypothalamic lesions in cats produce short-lasting behavioural and EEG arousal, but also paradoxical sleep episodes with atonia and electrographic changes, EEG desynchronization and erratic waves in the pons and lateral geniculate body.[164, 165]

These observations in animals are, on the whole, in keeping with the clinical evidence in man that lesions of the posterior hypothalamus produce sleepiness. Depending on the extent and exact site of the lesion, hypersomnia, coma or change in the circadian rhythmicity of sleep results.

FOREBRAIN AND ANTERIOR HYPOTHALAMUS

In addition to the well known serotonin raphe complex theory for sleep developed by Jouvet and his colleagues,[129, 130] there is the theory that forebrain areas contain powerful inhibitory and sleep-promoting mechanisms.[156] Anterior hypothalamic lesions in the pre-optic regions have opposite results to posterior hypothalamic lesions. Von Economo[222] found that lesions of the anterior hypothalamus in man produced, not somnolence, but insomnia, whereas lesions of the basal forebrain of animals may produce complete and terminal sleeplessness.[155] Bremer[72] showed that stimulation of this area had opposite effects to those of stimulation of the mesencephalic reticular formation, with inhibition of the activating reticular formation in animals and promotion of sleep.[166, 207, 208]

Stimulation experiments on the basal forebrain area have been numerous. The main effect is a short sleep latency, with subsequent involuntary sleep.[72, 162, 210] Stimulation of the basal forebrain, including the basal portion of the diagonal band of Broca, the suprachiasmatic and prechiasmatic areas, produces synchronization of the EEG with behavioural sleep in the unanaesthetized, freely moving cat,[207, 208] as well as entrainment of sleep–wake cycles in rodents. Opposite to the results of electrical stimulation of this area, lesion experiments produce experimental insomnia in animals, and also aphagia, adypsia, thermoregulatory disorders and temporary disturbances of REM sleep.[146, 209] The location of the cell bodies responsible for these behavioural effects is uncertain, and the whole area is very dense in fibre tracts.[156]

The latency to sleep following anterior hypothalamic stimulation is short, sometimes 5–30 s as compared with a minimum of 3 min for electrical thalamic stimulation; and the frequency of stimulation rate necessary to produce sleep is high, not low. High-frequency electrical stimulation in other areas, thalamus or brain stem, always produces arousal, not sleep. However, following high-frequency electrical stimulation to the basal forebrain and low-frequency stimulation to the thalamus, the immediate result is more often pre-sleep behaviour than sleep itself. The alert animal reclines, drops its head on its paws, and closes its eyes before the onset of EEG synchronization and behavioural sleep.[87]

CERVEAU ISOLÉ AND ENCÉPHALE ISOLÉ

Bremer[69] described the results of a midbrain transection just behind the third nerves in the cat (cerveau isolé). This leaves intact sensory input from the optic nerves and olfactory tract, and the motor output to the third nerve and preganglionic nerve cells of the oculomotor nucleus. The remainder of the sensory and motor pathways to the isolated cerebrum is divided. The EEG behaviour and ocular pattern in the cat is that of slow-wave sleep with intense meiosis (perhaps due to central inhibition of the Edinger–Westphal nucleus). However, the picture is more that of coma than of sleep. There is no alteration between sleep and waking, REM sleep is absent, sensory stimulation does not alert the animal, and a monotonous sequence of spindles occurs in the EEG.

In the chronic cerveau isolé preparation with a low section, wakefulness gradually returns. After 7–15 days, spontaneous periods of EEG desynchronization (but not REM sleep) occur, or may be produced by cooling the preparation or by olfactory stimulation.[128, 219]

The coma of the cerveau isolé animal contrasts with the normal sleep–wake cycle seen in low brain stem section at the cervical-medullary junction (encéphale isolé).[70, 71] From these results, Bremer suggested that a slight reversible sensory deafferentation was the cause of physiological sleep – although the cerveau isolé preparation was comatose, not asleep.

> The basic misconception was that coma could be used for the study of physiological sleep; as Sherrington and Magnus had assumed that the mechanisms of normal posture could be studied in the decerebrate animal. The correct conclusion to be drawn from Bremer's experiments is that the sleep–wake cycle is abolished by midbrain transection, and that some impulses arising above the spinal cord but below the midbrain are necessary to maintain the sleep–waking cycle.[162]

However, Bremer's observations are of direct relevance to human pathology, where high spinal injury (corresponding to the encéphale isolé preparation) disturbs sleep little if at all until respiratory paralysis occurs, whilst high brain stem posterior hypothalamic lesions (with some correspondence to the cerveau isolé) can result in a state of akinetic mutism, with prolonged or continuous unresponsiveness, more resembling coma than deep NREM sleep.

BRAIN STEM ACTIVATING SYSTEM

Bremer's fundamental observation that after experimental transection of the mesencephalon the brain lying ahead of the mid-collicular section in the cerveau isolé cat is in a state of coma or sleep was thought to have its basis in the interruption of ascending sensory pathways; and the conclusion from it, that sleep is due to de-afferentation of the cerebrum, was generally accepted.[150] However, Lindsley et al.[144] showed that medial mesencephalic lesions, which interrupted most of the midbrain reticular formation, but spared the classical ascending sensory pathways, resulted in sleep with a synchronized EEG, whereas large lateral lesions, which spared the reticular formation but interrupted the classic specific pathways, did not abolish sleep-waking cycles. This led to the important conclusion that the syndrome of the acute cerveau isolé was due to the interruption of a tonic flow of impulses arising from and coursing along the reticular formation.

The investigation of the reticular formation by Magoun and Moruzzi began with the chance observation that direct electrical stimulation of a portion of the brain stem induced changes in the EEG identical to those in awakening from sleep or in the electrocorticographic arousal reaction, alerting to attention. Arousal is most pronounced against a background of EEG synchrony, and little additional influence is apparent in the already aroused electrocorticogram. The area from which direct stimulation desynchronizes the EEG is distributed throughout most of the length of the brain stem in its central core. Electrical stimulation here, in addition to causing EEG and behavioural arousal, has a widespread influence on the activity of cortical and thalamic neurones, abolishes thalamic recruiting potentials, and has marked effects on cortical evoked potentials, as well as on perception.

There must be cross-connections between the brain stem activating reticular system and a medullary raphe nuclei deactivating system. In addition, there is both anatomic and physiological evidence that many reticular formation neurones project both caudally and rostrally.[75, 149]

Two fundamental systems can be recognized in this area of the brain stem: the first laterally placed ascending somatic and auditory pathways, the second extending from the reticular formation of the lower brain stem through the mesencephalic tegmentum and in the diencephalon, subthalamus and hypothalamus, and ventromedial thalamus to the internal capsule (the rostral continuation of the brain stem ascending reticular activity system was termed the diffuse thalamocortical projection system by Jasper).[120] Interruption of the second system only, which spares ascending sensory components, causes sleep.[161, 162]

Although highly complex, the main anatomical pathways of the reticular activating system and the neurotransmitters involved in these pathways can be visualized as follows. The ascending reticular activating system consists of the bulbar reticular formation, pontine and midbrain tegmentum, and sub- and hypothalamus. Excitatory impulses originating in this brain stem core lead to generalized desynchronization of neocortical activity either via a diffuse thalamic projection system to the entire cerebral cortex, or via an extrathalamic route. The brain stem tonic ascending projection system to the intralaminar nuclei and caudal hypothalamus consists of non-monoaminergic neurones.

These may be involved in cholinergic–cholinoceptive mechanisms.[136] Monoaminergic neurones from the dorsal raphe and locus coeruleus project to the same areas and to the entire cortex.

Anatomically, the name 'reticular formation' is applied to those parts of the lower brain stem which in the myelin stain are characterized by an interlacing network of fibre bundles. Olszewski and Baxter[170] delineated altogether 98 nuclei in the lower brain stem. These are very constant, and have a similar pattern of spatial arrangement in the rabbit, cat, monkey and man. These nuclei include the locus coeruleus, nucleus raphe pallidus and nucleus cuneiformis, possible sleep-related functions of which are considered below. Morphologically, the cytoarchitecture of this brain area shows great variety, with many different cell types, which show striking differences in size, shape, intensity of staining, position of nucleus and arrangement of Nissl substance, all within a few cubic centimetres of volume. The variation in cell type here is greater than in any other part of the central nervous system.

Respiratory, cardiovascular, vegetative and motor responses, as well as arousal responses, can be produced by electrical stimulation of this area. Pharmacologically, there is a great diversity of neurotransmitters: serotonin, mainly in mid-line raphe nuclei;[142] noradrenaline, in very high concentration in the locus coeruleus;[86] acetylcholine at the posterior hypothalamic level, clustering in neurones in the diagonal band of Broca and the nucleus basalis of Meynart, as well as the caudal locus coeruleus;[56] with also peptidergic[145, 211, 216] and dopaminergic[67] components.

The great functional importance of the reticular formation is shown by the effect of lesions of its cephalic parts which in general cause a chronic loss of wakefulness, stupor or coma, with a hypersynchronous EEG not affected by peripheral stimulation in either animals or man.[80, 102, 122, 123, 175, 212] Men, as well as monkeys, with acute lesions of this area, remain throughout survival in a comatose state, with absence of all behaviour associated with wakefulness. However, many of the studies dating from the pre-REM era did not differentiate sleep from coma, did not recognize the great diversity of sleep, or considered the reticular formation as a single functional unit, akin to the 'Organ des Wackens' which Purkinje had postulated[185] since 1846, but had wrongly localized in the cerebrum. The effect of lesions of the reticular formation upon wakefulness was considered, wrongly, to depend purely on their extent, or the rapidity of their evolution.

LOWER BRAIN STEM SLEEP SYSTEMS

The brain stem section just in front of the origin of the trigeminal roots – a few millimetres behind the usual level of postcollicular section – was found by Batini and his colleagues to cause a striking tendency to stay awake.[63, 64] The sleep–wake cycle was not completely abolished by this procedure, but the animal had true insomnia, with clear-cut ocular and EEG signs of alertness for most of the time. These experiments pointed to the presence of an active sleep-inducing structure at a level distal to the lesion, and situated in the lower part of the brain stem. The presence of such a lower brain stem hypnogenic centre was further suggested by lesions in the general area of the tractus solitarius, which lead to permanent wakefulness,[65, 148] whilst stimulation of this area is followed by sleep.[147] However, injection of sodium amylobarbitone into the vertebral artery does not cause any alteration of consciousness in humans, despite the occurrence of EEG desynchronization, whilst, in contrast, the introduction of barbiturates into the carotid artery causes both the abolition of consciousness and EEG slowing.[57, 58] Although there may be some animal evidence for an EEG synchronizing system localized to the caudal part of the brain stem, low focal medullary lesions do not generally prevent sleep in man.

The activity of the vagus nerve and the medullary area of the solitary tract nucleus, where the vagal afferents terminate, may influence sleep, either directly or via changes in a variety of autonomic functions. Thus electrical stimulation of carotid sinus and aortic vagal afferents induces slow-wave sleep, motor inhibition and the appearance of cortical spindles. Eguchi and Satoh[95] showed that cellular groups in the solitary tract nucleus fired during sleep, and Kukorelli and Juhasz[141] reported that intestinal stimulation increased sleep duration. However, these findings are somewhat variable, and the evidence that the carotid sinus plays any important part in sleep control mechanisms in man is uncertain.[184]

The ancients may have considered that the carotid artery was connected with sleep, as the name of the artery is derived from *karos* (heavy sleep) in Greek.[137] There is no definite evidence for this view. Cases quoted by Oswald[173] of subjects who abruptly fall asleep when twisting their neck to right or left while wearing a tight collar, because of distortion of the carotid wall, are perhaps instances of vertebro-basilar rather than carotid ischaemia, or of fainting rather than sleep; and sleep induction by the Balinese with carotid massage may be due more to monotony than carotid sinus stimulation. However, Bates[62] reported the association of narcolepsy–cataplexy with a salivary tumour involving the carotid artery, where the sleep disturbance was cured by surgery; and Møller and Ostenfeld[158] gave a second similar example.

RAPHE NUCLEI

The majority of the serotonin-containing neurones of the brain stem are located in the midline raphe nuclei, two long columns which extend from the upper medulla to the ponto-mesencephalic junction.[127–129] Jouvet considered that this area served as a brain stem deactivating system, in opposition to the brain stem activating reticular system, and was essential for the initiation of NREM sleep.

Jouvet and Renault[132] reported that the destruction of the raphe system of nuclei was followed by 3–4 days' insomnia. The degree of insomnia was dependent on the extent of the lesion. With total destruction, animals usually remained awake and did not sleep, whereas, with partial lesions, stage 3–4 NREM sleep was selectively abolished.[159] Sleep did appear later in these cats, but was strikingly reduced in duration, by as much as 80%. Moreover, sleep with a desynchronized EEG was not restored until the sleep phase characterized by EEG synchronization was well established.

Delorme et al.[92] showed that pharmacological synthesis inhibition of serotonin had a similar effect to raphe nuclei lesions, causing marked insomnia. (p-chlorphenylalanine (PCPA), like p-chlormethamphetamine, suppressed sleep.) The effect of serotonin synthesis inhibition could be reversed by the serotonin precursor 5-HTP. Production of insomnia by PCPA is delayed, not immediate, perhaps owing to initial preservation of endogenous serotonin; and in the doses that have been investigated in man, both PCPA and 5-HTP have little effect on sleep.

Raphe nuclei lesions in man, as in cats, can produce partial or complete insomnia. Freeman et al.[101] described the sleep of a patient with a localized infarct in the pons and mesencephalon. At necropsy, the raphe nuclei of the lower mesencephalon were damaged, but the laterally placed locus coeruleus was spared. In this patient, REM sleep was preserved, although the ability to look to the left, and REMs to the left during REM sleep, were abolished. NREM sleep was reduced. More severe bilateral midline raphe nuclei damage has been proposed with total insomnia in the subject with chorée fibrillaire de Morvan described on p. 243,[98] although at necropsy no specific or focal neuropathological lesion was discovered. The patient, a 27-year-old man, had a possible viral encephalitis and went four months without sleep. In spite of total lack of sleep, he never felt tired or sleepy, and had no memory or intellectual problem apart from dramatic hallucinatory experiences which occurred between 2100 and 2300 each day. High doses (2–12 g daily) of dl-5-HTP may have gradually restored some stage 3–4 NREM sleep, which occurred 50 min after drug administration. However, this effect was gradually lost and the patient died four months after the onset of his illness. (The nature of Morvan's fibrillary chorea is discussed on p. 243.)

Although brain stem lesions frequently cause insomnia, and may result in damage to raphe nuclei, insomnia cannot usually be attributed to specific damage to serotonin neurones. Animals with central tegmental tract lesions are insomniac, but do not show any evidence of serotonin depletion in forebrain or spinal cord regions.[125]

Neurones of the dorsal raphe nuclei appear to play an important role in the regulation of phasic events in REM sleep. Electrical stimulation of raphe nuclei causes suppression of PGO waves (see below) during REM sleep, and the spontaneous electrical activity of dorsal raphe neurones in the nucleus raphe pallidus shows an inverse relationship with PGO waves.[116] Simon et al.[204] demonstrated that midline lesions in the region of the raphe nuclei caused a transient increase in PGO-like waves which, unusually, occurred in both wakefulness and slow-wave, as well as during REM sleep. p-Chlorphenylalanine has a similar effect. Dement was the first to show that cats given PCPA had continuous PGO waves both in wakefulness and during slow-wave sleep. The appearance of these waves is blocked by 5-HTP.[94] According to these findings, the release of PGO waves into wakefulness by raphe lesions or PCPA is due to the removal of a tonic inhibitory influence on a PGO pacemaker mechanism from the raphe neurones. One function of the midline raphe system would thus be to confine PGO spikes to REM sleep.

PGO WAVES

Amongst the first signs of paradoxical sleep in the cat that can be recognized are large phasic potentials in the pons.[127, 128, 130] These can be recorded several minutes before the onset of cortical desynchronization. These pontine spikes are conducted rapidly to the lateral geniculate body, and from there to the occipital cortex – hence the terminology PGO waves (pons–geniculate body–occipital cortex). The occurrence of PGO spikes usually precedes or coincides with a burst of REM sleep, and the local discharge suddenly comes to an end when the paradoxical sleep episode is over (see also p. 16).

PGO spikes occur singly in the transition from NREM to REM sleep, and then in grouped bursts of three to six discharges.[160] In the cat, the PGO spike is a 150–200 µV biphasic wave of approximately 100–180 ms duration. A possible human analogue has been observed (see p. 79). Wilson and Nashold[226] recorded similar activity at the level of the dorsal pontine tegmentum, and Salzarulo et al.[198] over the occipital cortex. Pivik and Dement[179] suggested that the human K complex may be a cortical manifestation of PGO spikes, since phasic suppression of EMG and reflex activity are associated with pre-REM sleep K complexes as well as with PGO waves.

PGO spike generation is under the control of cell groups in the pons. Groups of neurones located in the caudal mesencephalic and rostral pontine tegmental area in the cat discharge in bursts of three to five trains of spikes lasting about 20 ms before the onset of PGO waves in the lateral geniculate nucleus. These executive neurones have been called PGO 'burst' or PGO 'on' neurones by Sakai and Jouvet.[196] Although initially the pontine pacemaker of REM sleep was considered to lie in the nucleus reticularis pontis oralis,[82] PS 'on' neurones are found in both the pons and the medulla.

Nelson et al.[167] have shown recently that PGO waves appear almost simultaneously in both lateral geniculate bodies in cats, but in each case one has a larger amplitude and precedes the other. During REM sleep, the larger primary wave is ipsilateral to the direction of rapid eye movements.

During REM sleep PGO 'on' cells fire in discrete bursts at fixed latencies before ipsilateral primary waves but almost never when the primary waves are contralateral. In wakefulness, PGO 'on' cells fire single spikes, not bursts. There is some anatomical evidence that these cells may project to the lateral geniculate body, the pulvinar-lateral posterior complex, or to the intralaminar nuclei; but do not project directly to the cerebral cortex. The diverse distribution of cortical PGO waves is accounted for by ascending projection systems arising from the lateral geniculate nucleus, pulvinar and the nucleus centralis lateralis.

PGO 'on' neurones do not contain monoamines – serotonin or noradrenaline (norepinephrine) – but contain high amounts of acetylcholinesterase.[195] Immunohistochemistry indicates that these same neurones may contain choline acetyltransferase.[136]

The brain structures involved in the ascending PGO activation system are directly innervated by noradrenaline-containing neurones of the locus coeruleus complex and by 5-HT-containing neurones of the dorsal raphe. Electrophysiological data shows that these neurones reduce or stop firing during paradoxical sleep.[196] As previously discussed, raphe neurone lesions result in the immediate appearance of PGO waves, and 5-HT synthesis inhibition by PCPA leads to the production of PGO waves outside paradoxical sleep. Neurones of the ventromedial medulla, in locus coeruleus and raphe nuclei, have therefore been considered as PGO 'off' neurones.[197]

PGO spikes can be elicited in several ways. In different species, PGO spikes can be produced by noise,[135] electrical stimulation of the mesencephalic reticular formation,[205] local injection of carbechol into the dorsal pontine tegmentum,[157] reserpinization[220] or REM deprivation.[117, 192]

PGO spikes (and REMs) are abolished by vestibular nuclei lesions when the medial descending vestibular nuclei of the cat are destroyed in their entire rostrocaudal extent; but not by de-afferentation of the vestibule, nor by cerebellectomy, nor by lesions of the superior and lateral vestibular nuclei. These facts, and electrophysiological studies on the lateral geniculate body, show that during REM sleep, PGO 'on' neurones trigger the medial and descending vestibular nuclei.[160, 180]

The PGO spikes of REM sleep are temporally related to eye movements, and appear to represent a non-retinal input to the visual system from the brain stem.[68] PGO waves also appear in the same regions when the awake cat moves its eyes.[76, 81, 121] The waves that occur in the two states, REM sleep and waking, are similar, but the PGO waves of REM sleep have several characteristics not shared by the waves of wakefulness.[77]

In the cat, PGO waves released into wakefulness by 5-HT synthesis inhibition are accompanied by random myoclonic twitching. Is any form of waking myoclonus in man the result of a comparable phenomenon? This may be the case in those examples of 5-HTP responsive myoclonus, and in which cerebrospinal fluid (CSF) 5-hydroxyindoleacetic acid (5-HIAA) levels are low,[84, 154] although sleep studies have not been reported in these patients.

The function of the PGO executive system is unknown. It must be remembered that most of the data on PGO waves derive from the cat, a sleepy animal in which PGO waves are frequent and prominent. PGO waves first occur tens of seconds before the onset of EEG desynchronization and atonia. PGO waves fire to the occipital cortex but also to the temporal and parietal cortices, corresponding to visual, auditory and association areas respectively. It is not known whether PGO waves occur in either the motor or somatosensory cortex.

1. The REMs themselves are likely to be epiphenomena. The need to generate random eye movement during sleep is not obvious, although reptiles such as the chameleon continue to scan the environment even when they are otherwise inactive. The idea that REMs, which resemble saccadic eye movements in wakefulness, result from, or are associated with, scene scanning in dreams is unlikely, for this would involve pursuit more than saccadic eye movement. Saccadic eye movements during wakefulness are generated by the frontal cortex and vision is suppressed during eye movement. The burst cells which generate PGO waves in sleep may be contiguous with or similar to those which generate saccadic eye movements in wakefulness. In pontine damage due to spinocerebellar degeneration, both REMs and saccadic eye movements are defective.[172]

2. The idea that PGO spikes represent endogenous activation of sensory analysers, and that high-density bursts may account for hypnagogic hallucinations, has often been suggested.[156] Cohen et al.[88] observed bizarre behaviour in the cat in conjunction with, and possibly as a response to, PGO spikes transferred from sleep to wakefulness by p-chlorphenylalanine, and referred to such behaviour in the cat as 'hallucinatory'.[94]

3. It has been suggested that PGO spikes are inhibitory to descending motor function and account for muscle atonia. However, there is no evidence that REM sleep atonia is causally associated with trains of PGO spikes.

4. Crick and Mitchison[89] have suggested that the random electrical bangs of PGO waves may improve cortical function, abolish unwanted memories but reinforce other mental processes. Unfortunately for this idea, REMs (and probably PGO waves) are lost in several chronic human diseases which destroy pontomesencephalic areas, although behaviour and memory may be entirely normal in some of these conditions (see the section on brain stem lesions and disturbances of sleep in man below).

5. The occurrence of random electrical discharges during REM sleep may be a partial explanation for sleep atonia, de-efferentation of the motor system preventing limb jerking. Alternatively, motor atonia during sleep may be a means of energy conservation.

LOCUS COERULEUS

The nucleus coeruleus of man is a large, darkly coloured region in the dorsolateral portion of the rostral mesencephalic and caudal mesencephalic tegmentum, shown in 1809 by Reil to contain a blue-black substance. The nucleus has been considered to be related to the trigeminal complex and thus a part of the somasthetic mechanism for the head; to be a portion of the mechanism of visceral sensibility; and to be a part of the regulatory mechanism for respiration. Russell concluded that the nucleus served an important relay function in the cortical and subcortical facilitation of central nervous control over general body vegetative function.

In initial studies of paradoxical sleep, neurones located within the pontine tegmentum were found to be crucial for the generation of REM sleep.[82, 127, 162] Subsequently, noradrenaline-containing locus coeruleus neurones within the pons were considered as the key elements for the organization of both tonic and phasic REM sleep components including desynchronization of the EEG, hippocampal theta waves, PGO waves, REMs, twitches of the limb and face, and postural atonia.[78, 130, 190, 191, 200] In particular, the middle third of the locus coeruleus was considered to be involved in triggering phasic events and EEG desynchronization during REM sleep. However, more recent experience indicates that the major involvement of locus coeruleus neurones in sleep control lies in the control of sleep atonia.

Electrical stimulation of the locus coeruleus area always induces wakefulness, not any significant increase in NREM or REM sleep,[100] whilst bilateral, electrolytic lesions of the dorsal noradrenergic bundle that ascends from the dorsal part of the locus coeruleus are followed by minor increases in both slow-wave sleep and paradoxical sleep.[177, 178] Cooling of the anterodorsal area around the locus coeruleus is immediately followed by slow-wave sleep and paradoxical sleep.[83] However, the main result of a 6-hydroxydopamine lesion, which selectively destroys catecholamine neurones of the ascending bundle from the locus coeruleus to the cerebral cortex, is to impair electrocortical, not behavioural, aspects of waking.[143]

In the last decade, studies of extensive lesions of the locus coeruleus nucleus and overlapping dorsolateral pontine tegmentum have not corroborated some of the earlier reported findings that destruction of this nucleus and region eliminates REM sleep.[126] Most locus coeruleus lesions which destroy paradoxical sleep also extend ventrally and medially into the tegmentum. Jones[124] demonstrated that it was lesions of the neighbouring gigantocellular and magnocellular tegmental field,[66] not lesions of the locus coeruleus, that abolish REM sleep.

Jones[124] showed that bilateral gigantocellular tegmental field lesions in the cat resulted in the complete elimination of paradoxical sleep. The phasic components, PGO waves and rapid eye movements did not occur in association with an activated EEG, as they do normally in paradoxical sleep, and the characteristic tonic muscular atonia was absent. Neural mechanisms in the pontine gigantocellular tegmental field thus appear to be critical for paradoxical sleep. These systems function during wakefulness in the coordination of eye, head and body movements.

The main effect of destruction of ventral areas around the locus coeruleus is the irreversible loss of normal REM sleep atonia (see below).[194] REM sleep atonia, but not other aspects of REM sleep, is abolished by bilateral lesions of the caudal third of the locus coeruleus.[131] Lesions of the pontine gigantocellular tegmental field have a similar result, perhaps due to interruption of a common central tegmental tract at two different levels, but in addition cause the loss of other aspects of REM sleep.

During REM sleep without atonia in cats, the animals may exhibit brief complex motor sequences resembling attacking, locomotion and orienting in the normal animal. REM sleep without atonia is produced by lesions of the rostal pontine tegmentum alone, but the additional release of these elaborate behavioural sequences, accompanied by phenomena of REM sleep, requires wider lesions.[109]

Loss of REM sleep atonia, similar to that resulting from localized locus coeruleus lesions in animals, but with preservation of other aspects of REM sleep, is occasionally reported as a result of brain stem lesions in man. Barros-Ferreira et al.[61] described an 8-year-old child with an infiltrating brain stem glioma. The child had no gross alteration in consciousness, and overall had normal sleep patterns. However, REM sleep was disorganized with, in particular, loss of normal muscle atonia. There was no relationship between the amount of rapid eye movements during sleep, and the absence, presence or intensity of axial muscle tone. The child reported having normal dreams. Based on a comparison with animal findings, the child was considered to have selective bilateral involvement of the caudal third of the locus coeruleus, although this was not demonstrated anatomically.

Pharmacological studies using catecholamine synthesis inhibitors and the catecholamine neurotoxin 6-hydroxydopamine have not supported the idea that noradrenaline neurones are involved, except perhaps in an inhibitory capacity in REM sleep mechanisms, and although monoamine neurones may modulate the sleep–waking cycle, they are probably not essential for sleep or wakefulness.[118, 124] Interruption of the central tegmental tracts, whilst interfering with sleep, does not affect noradrenaline levels in other areas. Non-monoamine neurones in the central magno- and gigantocellular tegmental field are important for a normal sleep cycle, and particularly for the state of paradoxical sleep.

SLEEP ATONIA

Motor inhibition is one of the most characteristic features of sleep. At sleep onset, voluntary muscle atonia commences in the eyelids, then the neck, and spreads in severity and extent until, during REM sleep, only the diaphragm is spared. Even patients who are severely spastic or rigid whilst awake become atonic when sleeping.[201] Atonia during REM sleep depends upon tonic excitation of a supraspinal inhibitory system which induces tonic post-synaptic inhibition of extensor and flexor spinal motor neurones. Sleep atonia depends on the activity of at least two brain stem areas: (1) pontine regions around the locus coeruleus, and (2) the medullary oblongata inhibitory area of Magoun and Rhines,[151] the nucleus reticularis magnocellularis.

There is considerable evidence for the existence of a cortico-bulbar-spinal motor inhibitory pathway which is tonically active during REM sleep, resulting in the inhibition of spinal motor neurones[181], with alteration in fusimotor activity and function.[104, 140] At a cortical level, stimulation of the orbital cortex with strychnine in the cat causes motor inhibition, and may precipitate a REM sleep-like state from wakefulness.[112] Orbital cortex and forebrain areas input into a motor inhibitory area of the pontine gigantocellular tegmental field.[85, 206]

Magoun and Rhines[151] showed that electrical stimulation of the rostral medullary reticular formation caused a strong inhibition of motor reflexes. These inhibitory influences appear to be due to inhibitory post-synaptic potentials in spinal motor neurones.[199] At the reticular formation level, there is input into the descending motor inhibitory pathway from the locus coeruleus. Lesions of the locus coeruleus cause, not paralysis and atonia characteristic of REM sleep, but *loss of motor inhibition* during REM sleep.[110, 111, 131] The motor inhibitory pathway descends from the medulla in the ventrolateral portion of the spinal cord, according to Jankowska *et al.*[119]

The neurotransmitters involved in the descending corticospinal motor inhibitory pathway are of more than academic interest, since this is the likely pathway for the motor inhibition of cataplexy, of drop attacks and atonic episodes, as well as of REM sleep. Carbachol injection into the region of the locus coeruleus or subcoeruleus induces a state very similar to cataplexy, but accompanied by PGO activity, nystagmus, salivation and panting in animals,[157, 203, 217] whilst muscarinic stimulation of the pontine reticular caudal and oral nuclei causes marked atonia and REM sleep-like characteristics, even in an alert animal.[105] This picture can be reversed by anticholinergic drugs, and these findings suggest that some portion of the pathway is cholinergic or cholinoceptive. Many of the drugs effective in cataplexy are predominantly anticholinergic or have anticholinergic effects (e.g. atropine in dogs,[91] tricyclics in man[79] – although anticholinergics are not very effective in human cataplexy; Guilleminault *et al.*[108] found that 0.5–4 mg atropine i.v. did not abolish status cataplecticus, and Thompson *et al.*[213] likewise found orphenadrine 300 mg daily had no anticataplectic effect). Tricyclic antidepressants such as imipramine, amitriptyline and clomipramine, which improve both human and canine cataplexy,[93, 99] in addition to their anticholinergic effects, block the re-uptake of serotonin and the catecholamines. This observation may indicate that the descending inhibitory motor pathway of sleep uses monoaminergic as well as cholinergic mechanisms. Also, all these drugs suppress other aspects of REM sleep.[182]

These findings are corroborated by histochemical findings in the cat. Atonia executive neurones do not seem to be monoaminergic. Kimura *et al.*[136] reported the presence of cholinergic–cholinoceptive neurones in those areas around the locus coeruleus and in magnocellular areas where carbachol or physostigmine injection will produce atonia. However, there are direct descending projections to the spinal cord from noradrenaline-containing locus coeruleus complex neurones as well as from 5-HT-containing neurones in the nucleus raphe dorsalis, magnus and pallidus. Sakai *et al.*[197] showed that these neurones ceased firing during REM sleep and, unless they have a defacilitatory effect, may not contribute to the generation of sleep atonia.

BRAIN STEM LESIONS AND DISTURBANCES OF SLEEP AND WAKEFULNESS IN MAN

Dorsal pontine tegmental lesions in man involve or destroy the reticular formation and result in loss of consciousness. In contrast, consciousness is preserved in *ventral pontine lesions* which do not involve the reticular formation. All recorded examples of dorsal pontine tegmental lesions which have resulted in complete loss of wakefulness in man have been bilateral (and most have involved ventral as well as dorsal pontine areas). Small unilateral lesions of the dorsal pontine tegmentum do not cause coma, although there may be minor alterations in sleep patterns. With ventral pontine lesions, although these are not usually well circumscribed, the ascending reticular activating system, if not its connections, is usually spared. Thus, consciousness may be preserved, although sleep is rarely entirely normal.

The effect of brain stem lesions in man upon sleep and wakefulness depends upon the exact areas of the reticular activating system involved, as well as the presence or absence of damage to REM sleep-generating mechanisms.

The exact localization and extent of the brain stem ascending reticular activating system in man is ill-defined, but there is clear evidence that the midbrain and pontine tegmental areas which are ventral to the ventricular system extending from the posterior hypothalamic area rostral to the lower third of the pontine tegmentum are critical to wakefulness in man.

The rostral continuation of the brain stem ascending reticular activating system (termed the diffuse thalamocortical projection system by Jasper[120]) extends to the subthalamus, hypothalamus and ventromedial thalamus to the internal capsule.

The caudal extent of structures critical to arousal may not be much lower than the level of trigeminal nerve entry in either man or animals. In animals, low areas of the reticular formation are not essential to sustained arousal. In cats, Jouvet reported that animals with brain stem transections at levels just rostral to the pontine-medullary junction had an alert appearance, and Batini et al.[64] (see p. 91) reported that animals with brain stem transections at midpontine levels appeared to be alert.

VENTRAL PONTINE LESIONS AND THE LOCKED-IN SYNDROME

In the ventral pontine, de-efferented, locked-in syndrome of Noiter de Villefort (a character in Dumas' *The Count of Monte Cristo*), sleep may be abnormal, although, in contrast to the coma of akinetic mutism, consciousness is largely preserved.[241, 269] In the locked-in syndrome, the usual pathological lesion is in the ventral pons, resulting in quadriplegia and anarthria,[255] but not any major sleep disturbance. However, the lesion is often very near to structures considered on the basis of animal experiments to be vital for sleep regulation. These patients may thus have sleep–wake cycles, but these, and sleep itself, are not normal, and in extreme cases sleep may be abolished.

The usual sleep pattern with ventral pontine lesions in man is one of hyposomnia with preserved sleep–wake cycles, despite chronic de-efferentation. The amount of slow-wave sleep is often reduced, and, when this falls below a certain critical level, REM sleep is abolished.[237, 261] The alternative picture, loss of NREM sleep without disturbance of REM sleep, does not occur, or is very uncommon.

PONTINE TEGMENTUM LESIONS

One single patient with an assumed pontine tegmental lesion but a highly atypical sleep pattern, a gross excess of REM sleep, but loss of NREM sleep, has been described. Hobson[246, 247] reported a 54-year-old man with signs of a brain stem lesion due to neuronal loss and demyelination, particularly of the pontine tegmental areas. His condition was reminiscent of narcolepsy, with frequent nocturnal arousals and daytime sleep attacks, with episodic lid-fluttering and eye closure, upward turning of the eyes, rapid eye movements and myoclonic twitching of all limbs lasting 1–2 min, followed by hallucinosis. There was no loss of postural muscle tone during these episodes, otherwise likened to REM sleep. In a sleep record, night sleep was found to consist almost entirely of REM sleep (although EMG tone was preserved) with virtually no NREM sleep.

Much more typically, localized pontine tegmental lesions in man reduce or abolish REM sleep.[236, 237, 240] Allowing for variability in anatomic extent of the lesion, speed and nature of the pathological insult, and variation in the period between brain stem damage and sleep recording, a fairly consistent picture emerges of the acute effects of brain stem tegmental lesions on sleep.[274] These lesions cause three major changes; reduction in total sleep time, alteration in NREM sleep, and reduction or abolition of REM sleep.

All sleep may be lost, or total sleep time severely truncated, in patients with sudden pontine infarction, traumatic basilar artery occlusion, with autopsy-verified lesions of the pontine and mesencephalic raphe nuclei.[240, 242, 276] Markand and Dyken[261] reported on seven patients with widespread bilateral pontine lesions causing a locked-in syndrome, tetraplegia, facial and pseudobulbar paralysis, and absence of conjugate horizontal gaze. In five patients, NREM sleep was reduced, absent or altered, with reduced vertex sharp waves and reduced sleep spindles during light NREM sleep; and REM sleep was entirely absent. The remaining two patients had less extensive lesions, little or no pontine tegmental involvement, and preservation of REM as well as NREM sleep. A decrease in total sleep time was the major abnormality in a patient in whom the clinical findings suggested brain stem involvement, and in whom a high CSF 5-HIAA level and clinical response to 5-HTP was assumed to be evidence for a lesion of the raphe system, described by Guilleminault *et al*.[245]

Decrease in REM sleep[263] or a condition resembling narcolepsy–cataplexy[228, 271] with pontine lesions has been linked to possible damage to the locus coeruleus, but the pathological localization of the lesion has rarely been exact. Damage to the locus coeruleus also occurs in idiopathic parkinsonism. Here REM sleep time is approximately halved in the late disease, although loss of the normal REM sleep atonia has not been described. A form of parkinsonism without damage to the locus coeruleus is known, due to toxic nigrostriatal damage,[234] but sleep patterns in this variety of parkinsonism have not yet been reported.

The reported absence of REM sleep in a group of patients with horizontal gaze paralysis due to pontine lesions may perhaps be due to difficulty in the recognition of this sleep phase. However, eye movements in REM sleep are as commonly vertical or oblique as horizontal,[250] and, although REMs during sleep are absent in some patients with gaze palsies, these subjects do have periodic low-voltage fast patterns during sleep which are characteristic of REM sleep episodes.[229]

The most obvious fact to emerge from the study of sleep in different brain stem diseases involving the pontine tegmentum is that despite a diversity of pathological processes the results are nearly identical. The occurrence of REM sleep is dependent on the degree of reduction of NREM sleep. It is unusual for the separate components of REM sleep (dreams, eye movements, a desynchronized EEG and sleep atonia) to be separated in man, although a desynchronized EEG without REMs has been described in Huntington's chorea.[272] Dreaming is occasionally preserved without other evidence of REM sleep,[233] and absence of REM sleep atonia, but with preservation of a desynchronized EEG with eye movements, has been reported.[230] In many of the degenerative and heredo-familial brain stem disorders that have been studied, changes in sleep are almost identical to those resulting from vascular lesions of the tegmental tracts of the pons.

The clearest documentation so far available of an exactly localized brain stem lesion with near total loss of REM sleep was given by Lavie et al.[258] in a 33-year-old lawyer who sustained a shrapnel injury at the age of 20. NREM sleep each night was short (an average of a little over 4 h), but NREM sleep structure was normal. In contrast, on three recording nights, there was no REM sleep, and on five other nights a total of less than 15 min REM sleep. Whenever REM sleep occurred, it appeared to be normal. Neurological abnormalities included signs of cerebellar as well as brain stem damage. The patient had bilateral abducens palsy, double elevator palsy in the right eye, opsoclonus, right central facial palsy, mild right hemiparesis with hyper-reflexia, severe cerebellar ataxia of the right limbs, dystonic postures of the right arm, and right hemisensory loss to pain, touch, vibration and position sense. Because of the ataxia, he could not stand or walk. The CT scan, and brain stem auditory evoked response studies, as well as the neurological examination, indicated a midpontine lesion with possible midbrain extension. There was also a small shrapnel fragment deep in the left cerebellar hemisphere. Despite almost complete absence of REM sleep, and a mild degree of hyposomnia, the patient had a relatively normal life.

RAMSAY HUNT SYNDROME

In a 13-year-old schoolgirl with the condition described by Hunt as dyssynergia cerebellaris myoclonica (generalized myoclonus, ataxia and tonic–clonic seizures), a highly unusual EEG pattern was reported by Bergamesco et al.[233] Waking, the EEG showed many multiple spike and wave bursts, which increased during drowsiness and stage 1–2 NREM sleep, but disappeared in stage 4 NREM sleep. During sleep, there was complete absence of REM activity, although the girl said that she dreamt every night, and had normal mental and psychic development. The authors considered that, .in this instance, spike and wave activity and myoclonic jerking was in some way related to REM sleep loss.

Pathology was not reported here, but one of the three original patients described by Hunt died 13 years after the onset of illness, and was found to have lesions within the pons, as well as widespread throughout the brain (this may have been an example of Wilson's disease).[249] Comparable clinical findings were reported in four further patients with dyssynergia cerebellaris myoclonica by Benassi et al.[232] but sleep staging is difficult in the Ramsay Hunt syndrome, and REM sleep loss is not always confirmed. Generalized clonic attacks lasting dozens of minutes sometimes occur on awakening from NREM sleep, and are accompanied by severe confusion.

SPINOCEREBELLAR DEGENERATION

Osorio and Daroff[265] and Yokoyama et al.[277] described the sleep of patients with spinocerebellar degeneration. Two subjects reported by Osorio and Daroff had the characteristic oculomotor disorder of this condition, slow saccadic but preserved pursuit eye movements, which is usually attributed to a lesion in the paramedian pontine reticular formation.[278] For seven recording nights, neither patient had any REM sleep. All aspects of REM sleep were lacking; there were no eye movements, no EEG desynchronization, no EEG atonia, no characteristic respiratory or heart rate changes, and no dream reports. Furthermore, REM sleep could not be provoked in either subject by 40 h of sleep deprivation. REM sleep loss was associated with a marked diminution of stage 3–4 NREM sleep. Osorio and Daroff[265] considered that the absence of REM sleep was due to a lesion of REM generating neurones, sited in the medial portion of the mid and low pons, whilst the absence of stage 3–4 NREM sleep was perhaps explained by a pontine raphe lesion. However, the most important suggestion was that saccadic eye movements and certain stages of sleep share the same neural circuitry.

Subjects with slow saccades characteristically have intact horizontal pursuit and intact vestibulo-ocular reflex eye movement, both of which require the integrity of specific neurones within the paramedian pontine reticular formation. Only isolated dysfunction of a specific pontine neuronal system, the 'burst' or 'pause' cell, can produce slow saccades with intact pursuit and vestibular-stimulated eye movements, as is the case in spinocerebellar degeneration.[279] Because of the combination of absent saccades and absent REM sleep, Osorio and Daroff[265] considered that 'burst' cells – or their driving neurones – could play an important role in the generation of REM sleep. (Despite loss of this system, PGO wave-like activity has been reported in the waking EEG of patients with spinocerebellar degeneration.[277]) However, in another condition characterized by the presence of slow saccades, Huntington's chorea, Starr[272] alluded to the presence of typical REM sleep, but with the exception of rapid eye movements.

No pontine lesion has been clearly documented in spinocerebellar degeneration.[270, 275] An extrapontine lesion, perhaps in the cerebellum, upper brain stem, thalamus or basal ganglia, may therefore account for sleep loss, although the saccadic REM abnormality is best attributed to a pontine lesion.

One important finding of the study of Osorio and Daroff lies not in the anatomical but in the behavioural sphere. These two REM-deprived patients were not demented, and their behaviour was entirely appropriate. Neither was psychotic, despite a loss of REM sleep for at least 11 years, the period during which symptoms had progressed.

OLIVOPONTOCEREBELLAR DEGENERATION

The special interest of olivopontocerebellar degeneration (OPCD) to sleep physiologists lies in the selective damage to brain stem structures derived from a single embryonic line, the cell bands of Essick, which gives rise to many pontine tegmental structures vital to sleep control, the locus coeruleus, the pontine lateral reticular nuclei and the gigantocellular tegmental field.[252] In addition, damage to the inferior olivary nuclei may indirectly affect REM–NREM sleep by interfering with the reception of afferent fibres from the central tegmental tract, and with transmission via efferent fibres through the inferior cerebellar peduncle to the vestibular nuclei. The middle cerebellar peduncles and the cerebellar cortex are involved in OPCD,[238, 256] but since cerebellar lesions by themselves do not greatly affect sleep (only motor control during sleep) OPCD provides a unique opportunity to study sleep mechanisms of pontine nuclei in humans.

Sleep in humans with the clinical diagnosis of OPCD is very similar to that of animals with lesions of the pontine tegmentum and locus coeruleus,[248, 253] and to patients with spinocerebellar degeneration.[254] Neil et al.[264] found in two patients with OPCD that the waking EEG was normal, but the sleep EEG was not: both delta and REM sleep were reduced. Even at a very early stage of the disease, there was a marked impairment of rapid eye movements during REM sleep, out of proportion to the loss of tonic components of REM sleep. The REM percent of total sleep time and the number of REM periods during a night's sleep were reduced, although REM cycles were prolonged and REM latency was normal. These REM abnormalities were accompanied by decreased or absent stage 3–4 NREM sleep, and sometimes by frequent awakenings and large spindles in light NREM sleep.

PROGRESSIVE SUPRANUCLEAR PALSY

Progressive supranuclear palsy (PSNP), like OPCD, affects brain stem structures important for human sleep, with degeneration of nuclei within the pontine and mesencephalic tegmentum. The locus coeruleus is almost invariably damaged, together with damage to the central grey core of the pons and mesencephalon, including areas occupied by raphe nuclei.[231, 273] The disease also damages other areas, but the cerebral cortex, white matter and thalamus are largely spared.

The constellation of sleep abnormalities in PSNP is very similar to that of vascular ventral tegmental lesions and also of OPCD. Patients with PSNP tend to have a late onset of sleep and wake early, with many spontaneous arousals throughout the night. This lack of sleep at night is not compensated for by day. At night, NREM sleep is very disorganized and REM sleep is absent or markedly reduced.[244, 257, 259, 266]

Observations on sleep in PSNP have shown occasionally that there is a dissociation between the electrographic and the behavioural manifestations of sleep. In PSNP, as much as half the time of behavioural sleep may be accompanied by the EEG pattern of partial wakefulness, and activity in the alpha frequency range may persist throughout sleep, intermixed with sleep spindles of 12–15 Hz.[244] This pattern is not specific for PSNP, however, and is probably due to poor, light sleep, with immobility and discomfort.

Idiopathic Parkinson's disease has common features with PSNP, severe damage to the locus coeruleus and motor retardation occurring in both disorders. Sleep changes are similar, although usually not as extensive in Parkinson's disease as in PNSP.[263] The late stage of PSNP may be accompanied by mental deterioration with, in particular, marked forgetfulness.[227, 262] The level of memory disturbance, however, is not closely related to the degree of impairment of REM sleep.[267]

AKINETIC MUTISM

Akinetic mutism, prolonged or continuous hypersomnia or coma, although with half-open eyes, usually results from a long-standing posterior hypothalamic–high brain stem lesion. The condition is usually considered to be one of coma, not of sleep, and the patient can not be aroused. However, self-sustained variations in behaviour and EEG pattern occur. The EEG sometimes corresponds closely to that of deep NREM sleep, although clear NREM–REM cycles are absent, and REM mechanisms may be damaged or disconnected. Despite the loss of both REM sleep and arousal mechanisms, the state of akinetic mutism has some similarity to deep NREM sleep. Certainly NREM sleep may be very deep, and arousal almost impossible in children who wake from delta sleep at night with night terrors or somnambulism, and it can be very difficult to arouse hypersomniacs with obstructive sleep apnoea. It should be remembered that deep NREM sleep with spontaneous arousal is contiguous with hibernation in some animals.

The condition of akinetic mutism resembles very closely animal behaviour in the recovering cerveau isolé preparation, although following eye movements may be partially preserved in humans. Patients with chronic high brain stem lesions may exist in a sleepy, stuporose or comatose state for months. The main varieties of loss of consciousness found by Cairns[235] with high brain stem and thalamic lesions were akinetic mutism, hypersomnia, and coma with tonic fits or decerebrate rigidity. These forms are interchangeable; for example, a patient with hypersomnia may progress to deep coma and decerebrate rigidity before death. Cairns found some change of awareness in 37 of 73 verified tumours of this region, hypersomnia or coma mainly being due to local lesions around the posterior walls of the third ventricle, not to raised intracranial pressure. In contrast to posterior lesions, colloid cysts, lesions of the upper and anterior part of the third ventricle rarely disturb consciousness except as a terminal event.

In akinetic mutism, EEG records generally show large irregular delta waves, interspersed with slightly faster sinusoidal and regular waves. As with the clinical state, the EEG does not greatly alter, despite strong sensory stimuli.

The seven sleepers of Ephesus, the Cretan poet Epemenides[239] who allegedly slept for 57 years in a cave, and the 78-year-old Italian village saint, Alfonso Cottini (*Sunday Times*, 8 November 1980, p. 9), may all have had posterior hypothalamic–high brain stem lesions, although the true state of awareness of some long sleepers, such as Victorine Doirat, described below, is doubtful.

> On January 31, 1897, the gates of Rochefort Hospital admitted a sleeper by the name of Victorine Doirat. She was carefully watched, and shamming was put out of the question. During a month, she was plunged more or less in sleep, remaining in a cataleptic condition for five consecutive days without eating or drinking or satisfying any of the wants of nature. The day on which she was taken to hospital, she had an attack of somnambulism, and she frightened her neighbours by going to them like an automaton with shut eyes. The morning after her admission, the chef de service going on his rounds found her asleep. By means of stimulants and suggestions, she was awakened and induced to take some soup and drink some milk. An hour afterwards, she fell into a sleep. The condition continued, interrupted by intervals of waking, which were very variable. Sometimes they occurred several times a day, at others after two or three days of sleep. She opened her eyes and asked for food; if not immediately satisfied, she fell asleep. In order to oblige her to take nourishment, she was awakened by stimulating the median and ulnar nerves, but her eyes closed again almost as soon as they opened. At 20 years of age, her excited condition obliged her family to put her in an asylum. At 28, she married a deaf and dumb man. Her appearance was healthy. The eyelids constantly trembled, the body was rigid, and the limbs remained for several hours in the position in which they were placed.
> (*Lancet*, 8 May, 1897)

Some other cases of trance or prolonged sleep that have been described illustrate the borderland between coma, akinetic mutism and deep sleep.

Pette[268] recorded the case of a man who lay for three months, from the onset of his illness to his death, in a state which resembled in a remarkable manner the lethargic condition seen in encephalitis lethargica. After death, an area of softening was found in the tegmentum between the substantia nigra and the aqueduct. This observation led Pette to conclude that the sleep centre itself lay in the grey matter in the floor of the third ventricle.

A year later, Lucksch[260] described a case of infective endocarditis in a man who slept almost continuously before his death. An embolic abscess was found in the caudal part of the third ventricle, and in the wall and surrounding parts of the beginning of the aqueduct.

Cairns[235] described an akinetic mute 14-year-old girl with a third ventricular epidermoid cyst. She lay inert, except that her eyes followed the direction of objects or could be diverted by sound. Swallowing movements and limb reflex withdrawal were preserved. The girl's third ventricular cyst was aspirated on several occasions. The first time the cyst was tapped, the child immediately aroused, and within 10 min could give her name, age and address correctly. Subsequent recovery, following further taps, was not, however, so prompt.

CONCLUSIONS FROM ANATOMICAL STUDIES

Studies in man indicate that the integrity of much of the brain stem, as well as the cerebral cortex, is necessary for normal sleep patterns, whilst neurones of the paramedian and dorsolateral pons are necessary for the generation of REM sleep. The sleep–wake rhythm itself seems likely to arise in the whole brain, the cerebrum as well as the brain stem, as shown by the recovery from coma in humans with high brain stem lesions, as well as in animals with a cerveau isolé preparation. However, it must be admitted that recovery is often slow and incomplete. Hypothalamic and midline thalamic areas may be of particular importance for determining pre-sleep behaviour and the slow conditioning necessary for sleep onset, whilst sleep onset itself is determined by a suprachiasmatic internal pacemaker, as well as by withdrawal of the influence of an ascending reticular system.

Activity of brain stem neuronal systems governs both sleeping and waking. In all human situations in which locked-in patients have been insomniac and have lacked REM sleep, pathological studies have indicated a lesion in the pontine tegmentum.[230, 237, 261, 265] In contrast, the corticospinal and corticobulbar pathways are not involved in sleep.

The separation of separate systems for wakefulness (a reticular activating system), NREM sleep (forebrain and pontine areas), REM sleep (more specific pontine nuclei) and circadian sleep control (suprachiasmatic nucleus) is somewhat artificial, for all these states are interdependent. Neurones of the pontine tegmental system may function during wakefulness in the coordination of eye, head and body movements, whilst neurones in the same region function during paradoxical sleep to produce rapid eye movements and PGO spikes in association with descending motor inhibition and total atonia of neck muscles. The fact that sleep is most severely affected in patients with brain stem lesions who have severe bilateral gaze palsies, or, as in olivopontocerebellar atrophy, loss of saccadic eye movements, suggests that the neural mechanisms concerned with sleep and certain aspects of eye movement are closely interrelated if not similar.[243] As a conclusion to many studies, although monoamine neurones of the pons may modulate the sleep–wake cycle, they are probably not essential for either sleep or wakefulness.[251, 252] There is conclusive evidence that brain stem structures are intimately involved in the generation of REM sleep in humans, but the transmitters by which these systems function have yet to be identified. The finding that subjects with loss of REM sleep may lead a normal life is difficult to reconcile with the results of sleep deprivation experiments and present views regarding the biological role of REM sleep.

HEAD INJURY AND SLEEP

Most cases of narcolepsy early this century were attributed to either encephalitis lethargica or head injury. As we have seen, occasionally encephalitis lethargica was followed by fairly typical narcolepsy–cataplexy, but this is never the case following head injury which, although resulting in coma, stupor, hypersomnolence or drowsiness, does not cause typical narcolepsy. The main importance of head injury to sleep physiologists is not the localization of the lesion, for this is rarely exact, but the pattern of slow recovery from unconsciousness, to severe sleep disturbance, to more normal awareness.

Blunt head injuries are often followed by coma, but yield little information on the cause of unconsciousness or severe sleep disturbance. In most cases coming to necropsy, either nothing is seen or the lesions are widely scattered. The cortical laceration so commonly found at the frontal and temporal poles after head injury is unlikely to be the cause of disordered awareness. Unlike blunt head injury, *gunshot wounds* of the brain are often not followed by loss of consciousness. When prolonged and severe coma does occur, Cairns[281] showed that the damage was widespread, or the situation was complicated by haemorrhage, meningitis or venous thrombosis.

During the slow recovery from coma following blunt head injury in both children and adults, patients are very sleepy throughout the entire 24 h period.[286] They fall asleep with monotony, but also during therapy, yawn a lot, and, as shown by Priganto *et al.*,[287] often describe a decrease in dreaming. However, the complaint of reduced or absent dreaming does not match with the time spent in REM sleep following injury. Recovery of normal wakefulness is slow, and sleep patterns may remain abnormal for as long as five years, with less stage 1–2 NREM sleep and a greater number of nocturnal awakenings than in normal subjects.

Following minor closed head injury, sleep may be disrupted for several months, and a number of non-specific EEG changes have been described, perhaps associated with brain damage, or even an initial lumbar puncture, which by itself may cause non-specific EEG abnormalities. These changes include a decrease of spindles and K complexes during NREM sleep, and a low level of REM activity.[282] These abnormalities may be due to minor brain stem rather than hemisphere damage, being of similar nature but less severe than the loss of deep sleep and loss of REM sleep reported after acute severe pontine lesions.[285]

Recovery of normal sleep patterns is a useful prognostic guide in post-traumatic coma. Overall, the appearance of typical polygraphic sleep–wake patterns indicates a good prognosis, and often accompanies other signs of improvement from coma.[280, 283, 284]

Do sleep abnormalities relate to cognitive function after head injury? Many studies have tried to relate improvement in cognition after acute closed head injury to recovery of REM sleep. Ron *et al.*[288] showed that, in the six months after head injury, steady improvement in cognitive function usually accompanied a steady increase in the time spent in REM sleep. However, an increase in REM sleep time is not essential for cognitive recovery. The second, but not the first, may occur after severe brain stem damage, perhaps dependent on the degree of separate injury to brain stem and to cortical structures.

REFERENCES

WAKING, SLEEP AND COMA

1. Adey, W.R., Bors, E. & Porter, W.R. Sleep EEG patterns after high cervical lesions in man, *Arch. Neurol.* (1968) **19**, 377–383.
2. Barros-Ferreira, M., Chodkiewicz, J.-P., Lairy, C.C. & Salzarulo, P. Disorganized relations of time and phasic events of REM sleep in a case of brain-stem tumour, *Electroenceph. Clin. Neurophysiol.* (1975) **38**, 203–207.
3. Brain, W.R. The cerebral basis of consciousness, *Proc. Roy. Soc. Med.* (1951) **44**, 37–42.
4. Bricolo, A., Gentilomo, A., Rosadini, G. & Rossi, G.F. Long-lasting post-traumatic unconsciousness. A study based on nocturnal EEG and polygraphic recording, *Acta Neurol. Scand.* (1968) **44**, 512–532.
5. Cairns, H. Disturbances of consciousness with lesions of the brain stem and diencephalon, *Brain* (1952) **75**, 109–146.
6. Cant, B.R. Somatosensory and auditory evoked potentials in patients with disorders of consciousness. In: Desmedt, J.E. (ed.) Clinical uses of cerebral, brain stem and spinal somatosensory evoked potentials, *Prog. Clin. Neurophysiol.* Vol. 7, Basel: Karger (1980) 282–291.
7. Chatrian, G.E., White, L.E. & Shaw, C.M. EEG patterns resembling wakefulness in unresponsive decerebrate state following traumatic brain stem infarct, *Electroenceph. Clin. Neurophysiol.* (1964) **16**, 285–289.
8. Cummings, J.L. & Greenberg, R. Sleep patterns in the 'locked-in' syndrome, *Electroenceph. Clin. Neurophysiol.* (1977) **43**, 270–271.
9. Foerster, O. & Spielmeyer, W. Die Pathogenese der epileptischen Krampfanfälle, *Deutsch. Z. Nervenheilk.* (1926) **94**, 15–58.
10. Jefferson, G., The nature of concussion, *Brit. Med. J.* (1944) **1**, 1–5.
11. Jones, B.E., Harper, S.T. & Halaris, A.E. Effects of locus coeruleus lesions upon cerebral monoamine content, sleep–wakefulness states and the responses to amphetamine in the cat, *Brain Res.* (1977) **124**, 473–496.
12. Jouvet, M. Recherches sur les structures nerveuses et les mécanismes responsables des différentes phases du sommeil physiologique, *Arch. Ital. Biol.* (1962) **100**, 125–206.
13. Jouvet, M. Neurophysiology of states of sleep, *Physiol. Rev.* (1967) **47**, 117–201.
14. Jouvet, M. The role of monoamine and acetylcholine containing neurones in the regulation of the sleep–waking cycle, *Ergebn. Physiol.* (1972) **64**, 166–307.
15. Lavie, P, Pratt, H., Scharf, B., Peled, R. & Brown, J. Localized pontine lesion: near total absence of REM sleep, *Neurology (NY)* (1984) **34**, 118–120.
16. Lindsley, D.B., Bowden, H.W. & Magoun, H.W. Effect upon the EEG of acute injury to the brain stem activating system, *Electroenceph. Clin. Neurophysiol.* (1949) **1**, 475–486.
17. Lindsley, D.B., Schreiner, L.L., Knowles, W.B. & Magoun, H.W. Behavioural and EEG changes following chronic brain stem lesions in the cat, *Electroenceph. Clin. Neurophysiol.* (1950) **2**, 483–498.
18. Loeb, C. & Poggio, G. Electroencephalograms in a case with ponto-mesencephalic haemorrhage, *Electroenceph. Clin. Neurophysiol.* (1953) **5**, 295–296.
19. Magoun, H.W. Ascending reticular activating system, *Res. Pub. Assoc. Nerv. Ment. Dis.* (1952) **30**, 480–492.
20. Mangold, R., Sokoloff, L., Connor, E., Kleinerman, J., Therman, P.-O. & Kety, S.S. Effects of sleep and lack of sleep on cerebral circulation and metabolism of normal young men, *J. Clin. Invest.* (1955) **34**, 1092–1100.
21. Moruzzi, G. The sleep–waking cycle, *Ergebn. Physiol.* (1972) **64**, 1–165.
22. Neil, J.F., Holzer, B.C., Spiker, D.G., Coble, P.A. & Kupfer, D.J. EEG sleep alterations in olivopontocerebellar degeneration, *Neurology* (1980) **30**, 660–662.
23. Orthner, H. Neuroanatomische Gesichtspunkte der Schlaf–Wach-Regelung. In: Jovanović, U.J. (ed.) *Der Schlaf*, Munich: J.A. Barth (1969) 49–84.
24. Osorio, I. & Daroff, R.B. Absence of REM and altered NREM sleep in patients with spinocerebellar degeneration and slow saccades, *Ann. Neurol.* (1980) **7**, 277–280.
25. Parmeggiani, P.L. & Rabin, C. Sleep and environmental temperature, *Arch. Ital. Biol.* (1970) **108**, 369–388.

26. Pavlov, I.P. Innere Hemmung der bedingten Reflexe und der Schlafen, *Skand. Arch. Physiol.* (1923) **44**, 42–58.
27. Pfurtscheller, G., Schwartz, G., Pfurtscheller, B. & List, W. Quantification of spindles in comatose patients, *Electroenceph. Clin. Neurophysiol.* (1983) **56**, 114–116.
28. Plum, F. & Posner, J.B. *The Diagnosis of Stupor and Coma*, Philadelphia, Pennsylvania: F.A. Davis (1980).
29. Reichardt, M. Hirnstamm und Psychiatrie, *Mschr. Psychiat. Neurol.* (1926) **68**, 470–506.
30. Ron, S., Algom, D., Hary, D. & Cohen, M. Time-related changes in the distribution of sleep stages in brain injured patients, *Electroenceph. Clin. Neurophysiol.* (1980) **48**, 432–441.
31. Rossi, G.F. Ricerche sulla natura della miosi nel sonno e nella narcosi barbiurica, *Arch. Sci. Biol. (Bologna)* (1957) **41**, 46–56.
32. Sakai, K. Central mechanisms of paradoxical sleep. In: Borbély, A. & Valatx, J.L. (eds.) *Sleep Mechanisms*, Berlin: Springer Verlag (1984) 3–18.
33. Sakai, K., Sastre, J.P., Kanamori, N. & Jouvet, M. State specific neurons in the ponto-medullary reticular formation with special reference to the postural atonia during paradoxical sleep in the cat. In: Pompeiano, O. & Ajmone Marsan, C. (eds.) *Brain Mechanisms and Perceptual Awareness and Purposeful Behaviour*, New York: Raven Press (1981) 405–429.
34. Sastre, J.P., Sakai, K. & Jouvet, M. Are gigantocellular tegmental field neurons responsible for paradoxical sleep? *Brain Res.* (1981) **229**, 147–161.
35. Siegel, J.M. & McGinty, D.J. Pontine reticular formation neurons: relationship of discharge to motor activity, *Science* (1977) **196**, 419–423.
36. Skinner, J.E. Electrocortical desynchronization during functional blockade of the mesencephalic reticular formation, *Brain Res.* (1970) **22**, 254–258.
37. Steriade, M. & Hobson, J.A. Neuronal activity during the sleep–waking cycle, *Prog. Neurobiol.* (1976) **6**, 155–376.
38. Villablanca, J. Behavioural and polygraphic study of 'sleep' and 'wakefulness' in chronic decerebrate cats, *Electroenceph. Clin. Neurophysiol.* (1966) **21**, 562–577.
39. Walker, J.M. & Berger, R.J. Sleep as an adaptation for energy conservation functionally related to hibernation and shallow torpor, *Prog. Brain Res.* (1980) **53**, 255–278.
40. Wieser, H.G. & Siegfried, J. Hirnstammableitungen (Makroelectroden) beim Menschen. 1. Elektrische Befunde in Wachzustande und Ganznachtschlaf, *Z. EEG–EMG* (1979) **10**, 8–19.

ENCEPHALITIS LETHARGICA AND SLEEP

41. Adie, W.J. Idiopathic narcolepsy: a disease sui generis; with remarks on the mechanisms of sleep, *Brain* (1926) **49**, 257–306.
42. Buzzard, E.F. & Greenfield, J.C. Lethargic encephalitis: its sequelae and morbid anatomy, *Brain* (1919) **42**, 305–338.
43. Gayet, M. Affection encéphalique (encéphalite diffuse probable) localisée aux étages supérieurs des pédoncles cérébraux et aux couches optiques, *Arch. Physiol.* (1875) **7**, 341–351.
44. Hirsch, E. Zur Frage der Schlafzentren im Zwischenhirn des Menschen, *Med. Klin.* (1924) **20**, 1322–1324.
45. Lhermitte, J. & Tournay, A. Rapport sur le sommeil normal et pathologique, *Rev. Neurol.* (1927) **1**, 751–887.
46. Mauthner, L. In: Protokoll der k.k. Gesellschaft der Aerzte in Wien, *Wien Klin. Wochenschr.* (1890) **3**, 445–446.
47. McAlpine, D. The anatomo-pathological basis of the parkinsonian syndrome following epidemic encephalitis, *Brain* (1926) **49**, 525–556.
48. Rail, D., Scholtz, C. & Swash, M. Post-encephalitic parkinsonism: current experience, *J. Neurol. Neurosurg. Psychiat.* (1981) **44**, 670–676.
49. Stolk, P.J. Adolf Hitler: his life and illness, *Psych. Neurol. Neurochir.* (1968) **71**, 381–398.
50. Symonds, C.P. Narcolepsy as a symptom of encephalitis lethargica, *Lancet* (1926) **ii**, 1214–1215.
51. Symonds, C.P. Cataplexy and other related forms of seizure, *Can. Med. Assoc. J.* (1954) **70**, 61.
52. Trömner, E. *Das Problem des Schlafs. Biologisch und psychophysiologisch betrachtet*, Wiesbaden: Bergmann (1912) 24–28.
53. von Economo, C. Schlaftheorie, *Ergebn. Physiol.* (1929) **28**, 312–339.
54. von Economo, C. Sleep as a problem of localization, *J. Nerv. Ment. Dis.* (1930) **71**, 249–259.

55. von Economo, C. *Encephalitis Lethargica. Its Sequelae and Treatment*, Newman, K.D. (trans.) London: Oxford University Press (1931).

ANATOMY OF SLEEP AND WAKING

56. Albanese, A. & Butcher, L.L. Acetylcholinesterase and catecholamine distribution in the locus coeruleus of the rat, *Brain Res. Bull.* (1980) **5**, 127–134.
57. Alema, G., Rosadini, G., Rossi, G.F. & Zattoni, J. Effetti clinici ed elettro-encefalografici della somministrazione di amobarbital sodium sul circolo vertebro-basilare dell'uomo, *Bull. Soc. Ital. Biol. Sper.* (1964) **40**, 835–838.
58. Alema, G., Rosadini, G. & Zattoni, J. Studio degli effetti selettivi dei barbituriei sul cervello anteriore e sul tronco dell 'encefalo mediante iniezione intracarotidea ed intravertebrale nell'uomo, *Minerva Anest.* (1964) **30**, 206–207.
59. Anden, N.E., Fuxe, K., Hamberger, B. & Hokfelt, T. A quantitative study on the nigro-striatal dopamine neuron system in the rat, *Acta Physiol. Scand.* (1966) **67**, 306–312.
60. Barret, R., Merritt, H.H. & Wolf, A. Depression of consciousness as a result of cerebral lesions, *Res. Publ. Assoc. Nerv. Ment. Dis.* (1967) **45**, 241–276.
61. Barros-Ferreira, M., Chodkiewicz, J., Lairy, G.C. & Salzarulo, P. Disorganized relations of tonic and phasic events of REM sleep in a case of brain stem tumour, *Electroenceph. Clin. Neurophysiol.* (1975) **38**, 203–207.
62. Bates, C.E.H. Mixed salivary tumour in the right tonsil fossa with narcolepsy and cataplexy, *Ann. Otol. Rhinol. Laryngol.* (1945) **54**, 812–817.
63. Batini, C., Magni, F., Palestini, M., Rossi, G.F. & Zanchetti, A. Neural mechanisms underlying the enduring EEG and behavioural activation in the midpontine pretrigeminal cat, *Arch. Ital. Biol.* (1959) **97**, 13–25.
64. Batini, C., Moruzzi, G., Palestini, M., Rossi, G.F. & Zanchetti, A. Effects of complete pontine transections on the sleep–wakefulness rhythm: the midpontine pretrigeminal preparation, *Arch. Ital. Biol.* (1959) **97**, 1–12.
65. Berlucchi, G., Maffei, L., Moruzzi, G. & Strata, P. Mécanismes hypnogènes du tronc de l'encéphale antagonistes du système réticulaire activateur. In: Jouvet, M. (ed.) *Aspects Anatomofonctionels de la Physiologie du Sommeil*, Paris: Centre National de Recherche Scientifique (1965) 89–105.
66. Berman, A.L. *The Brain Stem of the Cat. A Cytoarchitectonic Atlas with Stereotaxic Coordinates*, Madison, Wisconsin: University of Wisconsin Press (1968) 195.
67. Berod, A., Hartman, B.K., Keller, A., Joh, T.H. & Pujol, J.F. A new double labeling technique using TH and DBH immunohistochemistry: evidence for dopaminergic cells lying in the pons of the beef brain, *Brain Res.* (1982) **240**, 235–243.
68. Bizzi, E. & Brooks, D.C. Functional connections between pontine reticular formation and lateral geniculate nucleus during deep sleep, *Arch. Ital. Biol.* (1963) **101**, 666–680.
69. Bremer, F. Cerveau isolé et physiologie du sommeil, *C.R. Soc. Biol. (Paris)* (1935) **118**, 1235–1242.
70. Bremer, F. L'activité cérébrale au cours du sommeil et de la narcose. Contribution à l'étude du mécanisme du sommeil, *Bull. Acad. Roy. Med. Belg.* (1937) **4**, 68–86.
71. Bremer, F. L'activité électrique de l'écorce cérébrale et le problème physiologique du sommeil, *Bull. Soc. Ital. Biol. Sper.* (1938) **13**, 271–290.
72. Bremer, F. Preoptic hypnogenic area and reticular activating system, *Arch. Ital. Biol.* (1973) **111**, 85–111.
73. Bremer, F. & Terzuolo, C. Intéraction de l'écorce cérébrale et de la formation réticulée dans le mécanisme de l'éveil et du maintien de l'activité vigile, *J. Physiol. (Paris)* (1953) **45**, 56–57.
74. Bricolo, A. Sleep abnormalities following thalamic stereotactic lesions in man. In: Gastaut, H., Lugaresi, E., Berti-Ceroni, G. & Coccagna, G. (eds.) The abnormalities of sleep in man. Proceedings of the XVth European Meeting on Electrophysiology, Bologna 1967, Bologna: Auto Gaggi (1968) 135–138.
75. Brodal, A. *Neurological Anatomy*, 2nd edn., New York/London/Toronto: Oxford University Press (1969) pp. 314, 807.
76. Brooks, D.C. Waves associated with eye movement in the awake and sleeping cat, *Electroenceph. Clin. Neurophysiol.* (1968) **24**, 532–541.
77. Brooks, D.C. & Gershon, M.D. Eye movement potentials in the oculomotor and visual

systems of the cat: a comparison of reserpine-induced waves with those present during wakefulness and rapid eye movement sleep, *Brain Res.* (1971) **27**, 223–239.

78. Buguet, A. *Monoamines et Sommeils. V. Etude des relations entre les structures monoaminergiques du pont et les pointes ponto-geniculooccipitales du sommeil*, Lyon: Imprimerie des Beaux-Arts (1969) 216.

79. Cairncross, K., Gershon, S. & Gus, I. Some aspects of the mode of action of imipramine, *J. Neuropsychiat.* (1963) **4**, 224–231.

80. Cairns, H. Disturbances of consciousness with lesions of the brain stem and diencephalon, *Brain* (1952) **75**, 109–146.

81. Calvet, J., Calvet, M.C. & Langloise, J.M. Diffuse cortical activities waves during so-called desynchronized EEG patterns, *J. Neurophysiol.* (1965) **28**, 893–907.

82. Carli, G. & Zanchetti, A. A study of pontine lesions suppressing deep sleep in the cat, *Arch. Ital. Biol.* (1965) **103**, 751–788.

83. Cespuglio, R., Gomez, M.E., Faradji, H. & Jouvet, M. Alterations in the sleep–waking cycle induced by cooling of the locus coeruleus area, *Electroenceph. Clin. Neurophysiol.* (1982) **54**, 570–578.

84. Chadwick, D., Hallett, M., Jenner, P. & Marsden, C.D. Serotonin and action myoclonus – a review. In: Legg, N.J. (ed.) *Neurotransmitter Systems and their Clinical Disorders*, London: Academic Press (1978) 151–165.

85. Chase, M. & McGinty, D. Modulation of spontaneous and reflex activity of the jaw musculature by orbital cortical stimulation in the freely-moving cat, *Brain Res.* (1970) **19**, 117–126.

86. Chu, N.S. & Bloom, F.E. The catecholamine containing neurons in the cat dorsolateral pontine tegmentum: distribution of the cell bodies and some axonal projections, *Brain Res.* (1974) **66**, 1–21.

87. Clemente, C.D., Sterman, M.B. & Wyrwicka, W. Forebrain inhibitory mechanisms: conditioning of basal forebrain induced EEG synchronization and sleep, *Exp. Neurol.* (1963) **7**, 404–417.

88. Cohen, H., Ferguson, J., Henriksen, S., Stolk, J., Zarcone, V., Barchas, J. & Dement, W. Effects of chronic depletion of brain serotonin on sleep and behaviour, *Proceedings of the 78th Annual Convention APA* (1970) 831.

89. Crick, F. & Mitchison, G. The function of dream sleep, *Nature* (1983) **304**, 111–114.

90. Cunchillos, J.D. & de Andres, I. Participation of the cerebellum in the regulation of the sleep–wakefulness cycle. Results in cerebellectomized rats, *Electroenceph. Clin. Neurophysiol.* (1982) **53**, 549–558.

91. Delashaw, J.Jr., Foutz, A.S., Guilleminault, C. & Dement, W.C. Effects of pharmacological alterations of acetylcholine on cataplexy in dogs, *Sleep Res.* (1979) **8**, 180.

92. Delorme, F., Froment, J.L. & Jouvet, M. Suppression du sommeil par la *p*-chlorméthamphétamine et la *p*-chlorophénylalanine, *C. R. Soc. Biol. (Paris)* (1966) **160**, 2347–2351.

93. Dement, W.C., Carskadon, M.A. & Guilleminault, C. Narcolepsy, diagnosis and treatment, *Primary Care* (1976) **3**, 609–623.

94. Dement, W., Mitler, M. & Henriksen, S. Sleep changes during chronic administration of parachlorophenylalanine, *Rev. Can. Biol.* (1972) **31** (suppl.), 239–246.

95. Eguchi, K. & Satoh, T. Characterization of the neurons in the region of the solitary tract nucleus during sleep, *Physiol. Behav.* (1980) **24**, 99–102.

96. Eyzaguirre, C. & Fidone, S.J. *Physiology of the Nervous System*, 2nd edn., Chicago: Year Book Publishers (1975) 343–371.

97. Fadiga, E., Manzoni, T., Sapienza, S. & Urbano, A. Synchronizing and desynchronizing fastigial influences on the electrocortical activity of the cat, in acute experiments, *Electroenceph. Clin. Neurophysiol.* (1968) **24**, 330–342.

98. Fisher-Perroudan, C., Mouret, J. & Jouvet, M. Sur un cas d'agrypnie (quatre mois sans sommeil) au cours d'une maladie de Morvan. Effet favorable du 5-hydroxy-tryptophane, *Electroenceph. Clin. Neurophysiol.* (1974) **36**, 1–18.

99. Foutz, A.S., Delashaw, J.B. Jr., Guilleminault, C. & Dement, W.C. Monoaminergic mechanisms and experimental cataplexy, *Ann. Neurol.* (1981) **10**, 369–376.

100. Fredrickson, C.J. & Hobson, J.A. Electrical stimulation of the brain stem and subsequent sleep, *Arch. Ital. Biol.* (1970) **108**, 564–576.

101. Freeman, F.R., Salinas-Garcia, R.F. & Ward, J.W. Sleep patterns in a patient with a brain stem infarction involving the raphe nucleus, *Electroenceph. Clin. Neurophysiol.* (1974) **36**, 657–660.

102. French, J.D. Brain lesions associated with prolonged unconsciousness, *Arch. Neurol. Psychiat. (Chicago)* (1952) **68**, 727–740.
103. Gamper, E. Bau und Leistungen eines menschlichen Mittelhirnwesens (Arhinencephalie mit Encephalocoele) zugleich ein Beitrag zur Teratologie und Fasersystematik, *Z. Ges. Neurol. Psychiat.* (1926) **104**, 67–120.
104. Gassel, M. & Pompeiano, O. Fusimotor function during sleep in unrestrained cats, *Arch. Ital. Biol.* (1965) **103**, 347–368.
105. George, M., Haslett, W. & Jenden, D. A cholinergic mechanism in the brain-stem reticular formation: induction of paradoxical sleep, *Int. J. Neuropharmacol.* (1964) **3**, 541–552.
106. Goltz, F. Der Hund ohne Grosshirn – siebente Abhandlung über die Verrichtungen des Grosshirns, *Pflügers Arch. Ges. Physiol.* (1892) **51**, 570–614.
107. Guglielmino, S. & Strata, P. Cerebellum and atonia of the desynchronized phase of sleep, *Arch. Ital. Biol.* (1971) **109**, 210–217.
108. Guilleminault, C., Wilson, R. & Dement, W. A study of cataplexy, *Arch. Neurol.* (1974) **31**, 255–261.
109. Henricks, J.C., Morrison, A.R. & Mann, G.L. Different behaviours during paradoxical sleep without atonia depend on pontine lesion site, *Brain Res.* (1982) **239**, 81–105.
110. Henley, K. & Morrison, A. Release of organized behaviour during desynchronized sleep in cats with pontine lesions, *Psychophysiology* (1969) **6**, 245.
111. Henley, K. & Morrison, A. A re-evaluation of the effects of lesions of the pontine tegmental and locus coeruleus on phenomena of paradoxical sleep in the cat, *Acta Neurobiol. Exp.* (1974) **34**, 215–232.
112. Hernandez-Peon, R. & Drucker-Colin, R.A. A neuronographic study of cortico-bulbar hypnogenic pathways, *Physiol. Behav.* (1970) **5**, 721–725.
113. Hess, W.R. Stammganglion Reizversuche, presented at a Frankfurt meeting of the German Physiological Society. 27–30 September 1927, *Ber. Ges. Physiol.* (1927) **42**, 554–555.
114. Hirschkowitz, M., Thornby, J.L. & Karacan, I. Sleep spindles: pharmacological effects in humans, *Sleep* (1982) **5**, 85–94.
115. Hobson, J.A. The effects of chronic brain-stem lesions on cortical and muscular activity during sleep and waking in the cat, *Electroenceph. Clin. Neurophysiol.* (1965) **19**, 41–62.
116. Jacobs, B.L., Asher, R. & Dement, W.C. Electrophysiological and behavioural effects of electrical stimulation of the raphe nuclei in cats, *Physiol. Behav.* (1973) **11**, 489–495.
117. Jacobs, B.L., Henricksen, S.J. & Dement, W.C. Neurological basis of the PGO waves, *Brain Res.* (1972) **48**, 406–411.
118. Jacobs, B.L. & Jones, B.E. The role of central monoamine and acetylcholine systems in sleep–wakefulness states: mediation or modulation? In: Butcher, L.L. (ed.) *Cholinergic-Monoaminergic Interactions in the Brain*, New York: Academic Press (1978) 271–290.
119. Jankowska, E., Lund, S., Lundberg, A. & Pompeiano, O. Inhibitory effects evoked through ventral reticulospinal pathways, *Arch. Ital. Biol.* (1968) **106**, 124–140.
120. Jasper, H.H. Diffuse projection systems: the integrative action of the thalamic reticular system, *Electroenceph. Clin. Neurophysiol.* (1949) **1**, 405–409.
121. Jeannerod, M. & Sakai, K. Occipital and geniculate potentials related to eye movements in the unanesthetized cat, *Brain Res.* (1970) **19**, 361–377.
122. Jefferson, M. Altered consciousness associated with brain stem lesions, *Brain* (1952) **75**, 55–67.
123. Jefferson, G. & Johnson, R.T. The cause of loss of consciousness in posterior fossa compression, *Folia Psychiat. (Amst.)* (1950) **53**, 306–319.
124. Jones, B.E. Elimination of paradoxical sleep by lesions of the pontine gigantocellular tegmental field in the cat, *Neurosci. Lett.* (1979) **13**, 285–293.
125. Jones, B.E., Halaris, A.E. & Freedman, D.X. Innervation of forebrain regions by medullary noradrenaline neurons, a biochemical study in cats with central tegmental tract lesions, *Neurosci. Lett.* (1978) **10**, 251–258.
126. Jones, B.E., Harper, S.T. & Halaris, A.E. Effect of locus coeruleus lesions upon cerebral monoamine content, sleep–wakefulness states and the response to amphetamine in the cat, *Brain Res.* (1977) **124**, 473–496.
127. Jouvet, M. Recherches sur les structures nerveuses et les mécanismes responsables des différentes phases du sommeil physiologique, *Arch. Ital. Biol.* (1962) **100**, 125–206.
128. Jouvet, M. Neurophysiology of the states of sleep, *Physiol. Rev.* (1967) **47**, 117–177.
129. Jouvet, M. Biogenic amines and the states of sleep, *Science* (1969) **163**, 32–41.
130. Jouvet, M. The role of monoamine and acetylcholine containing neurons in the regulation of

the sleep–waking cycle, *Ergebn. Physiol.* (1972) **64**, 166–307.
131. Jouvet, M. & Delorme, J. Locus coeruleus et sommeil paradoxal, *C.R. Soc. Biol.* (1965) **159**, 895–899.
132. Jouvet, M. & Renault, J. Insomnie persistante après lésions des noyaux du raphé chez le chat, *C.R. Soc. Biol. (Paris)* (1966) **160**, 1461–1465.
133. Jovanovíc, U.J. (ed.) *Der Schlaf. Neurophysiologische Aspekte,* Munich: J.A. Barth (1969) pp. 67, 252.
134. Karacan, I., Schneck, L. & Hinterbuchner, L.P. The sleep–dream pattern in Tay-Sachs disease (preliminary observations). In: Aronson, S.M. & Volk, B.W. (eds.) *Inborn Errors of Sphingolipid Metabolism,* Elmsford, New York: Pergamon (1967) 413–421.
135. Kaufman, L.S. & Morrison, A.R. Spontaneous and elicited PGO spikes in rats, *Brain Res.* (1981) **214**, 61–72.
136. Kimura, H., McGeer, P.L., Peng, J.H. & McGeer, E.G. The central cholinergic system studied by choline acetyl transferase histochemistry in the cat, *J. Comp. Neurol.* (1982) **200**, 151–201.
137. Kleitman, N. *Sleep and Wakefulness,* Chicago: University of Chicago Press (1963) 241–242.
138. Kleitman, N. & Camille, N. Studies on the physiology of sleep. VI. The behaviour of decorticated dogs, *Am. J. Physiol.* (1932) **100**, 474–480.
139. Koella, W.A. *Sleep. Its Nature and Physiological Organization.* Springfield, Illinois: Charles C. Thomas (1967) 199.
140. Kubota, K. & Tanaka, R. The fusimotor activity and natural sleep in the cat, *Brain Res.* (1966) **3**, 198–201.
141. Kukorelli, T. & Juhasz, G. Sleep induced by intestinal stimulation in cats, *Physiol. Behav.* (1977) **19**, 355–358.
142. Leger, L., Wiklund, L., Descarries, L. & Persson, M. Description of an indolaminergic cell component in the cat locus coeruleus: a fluorescence histochemical and radioautographic study, *Brain Res.* (1979) **168**, 43–56.
143. Lidbrink, P. The effects of lesions of ascending noradrenaline pathways on sleep and waking in the rat, *Brain Res.* (1974) **74**, 19–40.
144. Lindsley, D.B., Bowden, H.W. & Magoun, H.W. Effect upon the EEG of acute injury to the brain stem activating system, *Electroenceph. Clin. Neurophysiol.* (1947) **1**, 475–486.
145. Ljungdahl, A., Hokfelt, T. & Nilsson, G. Distribution of substance P like immunoreactivity in the central nervous system of the rat. 1. Cell bodies and nerve terminals, *Neuroscience* (1978) **3**, 861–943.
146. Madoz Jáuregui, P. Influencia de la región preóptica en la regulación de la actividad électrica cerebral, *An. Anat.* (1969) **18**, 477–537.
147. Magnes, J., Moruzzi, G. & Pompeiano, O. Synchronization of the EEG produced by low-frequency electrical stimulation of the region of the solitary tract, *Arch. Ital. Biol.* (1961) **99**, 33–67.
148. Magni, F., Moruzzi, G., Rossi, G.F. & Zanchetti, A. EEG arousal following inactivation of the lower brain stem by selective injection of barbiturate into the vertebral circulation, *Arch. Ital. Biol.* (1959) **97**, 33–46.
149. Magni, F. & Willis, W.D. Identification of reticular formation neurons by intracellular recording, *Arch. Ital. Biol.* (1963) **101**, 681–702.
150. Magoun, H.W. The ascending reticular system and wakefulness. In: Dela Fresnaye, J.F. (ed.) *Brain Mechanisms and Consciousness,* Springfield, Illinois: Charles C. Thomas (1952) 1–20.
151. Magoun, H. & Rhines, R. An inhibitory mechanism in the bulbar reticular formation, *J. Neurophysiol.* (1946) **9**, 165–171.
152. Marchesi, G.F., Scarpino, O. & y Mauro, A.M. Studio poligrafico del sonno notturno in pazienti con sindrome cerebellare, *Arch. Psicol. Neurol. Psichiat.* (1977) **4**, 455–472.
153. Marchesi, G.F. & Strata, P. Climbing fibers of rat cerebellum: modulation of activity during sleep, *Brain Res.* (1970) **17**, 145–148.
154. Marsden, C.D., Hallett, M. & Fahn, S. The nosology and pathophysiology of myoclonus. In: Marsden, C.D. & Fahn, S. (eds.) *Movement Disorders,* London: Butterworth (1982) 196–248.
155. McGinty, D. & Sterman, M. Sleep suppression after basal forebrain lesions in the cat, *Science* (1968) **160**, 1253–1255.
156. Mitler, M.M. Toward an animal model of narcolepsy–cataplexy. In: Guilleminault, C., Dement, W.C. & Passouant, P. (eds.) New York: Spectrum Publications (1976) 387–409.
157. Mitler, M.M. & Dement, W.C. Cataplectic-like behaviour in cats after micro-injections of

carbachol in pontine reticular formation, *Brain Res.* (1974) **68**, 335–343.

158. Møller, E. & Ostenfeld, I. Studies on the cerebral carotid sinus syndrome and the physiological basis of consciousness, *Acta Psychiat. Neurol.* (1949) **24**, 59–80.

159. Morgane, P.J. & Stern. W.C. Monoaminergic systems in the brain and their role in the sleep states. In: Barchas, J. & Usdin, E. (eds.) *Serotonin and Behaviour*, New York: Academic Press (1973) 427–442.

160. Morrison, A.R. & Pompeiano, O. Vestibular influences during sleep. IV. Functional relations and lateral geniculate nucleus during desynchronized sleep, *Arch. Ital. Biol.* (1966) **104**, 425–458.

161. Moruzzi, G. Active processes in the brain stem during sleep, *Harvey Lect.* (1963) **58**, 233–297.

162. Moruzzi, G. The sleep–waking cycle, *Ergebn. Physiol.* (1972) **64**, 1–165.

163. Naitoh, P., Antony-Bass, V., Muzet, A. & Ehrhart, J. Dynamic relation of sleep spindles and K-complexes to spontaneous phasic arousal in sleeping human subjects, *Sleep* (1982) **5**, 58–72.

164. Naquet, R., Denavit, M. & Albe-Fessard, D. Comparaison entre le rôle du subthalamus et celui des différentes structures bulbo-mésencéphaliques dans le maintien de la vigilance, *Electroenceph. Clin. Neurophysiol.* (1966) **20**, 149–164.

165. Naquet, R., Lanoir, J. & Albe-Fessard, D. Altérations transitoires ou définitives de zones diencéphaliques chez le chat. Leurs effets sur l'activité électrique corticale et le sommeil. In: Jouvet, M. (ed.) *Aspects Anatomo-Fonctionnels de la Physiologie du Sommeil*, Paris: CNRS (1965) 657.

166. Nauta, W.J.H. Hypothalamic regulation of sleep in rats. Experimental study, *J. Neurophysiol.* (1946) **9**, 285–316.

167. Nelson, J.P., McCarley, R.W. & Hobson, J.A. REM sleep burst neurons, PGO waves, and eye movement information, *J. Neurophysiol.* (1983) **50**, 784–797.

168. Niakin, E., Belluomini, J., Lemmi, H., Summitt, R.L. & Ch'ien, L. Disturbance of rapid-eye-movement sleep in three brothers with Pelizaeus-Merzbacher disease, *Ann. Neurol.* (1979) **6**, 253–257.

169. Nielson, J.M. & Sedgwick, R.P. Instincts and emotions in an anencephalic monster, *J. Nerv. Ment. Dis.* (1949) **110**, 387–394.

170. Olszewski, J. & Baxter, D. *The Cytoarchitecture of the Human Brain Stem*, Philadelphia: Lippincott (1954).

171. Orthner, H. Neuroanatomische Gesichtspunkte der Schlaf–Wach–Regelung. In: Jovanović, U.J. (ed.) *Der Schlaf*, Munich: J.A. Barth (1969) 49–84.

172. Osario, I. & Daroff, R.B. Absence of REM and altered NREM sleep in patients with spinocerebellar degeneration and slow saccades, *Ann. Neurol.* (1980) **7**, 277–280.

173. Oswald, I. *Sleeping and Waking: Physiology and Psychology*, Amsterdam: Elsevier (1962) 232.

174. Passouant, P. Introduction à l'étude des hypersomnies, *Rev. Neurol.* (1967) **116**, 467–470.

175. Penfield, W. The cerebral cortex in man. 1. The cerebral cortex and consciousness, *Arch. Neurol. Psychiat. (Chicago)* (1938) **40**, 417–442.

176. Penfield, W. & Jasper, H.H. Highest level seizures, *Assoc. Res. Nerv. Ment. Dis. Proc.* (1947) **26**, 252–271.

177. Petitjean, F., Sakai, K., Blondaux, C. & Jouvet, M. Hypersomnie par lésion isthmique chez le chat. II. Étude neurophysiologique et pharmacologique, *Brain Res.* (1975) **88**, 439–453.

178. Petitjean, J.J., Ternaux, J.P., Foutz, A.S. & Fernandez, G. Les stades de sommeil de la préparation encéphale isolé. 1. Déclenchement des pointes ponto–geniculo–occipitales et du sommeil phasique à ondes lentes. Rôle des noyaux du raphé, *Electroenceph. Clin. Neurophysiol.* (1975) **37**, 569–576.

179. Pivik, T. & Dement, W. Phasic changes in muscular and reflex activity during non-REM sleep, *Exp. Neurol.* (1970) **27**, 115–124.

180. Pompeiano, O. The neurophysiological mechanisms of the postural and motor events during desynchronized sleep, *Res. Publ. Assoc. Nerv. Ment. Dis.* (1967) **45**, 351–425.

181. Pompeiano, O. Mechanisms of sensorimotor integration during sleep, *Prog. Physiol. Psychol.* (1970) **3**, 1–179.

182. Polc, P., Schneeberger, J. & Haefely, W. Effect of several centrally active drugs on the sleep wakefulness cycle of cats, *Neuropharmacology* (1979) **18**, 259–267.

183. Puech, P., Guilly, P., Fishgold, H. & Bounes, G. Un cas d'anencéphalie hydrocéphalique. Étude electroencéphalographique, *Rev. Neurol.* (1947) **79**, 116–124.

184. Puizzilout, J.J., Gaudin-Chazel, G. & Bras, H. Vagal mechanisms in sleep regulation. In: Borbély, A. & Valatax, J. (eds.) *Sleep Mechanisms*, Berlin: Springer Verlag (1984) 19–38.

185. Purkinje, J.E. Wachen, Schlaf, Traum und verwandte Zustände. In: Wagner, R. (ed.) *Handwörterbuch der Physiologie*, 9 Bände, Bd 3, Abt 2, Braunschweig: Friedr. Vieweg & Sohn (1846) 412–480.
186. Purpura, D.P. & Yahr, M.D. (eds.) *The Thalamus*, New York/London: Columbia University Press (1966) 438.
187. Ranson, S.W. Somnolence caused by hypothalamic lesions in the monkey *Arch. Neurol. Psychiat. (Chicago)* (1939) **41**, 1–23.
188. Reil, J.C. *Reil's Arch. Physiol.* (1809) **9**, 511.
189. Rossi, G.F. Electrophysiology of sleep. In: Gastaut, H., Lugaresi, E., Berti Leroni, G. & Coccagna, G. (eds.) *The Abnormalities of Sleep in Man*, Bologna: Aulo Gaggi (1968) 13–23.
190. Roussel, B. *Monamines et sommeil. IV. Suppression du sommeil paradoxal et diminution de la noradrénaline cérébrale par lésions des noyaux locus coeruleus*, Lyon: Imprimerie des Beaux-Arts (1967) 141.
191. Roussel, B., Buguet, A., Bobillier, P. & Jouvet, M. Locus coeruleus, sommeil paradoxal, et noradrénaline cérébrale, *C.R. Soc. Biol.* (1967) **161**, 2537–2541.
192. Ruch-Monachan, M.A., Jalfie, M. & Haefely, W. Drugs and PGO waves in the lateral geniculate body of the curarized cat, *Arch. Int. Pharmacodyn. Ther.* (1976) **219**, 251–346.
193. Russell, G.V. The nucleus locus coeruleus (dorsolateralis tegmenti), *Tex. Rep. Biol. Med.* (1955) **13**, 939–988.
194. Sakai, K. Some anatomical and physiological properties of ponto-mesencephalic neurons with special references to the PGO waves and postural atonia during paradoxical sleep in the cat. In Hobson, J. & Brazier, M. (eds.) *The Reticular Formation Revisited*, New York: Raven Press (1980) 427–447.
195. Sakai, K. Central mechanisms of paradoxical sleep. In: Borbely, A. & Valtax, J.-L. (eds.) *Sleep Mechanisms*, Berlin: Springer Verlag (1984) 3–18.
196. Sakai, K. & Jouvet, M. Brain stem PGO – on cells projecting directly to the cat dorsal lateral geniculate nucleus, *Brain Res.* (1980) **194**, 500–505.
197. Sakai, K., Vanni-Mercier, G. & Jouvet, M. Evidence for the presence of PS-OFF neurons in the ventromedial medulla oblongata of freely moving cats, *Exp. Brain Res.* (1983) **49**, 311–314.
198. Salzarulo, P., Lairy, G.C., Bancaud, J. & Munari, C. Direct depth recording of the striata cortex during REM sleep in man: are there PGO potentials? *Electroenceph. Clin. Neurophysiol.* (1975) **38**, 199–202.
199. Sasaki, K., Tanaka, R. & Mori, K. Effects of stimulation of pontine and bulbar reticular formation upon spinal motorneurones of the cat, *Jap. J. Physiol.* (1962) **12**, 45–62.
200. Sastre, J.P. *Effets des lésions du tegmentum pontique sur l'organisation des états de sommeil chez le chat*, doctoral thesis, Lyon: University of Lyon (1978) 256.
201. Schaltenbrand, G. Über die Beziehungen zwischen krankhaften Steigerungen des Muskeltonus und dem Schlaf, *Pflüg. Arch. Ges. Physiol.* (1941) **224**, 610–621.
202. Scheibel, M.E. & Scheibel, A.B. Structural substrates for integrative patterns in the brain-stem reticular core. In: Jasper, H.H. (ed.) *Reticular Formation of the Brain*, Boston/Toronto: Little, Brown & Co. (1958) 31–55.
203. Silberman, E.K., Vivaldi, E., Garfield, J., McCarley, R.W. & Hobson, J.A. Carbachol triggering of desynchronized sleep phenomena: enhancement via small volume infusions, *Brain Res.* (1980) **191**, 215–224.
204. Simon, R.P., Gershon, M.D. & Brooks, D.C. The role of raphe nuclei in the regulation of ponto-geniculo-occipital wave activity, *Brain Res.* (1973) **58**, 313–330.
205. Singer, W. & Bedworth, N. Correlation between the effects of brain stem stimulation and saccadic eye movements on transmission in the cat lateral geniculate nucleus, *Brain Res.* (1974) **72**, 185–202.
206. Sterman, M., McGinty, D. & Iwamura, Y. Modulation of trigeminal reflexes during the REM state in brain transected cats, *Arch. Ital. Biol.* (1974) **112**, 278–297.
207. Sterman, M.B. & Clemente, C.D. Forebrain inhibitory mechanisms: cortical synchronization induced by basal forebrain stimulation, *Exp. Neurol.* (1962) **6**, 91–102.
208. Sterman, M.B. & Clemente, C.D. Forebrain inhibitory mechanisms: sleep patterns induced by basal forebrain stimulation in the behaving cat, *Exp. Neurol.* (1962) **6**, 103–117.
209. Sterman, M.B. & Clemente, C.D. Basal forebrain structures and sleep, *Acta Physiol. Lat. Am.* (1968) **14**, 228–244.
210. Sterman, M. & Fairchild, M. Modification of locomotor performance by reticular formation and basal forebrain stimulation in the cat: evidence for reciprocal systems, *Brain Res.* (1966) **2**, 205–217.

211. Strahlendorf, H.K., Strahlendorf, J.C. & Barnes, C.D. Endorphin mediated inhibition of locus coeruleus neurons, *Brain Res.* (1980) **191**, 284–288.
212. Thompson, G.N. & Nielson, J.M. Area essential to consciousness: cerebral localization of consciousness as established by neuropathological studies, *J. Am. Med. Assoc.* (1948) **137**, 285.
213. Thompson, C., Schachter, M. & Parkes, J.D. Drugs for cataplexy, *Ann. Neurol.* (1982) **12**, 63–64.
214. Tinbergen, N, *The Study of Instinct*, 2nd edn., Oxford: Clarendon Press (1955) 228.
215. Trulson, M.E., Preussler, D.W. & Howell, G.A. Activity of substantia nigra units across the sleep–waking cycle in freely moving cats, *Neurosci. Lett.* (1981) **26**, 183–188.
216. Uhl, G.R., Goodman, R.R. & Snyder, S.H. Neurotensin-containing cell bodies, fibers and nerve terminals in the brain stem of the rat: immunochemical mapping, *Brain Res.* (1979) **167**, 77–91.
217. Van Dongen, P.A.M., Broekkamp, C.L.E. & Cools, A.R. Atonia after carbachol microinjections near the locus coeruleus in cats, *Pharmacol. Biochem. Behav.* (1978) **8**, 527–532.
218. Villablanca, J. Electroencephalogram in the permanently isolated forebrain of the cat, *Science* (1962) **138**, 44–46.
219. Villablanca, J. The electrocorticogram in the chronic cerveau isolé cat, *Electroenceph. Clin. Neurophysiol.* (1965) **19**, 576–586.
220. Vimont-Vicary, P. La suppression des différentes états de sommeil. Etude compartémentale, EEG, et neuropharmacologie chez le chat, thesis, Lyon: University of Lyon (1965) 95.
221. von Economo, C. Schlaftheorie, *Ergebn. Physiol.* (1929) **28**, 312–339.
222. von Economo, C. Sleep as a problem of localization, *J. Nerv. Ment. Dis.* (1930) **71**, 249–259.
223. von Economo, C. *Encephalitis Lethargica: Its Sequelae and Treatment*, K.D. Newman (trans.) London: Oxford University Press (1931).
224. Whitlock, D.G., Aruini, A. & Moruzzi, G. Microelectrode analysis of pyramidal system during transition from sleep to wakefulness, *J. Neurophysiol.* (1953) **16**, 414–429.
225. Wilkus, R.J. & Farrell, D.F. Electrophysiological observations in the classical form of Pelizaeus–Merzbacher disease, *Neurology (Minneap.)* (1976) **26**, 1042–1045.
226. Wilson, W. & Nashold B. The sleep rhythms of subcortical nuclei: some observations in man, *Biol. Psychiat.* (1969) **1**, 289–296.

BRAIN STEM LESIONS AND DISTURBANCES OF SLEEP AND WAKEFULNESS IN MAN

227. Albert, M.L. Subcortical dementia. In: Katzman, R., Terry, R.D. & Bick, K.L. (eds.) Alzheimer's disease: senile dementia and related disorders, New York: Raven Press (1979) 173–180.
228. Anderson, M. & Salmon, M.V. Symptomatic cataplexy, *J. Neurol. Neurosurg. Psychiat.* (1977) **40**, 186–191.
229. Appenzeller, C. & Fischer, A.J., Jr., Disturbances of rapid eye movement during sleep in patients with lesions of the nervous system, *Electroenceph. Clin. Neurophysiol.* (1968) **25**, 29–32.
230. Barros Ferraira, M., Chodkiewicz, J., Lairy, G.C. & Slazarulo, P. Disorganized relations of tonic and phasic events of REM sleep in a case of brain stem tumour, *Electroenceph. Clin. Neurophysiol.* (1975) **38**, 203–207.
231. Behrman, S., Carroll, J.D., Janota, I. & Matthews, W.B. Progressive supranuclear palsy. Clinico-pathological study of four cases, *Brain* (1969) **92**, 663–678.
232. Benassi, E., Abburzzese, M., Ottonello. G.A. & Tananelli, P. Sleep abnormalities in four cases of dyssynergia cerebellaris myoclonica of Ramsey–Hunt, *Ital. J. Neurol. Sci.* (1981) **2**, 159–163.
233. Bergamasco, B., Bergamini, L. & Mutani, R. Lack of paradoxical sleep phase in a case of Ramsey–Hunt disease. In: Gastaut, H., Lugaresi, E. & Berti-Ceroni, G. (eds.) *The Abnormalities of Sleep in Man*, Bologna: Aulo Gaggi (1968) 303–310.
234. Burns, R.S., Markey, S.P., Philips, J.M. & Chiueh, C.C. The neurotoxicity of 1-methyl-4-phenyl-1,2,3,6-tetrahydropyridine (MPTP) in the monkey and man, *Can. J. Neurol. Sci.* (1984) **11** Suppl, 166–168.

235. Cairns, H. Disturbances of consciousness with lesions of the brain stem and diencephalon, *Brain* (1952) **75**, 109–146.
236. Chase, T.N., Moretti, L. & Prensky, A.L. Clinical and electroencephalographic manifestations of vascular lesions of the pons, *Neurology* (1968) **18**, 357–368.
237. Cummings, J.L. & Greenberg, R. Sleep patterns in the 'locked-in' syndrome, *Electroenceph. Clin. Neurophysiol.* (1977) **43**, 270–271.
238. Eadie, M.J. Olivo-ponto-cerebellar atrophy (Menzel type). In: Vinken, P.J. & Bruyn, G.W. *Handbook of Clinical Neurology*, Vol. 21, Amsterdam: North Holland (1975) 443–449.
239. Epemenides. In: *Encyclopaedia Britannica*, Chicago: Encyclopedia Britannica (1966) **8**, 646.
240. Feldman, M.H. Physiological observations in a chronic case of 'locked-in' syndrome, *Neurology (Minneap.)* (1971) **21**, 459–478.
241. Freeman, F.R. Akinetic mutism and bilateral anterior cerebral artery occlusion, *J. Neurol. Neurosurg. Psychiat.* (1971) **34**, 693–698.
242. Freeman, F.R., Salinas-Garcia, R.F. & Ward, J.W. Sleep patterns in a patient with a brain stem infarction involving the raphe nucleus, *Electroenceph. Clin. Neurophysiol.* (1974) **36**, 657–660.
243. Goebel. H.H., Komatsuzaki, A. & Bender, M.B. Lesions of the pontine tegmentum and conjugate gaze paralysis, *Arch. Neurol.* (1971) **24**, 431–440.
244. Gross, R.A., Spehlmann, R. & Daniels, J.C. Sleep disturbances in progressive supranuclear palsy, *Electroenceph. Clin. Neurophysiol.* (1978) **45**, 16–25.
245. Guilleminault, C., Cathala, H.P. & Castaigne, P. Effects of 5-hydroxytryptophane on sleep of a patient with a brain stem lesion, *Electroenceph. Clin. Neurophysiol.* (1973) **34**, 177–184.
246. Hobson, J.A. Brain-stem signs, sleep attacks, and REM sleep enhancement, *Psychophysiology* (1970) **7**, 310.
247. Hobson, J.A. Dreaming sleep attacks and desynchronized sleep enhancement. Report of a case of brain stem signs, *Arch. Gen. Psychiat.* (1975) **32**, 1421–1424.
248. Hobson, J.A., McCarley, R.W. & Wyzinski, P.W. Sleep cycle oscillation: reciprocal discharge by two brainstem neuronal groups, *Science* (1975) **189**, 55–58.
249. Hunt, J.R. Dyssynergia cerebellaris progressiva – a chronic progressive form of cerebellar tremor, *Brain* (1914) **37**, 247–268.
250. Jacobs, L., Feldman, M. & Bender, M.B. Eye movements during sleep. 1. The pattern in the normal human, *Arch. Neurol.* (1971) **25**, 151–159.
251. Jacobs, B.L. & Jones, B.E. The role of central monoamine and acetylcholine systems in sleep–wakefulness states: mediation or modulation? In: Butcher, L.L. (ed.) *Cholinergic–Monoaminergic Interactions in the Brain*, New York, Academic Press (1978) 271–290.
252. Jones, B.E. Elimination of paradoxical sleep by lesions of the pontine gigantocellular tegmental field in the cat, *Neurosci. Lett.* (1979) **13**, 285–293.
253. Jouvet, M. The role of monoamines and acetylcholine-containing neurons in the regulation of the sleep–waking cycle, *Ergebn. Physiol.* (1972) **64**, 166–307.
254. Kazukawa, S. A polygraphic study on nocturnal sleep of patients with spino-cerebellar degeneration – a comparative study of Marie's ataxia and OPCA, *Seishin Sinkeigaku Zasshi* (1982) **84**, 135–161.
255. Kemper, T.L. & Romanul, F.A.C. State resembling akinetic mutism in basilar artery occlusion, *Neurology (Minneap.)* (1967) **17**, 74–80.
256. Konigsmark, B.W. & Weiner, L.P. The olivopontocerebellar atrophies. A review. *Medicine (Baltimore)* (1970) **49**, 227–241.
257. Laffont, F., Autret, A., Minz, M., Beillevaire, T., Gilbert, A., Cathala, H.P. & Castaigne, P. Etude polygraphique du sommeil dans neuf cas de maladie de Steele–Richardson, *Rev. Neurol.* (1979) **135**, 127–142.
258. Lavie, P., Pratt, H., Scharf, B., Peled, R. & Brown, J. Localized pontine lesion: nearly total absence of REM sleep, *Neurology (Cleveland)* (1984) **34**, 118–120.
259. Leygonie, F., Thomas, J., Degos, J.D., Bouchareine, A. & Barbizet, J. Troubles du sommeil dans la maladie de Steele–Richardson, *Rev. Neurol.* (1976) **132**, 125–136.
260. Lucksch, F. Ueber das 'Schlafzentrum' *Z. Ges. Neurol. Psychiat.* (1924) **93**, 83–94.
261. Markand, O.N. & Dyken, M.L. Sleep abnormalities in patients with brain stem lesions, *Neurology (Minneap.)* (1976) **26**, 769–776.
262. McHugh, P.R. & Folstein, M.F. Subcortical dementia. Address to the American Academy of Neurology, Boston, April 1973 (unpublished).
263. Mouret, J. Differences in sleep in patients with Parkinson's disease, *Electroenceph. Clin. Neurophysiol.* (1975) **38**, 653–657.

264. Neil, J.F., Holzer, B.C., Spiker, D.G., Coble, P.A. & Kupfer, D.J. EEG sleep alterations in olivopontocerebellar degeneration, *Neurology* (1980) **30**, 660–662.

265. Osorio, I. & Daroff, R.B. Absence of REM and altered NREM sleep in patients with spinocerebellar degeneration and slow saccades, *Ann. Neurol.* (1980) **7**, 277–280.

266. Perret, J.L. & Jouvet, M. Etude du sommeil dans la paralysie supra-nucléaire progressive, *Electroenceph. Clin. Neurophysiol.* (1979) **47**, 323–329.

267. Perret, J.L., Tapissier, J. & Jouvet, M. Insomnia and memory. A propos of a case of striato-nigral degeneration, *Electroenceph. Clin. Neurophysiol.* (1979) **47**, 499–502.

268. Pette, H. Die epidemische Encephalitis in ihren Folgezustanden, *Deutsch. Z. Nervenheilk.* (1923) **56**, 1–71.

269. Plum, F. & Posner, J.B. *The Diagnosis of Stupor and Coma,* Philadelphia: F.A. Davis (1980).

270. Sears, E.S., Hammerberg, E.K. & Norenberg, M.D. Supranuclear ophthalmoplegia and dementia in olivopontocerebellar atrophy: a clinicopathologic study, *Neurology (Minneap.)* (1975) **25**, 395.

271. Stahl, S.M., Layzer, R.B., Aminoff, M.J., Townsend, J.J. & Feldon, S. Continuous cataplexy in a patient with a midbrain tumour: the limp man syndrome, *Neurology (Minneap.)* (1980) **30**, 1115–1118.

272. Starr, A. A disorder of rapid eye movements in Huntington's chorea, *Brain* (1967) **90**, 545–564.

273. Steele, J.C., Richardson, J.C. & Olszewski, J. Progressive supranuclear palsy. A heterogeneous degeneration involving the brain stem, basal ganglia and cerebellum with vertical gaze and pseudobulbar palsy, nuchal dystonia and rigidity, *Arch. Neurol. (Chic.)* (1964) **10**, 333–359.

274. Tamura, K., Karacan, I., Williams, R.L. & Meyer, J.S. Disturbances of the sleep–waking cycle in patients with vascular brain stem lesions, *Clin. Electroenceph.* (1963) **14**, 35–46.

275. Wadia, N.H. Heredo-familial spinocerebellar degeneration with slow eye movements – another variety of olivopontocerebellar degeneration, *Neurol. India* (1977) **25**, 147–160.

276. Wilkus, R.J., Harvey, F., Moretti Djeman, L. & Lettich, E. Electroencephalography and sensory evoked potentials, *Arch. Neurol.* (1971) **24**, 538–544.

277. Yokoyama, S., Katayama, S., Tsunashima, Y., Kimura, T., Araki, M., Yamano, K. & Ishii, S. PGO wave-like EEG in a patient with spino-cerebellar degeneration, *Folia Psychiat. Neurol. Jap.* (1981) **35**, 399.

278. Zee, D.S., Optican, L.M., Cook, J.D., Robinson, D.A. & King Engel, W. Slow saccades in spinocerebellar degeneration, *Arch. Neurol.* (1976) **33**, 243–251.

279. Zee, D.S. & Robinson, D.A. A hypothetical explanation of saccadic oscillations, *Ann. Neurol.* (1979) **5**, 405–414.

HEAD INJURY AND SLEEP

280. Bergamasco, B., Bergamini, L., Doriguzzi, T. & Fabiani, D. EEG sleep patterns as a prognostic criterion in post-traumatic coma, *Electroenceph. Clin. Neurophysiol.* (1968) **24**, 374–377.

281. Cairns, H. Disturbance of consciousness with lesions of the brain stem and diencephalon, *Brain* (1952) **75**, 109–146.

282. Harada, M., Minani, R., Hattori, E., Nakamura, K., Kabashima, K., Shikai, I. & Sakai, V. Sleep in brain damaged patients: an all night study of 105 cases, *Kumamoto Med. J.* (1976) **29**, 110–127.

283. Jouvet, D., Valatz, L. & Jouvet, M. Etude polygraphique du sommeil du chat, *CR Soc. Biol. (Paris)* (1961) **155**, 1313–1316.

284. Lesard, E.S., Sarces, A. & Larson, S.J. Period analysis of EEG signals during sleep and post-traumatic coma, *Aerospace Med.* (1974) **45**, 664–668.

285. Markand, O.N. & Dyken, M.L. Sleep abnormalities in patients with brain-stem lesions, *Neurology (Minneap.)* (1976) **26**, 769–776.

286. Newcombe, F. & Ratcliff, G. Long-term psychological consequences of cerebral lesions. In: Gazzaniga, M.S. (ed.) *Handbook of Behavioural Neurology, Vol. 2, Neuropsychology,* New York: Plenum Press (1979).

287. Prigatano, G.P., Stahl, M.L., Orr, W.C. & Zeiner, H.K. Sleep and dreaming disturbances in closed head injury patients, *J. Neurol. Neurosurg. Psychiat.* (1982) **45**, 78–80.

288. Ron, S., Algom, D., Hary, D. & Cohen, M. Time related changes in the distribution of sleep stages in brain injured patients, *Electroenceph. Clin. Neurophysiol.* (1980) **48**, 432–441.

CHAPTER 3

CIRCADIAN RHYTHMS AND SLEEP

GLOSSARY

Circadian: about one day, i.e. approximately 24 h.

Ultradian: beyond, outside, more or less than one day.

Free-running: a term applied to subjects in temporal isolation, without any external time cues.

Entrainment: synchronization to external time cues.

Masking: the hiding of one rhythm (e.g. temperature) by another interlinked rhythm (e.g. sleep–waking).

Zeitgeber (German neologism): environmental time marker.

Internal desynchronization: the separation of sleep–wake from temperature rhythms during temporal isolation.

Temporal isolation: separation from all external time markers, e.g. in a special laboratory, cave or cellar free of all time cues.

Phase-trapping, relative entrainment: quasi-rhythmic phase shifts between temperature and sleep cycles during free-running conditions. Sometimes a precursor of internal desynchronization.

Suprachiasmatic nucleus: should this be suprachiasmatic nuclei? The terminology is confusing. Individual brain nuclei, such as the nucleus accumbens, are usually referred to in the singular, although they are paired; whilst nuclear groups such as those of the thalamus and brain stem raphe are usually referred to in the plural, e.g. raphe nuclei. The term suprachiasmatic nucleus is used here to refer to the paired left and right cell complexes.

CIRCADIAN RHYTHMS

All living organisms, including plants and marine algae, as well as man, show regular cycles of rest and activity. The cycle length may be very short, seconds only (e.g. the period of the sino-atrial node); or extend over hours (e.g. eating, hunger), days (sleep–waking, rest–activity), months (the menstrual cycle), or years (weight change in cyclical depression).

Each individual cycle is determined by a number of cues. The coming in and the going out of the tide determines the luminescence cycle of some marine algae, the change in season causes the squirrel to lay up nuts and hibernate, sunshine and darkness give the cue for melatonin synthesis and determination of the correct breeding season for many farm and wild animals, and the cockerel is the morning alarm for countrymen. Circadian periodicity is largely imposed by a light–dark environment due to the rotation of the earth. One might expect most, if not all, important biological cycles related to rest and activity to have an exact 24 h period, and be entirely determined by external cues. However, this is not the case. Exact timekeeping in both animals and man, as well as being dependent on external time markers (zietgebers) is determined by internal clocks.

A Frenchman and a Swiss were the first to show that internal clocks as well as outside changes in the environment determine timekeeping. The concept of an endogenous clock was born when the French astronomer, Jean-Jacques d'Ortous de Mairan, discovered in 1729 that a heliotrope plant, which regularly opens its leaves in the morning light and closes them at dusk, continued this cycle for a while under conditions of unchanging light when the plant was placed in his closet.[8] The botanist Alphonse de Candolle added a second important piece of evidence when he showed, in 1832, that the precise period of daily leaf movements in a flowering plant was not exactly 24 h, but nearer to 26 with a progressive phase advance of 1.5–2 h each day.[7] This non-24 h cycle is also found in animals. When separated from all external time cues, man initially has a daily sleep–wake and also a temperature cycle time nearer to 25 h than 24. Why this is so is a mystery, since man has a striking ability for exact internal timekeeping and can adjust the alteration between sleep and wakefulness to exact limits even in a time cue-free environment.[25] Perhaps, as Pittendrigh and Daan[15] suggest, to enable animals and man to adapt precisely to seasonal changes in day length, some mechanism of adjustment is necessary if internal circadian rhythms are to have a stable relationship with the outside 24 h world.[13]

Aschoff[1] has described more than 100 biological functions in man that vary between maximum and minimum levels over a 24 h period (See Fig. 3.1).

The most obvious of these is the sleep–wake cycle, but there are also marked variations in the degree of mental alertness throughout the day, glandular activity by day and night, respiration, activity of the stomach, liver and intestines, urinary excretion, the composition of the blood, body temperature, and the ability to metabolize and excrete drugs. Both the toxicity and the effectiveness of cytotoxic drugs may depend on circadian variation in the rate of DNA synthesis in susceptible tissue.

The temperature rhythm is extremely stable. Over 24 h, the temperature falls in the late afternoon, is lowest during the second third of the sleep period and rises before morning awakening.

Hormonal rhythms depend on circadian factors as well as age. In pre-pubertal children, a single pulse of growth hormone secretion occurs after sleep onset. The episodic pattern of cortisol release is well known, with maximum plasma concentrations between 0400 and 0800. The rate of urinary potassium excretion varies five-fold in normal subjects across the day, and is independent of light–dark changes, activity, posture or food.[12] The activity of hepatic drug-metabolizing enzymes varies in a clear circadian fashion,[16] and likewise the rate of drug excretion.[2] In some instances the exact circadian

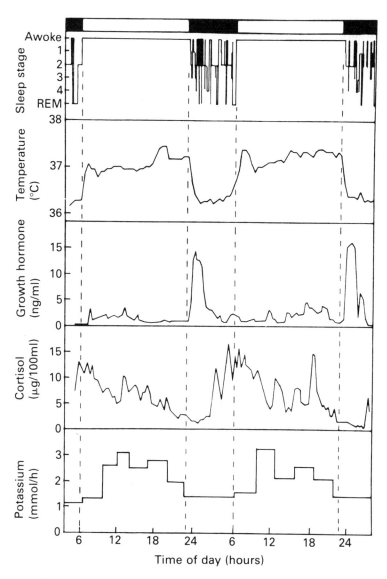

Figure 3.1.   *Circadian rhythms in sleep, body temperature, plasma concentrations of growth hormone and plasma cortisol, and urinary excretion of potassium measured over 48 h in a normal human subject. Sleep stages include REM sleep and NREM sleep, stages 1–4. Body temperature was measured rectally. The light–dark cycle is indicated by the horizontal bar at the top. Reprinted with permission from Moore-Ede et al.[13]*

timing of drug administration may be of practical importance because of changes in metabolism and excretion with the time of day.

The pattern of circadian rhythms in man is established in the first year of life and is then surprisingly stable although, with increasing age, the clock – or clocks – may slow down a little. First appearance of anything approaching normal adult sleep–wake, rest–activity cycles in infancy may depend on the establishment of retinal connections to the hypothalamic suprachiasmatic nucleus, the present main contender for the role of internal pacemaker in man. In animals, the development of these connections is linked to the development of circadian rhythms. In rodents, the suprachiasmatic nucleus is relatively undifferentiated at birth, but rapidly develops during the first post-natal days, and the retino-hypothalamic fibres develop synaptic connections with supra-chiasmatic nucleus neurones at the same time as circadian rhythms develop.[17, 18]

In human infants, the normal development of an entrained 24 h day after birth takes 3–4 months to establish. The initial four months are taken up by ultradian rest–activity cycles, waking about every 4 h. This is then followed by a steady coalescence of waking periods, which appear to free-run for some time until proper entrainment to a 24 h day occurs.[11, 27]

Do internal clocks run down in old age? Old people tend to go to bed earlier than young people, wake up earlier and have a shorter total sleep time and more arousals at night. Weitzman et al. (1983) considered that all these changes might be due to ageing of circadian oscillators. Data on this point from animal studies are conflicting. Pittendrigh and Daan reported that the length of the rest–activity cycle in rats decreased with advancing age,[15] but Wax found the reverse.[21]

Although circadian rhythms are intrinsically stable, shifts can be produced by a number of factors. Thus prolonged sleep deprivation, large temperature changes, alteration in plasma melatonin concentration, and tricyclic drugs have all been shown to alter circadian time-keeping. The effects of these are usually minor. Internal clocks are temperature-compensated, and large temperature increases in animals do not greatly affect rest–activity cycles and may even result in over-compensation. The monoamine oxidase inhibitor clorgyline and the tricyclic drug imipramine both lengthen the period of the free-running rest–activity cycle in animals and also, possibly, in man.[23, 26, 28]

In manic-depressive psychosis the switch from mania to depression and vice-versa has been associated with a major alteration in sleep–wake rhythm timing, and during this shift there may be a period of 48 h without any sleep. Wehr et al. showed that the normal coupling of sleep–wake and temperature rhythms was abolished at this period, even in subjects not in temporal isolation where internal desynchronization is an expected finding.[23] These observations have led to speculation that the promotion by antidepressant drugs of the switch from depression to mania may be associated with drug-induced changes in circadian rhythmicity. Thus stabilization of manic-depressive illness by lithium may depend on circadian effects; lithium has been shown to alter circadian periodicity.[9, 10]

As well as antidepressant drugs, sex hormones alter circadian rhythmicity. In animals, castration lengthens, and testosterone and oestradiol shorten, circadian periods.[6, 14]

The circadian pacemakers and the regulatory mechanisms of sleeping and waking are postulated to be structurally separate. The circadian sleep–wake rhythm is largely independent of sleep homeostasis (i.e. the structure and length of sleep). However, sleep deprivation causes a subsequent slight circadian delay in the next cycle; and early onset REM sleep is a characteristic feature of free-running circadian sleep–wake cycles in subjects in temporal isolation. A similar pattern of early onset REM sleep is seen in infancy, before normal circadian periodicity is established. The compensatory increase in slow-wave sleep that occurs after sleep deprivation during the next NREM–REM cycle is independent of circadian factors.[4, 22] This is also the case with the lowering of sleep propensity after excessive sleep. Thus, the system in the brain which measures and regulates the proper proportions and length of sleep is not greatly influenced by internal clocks. Even when circadian rhythmicity is abolished, as happens after suprachiasmatic nucleus lesions in the monkey, an increase in both slow-wave and REM sleep still occurs after sleep deprivation.[3]

The sensitivity of circadian timekeeping and sleep–wake alternation is exquisite. Wever[25] has recently shown in subjects living in temporal isolation that every distortion in the sleep–wake rhythm is rapidly corrected. Essentially any chance variation in the duration of a sleep–wake cycle is corrected within the next and, to a smaller amount, in the next but one cycle. A wake episode determines the duration of the following sleep episode; and a sleep episode determines the duration of the following wake period.

Perhaps the most surprising of Wever's demonstrations of the fundamental properties of the human sleep–wake cycle in temporal isolation is the finding that the total mean length of the sleep–wake cycle of females is shorter than that of males, on the average by 28 min. There is also a sex difference in the fraction of sleep in each sleep–wake period; on average, the wake episode is shorter by 1 h 49 min and the sleep episode is longer by 1 hr 21 min in females than in males, i.e. the fraction of sleep is longer by 18% in women than in men.[25]

Physiological rhythms may be affected by or associated with biochemical changes in the brain; and both generalized and regional changes in brain noradrenaline and serotonin content have been demonstrated over a 24 h period. The activity of catecholamine and 5-HT synthesizing enzymes, monoamine oxidase, tryptophan hydroxylase and tyrosine hydroxylase, varies with sleep and waking, rest or activity, light or dark over a 24 h period. There is a circadian rhythm of tryptophan hydroxylase in the pineal body in an opposed phase to the 5-HT rhythm,[20] perhaps explained by insufficient production to keep pace with the increased activity of tryptophan hydroxylation. There are also alleged differences in human pineal content of melatonin by day and night, as determined by human post mortem pineal specimens, with highest levels in nocturnal demise.[5] In the suprachiasmatic nucleus of the rat brain, noradrenaline shows a circadian rhythm with a peak value at the beginning of the light period, which suggests that a noradrenergic mechanism may be involved in oscillating biological rhythms in rats. In some brain stem nuclei, (nucleus raphe dorsalis and nucleus raphe medialis), 5-HT and 5-HIAA increase during the light period. The 5-HT rhythm in the nucleus raphe dorsalis is maintained even under constant dark conditions, and may be endogenous.[19]

THE SUPRACHIASMATIC NUCLEUS

Timekeeping in man depends on the central nervous system, not anywhere else. The idea of an internal pacemaker is conceptually attractive, but needs experimental substantiation. The search for a biological clock described by Moore-Ede et al.[47] has focussed on the visual pathways since, in adult animals in temporal isolation, the rest–activity cycle is synchronized by light–dark cycles but not by extraretinal stimulation. Richter[48, 49] initially showed that the circadian activity of blinded rats was not influenced by removal of the adrenals, pancreas, pituitary, thyroid, pineal glands or gonads; and alcoholic stupor, electroshock, convulsions and prolonged anaesthesia likewise had no effect. With brain lesions, Richter found that the only effective site where a lesion inhibited spontaneous activity rhythms was in the hypothalamus. A general area of the ventral hypothalamus was identified where lesions interfered with the timing of activity, drinking and feeding. This work finally led up to the identification of a sleepiness–activity timing mechanism in the paired suprachiasmatic nuclei (SCN) of the hypothalamus. These lie astride the optic chiasma, and comprise two clusters of small nerve cell bodies, each nucleus situated just lateral to the third ventricle. The presence of an SCN is common to birds and mammals, including primates and probably man.[41] However, most of the data refer to nocturnal mammals.

Some of the SCN small-diameter cells may have a neurosecretory function since neurosecretory material is present.[51] However, the rhythm-controlling function depends on neuronal activity, not on neuromodulator release, since circadian rhythmicity is abolished by SCN isolation with a circular cut that produces SCN disconnection from efferent and afferent pathways.[40]

Two specific substances have been identified as being produced by SCN neurones, the peptides vasopressin and vasoactive intestinal polypeptide (VIP). In addition, somatostatin occurs in the same general area. Vasopressin neurones comprise approximately 30% of SCN neurones in the human. VIP neurones are concentrated in the more ventral portion of the rodent SCN: there appear to be fewer VIP than vasopressin neurones. None of the other currently known neuropeptides have, to date, been reported in SCN neurones.[54]

The SCN are linked to the retina by the retino-hypothalamic tract. In the mammalian visual system, the major visual projection passes via the optic nerves, optic chiasma and optic tract to the lateral geniculate complex, the dorsal division of which gives rise to a prominent projection to the visual cortex. A second retinal pathway terminates in the tectal and pretectal areas. Lesions of the terminal parts of these optic pathways do not alter circadian rhythmicity or cause any loss of entrainment to light–dark stimulation. Similarly, lesions of the optic system to the midbrain tegmentum leave the entrainment of circadian rhythms undisturbed. In contrast, lesions of the retino-suprachiasmatic pathways abolish light entrainment of circadian rhythms.

A direct monosynaptic retino-suprachiasmatic nucleus pathway has been shown by tritium studies. Radioactive aminoacids injected into the vitreous humour of the eye are taken up by retinal ganglion cells and then transported through the neural projections from the retina terminating in the SCN.[42, 46] This retino-hypothalamic tract has been identified in a number of species, but not yet in man. It starts in the left and right retinal ganglion cells, and ramifies with mixing in the left and right SCN.[42] Bilateral, but not unilateral, lesions abolish light entrainment of circadian activity.

The SCN of rats projects to the ventromedial, dorsomedial and arcuate nuclei of the hypothalamus. A single projection from the SCN to the brain stem has also been identified. This terminates in the central peri-aqueductal grey matter.[33] The SCN also projects indirectly to the pineal via the inferior optic tract, superior cervical ganglia and the sympathetic fibres of the nervi conarii.[29, 45, 58] This pathway is important for retino-hypothalamic control of pineal melatonin synthesis.

There is a lot of evidence which supports the conclusion that the control of sleep–wake timing and other circadian rhythms in mammals is determined by the SCN. Three broad lines of investigation all point to this conclusion: (1) these nuclei are sensitive to overall levels of luminescence, (2) their destruction interferes with circadian rhythms, and (3) the development of SCN connections in infancy occurs in relation to the development of circadian timekeeping.

The activity of SCN neurones is increased by visual stimulation. This in turn alters the activity of sympathetic neurones that supply pinealocytes. Single SCN neurones in rodents and cats respond to visible light striking the eye in rough proportion to log light intensity.[52] This response is different from that seen in the primary visual area neurones which are affected by the spatial and temporal gradients of light intensity. Thus the SCN appears to respond to the overall luminescence level.

Lesions of the SCN have two major effects. Circadian rhythmicity of functions such as drinking, feeding, motor activity and sleep–wakefulness are reduced or abolished, but in addition the ability to synchronize these functions to light–dark shifts is lost.[30] This effect of SCN lesions is different from that produced by lesions of the retino-hypothalamic tract which cause loss of light entrainment but not the abolition of circadian rhythms themselves.

Destruction of the SCN causes loss of several different circadian rhythms. In the hamster there is loss of eating, drinking, locomotor and adrenal cortisone rhythms,[44, 55] whilst bilateral SCN lesions in the rat cause complete and permanent loss of many circadian rhythms including that of sleep and wakefulness. In primates, SCN lesions may have more selective effects from those in lower mammals and Fuller et al.[34] found that although SCN lesions in squirrel monkeys caused abolition of the sleep–wake cycle, the temperature cycle was undisturbed.

Suprachiasmatic nucleus destruction abolishes the normal circadian distribution of the rest–activity, sleep–wake cycle whilst electrical stimulation of the nucleus will entrain rest–activity cycles in a similar manner to the effect of light–dark cycles. Also, electrical stimulation of the retino-hypothalamic tract alters the firing rate of SCN neurones.[38] However, the total 24 h sleep time and the time spent in each sleep phase is unaltered.

In addition to light-imposed rhythms, SCN neurones possess an inherent rhythmicity of their own. The aggregate firing of SCN cells increases and decreases ten-fold with the circadian period in animals in constant light environmental conditions. This rhythmicity persists even when the SCN is isolated from all neuronal connections.[40] Recent studies have further demonstrated that there is a persistent circadian rhythm of neural activity in in vitro SCN tissue.[35] Unlike other hypothalamic tissue, 2-deoxyglucose uptake studies have shown that there is a circadian pattern of glucose uptake in SCN tissues in rodents under both cyclic and constant light conditions.[53] The intrinsic period of the SCN pacemaker may be altered by factors other than light. Thus oestradiol will shorten the period in female hamsters, and intraventricular carbachol will mimic the phase-shifting effect of light on the circadian rhythm of motor activity in rodents.

In ontogeny, the development of circadian rhythms goes hand in hand with the development of SCN connections. If the retinal connections are destroyed, then the SCN does not develop and circadian rhythmicity fails to become established.[50, 51]

If the SCN is indeed an internal clock, some such mechanism as envisaged by Enright[32] may be necessary to produce exact timekeeping. Enright suggested that a large number of rhythmic neuronal timers may be capable of greatly enhanced precision by their collective action, with entrainment of the minor fluctuations of each separate component.[56, 57]

As already stressed, the circadian pacemaker of the sleep–wake cycle and the regulatory mechanisms of sleep may be structurally separate, and sleep deprivation experiments carried out on SCN-lesioned rats show the normal clear increase in both slow-wave and REM sleep following sleep deprivation.[31, 37] The anatomical substrate of sleep homeostasis mechanisms is unknown but efferent pathways from the SCN must be involved in sleep-onset regulation.

The pathways through which the SCN impose their circadian rhythms on the rest–activity or sleep–wake cycle are unknown. Pinealectomy or hypophysectomy do not abolish the sleep–wake rhythm, and this is not primarily determined by light-imposed SCN-mediated changes in melatonin synthesis. Surprisingly, lesions of the caudal SCN projection to the brain stem, which might be expected to alter the control of sleep and waking, are also without effect. Groos[36] suggested that the dorsocaudal SCN projections which terminate in the paraventricular region of the diencephalon and rostral mesencephalon are the most likely candidates to couple the SCN to the other structures which control sleep.

Most of the experiments on circadian rhythmicity and function of the SCN have used nocturnal rodents, rats and hamsters. However, other nocturnal (mice, voles) and diurnal (ground squirrels) animals have been investigated with comparable results, as well as diurnal primate species. Is there a functional SCN pacemaker in man? Blind subjects sometimes have absence or inversion of the normal light–dark entrainment of melatonin rhythms, and a 24.9 h, not 24 h, day has been reported in one blind subject, despite the presence of normal environmental time cues other than light–dark cycles.[43] Arrhythmic or prolonged sleep–wake cycles have also been described following head injury, during recovery from coma and drug and alcohol intoxication, as well as in hepatic encephalopathy. The Kleine–Levin syndrome (see p. 318) may be primarily due to a disturbance of circadian rhythms; endogenous depression and the switch from depression to mania are accompanied by non-24 h sleep–wake cycles or disturbance in timing of REM sleep; and this also occurs in subjects in temporal isolation. The maintenance of semi-comatose patients in highly artificial surroundings with lack of the normal external 24 h time cues may be partly responsible for apparent loss of sleep–wake cycle activity in these subjects. Rare examples of disturbance of 24 h sleep–wake rhythms after hypothalamic parapituitary lesions with the potential for producing SCN damage[39] do not constitute definite evidence for the presence of a functional SCN pacemaker in man. The critical experiment, that of restoration of lost rhythmicity by SCN transplant, has not and is not likely to be achieved in either animals or man, since neuronal, rather than neurohormonal connections, are required for pacemaker function. However, the present evidence strongly indicates that there is a hypothalamic pacemaker in man. Indirect evidence for this may date back to von Economo, who found that encephalitis lethargica, in addition to producing hyposomnia and hypersomnia, sometimes causes the loss of regular sleep–wake cycles.

HOW MANY CLOCKS?

Does man have one or more clocks in the brain? Lydic et al.[67] have identified in man a structure analogous to the SCN of animals. This is a likely candidate for the role of central pacemaker,[70] and much importance centres on the recent demonstration of melatonin light sensitivity in the human[66] as evidence for the existence of light entrainment systems in man. Humans are much less sensitive to melatonin light entrainment than are other mammals, but the presence of any response argues for a functional retinal–SCN–pineal pathway.

In squirrel monkeys, SCN lesions destroy activity, feeding and drinking, but not temperature rhythms.[63, 69] Since an area much larger than the SCN is destroyed in these animals, a second (temperature) pacemaker may lie outside the hypothalamus. Other clues to the presence of a non-SCN pacemaker are the finding of a persistent circadian rhythm of cortisol in the cerebrospinal fluid of the rhesus monkey after total SCN ablation[71] and the dissociation of sleep and temperature rhythms during temporal isolation in man.

One major conclusion from temporal isolation experiments in man has been that, under free-running conditions, different variables develop different and independent cycle lengths.[73] Sleep–wake and temperature cycles are normally coupled. In subjects in temporal isolation, sleep–wake and temperature cycles may uncouple and run with their own natural frequency. When Aschoff and Wever[60] discovered the fact that sleep–wake cycles in humans need not remain synchronized with temperature rhythms, they suggested that two relatively independent clocks were present, only one of which was associated with the temperature rhythm. According to the two-model hypothesis of Wever[75] there are two clocks, a strong oscillator that controls body temperature and a second weaker oscillator that controls the sleep–wake cycle.

With the occurrence of desynchronization of sleep–wake cycles from temperature rhythms in subjects in temporal isolation, other rhythms tend to follow either temperature or rest–activity. The body temperature or *x standard* is followed by REM sleep and cortisol secretion whilst the rest–activity or *y standard* is followed by slow-wave sleep and sleep-onset growth hormone release. The situation is, however, extremely complex to decipher in man, in whom continuous temperature data recording is difficult and in whom hormonal cycles have many separate components. At least two components of the plasma cortisol circadian curve can be demonstrated during free-running conditions. One component follows sleep onset, with a sharp inhibition of cortisol secretion during the first 2–3 h sleep, whilst a second component has a phase advance of 6–8 h before sleep onset. On the other hand, growth hormone release is intimately related to the first hour of sleep onset in almost all sleep periods.

Kronauer et al.[65] interpreted internal desynchronization as the consequence of a small progressive change in the activity of one of two pacemakers, with a slow regular increase in the intrinsic period of the oscillator governing the sleep–wake cycle during free-run conditions. Mathematical models have been developed to explain the performance of such a system of multiple oscillators which are normally synchronized with each other, but may separate under free-running conditions.[65, 74] However, Winfree[76, 77] and Eastman[62] still doubt the existence of a second clock and argue that a single circadian clock in man determines the temperature rhythm, and that sleep habits, although affected by temperature changes, have no inherent rhythmicity of their own.

The relationship between temperature and sleep is extremely complex. Zulley[79] and Czeisler et al.[61] discovered that people in temporal isolation awaken spontaneously at a definite phase of the temperature rhythm. This is predictable within an hour or so by knowing the phase at which sleep began. However, the sleep–wake cycle may not be greatly altered by changes in body temperature. Moore-Ede et al.[69] stressed the observation that in animals circadian rhythms are temperature compensated[64, 72] and do not speed up with marked increases in body temperature as much as some other metabolic processes. It is not clear if the temperature rhythm in humans can be entrained by the forced scheduling of sleep or waking, while other factors are held constant.

Wever[75] believes that the light–dark cycle affects the temperature cycle and the sleep–wake cycle independently, although the sleep–wake cycle time period is only slightly sensitive to changes in light intensity in nocturnal species and insensitive in diurnal mammals.[59]

CAVES AND CELLARS

Much of our knowledge of circadian rhythms in man has come from experiments in which normal volunteers have lived for prolonged periods in caves in Bavaria, hospital cellars in Munich or specially constructed laboratories in the Bronx where all normal external time cues, sunshine, wrist watches, alarm clocks and fixed meal times are abolished. To date, at least 500 subjects have been studied living in temporal isolation for periods as long as six months.[92] These experiments have yielded more information about circadian rhythmicity than the study of man in the Arctic where, although 24 h light–dark cycles may be absent, the harsh and stressful environment, as well as the presence of other time cues, and the difficulty in exact continuous documentation of physiological variables, make it difficult to assess the effect of external factors on internal timekeeping.

Commencing with Aschoff and Wever,[88] who isolated normal subjects in a deep cellar beneath a Munich hospital for 8–19 days, and with Siffre et al.[95] who used an underground cave in the French Alps, all the isolation experiments have given essentially similar results.[90, 91, 96, 98] The major conclusions were summarized by Weitzman et al.[97] as follows:

1. During free-running conditions, different variables develop different cycle lengths.
2. In some, but not all subjects, a change in the phase relationship between body temperature and rest time may develop.
3. Some humans develop very long (30–50 h) rest–activity rhythms.
4. 'Social' rather than light–dark cues are important for sleep–wake cycle entrainment in man.

Non-24 h sleep–wake cycles develop within a few days of starting temporal isolation.[93, 94] Humans, on average, have a 24.7–25 h free-running sleep–wake cycle. For normal entrainment to a 24 h world, therefore, there must be a

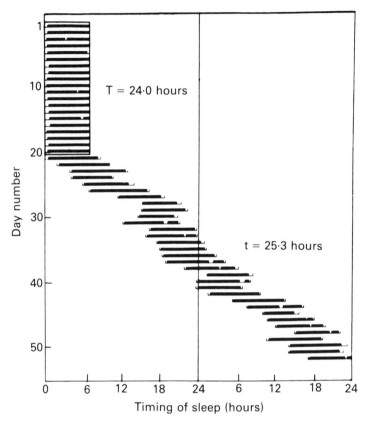

Figure 3.2. *55-day recording of circadian sleep–wake cycle in a normal human subject in a schedule-free environment.*
T: mean length of sleep–wake cycle under entrained conditions, t: mean length of sleep–wake cycle in schedule-free environment. Reprinted by kind permission from Moore-Ede et al., New Engl. J. Med. (1983) 309, 470.

40–60 min advance in the setting of any internal pacemaker each day (Fig. 3.2). With prolonged isolation, the sleep–wake cycle length may be substantially increased beyond 25 h and very long rest–activity periods of between 30 and 50 h sometimes develop.[90, 91]

Major changes in the sequential hourly timing of REM sleep during the course of the subject's sleep episodes occur under free-running conditions. REM sleep shifts to an earlier time during the 'daily' sleep episode and REM latency is sometimes less than 10 min after sleep onset. However, the total REM amount and the percentage of REM sleep in each sleep episode remain constant. Unlike REM sleep, the timing of stage 3–4 NREM sleep within the sleep episode is similar in entrained and in free-running conditions.[98] Because of this finding, Weitzman considered that NREM, but not REM, sleep was directly linked to the initiation and maintenance of the sleep process. Despite changes in the length of the sleep–wake cycle in free-running conditions, the ratio of the sleep time to total sleep–wake cycle time remains remarkably constant, at about 0.3:1.

Spontaneous awakening during free-running conditions may occur 'too early', after only a short sleep period, and be followed by a further brief, fragmented sleep period, or by full arousal with inability to fall asleep again. Despite occasional 'early wakening', the waking-up time is usually predictable from the sleep-onset time, although the sleep-onset time is not always predictable from the previous wake-up time. The transition from sleeping to waking, and from waking to sleeping may therefore be determined by different mechanisms.

Temperature and sleep–wake rhythms are almost synchronized at the start of temporal isolation, with closely matched mean day lengths. Subsequently, shifts of phase between temperature and sleep–wake cycles occur when mid-low temperature and mid-sleep times are compared. The temperature cycle length is usually more stable than the sleep cycle length. Under normal conditions, sleep onset usually precedes the lowest temperature by about 6 h but, in temporal isolation, sleep onset may begin close to the temperature low. When external entrainment factors are lacking, subjects may select sleep onset when the circadian temperature approaches its lowest values for the day. Under normal entrained conditions, there is a well described fall of 0.5–1 °C in rectal temperature following the onset of sleep, with a rise of temperature at the end of the sleep period. In free-running conditions, there is a change in both phase and shape of the temperature curve. Temperature starts to fall 6–8 h before sleep onset, with low values at sleep onset and then occasionally a subsequent minor further fall (0.25 °C) during sleep.

Some free-running subjects who develop long sleep–wake cycles also develop a long temperature cycle, but additional small amplitude (0.5 °C) 24 h temperature changes usually remain obvious.

As with sleep–wake cycles and body temperature cycles, shifts in the pattern of excretion of urinary electrolytes and pituitary pineal and adrenal hormones occur under conditions of temporal isolation.[81–83, 86, 89]

Separation of the sleep–wake and temperature cycles (*internal desynchronization*), with the development of different and independent cycle lengths, and a change in phase angle relationship between the two physiological variables has been documented unambiguously in at least 44 human subjects in temporal isolation.[101] Whether internal desynchronization would occur in all subjects if kept long enough in temporal isolation is not known. Wever[100] has shown an increased tendency for desynchronization to occur in older subjects. The temperature cycle is relatively stable in time and form and usually remains in the circadian range with a free-run period of about 25 h, but the rest–activity rhythm cycle can lengthen to 30–50 h.[80, 82, 84, 87, 97, 99]

The shift from free-running but regular circadian rhythms to the more chaotic pattern of internal desynchronization occurs in different ways in different subjects. The transition from synchronization to desynchronization is often abrupt but in a minority of subjects is preceded by 'phase trapping' with advance of sleep onset relative to temperature cycle, so that mid-sleep occurs towards the end of the low-temperature sector. The time of onset of internal desynchronization, after the commencement of temporal isolation, is also very variable but usually this occurs 30–60 days after the start of free-running periods (Fig. 3.3).

The sleep–wake cycle varies considerably in length during internal desynchronization, with alternation between several short sleep episodes (6–10 h) and one or two long sleep episodes (10–15 h). The occurrence of long sleep episodes tends to be rhythmic, being seen about once every five subjective days.

'Social' factors have been demonstrated by Aschoff et al.[85] to be more important in temporal isolation, as in a normal environment, than light–dark cues for entrainment of the sleep–wake cycle. Under both normal and free-running conditions the organization of biological time depends on the presence of external time markers or zeitgebers.

Internal desynchronization may bode ill for those experiencing it. Most subjects report feeling poorly when this happens. Insect experiments suggest that internal desynchronization caused by continued scheduling irregularities

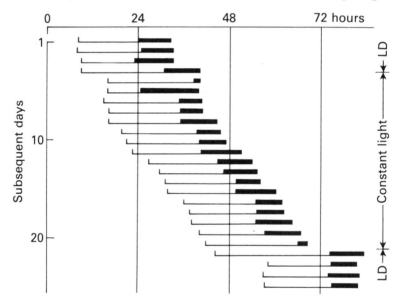

Figure 3.3. *Entrained and free-running sleep–wakefulness rhythm in an isolated human subject. Each sleep–wakefulness cycle in this record is represented by a dark bar (sleep) and a line (wakefulness). The first cycle is at the top. During the first three days of the experiment the subject was exposed to an artificial 12-h light–dark cycle (LD), to which he entrained normally. On the fourth day he was exposed to constant light. The subject develops a free-running sleep–wake cycle with a period longer than 24 h. On day 22, the previous light–dark cycle is reinstated, and following one long sleep–wake cycle the subject is again entrained. Reproduced by kind permission from Groos, G.A.* Sleep, Normal and Deranged Function, *Boerhaave Course, State University, Leiden (1981) p. 58.*

may shorten the life span, although stress is probably the causative factor here. About 20% of individuals who manifest internal desynchronization under conditions free of time cues show more neuroticism on psychometric testing and complain more about physical symptoms than do those whose physiological clocks remain mutually synchronized, but there is no conclusive evidence that neuroticism or hypochondriasis are in any way dependent on the activity of internal clocks.

ZEITGEBERS

The time period for internal clocks varies slightly from the exact 24 h necessary to maintain synchronization of the rotation of the earth with light–dark cycles. Moore-Ede et al.[104] point out that in some species (e.g. mice) free-running periods are less than 24 h in duration, so that periods must be lengthened, whilst in organisms with periods longer than 24 h (e.g. humans) each cycle must be shortened.

The light–dark cycle, dawn and dusk, is probably the strongest time marker in most organisms.[107] Light–dark cycles can successfully entrain human circadian rhythms,[103] but social factors and learned behaviour appear to be more important determinants of both circadian and ultradian rhythms in man. Powerful zeitgebers in man include compulsory sleep,[109] waking time and in particular alarm clocks,[108] knowledge of the time of day,[102] food and stimulants,[105] social contacts,[106] extremely low-frequency electromagnetic fields,[109] or even, as recounted by Winfree,[110] a young man's delight in receiving illicit daily letters whilst confined to temporal isolation and whilst the professor was out of town. Many other indices of environmental time are used by other animals;[104] marine organisms, for example, use tidal cycles as zeitgebers.

In normal healthy people, the wake-up time is probably the most powerful entrainment control point. Variation in this, at weekends and on holidays, may disrupt subsequent sleep–wake cycles. With the development of artificial lighting, day length and the duration of each illumination cycle is comparatively unimportant in man. However, most inhabitants of northern Norway sleep a little longer in the permanent dark of winter than in the permanent daylight of summer despite the occurrence in some subjects of midwinter insomnia.

PHASE–RESPONSE CURVES

The range of entrainment between zeitgebers and biological clocks is limited. In man, the period of adjustment possible is approximately ±1.5–2 h in a central clock time of 25 h; that is, between 23.5 and 26.5 h a day.[115] This phase shift will easily encompass minor variations in daily routine. However, the capacity is somewhat limited and any more prolonged variation of day length due to, for example, shiftwork or rapid time-zone travel, can cause a number of different synchronization failure disorders. The asymmetry from 24 h clock time of the adjustment that can be made is the likely explanation for the finding that eastbound meridian flight is more disruptive than westbound. Most people compensate better to westbound travel (phase delay) than to eastbound travel (phase advance). If the phase delay is greater than 2–3 h or the phase advance is greater than 1–2 h, more than one day may be required for resynchronization.[115] In some people who are subjected to long phase shifts the circadian system may adjust the wrong way round the clock (i.e. instead of an 8 h advance, a 16 h delay), resulting in severe and prolonged jet lag.[114]

How do external time markers affect endogenous circadian pacemakers? Light entrainment of melatonin rhythms may signal to the animal differing day lengths; and the melatonin itself will alter the intrinsic circadian rhythmicity of hormonal cycles in animals[117] and possibly man.[111] Moore-Ede et al.[115] stress the major advances in understanding of the mechanism of entrainment due to the experiments of Hastings and Sweeney,[113] de Coursey[112] and Pittendrigh.[116] These experiments have shown that the effect of a light pulse or other phase-shifting stimulus, such as electrical stimulation of the SCN[118] on circadian rhythms, is dependent upon the phase of the circadian cycle at which the stimulus occurs. Thus a standard light pulse given early in the night results in a subsequent phase delay, whilst if the same pulse is given late at night the result is phase advance. A similar light pulse, if given in the middle of the day, does not alter circadian rhythmicity. Sometimes, if the light pulse is too short to produce absolute synchronization of circadian rhythms, the magnitude of the phase shift achieved is found to depend on the size of the stimulus given. Different organisms achieve 24 h entrainment in different ways: in marine algae, RNA synthesis–inhibition with anisomycin will shift the phase of bioluminescence rhythms.[119] Moore-Ede et al.[115] suggest that although detailed studies of the phase–response curve have not been reported in humans, characteristics of mammalian response curves probably equally apply to the sleep–wake cycle of man.

DEPRESSION AND CIRCADIAN TIMEKEEPING

Normal subjects show some dysphoria after the loss of a night's sleep but, in contrast, depressed patients may become euphoric: bipolar depression has been linked with disturbed circadian timekeeping,[129] and alteration in the normal timing of REM sleep. According to this view, the sleep–wake disturbance seen in depression and in mania may not be secondary to insomnia, anxiety or drugs, but is a fundamental part of the illness. The evidence for this view is as follows. (1) The sleep pattern of endogenous bipolar depression is characteristic, with waking at 0300–0400; and most patients with bipolar illness sleep more when they are depressed and less when they are manic.[126] (2) The change from depression to mania can temporarily double the sleep–wake cycle. Wehr *et al.*[139] found that 13 of 15 manic-depressive patients had one or more nights of total insomnia when they switched from depression to mania, although subjects do not really like to entrain at a double period to their normal rhythm. (3) The normal NREM–REM sleep sequence is destroyed and replaced by early sleep-onset REM–NREM cycles; moreover, REM distribution in the first part of the night is bimodal, not unimodal, in patients with severe endogenous depression.[135] (4) Hormonal and temperature rhythms as well as sleep rhythms are disturbed in endogenous depression with a phase advance in cortisol release.[122, 139]

There is some evidence that antidepressant drugs alter circadian timekeeping. Lithium, tricyclic drugs and monoamine oxidase inhibitors all cause, after a 2–3 week delay, a delay in the timing of sleep–wake and rest–activity cycles in animals.[128, 139, 142] This period of 2–3 weeks delay corresponds with their antidepressant latency in man. Also, drug-induced improvement in depression is associated with a return to normal sleep–wake and cortisol rhythms.[123]

The evidence that endogenous depression is strongly linked to an upset of circadian mechanisms is far from conclusive. Although changes in circadian timekeeping are present in some depressed patients, these are not universal. The periodicity of sleep–wake behaviour is affected ultimately by any continuous disturbance of initiating or maintaining sleep. This fact alone may account for circadian misalignment in affective disorders. REM deprivation treatment of depression is not always effective, and antidepressant drugs have many actions besides their effects on circadian rhythmicity.

Severe endogenous depression is usually accompanied by difficulty in staying asleep and early morning arousal,[125] but without necessary delay in sleep onset, whilst in mania and hypomania the onset of sleep is delayed and sleep is short. Unusually in some instances, the depressive phase is associated with excessive, not reduced, total sleep length;[132] or sleep may be entirely normal.[127]

Vogel[135] has described a specific set of three REM sleep abnormalities in endogenous depression: (1) short REM latency, (2) high REM frequency, and (3) abnormal temporal distribution of nocturnal REM sleep. The most striking of these abnormalities is early onset REM sleep in patients with severe insomnia associated with endogenous depression, present in perhaps 60% of all such subjects.[121, 131] The first sleep REM period may occur 5–10 min after sleep onset and be longer than usual. There is an increase in REM sleep in the first third of the night and a decrease in the last third of the night so that the normal skew distribution of REM sleep across the night is lost in patients with severe depressive illness.[124] Also, the pattern of eye movements during REM sleep may be abnormally intense.[129–131] In some subjects with severe bipolar illness there is an increase in REM sleep time during depression and a decrease in REM sleep time during mania. None of these changes are found in secondary or reactive depression, and thus Vogel considered that the REM profile may indicate the likely pathogenesis of depression as well as predict the likely drug response.

Vogel[135] considered that the REM sleep changes of endogenous depression were unique since the combination of low REM sleep latency, high REM frequency and abnormal temporal distribution of nocturnal REM sleep is not encountered in other psychiatric disorders or medical conditions. Wehr et al.[140] suggested that the intrinsic rhythms of circadian pacemakers could be abnormally fast in endogenous depression, and that the pattern of sleep in the second half of the night might initiate and sustain depressive illness, since attempts to shift the REM sleep phase sometimes resulted in improvement of mood. Others have likened the pattern of REM sleep in endogenous depression to that seen after sleep deprivation or that occurring in free-running subjects living in temporal isolation. Weitzman et al.[141] stressed the similarity between the sleep of normal subjects whose sleep period is shifted experimentally later relative to their REM sleep rhythm, and depressed patients whose REM sleep is shifted earlier relative to their sleep period. Perhaps all the sleep abnormalities found in endogenous depression are secondary to a previous sleep deficit.[138]

In contrast to REM sleep changes in depressive illness, NREM sleep changes are much less marked, although Kupfer et al.[131] found that delta sleep is reduced in most forms of depression and some patients with major depressive symptoms or who have bipolar disorders of psychotic proportion have no stage 3 and 4 NREM sleep at all. NREM sleep loss is non-specific, and sometimes (in secondary depression) related to a primary medical illness.

The attempts that have been made to treat depressive illness with sleep deprivation and REM sleep deprivation have met with varying success.[133, 136, 137] Some of these studies have not been replicated but total sleep deprivation, or alternatively partial sleep deprivation in the second half of the night, can temporarily switch patients from a depressed to a euthymic or manic phase. Like antidepressant drugs, REM sleep deprivation may take 2–3 weeks to work (see p. 38).

Is the action of antidepressant drugs dependent upon REM sleep suppression? Most effective antidepressants cause a large and sustained reduction in REM sleep by at least 50% – from 20% to less than 10% of total sleep time.[135] Other drugs, less or non-effective in the treatment of depression, although reducing REM sleep, are much less effective at this than conventional tricyclic drugs. The combination of a delay in the timing of sleep–wake cycles with REM sleep suppression may partly account for the action of antidepressant drugs. However, ECT, which is effective in the treatment of endogenous depression, does not alter REM latency.

In endogenous depression, changes in both the timing and the control of cortisol release have been reported in up to 70% of all subjects.[134, 138] The usual findings are an overall increase in mean 24 h urinary free cortisol concentration and an increase in the degree of diurnal variation of plasma cortisol level. In addition, Doig et al.[122] found that the daily onset of cortisol secretion was abnormally advanced in endogenous depression. Peak plasma cortisol levels may occur 3–4 h earlier than usual (e.g. 0300 instead of 0700) and the nadir timing may be advanced a similar amount.

Dexamethasone suppression of cortisol release is sometimes impaired in subjects with endogenous depression. This impairment may be related to circadian factors. Ceresa et al.[120] found that high (above 2 mg) intravenous doses of dexamethasone given at any time caused a suppression of urinary 17-hydroxycorticosteroid output in normal subjects, but low dexamethasone doses achieved this only when given from 0400 to 0800. Failure of dexamethasone to inhibit cortisol secretion in endogenous depression may therefore be associated with the circadian advance in cortisol secretion in depressed patients. Whatever the mechanism, variations in plasma cortisol concentration and results of dexamethasone suppression in endogenous depression return to normal timing and amplitude with treatment and recovery. Whether the abnormal cortisol biorhythms are simply the result of sleep disturbance, previous sleep disruption or insomnia, or are linked to temporal advances in other rhythms in endogenous depression is not at present clear.

Perhaps the most striking change in depressive illness is not the hormonal or REM changes, but the early morning despair, lethargy and total misery. Similar, although much less severe, depression has been described in up to 20% of all narcoleptics who also have sleep onset REM periods. However, sleep-onset REM periods (see following section) are very unlikely to be a biological cause of depression, for this is the normal pattern of sleep in infancy as well as following sleep deprivation.

SLEEP ONSET RAPID EYE MOVEMENTS (SOREMS)

Under normal circumstances, REM sleep almost always follows rather than precedes NREM sleep, and in experimental insomnia REM sleep disappears if NREM sleep is reduced below a critical level. In normal human adults the latency from sleep onset to the first appearance of REM sleep is about 60–90 min, and the NREM–REM cycle is repeated five or six times regularly each night. This normal adult NREM-REM cycle is reversed very rarely. The exceptions are temporal isolation, narcolepsy and endogenous depression.[149, 151, 153] However, in the first month of life, more than half all sleep periods commence with REM activity.[150]

When sleep does start with REM activity, a bimodal distribution of REM peaks is often found, with a first peak at 10–20 min after sleep onset and a second at 60–90 min. This bimodal distribution has been observed in depression,[153] in infancy[152] and in narcolepsy.[149]

Disturbance of circadian rhythms often results in SOREM periods. These occur in subjects living on a very short (90–180 min) sleep–wake cycle[143, 158] and in others living on a long 48 h day.[148] Rapid time-zone shifts[145] as well as temporal isolation from normal time cues[144, 159] also sometimes result in SOREM periods.

In all these conditions, reversal of the normal NREM–REM sleep sequence has no known consequence and perhaps surprisingly there is no evidence of any change in performance, mood, memory or other aspect of physical or mental function attributable to the occurrence of REM activity at sleep onset.

The neurochemical control of REM sleep latency has been investigated by a number of authors. Sitaram et al.[154] showed that increased cholinergic activity (e.g. physostigmine, arecoline) reduced REM sleep latency. However, the majority of others drugs, although having powerful effects on REM sleep time, do not greatly alter REM sleep latency.

Circadian factors appear to be paramount in determining the occurrence of SOREMs. The propensity for REM sleep varies with the time of day/night.[146, 147, 157, 158] Thus, in narcolepsy, afternoon or evening naps are accompanied more often than morning naps by SOREM periods. The propensity for REM sleep to occur and the distribution of REM sleep within the total day–night sleep time depends on the phase relationship between bed-rest and body-core temperature.[160, 161] Usually the peak circadian distribution of REM sleep coincides with the trough of circadian body temperature rhythm.

There must be a mechanism inside the brain which determines REM rebound after REM sleep deprivation. Under appropriate experimental conditions, REM rebound can be delayed for up to five days. The concept of REM pressure, with an initial deficit of REM sleep being followed by subsequent build-up of this sleep phase, has been used to explain the SOREM activity which occurs in endogenous depression.[155]

REM deprivation is followed by REM pressure in normal subjects, but this mechanism may be faulty in narcoleptics. Spielman et al.[156] studied four male narcoleptic subjects who were REM sleep-deprived by multiple awakenings throughout the night. To achieve this, narcoleptics required many more arousals (25–38) than normal subjects. Even in narcoleptics who were prevented from taking day naps, the expected REM rebound did not occur on the recovery night.

SLEEP DISORDERS DUE TO CIRCADIAN RHYTHM DISTURBANCES

A number of sleep disorders in man have been attributed to wrong circadian timekeeping. This may be due to entrainment failure, loss of central rhythmicity, or to abnormal rhythm amplitude.[171] Perhaps some 10% of all insomniacs have a circadian disturbance of sleep–wake rhythm.[173]

Entrainment failure may be due to blindness or damage to the retino-hypothalamic tract, but also occurs in normally sighted subjects.[162, 170, 174] Most blind men retain normal sleep–wake cycle timing, due to the presence of normal social cues, but, as would be expected, many lose melatonin rhythmicity and a few have day lengths greater than 24 h.

Loss of central rhythmicity can result from damage to pacemaker structures in the hypothalamus. Some patients with hypothalamic tumours give a history of sleep–wake cycle disturbance.[163, 164] Abnormal urinary electrolyte rhythms have been documented with hypothalamic disease,[166] abnormal body temperature rhythm has been associated with third ventricular obstruction,[172] and a subject described by Moore-Ede *et al.*,[171] who was unable to synchronize his sleep–wake cycles to normal environmental cues, subsequently proved to have a pituitary tumour. A totally irregular sleep–wake pattern, lacking any inherent rhythmicity, is occasionally seen following head injury.[165]

Disorders of rhythm amplitude are described only very rarely, perhaps because they are so difficult to quantitate. Eskimos and polar explorers exposed to continuous winter dark or summer sun are the obvious candidates for investigation, and here the seasonal pattern of urinary electrolyte excretion is said to be of low amplitude.[168, 169, 171] This evidence is not very convincing. Arctic explorers in North Greenland and Japanese explorers in the Antarctic have frequent disturbances of sleep–wake timing not due primarily to circadian factors.[167, 178]

Weitzman and his colleagues have identified a group of insomniacs with an unusual phase-lag syndrome, the *delayed sleep-phase syndrome*.[175, 176] The condition is described on p. 256.

The delayed sleep phase syndrome has been viewed as the result of ineffective entrainment to normal zeitgebers. In these subjects any occasional increase in the length of sleeping or waking periods, which is unavoidable from time to time, results in a delay in the sleep phase which is very difficult or impossible to overcome.[175, 176] If this explanation is correct, however, a progressive rather than stable time of sleep onset might be expected (Fig. 3.4).

The antonym to the delayed-sleep phase syndrome, an *advanced sleep phase syndrome,* with sleep onset at 2000–2100 and waking at 0300–0500, has been recognized, but is much less common. It is not clear whether this represents a constant and involuntary dissociation of clock time and personal sleep–wake schedule, or whether the condition is primarily due to a depressive illness or laziness.[173] In any case, early-onset sleep and waking cause much less social and work disruption than the opposite pattern.

Non-24 h sleep–wake syndromes are very rare. Time keeping may correspond closely to the sleep pattern of normal subjects in temporal isolation, with a free-running periodicity of over 24 h. This results in an incremental delay in sleep-onset time and wake time to a successively later period each day. Only a handful of such cases has been described and most are in people blind for many years.[170] One subject had been followed up for 18 months without ever achieving normal sleep–wake cycles.[174, 177] There is no effective treatment, and attempts to maintain a stable 24 h cycle lead only to periods of sleep deprivation.

Totally irregular sleep–wake patterns, without any clear 24 h life cycle and no recognizable rest–activity rhythm or defined meal time, have been described by Hauri[165] in association with the combination of organic and psychiatric

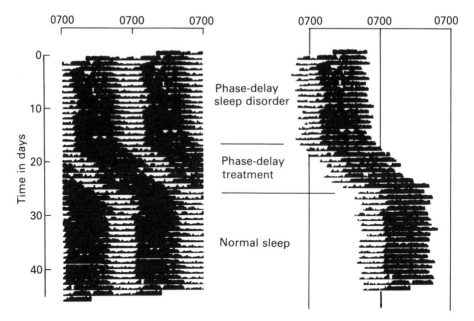

Figure 3.4.   *Rest–activity cycle as measured by a small computer-based activity monitor worn continuously on the wrist in a subject with phase-delay sleep disorder, before and after phase-delay treatment. Reprinted with permission from Wirz-Justice, A., Wehr, T.A. & Gillin, J.C. Sleep disturbance in relation to circadian rhythms. In: Kubicki, S. (ed.)* Methods of Sleep Research, *Stuttgart: Fischer (1984) 155.*

illness, head injury and severe depression, together with hypnotic drug dependency. In such a multifactorial situation, normal time cues are ignored, sleep is poor and irregular both by day and by night, and any clear pattern of circadian temperature or endocrine rhythm is absent.

Clear 24 h sleep–wake rhythms are also abolished in a number of conditions, most notably following recovery from coma and severe head injury, but also during the recovery phase from drug and alcohol intoxication. Here the maintenance of comatose patients in highly artificial environments, with lack of external zeitgebers, may be partly responsible for the apparent loss of sleep–wake cyclical activity.

Sleep reversal, asleep by day and awake by night, is sometimes described although poorly documented in elderly patients with Alzheimer's disease or related forms of senile dementia, as well as in multi-infarct dementia, although not in psychiatric disorders. Many demented subjects are extremely restless by night, very agitated and, if able to sleep at all, have very frequent awakenings. This may all be due to the combined effects of disorientation in the dark, other environmental factors, sleep apnoea, hypnotics, discomfort with joint disease, prostatism in males, normal poor sleep in the elderly, and partial loss of circadian rhythmicity rather than being a true reversal of the 24 h sleep–wake cycle. However, sleep reversal has also been described in the end stages of

South African trypanosomiasis in which the increasing colonization of the choroid plexus and neighbouring brain by the parasites of sleeping sickness may be accompanied by profound drowsiness during the day but alertness at night.

SHIFTWORK AND SLEEP

Frequent changes of sleep–wake schedule are part of modern society. A recent American health survey has indicated that over 27% of male workers and 16% of female workers have some kind of work-shift rotation.[185] Junior hospital doctors may be on continuous call for three nights and then work one night in two, and highly unusual work schedules occur in many other professions.[189, 197] Armed forces personnel are particularly at risk; American nuclear submarine crews keep an 18 h day; 6 h on watch and 12 h off.[198] There is no doubt that in all these situations mood, performance and vigilance suffer. Humans function best in a 24 h way of life.

Up to 80% of shiftworkers have been shown to develop serious sleep problems, particularly sleepiness at work and insomnia at home.[183] The sleep disorders related to shiftwork are very much determined by changes in circadian rhythms, as well as by the relative flexibility of the individual to adapt.[190]

The overall degree of disruption depends on the number of hours shifted, the frequency of the shifts, and the amount of time allowed for stable sleep–wake cycles to develop. Overall, a sudden shift from day to nightwork causes immediate sleepiness and poor performance at work and this lasts at least a week. With continued nightwork, symptoms rapidly improve, but even in the long-term reversed but otherwise completely normal sleep–wake patterns seldom develop.

The major symptoms of frequent changes of sleep–wake schedule are insomnia and sleepiness at the wrong times, overall poor performance and difficulty in realizing normal sleep–wake cycles. In European industrial workers on nightshifts during the First World War, there was a marked tendency for peptic ulcers to develop, but here several factors other than shiftwork may have been involved. However, there is no doubt that stress, severe mood changes, hypnotic dependence and alcoholism are more frequent amongst nightworkers than amongst dayworkers.

With any abrupt change in work shift, a minority of subjects can adjust their total sleep, REM time and NREM time quickly to the new sleep–wake schedule. The majority take at least a week to adjust, and sleep may even progressively worsen for a short period before adjustment starts. After shift inversion, body temperature cycles may take three or more weeks to establish a 'normal' pattern.[194] A nightworker who constantly goes to bed at 0800 and learns to stay asleep until 1600 eventually develops a low body temperature at noon and a high temperature at midnight.[192] The body temperature may be of particular importance in relation to vigilance cycles. Foret and Benoit[187] showed that the time of arousal, the time of peak vigilance and the temperature peak are all related, although the temperature peak time is more closely associated with the time for wakening than with the time of peak vigilance.

Why do some people adapt to shiftwork much better than others? Many factors seem to be involved here. As well as the nature of the shift, whether stable or rotating, and the degree of time change involved, the ability to adapt varies with age, personality and previous sleep habits. Of all these factors, the most important is the pattern of shiftwork and the regularity or irregularity of the work schedule involved.[199] However, there is such a great degree of individual variability involved that it is impossible to predict the likely degree of tolerance to changes in work shift in any single individual.[186]

Rotating shiftwork patterns are much more disruptive than fixed shift changes. As Dahlgren[184] has shown, in the long term, rotating shiftworkers have more disturbances of sleep than permanent nightworkers and very poor adjustment of body temperature rhythms. Despite this, rotating 8 h (night–evening–day) shifts are common in industry with the need for a weekly 8 h advance. As Czeisler et al.[183] point out, these shifts are in the wrong direction and involve too great time jumps. Phase delay, not phase advance, is necessary to achieve a smooth transition; and the maximum time shift that can be achieved without disruption in any single 24 h period is usually no greater than 2 h. Czeisler and his colleagues stress the importance of application of simple circadian factors to the planning of all work shifts.

After the pattern of work shift, age is the next most important factor in determining the ability for shiftwork. Young people adapt much better than old. Some studies have even indicated that there may be no long-term adaptation to shiftwork in elderly subjects.[188] The forties are the critical period, although very occasionally work schedules that require a phase advance may be tolerated better by old than by young subjects.[179]

Individual differences in the approach to shiftwork, personality traits[181, 182, 195] and normal sleep habits play a large part in determining the ability to adapt to shiftwork. Important factors documented to date include the normal distribution of spontaneous sleep[191] and the 'morningness' or 'eveningness' type.[193]

Horne and Ostberg[193] developed their morningness–eveningness ('lark–owl') scale to indicate both activity schedules and subjective feelings of activation. This index is strongly associated with bed and arising times, and, to a lesser extent, with temperature peak times.[187] Webb and Bonnet[200] demonstrated that larks – or morning types – have a less variable sleep and awakening time than owls, and also a different ability to adapt to work-shift changes.

Day sleep is unusual in normal subjects carrying out their daytime activities, but may follow sleep deprivation and is characteristic of narcolepsy, sleep apnoea and a variety of psychiatric disorders, depression, schizophrenia and obsessive–compulsive disorders. In all these conditions, day sleep may have a characteristic and different structure from night sleep;[201] but the evidence that day sleep in nightworkers is in any way unusual or poorer in quality, as compared to normal night sleep, is uncertain.

Some observers suggest that shiftworkers or people committed to schedule reversal are unable to sleep as long during the day as they habitually sleep at night[186] and sometimes day sleep is not considered to be so 'good' as sleep at night. This is probably due to environmental factors, particularly noise and light, rather than to any fundamental difference in the quality of day and night sleep. However, with early morning sleep onset, a short total sleep period and a displacement of REM sleep over the sleep period is common. This is not found when sleep starts in the early afternoon.

Circadian sleep disorders due to shiftwork may improve with reinforcement of new social time cues as well as less frequent shift changes or rescheduling of time shifts. Despite all these, many subjects and particularly the elderly are unable to tolerate any form of shiftwork. Others become chronically dependent on hypnotics.

Daytime hypnotics for use at unusual times by shiftworkers have been the subject of very few studies, and the effectiveness of these drugs for afternoon sleep and nighttime activity possibly varies from their usual effects. Nicholson and Stone[196] demonstrated that diazepam and its hydroxylated metabolites, temazepam and oxazepam had slightly different effects on day and on night sleep. Temazepam and oxazepam were less active during the day than the night. Presumably, to promote day sleep, relatively rapid drug kinetics with a limited duration of action are desirable. Flunitrazepam (0.25–0.5 mg) and triazolam in the same dosage should be successful. Bilwise et al.[180] studied the nighttime and daytime efficacy of flurazepam and oxazepam in chronic insomnia. Flurazepam produced substantial daytime sleepiness, but oxazepam did not. Oxazepam therefore, although less active during the day than the night, may be of value in the control of daytime insomnia in night shiftworkers.

JET LAG

In a study of 315 senior executives in 29 British and 20 American companies, some 87% reported sleep disturbance following air travel.[203] Jules Verne's hero took 80 days to travel round the world in 1878, Wiley Post actually flew round the world in 8 days in 1930, whilst American astronauts circled the earth in 88 min in 1965.[207] Wiley Post was one of the first to take into account the effect of time-zone travel on body rhythms. He allowed for the effect of altered sleep–wake cycles on his flying efficiency, and worked out a programme to break his habitual patterns.

Jet lag is caused, not primarily by sleep deprivation, but by desynchronization between outside clock time and internal body rhythms, including temperature and hormonal as well as sleep–wake cycles.[204] The symptoms are, however, those of sleep lack, with sleepiness and fatigue during waking periods and insomnia during sleep periods. After rapid travel across many time zones, the syndrome is universal, and symptoms may last 1–3 weeks. The severity of fatigue increases with the number of time zones crossed, especially in older subjects. Outward journeys may be more disruptive than homebound travel.[208]

There are large individual variations in the susceptibility to jet lag, although these differences may be due partly to the effect of alcohol consumption. Most airlines compensate for monotony on long trips with movies, music and a lot of alcohol. The combined effect of alcohol and high altitude may be considerable. McFarland[206] established that at 10 000–12 000 feet the alcohol in two or three cocktails had the physiological effect of four or five drinks at sea level.

Westbound flights, involving a phase delay, are less disruptive than eastbound flights which cause a phase advance. North–south flights, and return, in which time zone changes are not a factor, do not alter circadian rhythms or impair psychological performance, although they do cause subjective fatigue.

In comparison of westbound and eastbound flights, Klein et al.[205] showed that there were large individual differences in adaptation. The time taken to resynchronize sleep–wake schedules after a westbound flight phase delay of 6 h from Brussels to Chicago was up to 6 days, but after a flight the other way three of 14 subjects took 14–18 days to compensate fully. The ability to compensate for phase delay better than phase advance has been explained by the natural period of the human biological clock being set nearer to 25 than to 24 h. It seems probable that subjects who compensate well to jet leg are also able to adjust well to frequent changes in work shift.

All seasoned travellers have their own remedy for jet lag. Medium- or long-acting benzodiazepines may increase total sleep time without improving wellbeing. After a westbound flight from London to New York, a short-acting benzodiazepine with rapid onset of action, such as triazolam, taken at the new New York bedtime of 2200 and rising at 0600 may help promote a good night's sleep and rapid adjustment. Too much alcohol will interfere with sleep in any case. Many unusual methods to prevent jet lag have been proposed (e.g. 'I fly across the Atlantic every six weeks or so and I have now found a very successful way of resetting my rhythms using dexamethasone and colchicine').[209] Melatonin will cross the blood–brain barrier and is absorbed both orally and parenterally.[202] Melatonin given orally or intramuscularly will entrain rest–activity cycles in rats, the oestrus cycle in ewes and antler growth in deer, but whether it will increase the effective 'night' length and prevent jet lag after eastbound flight remains to be determined.

HORMONES AND SLEEP

There has been a recent explosion of knowledge about endocrinology in relation to sleep and the brain. The inter-relationships between hormones, sleep and circadian rhythms are discussed here for three main reasons. (1) The clinical diagnosis and investigation of endocrine disorders is often dependent on correct interpretation of circadian changes in plasma hormone levels. (These are of great importance also in considering the possible relationship between cortisol rhythms and depressive illness.) (2) The relationships between external factors (day–night, light–dark and internal clocks) and sleeping and waking and other body rhythms are controlled largely by hormonal mechanisms. (3) There is an extraordinary association between hormonal changes during sleep and the development of puberty in man.

Anterior pituitary hormones, the pineal hormone melatonin, and cortisol (under the influence of adrenocorticotrophic hormone, ACTH) are released in approximately sinusoidal fashion over a 24 h period. Hormonal circadian rhythms are determined by the activity of the central nervous system, feedback mechanisms, environmental factors, light–dark changes, food intake, temperature and social factors. In addition, the release of some, but not all, hormones is determined by the sleep–wake cycle (Table 3.1).

Table 3.1. *Circadian hormonal and catecholamine changes*

	Effect of sleep	Possible implications
Growth hormone	Sleep-onset release in man	Brain, not body, restitution?
Prolactin	Sleep-dependent Highest concentration in late sleep (0500–0700)	Unknown
ACTH Cortisol	Sleep inhibition? Highest plasma concentration in late sleep, early waking	No primary brain function?
LSH FSH Testosterone	Sleep, puberty and age-related	Initiation and maintenance of puberty?
Melatonin	Light–dark dependent	Light-entrainment of breeding seasons in animals. Sexual function in man not established, but melatonin levels vary with puberty
Serotonin	20-fold higher CSF and 1.5-fold higher brain concentration sleeping than waking (rhesus monkey)	Control of pituitary hormonal release?
Catecholamines	Circadian changes in plasma and urine adrenaline	Related to autonomic function?
Insulin	Sleep-independent	Sleep not time of body tissue repair?

The importance of the cortical mechanisms for hormone release was shown by studies in decorticate subjects by Ratge *et al.*[219] who demonstrated that an intact connection between the cortex and the brain stem, as well as an intact hypothalamic-pituitary axis, is necessary for the existence of cortisol, prolactin and catecholamine rhythms.

SLEEP IN ENDOCRINE DISORDERS

In many endocrine disorders, the pattern of sleep, as well as the pattern of 24 h hormonal release, is abnormal. There are reports of poor sleep or a decrease in REM sleep in Cushing's syndrome,[215] alterations in sleep in myxoedema, thyrotoxicosis and acromegaly, and menstrual-related changes in sleep patterns in normal women, as well as in narcolepsy and sleep apnoea. However, there is little evidence for any major effect of any hormone on sleep itself. The changes described are usually minor or inconstant and, in some instances, the explanation sometimes given (e.g. that growth hormone in acromegaly may cause 'narcolepsy' by a central effect on sleep mechanisms) may not be correct.

Mendelson et al.[216] found that the repeated administration of *growth hormone* had no effect on human sleep in normal volunteers. The evidence linking *progesterone* with sleep induction is inconclusive. With *ACTH*, both an increase and a decrease of sleep have been reported.[212, 215, 217]

WHY HORMONE RELEASE DURING SLEEP?

Thus, in most instances, hormones have little or no effect on sleep itself. However, sleep (or light–dark cycles) affects the release of most pituitary hormones and of melatonin. In no case is the function of sleep hormone release obvious. Arguments based on the possible function of pituitary hormone release during sleep in different animal species may not apply to man, and there are marked species differences in the timing, amplitude and trigger factors that determine pituitary hormone release during sleep. (1) Man, alone amongst higher mammals, has been shown convincingly to have sleep-onset growth hormone release. (2) In the rhesus monkey, growth hormone release is dependent not upon sleep onset but rather upon waking, and (3) in the rat growth hormone release is probably dependent upon light–dark cycles, not sleep itself.[218] (4) A major difference in growth hormone systems in animals and man lies in the central control mechanisms involved; dopamine does not elevate growth hormone levels in animals, but is a major stimulant in man. (5) In the rat, adrenaline is the most important catecholamine for growth hormone stimulation and GABA (gamma-aminobutyric acid) has a major inhibitory role.[221] (6) All mammals show nocturnal melatonin release, but the amplitude of this rhythm is much lower in man than in other species and light-entrainment is more difficult to produce. (7) Light inhibition or dark stimulation of melatonin release may be important cues to seasonally breeding animals, but this is unlikely to be the case in man.

Thus, sleep-determined hormonal release has different characteristics and probably different functions in different species. Most of these functions are undetermined in man, but pulsatile sleep-related release of growth hormone, LH and melatonin at pubescence indicate that these changes may be important for adolescent growth and the initiation and maintenance of puberty.

HORMONE CONTROL DURING SLEEP

The control of pituitary and pineal hormonal release during sleep is dependent on brain and possibly CSF amine mechanisms, and on hormonal negative feedback loops.

There is a circadian rhythm of serotonin release, reflected in brain, CSF and plasma concentration and urinary excretion, but this has not been demonstrated so well as changes in growth hormone, cortisol or prolactin release.[222, 223] However, a nocturnal light-regulated flooding of serotonin throughout the cerebroventricular system plays an important role in the neuroendocrine rhythm of growth hormone, prolactin and follicle stimulating hormone.[210, 220] In the rhesus monkey, nocturnal CSF serotonin concentration is 20 times greater than the diurnal concentration. Circadian changes in brain serotonin concentration are less pronounced than those found in the CSF, but may be equally important in pituitary hormone control.[220] The normal night-time increase in plasma and CSF prolactin concentration can be duplicated in daylight hours by giving serotonin intraventricularly, or by the peripheral administration of the serotonin precursors l-tryptophan and 5-HTP.[214]

Little is known of any variation in brain, CSF and plasma catecholamine concentration with sleep and waking, and most of the available evidence is based on urinary catecholamine analysis. There are marked circadian variations in urinary adrenaline (epinephrine) but not in noradrenaline excretion. Adrenaline usually peaks in the early afternoon, and night values are very low, even if the subject is awake. In experiments with adrenaline infusion, Hjemdahl *et al.*[213] reported that sleep is terminated at infusion levels of $0.18 \text{ nmol kg}^{-1} \text{ min}^{-1}$ (yielding levels of 0.7 nmol in venous plasma); but, at this level in awake subjects, diastolic blood pressure has fallen and subjects begin to report increased subjective unpleasantness (Table 3.1).

GROWTH HORMONE

The term sleep-*onset* growth hormone *release* is used in this section. The latency from growth hormone releasing *stimulus* (e.g. electrical stimulation of hypothalamic nuclei in animals, or oral levodopa in man) to *peak* plasma growth hormone level is between 10 and 60 min. During sleep, the growth hormone peak usually occurs during the first 60 min of overnight sleep during the first NREM stage 3–4 cycle. Thus the stimulus to growth hormone release may accompany sleep onset, whilst growth hormone peak levels occur during NREM stage 3–4 sleep.

GROWTH HORMONE RELEASE AND SLEEP

Growth hormone (GH) release from the pituitary is episodic (Fig. 3.5). Approximately 1–2% of the total pituitary content is released in a single burst,

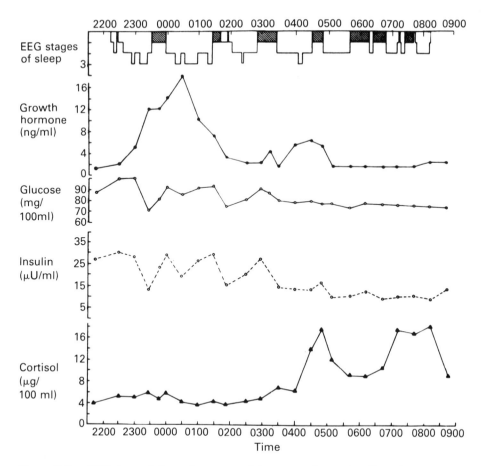

Figure 3.5. *EEG stages of sleep, plasma growth hormone, glucose, insulin and cortisol levels during a normal night's sleep in a 27-year-old man. Shaded areas are periods of REM. Reproduced with permission from Takahashi et al.*[256]

with a total of 0.5 mg GH secreted per 24 h in an adult. GH release occurs with exercise, physical stress, insulin hypoglycaemia or arginine infusion, and is suppressed by glucocorticoids. Levodopa causes a considerable rise in plasma GH concentration in man, and, in addition, somatostatin (growth hormone release-inhibiting factor, GHRIF), growth hormone releasing factor (GHRF), other peptides, metencephalin, angiotensin, histamine and GABA, all have a direct or modulatory effect on GH release.[255] However, the main stimulus for GH release in man is sleep. Sleep accounts for between 70 and 90% of the total 24 h output in a child, slightly less in an adult.

Sleep-related GH release is independent of changes in insulin or cortisol secretion[245] and mainly occurs 30–60 min after sleep onset. Following the initial peak, there are a number of secondary peaks throughout the night. Over the whole sleep period, 43% of peaks accompany slow-wave sleep.[256]

SLEEP-RELATED GROWTH HORMONE RELEASE AND AGE

Growth hormone release during sleep is dependent upon age. Below the age of 3 months, sleep-related GH peaks are not found. Between infancy and puberty, children release GH mainly, if not entirely, during sleep, with few if any spontaneous waking peaks, and a mean secretion rate of around 90 µg/ 24 h. There is a six- to seven-fold increase in this rate by adolescence, with up to 600 µg/24 h secretion rates, and frequent spontaneous GH peaks occur waking as well as sleeping. Secretion rates are somewhat lower in young adults, and in a small minority of elderly subjects no spontaneous waking or sleeping GH release can be detected, although waking responses to pharmacological stimuli are retained.[249] There are large individual variations in GH release at all ages. Age-related changes in GH release are associated with the initial increase and then decline of slow-wave sleep with age. Other factors, changes in diet, weight, and differences in catecholamine metabolism, are less important.[228, 261]

SOMATOMEDINS AND SLEEP

It takes several hours for the liver to synthesize growth hormone factors (somatomedins) under the stimulus of GH. Plasma levels of these are usually highest in the day and lowest at night, with a long lag between the peak sleep-onset GH concentration and peak morning somatomedin levels. These occur around 2300–0000.[243] Waking and sleeping somatomedin formation and clearance rates have not yet been determined in humans.

SLEEP ONSET DETERMINES GROWTH HORMONE RELEASE

GH release during sleep is determined by sleep onset, and not by circadian rhythms. No other independent human biological GH rhythm has been detected.[254] Sleep-onset GH release occurs in subjects with both normally entrained and free-running sleep cycles.[264] The effect of light–dark cycles or changes of illumination level at sleep onset appears to make no difference. Sleep secretion of GH is similar in both summer and winter in the inhabitants of northern Norway despite the absence of any sunlight during the winter.[265] However, loss of sleep-onset GH release has been reported in two blind subjects, both of whom retained arginine responsiveness.[234]

What causes sleep-onset GH release? Plasma dopamine concentrations do not greatly alter with sleep onset, and other circadian hormonal changes have little effect on GH release. Melatonin, and also sex steroids, have no effect on GH release in man.[263] The acute administration of corticosteroids does not prevent sleep-related GH release; and neither fasting nor temperature changes alter GH release during sleep.[233, 245, 252, 264] However, GH levels and cortisol levels appear to be inversely related, on waking, with GH inhibition and cortisol enhancement.[264] The system that triggers sleep onset also appears to trigger GH release. This trigger effect of sleep is seen with normal sleep onset but also in connection with the return to sleep after transient awakenings, any major phase shift of sleep, and non-24 h sleep–wake schedules. In addition, GH secretion is often disturbed in primary sleep disorders. A compensatory increase in GH secretion is observed during the eventual recovery sleep following sleep deprivation.

SLOW-WAVE SLEEP, REM SLEEP AND GROWTH HORMONE RELEASE

The release of GH is most prominent in about 95% of adult subjects in the first hour or two of the night, and highest plasma concentrations occur at a time of maximum NREM stage 3–4 sleep. However, NREM stage 3–4 sleep is not invariably related to GH peaks, and, conversely, GH release may be unaccompanied by NREM stage 3–4 sleep.[256] Weitzman and his colleagues have shown that sleep GH release may be related not to NREM stage 3–4 sleep duration but to sleep onset, although GH release occurs only when sleep episodes last longer than 36 min, when the normal sleep–wake cycle is divided into eight 1 h separate sleep periods over 24 h.

The independence of NREM stage 3–4 sleep and GH release has been shown in pharmacological studies. Drugs that reduce NREM stage 3–4 sleep do not necessarily reduce sleep GH release and vice versa. Thus, benzodiazepines reduce NREM stage 3–4 sleep, but do not alter sleep-related GH release,[253] and conversely imipramine, medroxyprogesterone acetate and free fatty acids all blunt or abolish GH release, but do not alter NREM stage 3–4 sleep.[235–237] Acute alcohol consumption causes an increase in NREM stage 3–4 (and reduction of REM) sleep but a suppression of growth hormone release.[250]

LOSS OF SLEEP GH RELEASE

An abnormal sleep GH release pattern is found in several diseases.

Acromegaly
In acromegaly, sleep-related GH peaks are usually, but not always, abolished.[225, 262] The situation in acromegaly may be comparable to that found in animal experiments in which the hypothalamus is isolated from the brain. In these animals, all episodic GH secretion is lost.[232] In acromegaly it is possible that the degree of hypothalamic control and the degree of tumour autonomy may influence both sleep-related GH release as well as the response to dopamine agonist drugs.

Hypothalamic disorders and obesity
Sleep GH responsiveness is reduced or lost in hypothalamic disorders (see Martinez-Campos et al.[238] for a review of GH secretion in neurological disorders). The observation[251] that obese persons have diminished or absent sleep-onset GH peaks suggests that some metabolic or emotional factor may be

involved in obesity. In contrast, sleep GH levels are sometimes high in malnutrition and kwashiorkor.[247]

Narcolepsy
In REM narcolepsy, there is a diminution in both the total NREM stage 3–4 sleep time and the total GH output during nocturnal sleep,[257] although, allowing for episodic GH release during long day naps and possibly also in response to amphetamine treatment, overall 24 h GH release is normal.

Growth hormone deficiency in children
In normal children, sleep-related GH release is slightly more consistent than the waking GH response to pharmacological stimuli (arginine, levodopa and insulin hypoglycaemia). These waking responses are occasionally absent in children with preserved sleep-onset GH release.[260] In children with low, but not absent, GH levels, due to congenital GH deficiency or acquired hypothalamic and pituitary lesions, including craniopharyngiomas, the opposite situation is sometimes seen, with preservation of some degree of waking insulin hypoglycaemia GH response, but loss of sleep-onset GH release.[230, 258] In a few children with extracranial (as well as intracranial) disease, both sleep and insulin-induced GH responses may be reduced or lost.[227]

Emotional as well as physical factors may blunt sleep-onset GH release. This is reduced or absent in some emotionally deprived children[248] and may be one factor accounting for short stature here.

GROWTH HORMONE CONTROL DURING SLEEP

The GH response to pharmacological stimuli is possibly different during sleep and during waking; and there may be dual-control mechanisms for GH release in the different states of consciousness. However, any differences are likely to be due to differences in drug metabolism or secondary to changes in brain amine and other neurotransmitters accompanying sleep and waking, not to fundamentally different mechanisms or pathways of GH control sleeping and waking.

In the waking state, the magnitude of the GH response to a standard stimulus is somewhat variable. Chambers and Brown[226] found a clear GH dose–response relationship to intravenous *dopa*; whereas Jacoby et al.[231] found that the response was independent of the dose. Minor differences in the sleeping and waking GH response to adrenergic, cholinergic and serotoninergic stimuli have sometimes been shown, but the GH responses to *ACTH, corticosteroids* and elevated *free fatty acid levels* are usually similar sleeping and waking.[235, 244]

Lucke and Glick[236, 237] found that sleep-related GH release was usually unaffected by acute peripheral *α or β receptor blockade* using phentolamine and propranolol. (These drugs respectively increase and decrease insulin-dependent GH release in the waking state.) With *cholinergic* responses,

Mendelson *et al.*[242] showed that piperidine facilitated both sleep-related and waking (insulin-induced) GH release. However, cholinergic inhibition with methscopolamine causes a large increase in sleep-related GH release, but only a minor change in the insulin GH response.[241] Differences in the waking and sleeping GH responses to *serotonin* have been deduced from the finding that methysergide increases sleep-related, but inhibits insulin-provoked, GH release.[240]

Growth hormone release in response to insulin hypoglycaemia, α and β adrenergic stimulation, levodopa and sleep in man is mediated by a final catecholamine pathway, which regulates the release of GHRIF and GHRF. GH inhibition can be prevented by pretreatment with anti-somatostatin antibodies.[259]. The GH response to dopamine, a major physiologic stimulant of GH secretion in man, is similar during sleep and wakefulness and probably depends on both pituitary-hypothalamic and central stimulation.[224] The feedback suppression of GH release by GH itself is similar both sleeping and waking.[239]

FUNCTION OF GROWTH HORMONE RELEASE DURING SLEEP

Sleep-onset GH release is rare among mammals, and of unknown purpose. The idea that GH release is necessary for body tissue repair during sleep may be false, although the reparative actions of fibroblasts are dependent on the presence of GH. Horne[229] stresses the possibility that sleep may be a time of tissue degradation, not repair, owing to the night-time fast; and that the primary target of GH release during sleep may be the brain, not the body.

PROLACTIN

Prolactin is important for the initiation and maintenance of lactation, but as many as 80 other actions have been suggested, including sperm transport in the seminiferous tubules in males. Prolactin levels in males are approximately 40% lower than those in females. In both sexes, prolactin release is episodic, pulsatile and sleep-related. Prolactin is synthesized in anterior pituitary lactotroph cells and has a close structural similarity with growth hormone. Despite the similar pituitary origin and molecular size, prolactin release in sleep follows rather than accompanies GH release, and under normal circumstances dopamine inhibits prolactin but causes stimulation of GH release, both sleeping and waking.

PROLACTIN RELEASE

Prolactin synthesis and release are under predominantly inhibitory control. The major physiologically active prolactin inhibitory factor is dopamine. Non-catecholamine releasing and release-inhibiting factors have not yet been identified. However, hypoglycaemia, mental and physical stress, and TRH (thyrotrophin-releasing hormone), which directly stimulates the lactotroph cell, all cause prolactin release. Histamine, cimetidine, corticosteroids, endorphins, and serotonin modulate the prolactin response to dopamine.[270-274] Prolactin, unlike GH, is not influenced by cholinergic drugs. Neither methscopolamine nor piperidine alters sleep-related prolactin release.[268, 269]

SLEEP AND PROLACTIN

For over a decade it has been known that prolactin, like GH, has a prominent circadian rhythm, with in both cases a strong relationship between hormonal secretion and sleep. Partial or complete inversion of the sleep–wake cycle causes an immediate shift of prolactin secretion.[274] The association between sleep and prolactin release is also shown by the finding of prolactin surges during daytime naps.[271] It has been reported that prolactin secretion is related to the end of REM periods,[268, 271] but this appears to be an artefact. When sleep is abolished, there is a compensatory increase in prolactin during recovery sleep.

Over a 24 h period, plasma prolactin levels are highest during late night sleep, usually at 0500–0700, with a fall to lower values on waking. A separate prolactin pulse may occur 40–60 min after the initial sleep-onset GH release. Waking (or possibly the physical activity of arousal) sometimes results in a brief pulse of prolactin release. Pulsatile release and rapid metabolism (prolactin is rapidly metabolized with a half-life of about 20 min) result in very uneven plasma concentration over the 24 h period. Prolactin enters the CSF via the choroid plexus. Cerebrospinal fluid mean prolactin levels are similar to those observed in the serum, with low levels (2 ± 0.3 ng/ml) during daytime and higher levels (3.3 ± 0.1 ng/ml) at night.

Elevation of sleeping, as well as waking, prolactin levels occurs with phenothiazines, butyrophenones and other long-acting dopamine antagonists. In contrast, levodopa, with a plasma half-life of 90–120 min, causes only a brief depression of prolactin levels, although dopamine agonist ergot drugs (bromocriptine, lisuride and pergolide) bind irreversibly to the receptor on the lactotroph, and cause night-long prolactin suppression after a single evening dose.

The normal circadian rhythm of prolactin secretion may be damped in the presence of physiological hyperprolactinaemia (pregnancy, lactation), as well as in pathological hyperprolactinaemia (due to a pituitary prolactinoma, liver and kidney disease, hypothyroidism or drugs). In these conditions, waking prolactin levels may be as high as sleeping levels, but frequent sampling usually reveals some evidence of episodic hormonal secretion.[267, 270] With very high plasma prolactin concentrations, and with large prolactinomas, variation in plasma level sleeping and waking may be difficult to detect. In primary sleep disorders, the normal pattern of prolactin secretion may be disturbed and, on the whole, prolactin and GH secretion have somewhat similar patterns in the sleep–wake cycle.

CORTISOL AND ACTH

CIRCADIAN PATTERN OF CORTISOL RELEASE

Cortisol release is episodic, with an average of 9–11 bursts spread over a 24 h period, closely following bursts of ACTH secretion,[277, 278, 289] although the physiological morning peak of cortisol release may not depend on previous pituitary ACTH secretion. The pattern of cortisol release is asymmetric over 24 h, since the amplitude and frequency of cortisol bursts are greater in late sleep and early waking than at other times. Because of this, mean plasma cortisol levels are generally highest between 0600 and 0800 and lowest from 0000 to 0200. There may be no release at all of cortisol between 2200 and 0200 (as well as at other times). Diurnal cortisol levels, unlike GH, do not greatly alter with age, and are similar in young and old people.

The circadian pattern of ACTH release is closely similar to that of cortisol release, being lowest in the initial hours of sleep, and highest in late sleep.[284] Pulses of cortisol release are either endogenous and due to a programmed circadian pattern of ACTH release, or result from meals, physical or emotional stress, or temperature changes.[287] In normal subjects there is some correlation between episodic cortisol and aldosterone release, which is preserved even in subjects with primary aldosteronism.[280–282]

CORTISOL RELEASE DEPENDS ON CIRCADIAN RHYTHMS MORE THAN SLEEP

Although most cortisol and ACTH bursts occur in late sleep and early waking, and at times when REM sleep is maximal,[284] the basic circadian rhythm of ACTH and cortisol secretion is not closely related to the sleep–wake cycle. Indeed, sleep may inhibit cortisol release. Interestingly, cortisol inhibition may coincide with GH release. Recently, Weitzman et al.[293] have shown in normal subjects in temporal isolation that cortisol secretion is reduced during sleep, even when sleep occurs at times when the subject would usually be awake. Sleep deprivation studies have not given consistent results, but both ACTH and cortisol release are independent of changes in the REM–NREM cycle, and are not altered by 1–2 nights of sleep deprivation.[285] Inversion of the sleep–wake cycle in man does eventually cause a shift in plasma cortisol level, but this does not occur until 1–2 weeks after the sleep shift.[290] Further evidence of independence of the diurnal ACTH rhythm and the sleep–wake cycle is shown by the finding that there is a lag of several days for the ACTH cycle to shorten or lengthen in response to shortening or lengthening of the sleep–wake cycle. However, normal subjects placed on a 3 h sleep–wake cycle for 10 days retain a 3 h cycle of cortisol secretory episodes which is entrained to the 3 h sleep–wake cycle, although this does not alter the average 24 h cortisol output, the number of secretory episodes or the total secretory time.[291] In some of these subjects, sleep had a minor inhibitory effect on cortisol secretion.

In attempts to separate the effects of sleep–wake and light–dark cycles on the release (or inhibition of release) of ACTH and cortisol, blind people have been investigated. These studies indicate that the change from sleep to waking, but not that from waking to sleeping or from light to dark, is of importance, and most blind people retain a normal and definite circadian pattern of cortisol secretion.[292] In free-running subjects in temporal isolation, the episodic pattern of cortisol secretion is linked to the body temperature rhythm as well as to the sleep–wake cycle.[288] Spontaneous cortisol release depends on stable repetition of body rhythms, and not on the sleep–wake cycle itself.

There is a close correlation between the circadian patterns of cortisol and β-endorphin release. In normal young subjects. lowest levels of plasma β-endorphin concentration occur between 2200 and 0300 and highest levels between 0400 and 1000. ACTH and β-endorphin are derived from a common precursor, proopiocortin, and concomitant secretion of the two hormones occurs in Cushing's disease and Nelson's syndrome. No relationship between β-endorphin release and any sleep stage has been discovered.[276]

DIURNAL CORTISOL SECRETION IN DISEASE

Addison's disease
In Addison's disease, despite reduction of cortisol secretion or diurnal cortisol variation, episodic ACTH release continues.[283]

Adrenal neoplasm and hyperplasia
In hypercortisolaemia due to adrenal neoplasm or hyperplasia, ectopic hormonal production, anorexia nervosa or prostatic carcinoma in men, the plasma concentration of cortisol is usually increased throughout the 24 h period. In these conditions, cortisol may still be secreted episodically, but a loss of circadian rhythmicity or reduction in the rhythm amplitude (the variation between day and night cortisol levels) is usually found. In non-ACTH responsive adrenal hyperplasia or adenoma, in most instances all circadian rhythmicity is lost, although cortisol continues to be secreted in irregular episodes. In a minority of patients with proven adrenal cortical adenomas, a minor variation between day and night levels is retained but the range of cortisol values over 24 h is very narrow.[286]

Cushing's disease
Boyar et al.[275] demonstrated that although patients with proven pituitary ACTH-secreting tumours had higher plasma cortisol levels than normal by day and night, the coefficient of variation between day and night values was decreased. However, very occasionally in Cushing's disease the 24 h rhythm of cortisol secretion is retained, or even sometimes exaggerated.

Cyclical Cushing's syndrome
Cyclical Cushing's syndrome is a rare disorder in which rhythmic fluctuations

of ACTH secretion result in a more or less predictable cyclic variation of adrenal steroid production.[279] Cyclical Cushing's syndrome has been reported in patients with pituitary tumour and bronchial carcinoma, as well as in adrenal hyperplasia. The cycle periods generally range from 7 to 18 days, but one unusual patient with a cycle length of approximately 88 days has been reported. These different cycle lengths can cause difficulty in interpreting diagnostic tests to differentiate the various causes of Cushing's syndrome. In a 57-year-old woman with Cushing's syndrome studied by Jordan et al.[279], two abnormal ACTH biorhythms were present; a circadian rhythm with peak ACTH and cortisol values in the afternoon (1200) in contrast to the normal early morning peak, but also a 1–6 day cycle which averaged 4.4 days.

MELATONIN

Melatonin occurs in the retina, some brain stem nuclei, and the pineal gland.[339] The human pineal gland contains between 24 and 6860 pmol/g melatonin.[299] Melatonin is released at night, but this depends on illumination level rather than on sleep. Human subjects have low blood levels (0–50 pg/ml) during the day, and high levels (80–200 pg/ml) at night, the highest concentration occurring between 0100 and 0500. These variations are also found in the CSF and urine.[342] Comparison of nocturnal plasma and urinary melatonin (and metabolite) levels shows a good correlation, with a characteristic urinary circadian melatonin excretion rhythm, which is highest at 2300–0300.[323]

MELATONIN AND AGE

The 24 h melatonin profile in humans changes with age and puberty, although morning levels do not alter with sexual maturation or with age. Nocturnal secretion is established in infancy. Initial reports indicated a two- to three-fold increase in nocturnal secretion at the time of puberty.[308, 311, 333] However, sensitive assays have shown that night-time serum melatonin levels may be very high at an earlier age, with levels above 200 pg/ml in pre-pubertal children younger than 7 years of age, with a fall to 120 pg/ml in older children, and a further reduction to 50 pg/ml in young adults. Nocturnal plasma concentrations of luteinizing hormone (LH) tend to vary inversely with those of melatonin.[346]

MELATONIN IN THE CSF

As with plasma melatonin levels, the concentration of melatonin in the CSF at night decreases in the elderly.[301] Melatonin is released into the blood, and reaches the CSF compartment secondarily, despite the proximity of the pineal to the third ventricle.[342]

CIRCADIAN MELATONIN RELEASE

A circadian rhythm of melatonin release has been found in all animals studied (even in the nine-banded armadillo, which lacks a distinct pineal gland[314, 315]) with low melatonin levels by day and high levels by night.[337] The degree of nocturnal melatonin elevation is much higher in some species, and particularly in nocturnal mammals such as the rat, than in man, although the time at which maximum elevation of plasma melatonin concentration occurs (about 2.5 h after exposure to darkness, and 1.5 h after sleep onset) is comparable in many species.

MELATONIN AND LIGHT

The major factor controlling the melatonin rhythm appears to be the total hours and illumination level of daylight, rather than the sleep time. Other factors, including physical stress, do alter plasma melatonin concentration, but are of minor importance. Levels change somewhat with the menstrual cycle[347], as well as with the season of the year,[297] although here the effect of different day lengths may be all-important. The effects of sleep alone on the melatonin rhythm are minor. A circadian pattern of melatonin persists for at least several days of wakefulness.[319]

Sunlight, very high levels of artificial illumination and changes in day length affect melatonin release in man. An increase in day length during a westbound jet flight from Brussels to Chicago causes a decrease in total 24 h melatonin secretion (sleeping and waking), although some rhythmicity is maintained. Eastbound flights, with shortening of day length, cause more disruption, and all rhythmicity of melatonin release may be lost. It can take up to 11 days after both westbound and eastbound flights for melatonin acrophases to adapt to local time.[312]

There is a fairly consistent 6 h difference between melatonin and cortisol rhythms in man. This is abolished by meridian shifts, and ACTH rhythms take 2–3 days longer than melatonin rhythms to adapt to time-zone travel (an average of 14 as compared to 11 days). This temporal dissociation indicates separate control of ACTH and melatonin release.[312]

The human pineal is light-sensitive, but only at intensities and frequencies similar to those of daylight.[326] Blind men have very variable patterns of melatonin release over 24 h. Abnormal melatonin rhythms were discovered in six out of ten blind subjects investigated by Lewy and Newsome.[325] One of these subjects released melatonin by day, not by night, and another had a free-running melatonin period of 24.7 h, not 24 h.

These results indicate that the circadian periodicity of plasma melatonin peak levels in the night is primarily determined by the light–dark cycle, with less dependence on the sleep–wake cycle and no dependence on changes in sleep stage.[328, 343–345, 349]

MELATONIN SYNTHESIS

Serotonin is converted to melatonin in the pineal gland by a two-step process which involves the enzyme serotonin N-acetyltransferase (NAT) and hydroxyindole O-methyltransferase (HOMT). The activity of NAT is thought to rate-limit the amount of melatonin formed. Both the activity of NAT and HOMT and the pineal content of melatonin show a pronounced daily rhythm, with a 30- to 60-fold nocturnal increase in NAT and a 10- to 20-fold increase in pineal melatonin in the rat.[335] HOMT activity in the pineal gland remains unaltered with age,[348] but is altered by sleep and darkness.[318, 349]

As with melatonin, there is a large diurnal rhythm for serotonin, which in the rhesus monkey reaches 20–70 times higher peaks in the CSF by night than by day. The concentration of CSF serotonin at night exceeds that of melatonin 50-fold, and may contribute to some of the effects attributed to melatonin.

The light–dark cycle may affect the synthesis of serotonin as well as of melatonin. Both light and propranolol suppress the nocturnal elevation of serotonin in the CSF of rhesus monkeys.[313]

ANATOMICAL BASIS OF LIGHT ENTRAINMENT OF MELATONIN RHYTHMS

Pinealectomy abolishes the plasma melatonin rhythm but does not alter normal diurnal changes in retinal melatonin concentration.[350] The neural organization behind this rhythm is situated in the retina and hypothalamus. Lesions of the suprachiasmatic nucleus of the hypothalamus, but not other areas, result in loss of the melatonin rhythm in both rats and monkeys.[322, 338] The effect of light is mediated by the retino-hypothalamic tract, which extends from the retina to the suprachiasmatic nucleus.[330] There appears to be no negative feedback effect of melatonin on its own synthesis and release.[320, 321]

ALTERATIONS IN PLASMA MELATONIN LEVELS WITH DRUGS AND DISEASE

Interference with 5-HT synthesis alters plasma melatonin levels. Increase in 5-HT levels following the use of 5-HTP causes an increase in plasma melatonin level,[331] whereas the beta blocker atenolol, probably other beta blockers, and extracerebral decarboxylase inhibition with benserazide (used in combination with levodopa in the treatment of parkinsonism) result in low 24 h melatonin levels.[305, 316]

Hypothalamic-pineal disease causes marked changes in plasma 24 h melatonin levels. Destructive hypothalamic and pineal lesions usually cause low or absent levels, with high levels in hepatic disease due to failure of metabolism. Ten-fold increases above normal in plasma melatonin level may occur in hepatic failure, with failure of melatonin degradation to 6-hydroxymelatonin. Melatonin levels are also increased in patients with pineal tumours.[298] In functional hypothalamic disorders, extreme obesity, premature as well as delayed puberty, the Prader–Willi syndrome (extreme obesity and delayed puberty) and the Kleine–Levin syndrome, day–night melatonin levels are usually normal, an argument against any dysfunction of the suprachiasmatic nucleus of the hypothalamus in these conditions.[341] However, there are minor changes in melatonin secretion, with increase in body weight, following meals and after fasting.[294]

Abnormal melatonin rhythms, with both high and low nocturnal release, have been described in a wide variety of psychiatric illnesses, but results are inconsistent and have no definite relationship to possible changes in circadian rhythm in either schizophrenia[310] or depressive illness.[347]

ACTIONS OF MELATONIN

The pineal appears to be an intermediary between the environment and the neurohormonal system. It acts as a transducer of photoperiod information, and may give seasonal time clues.[327, 336] These functions seem unlikely to be of importance in man, but may be vital in animals which need this information to regulate breeding. There is convincing proof that the pineal melatonin level of seasonally breeding animals affects the gonadal status, but there is little evidence for any reproductive function of melatonin in man. Abnormal (both high and low) plasma melatonin levels have been reported in idiopathic precocious and delayed puberty in humans, but the range of individual variation in plasma melatonin concentration is considerable in normal subjects. Also, sometimes these results may be due to unsuspected pinealomas.[304]

The reproductive effects of melatonin in animals (but not demonstrated in man) include the regulation of prostatic androgen metabolism, gonadal responsiveness to luteinizing hormone, maintenance of ovulation, and modulation of pituitary control mechanisms. Non-reproductive actions of melatonin reported in animals include changes in carbohydrate metabolism, control of heat production and adipose tissue formation, prostaglandin release, production of analgesia, and inhibition of dopamine mechanisms.

Pavel et al.[332] suggested that melatonin could induce REM periods at sleep onset in narcolepsy. In an uncontrolled study, 50 mg melatonin i.v. given to three narcoleptics was followed by an increase in REM sleep and reduced REM sleep latency compared with melatonin given to normal volunteers. However, there is little evidence that melatonin has a primary role in sleep regulation (see below).

MELATONIN AND ANIMAL REPRODUCTION

The use of melatonin as a seasonal time cue is now a commercial story.[327] Oral administration of melatonin to animals in water or in their feed, or as a small subcutaneous implant, will cause high or constant levels of melatonin and alter breeding season in ewes, other farm animals, and deer.[296, 302] Oral administration of melatonin will induce antler maturation and rutting behaviour in male deer, and Kennaway et al.,[320, 321] working in Adelaide, have shown that giving sheep 2 mg of melatonin produces a physiological 'night-time' increase in the blood level of melatonin lasting up to 8 h. This will induce a short-day response in the animal, even when given in prolonged daylight, and alter the oestrus cycle.

Two problems remain. Prolonged treatment with melatonin in animals leads to refractoriness; and, although giving melatonin is a convenient way of inducing winter changes in the summer, the reverse has not yet been achieved. However, a blocker of melatonin synthesis such as benserazide[316] or a melatonin antiserum might achieve these results.[327]

MELATONIN AND SLEEP

Melatonin has a number of minor actions on sleep. These are species-dependent. Pinealectomy or injection of melatonin does not alter circadian activity rhythms of the rat,[303] but melatonin does cause dose-dependent reduction in sleep latency and the time spent awake, with an increase in both slow-wave sleep and REM sleep, without any overall change in EEG pattern in some species. There is anecdotal evidence that melatonin causes mild sleepiness or sedation in man,[324] but reports of EEG changes in man are conflicting. Cramer et al.[306, 307] reported that melatonin caused a reduction in sleep latency, but no other specific change, whereas Fernandez-Guardiola and Anton-Tay[309] found that melatonin caused a large increase in light sleep (NREM 2) at the expense of deep sleep (NREM 3 and 4), with an increase in the number of awakenings throughout the night.

How might melatonin promote sleep? Holmes and Sugden[317] reported that melatonin did not elevate brain serotonin levels, or alter noradrenaline or dopamine levels in the rat, and concluded that, although subtle changes in these amines may not have been detected, the sedative effect of melatonin was likely to be due to other causes, perhaps through an interaction of melatonin with benzodiazepine receptors. In support of this idea is the finding that melatonin can inhibit the binding of ^{3}H-diazepam to synaptosomal preparations.[329] The melatonin metabolite N-acetyl-5-methoxykynurenamine (AMK) is ten times more potent than melatonin in this respect. Not only do benzodiazepines and melatonin promote sleep, but melatonin at high doses shares the muscle relaxant and anticonvulsant properties of the benzodiazepines.[340] Holmes and Sugden[317] stressed the structural similarities between AMK and the ß-carbolines, one of which may be an endogenous ligand for the benzodiazepine receptor.[300] Perhaps the psychopharmacological effect of melatonin is due to an action as a ligand at benzodiazepine receptors. However, the brain concentration of melatonin is very low, and melatonin is unlikely to be an endogenous sleep-promoting factor.

Can melatonin alleviate jet lag? In rats, melatonin may act as a zeitgeber or synchronizer of the rest–activity cycle.[334] A similar action has not yet been demonstrated in man, although Arendt and Marks[295] have speculated that melatonin may hasten the resynchronization of human 24 h rhythms disturbed by time-zone changes.

SLEEP AND THE KIDNEY

Secretion of hormones influencing water and electrolyte balance – antidiuretic hormone (ADH), aldosterone, renin and prolactin – shows, with the exception of prolactin, few sleep-related changes. Urine volume decreases and osmolarity increases during the night, but there is little evidence that this is due to sleep-related ADH release, but more to decreased glomerular filtration, as well as to a possible rhythm of renin release.[352]

ADH is released in a pulsatile, episodic manner, both sleeping and waking, with no overall relation to sleep stage or time of night.[356] One early study of renal activity during sleep in elderly men showed that urine volume decreased and osmolarity increased in conjunction with REM sleep,[353] but there is no convincing evidence of REM sleep-related ADH release. Changes in posture, reduced fluid intake and neural factors other than ADH release influence urine volume during sleep.

A *low-sodium diet* may be associated with disturbed sleep patterns. Vitiello *et al.*[357] found that normal men eating less than 500 mg per day of sodium in the diet had increased wakefulness and decreased slow-wave and REM sleep. Since these sleep changes are similar to those of normal aged subjects, who also have elevated daytime and nighttime plasma noradrenaline, the authors considered that therapies altering sympathetic activity may affect sleep.

Interest in the Brattleboro *diabetes insipidus rat* with a chronic lack of vasopressin (ADH) has resurged with the interest in brain peptides and the impaired ability of these animals for memory consolidation. Danguir[351] reported a 38% reduction in paradoxical sleep time in the Brattleboro rat. This was restored to normal by vasopressin, but also by changes in daily water intake, indicating that the paradoxical sleep defect was not due to the absence of vasopressin, but more probably to the need for these animals to rehydrate themselves continuously.

No consistent circadian or ultradian rhythm of *renin* release has been observed with marked variability by day and night, waking and sleeping. However, minor nocturnal variations in plasma renin activity have been linked with changes in the state of sleep. Mullen *et al.*[354] showed that REM sleep was associated with a virtual cessation of renin production. The onset of REM sleep was followed by a decrease in plasma renin activity, which continued throughout this sleep phase. No association between the specific stages of sleep and *aldosterone* has been found.[355]

THYROID HORMONE AND SLEEP

Thyroid stimulating hormone (TSH) levels show a circadian pattern with high levels in the evening before sleep onset.[363] With very frequent plasma sampling, circadian variation in serum T_3 and T_4 levels is also apparent in normal subjects with highest concentrations during sleep,[358, 362, 364] although T_3 and T_4 levels do not exhibit exactly the same patterns as TSH. When sleep is displaced, the TSH evening increase usually continues past the habitual peak and is broken either by sleep onset or by the daytime circadian decline. Sleep or sleep onset may exert a direct inhibitory effect on TSH secretion, modulated by its own stimulatory hypothalamic hormone, TRH, and possibly by somatostatin (GHRIF).[360]

In children aged 6–10 there is a circannual rhythm of TSH secretion, with an annual crest in December in Italy (Fig. 3.6).[359]

Physical exertion, rather than sleep, in combat exercise studies in Norwegian military personnel is a major stimulant to the thyroid hormones (T_4, FT_4, T_3, rT_3). Sleep deprivation does not usually have any significant influence on thyroid hormone serum levels, despite causing considerable alterations in other endocrine functions.[361]

GONADOTROPHINS AND SLEEP

Luteinizing hormone and testosterone are released episodically and at frequent intervals by both day and night. Pulsatile follicle stimulating hormone (FSH) release also occurs but has not been well characterized in any species. The pattern of release during sleep varies with age, and is related to the sleep stage. Hormonal release during sleep seems to be involved in the initiation and maintenance of puberty.

Before puberty, the mean serum and urine gonadotrophin levels slowly increase from age 5 to 10.[374, 380] At this stage of development, mean gonadotrophin levels are similar, sleeping and waking. LH release occurs with high frequency but low amplitude throughout wakefulness, with higher amplitude pulses at lower frequency rates. LH release at 70–90 min intervals has been detected during sleep, sometimes matching the temporal sequence of NREM–REM cycles, although the distribution is mainly random.

In early puberty, high-amplitude periodic episodes of LH release occur much more often during sleep than during waking in both boys and girls.[365] During late adolescence and in adult life, LH release occurs during wakefulness as well as during sleep, so that, as in early childhood, the total hormonal release during sleeping and waking is approximately equal although there are some differences in LH release during sleep in adult men and women. In adult males, random LH peaks occur both sleeping and waking. In adult females, LH release is slightly more rhythmic over 24 h than in men,[371] although the size of the pulse varies in relation to the stage of the menstrual cycle, and in some women the mid-cycle ovulatory LH surge is most obvious during the late hours of sleep or just after waking. In normal women, sleeping and waking LH secretion is modulated by progesterone.

Sleep inversion causes an immediate shift of nocturnal LH release in pubertal children.[371]

In adult women, sleep-dependent LH release is not determined by oestrogen feedback or by ovarian function, since patients with gonadal dysgenesis (Turner's syndrome) retain pulsatile sleep-related LH secretion,[366] although, in

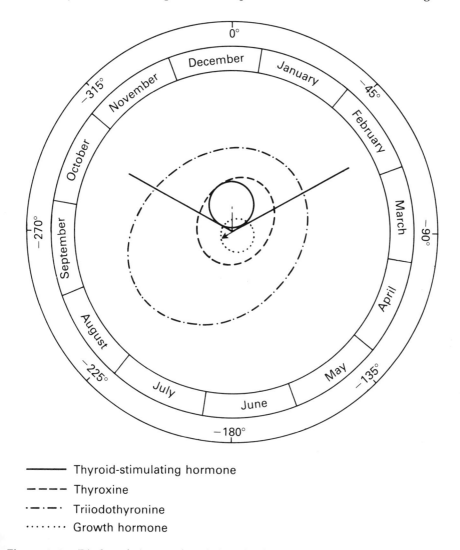

———— Thyroid-stimulating hormone

- - - - Thyroxine

·—·—· Triiodothyronine

········ Growth hormone

Figure 3.6. *Display of circannual variations in thyroid-stimulating hormone, thyroxine, triiodothyronine and growth hormone concentration. Reproduced with permission from Bellastella et al.* [359]

hypogonadal males, the amplitude of sleep-related gonadotrophin pulses is increased.

It is not clear whether FSH possesses a diurnal rhythm in adults, but frequent sampling every 20–30 min has not revealed a definite circadian or ultradian rhythm.[378] During puberty, however, FSH behaves somewhat like LH.

The role of the CNS in the control of sleep-related gonadatrophin release may be particularly important in children with abnormal sexual development,[373] many of whom have abnormal nocturnal gonadotrophin secretory patterns. Pubertal gonadotrophin secretion may be absent in girls with the McCune–Albright syndrome (café au lait skin pigmentation, fibrous dysplasia of bone and precocious puberty). Sleep LH release is abnormal in rhythm or amplitude in some children with other forms of precocious puberty, and also in young girls with the polycystic ovary syndrome. Some patients with hyperprolactinaemia have unusually low nocturnal (as well as daytime) LH secretion.[372] Sleep-related episodic LH release has been demonstrated as early as 18 months[365, 369] in children with precocious puberty, and long-term suppression of gonadotrophin release is effective treatment for central precocious puberty. In teenage girls with the polycystic ovary syndrome, daily, non-ovulatory, waking rather than sleeping, LH surges occur 7–8 h later than normal.[381] Perhaps polycystic ovaries are the result of a central nervous system disorder. There is some evidence of decreased endogenous dopamine and opioid inhibitory influences on LH secretion in the polycystic ovary syndrome, so perhaps a hypothalamic defect in endogenous dopamine or opioid control may be responsible.[367] This is a possible explanation for the occasional effect of the dopamine agonist bromocriptine in this disorder. Bromocriptine causes a subjective improvement in hirsutism, increase in the frequency of menstruation, restoration of cyclic ovarian function and reduced androgen synthesis.

TESTOSTERONE

In males, testosterone release occurs mainly at night, sometimes in conjunction with REM sleep[368] and the transition from NREM to REM sleep may have a close relation to testosterone release. Overall, modulation of testosterone release with sleep stage changes contributes little to the total 24 h variation, and sleep has much less effect on testosterone release than on GH or prolactin. Maximum testosterone levels occur at about 0700–0800.[375, 376] Weitzman[379] suggested that this testosterone release was the result of alterations in testicular blood flow during sleep: the testosterone was of testicular origin, and not associated with cortisol-correlated pulses of androstenedione and dehydro-3-epiandrosterone.[377] At the time of puberty, and also in young adults, testosterone release is sometimes modulated by a previous LH pulse, and the control of nocturnal episodic testosterone secretion during puberty may be related to LH secretion. Acute changes in the sleep–wake cycle cause an immediate shift in testosterone release, as well as in LH release in pubertal boys, and testosterone is strongly reduced by sleep deprivation.

REFERENCES

CIRCADIAN RHYTHMS

1. Aschoff, J. Exogenous and endogenous components in circadian rhythms, *Cold Spring Harbour Symp. Quant. Biol.* (1960) **25**, 11–28.
2. Beckett, A.H. & Rowland, M. Rhythmic urinary excretion of amphetamine in man, *Nature* (1964) **203**, 1203–1204.
3. Borbély, A.A. Circadian rest–activity and sleep–wake rhythms. In: Koella, W.P. (ed.) *Sleep 1980* Basel: S. Karger (1981) 40–42.
4. Borbély, A.A., Baumann, F., Frandeis, D., Strauch, I. & Lehmann, D. Sleep deprivation: effect on sleep stages and EEG power density in man, *Electroenceph. Clin. Neurophysiol.* (1981) **51**, 483–493.
5. Carmen, J.S., Post, R.M., Buswell, K. & Goodwin, F.K. Negative effects of melatonin on depression, *Am. J. Psychiat.* (1976) **133**, 1181–1184.
6. Daan, S., Damassa, D., Pittendrigh, C.S. & Smith, E.R. An effect of castration and testosterone replacement on a circadian pacemaker in mice (*Mus musculus*), *Proc. Nat. Acad. Sci. USA* (1972) **72**, 3744–3747.
7. de Candolle, A.P. *Physiologie végétale*, Paris: Bechet Jeune (1832).
8. de Mairan, J. *Observation Botanique*, Histoire de l'Académie Royale des Sciences (1729) 35–36.
9. Johnsson, A. & Engelmann, W. Effect of lithium ions on human circadian rhythms, *Z. Naturforsch. (C)* (1980) **35**, 503–507.
10. Johnsson, A., Pflug, B., Engelman, W. & Klemke, W. Effect of lithium carbonate on circadian periodicity in humans, *Pharmakopsychiat. Neuropsychopharmakol.* (1979) **12**, 423–425.
11. Kleitman, N. (1963), cited by Wirz-Justice.[27]
12. Moore-Ede, M.C., Brennan, M.F. & Ball, M.R. Circadian variation of intercompartmental potassium fluxes in man, *J. Appl. Biol.* (1975) **38**, 163–170.
13. Moore-Ede, M.C., Czeisler, C.A. & Richardson, G.S. Circadian timekeeping in health and disease. In: Basic properties of circadian timekeepers, *New Engl. J. Med.* (1983) **309**, 469–476.
14. Morin, L.P., Fitzgerald, K.M. & Zucker, I. Estradiol shortens the period of hamster circadian rhythms, *Science* (1977) **196**, 305–307.
15. Pittendrigh, C.S. & Daan, S. Circadian oscillations in rodents: A systematic increase of their frequency with age, *Science* (1974) **186**, 548–550.
16. Radzialowski, F.M. & Bousquet, W.F. Circadian rhythm in hepatic drug metabolizing activity in the rat, *Life Sci.* (1967) **6**, 2545–2548.
17. Rietveld, W.J. & Groos, G. In: Scheving, L.E. & Halberg, F. (eds.) *Chronobiology: Principles and Applications to Shifts in Schedules*, Alphen aan de Rijn: Sijthoff and Noordhoff (1980) 189.
18. Rusak, B. & Zucker, I. Neural regulation of circadian rhythms, *Physiol. Rev.* (1979) **59**, 449–526.
19. Semba, J., Toru, M. & Mataga, N. Twenty-four hour rhythms of norepinephrine and serotonin in nucleus suprachiasmaticus, raphe nuclei and locus coeruleus in the rat, *Sleep* (1984) **7**, 211–218.
20. Shibuya, H., Toru, M. & Watanabe, S. A circadian rhythm of tryptophan hydroxylase in rat pineals *Brain Res.* (1977) **138**, 364–368.
21. Wax, T.M. Effects of age, strain and illumination intensity on activity and self-selection of light–dark schedules in mice, *J. Comp. Physiol. Psychol.* (1977) **91**, 57–62.
22. Webb, W.B. & Agnew, H.W. Stage 4 sleep: influence of time course variables, *Science* (1971) **174**, 1354–1356.
23. Wehr, T.A., Goodwin, K.F., Witz-Justice, A. & Lewy, A.J. Uncoupling of circadian oscillators in manic-depressive illness. Cited in: Witz-Justice, A. Uncoupling of circadian rhythms in hamsters and men. In: Koella, W.P. (ed.) *Sleep 1980*, Basel: S. Karger (1981) 71.
24. Weitzman, E.D., Czeisler, C.A., Zimmerman, J.C., Moore-Ede, M.C. & Ronda, J.M. Biological rhythms in man: internal physiological organization during non-entrained (free-running) conditions and application to delayed sleep phase syndrome. In: Chase, M.H. & Weitzman, E.D. (eds.) *Sleep Disorders: Basic and Clinical Research*, New York: Spectrum (1983) 153–171.
25. Wever, R.A. Properties of human sleep–wake cycles: parameters of internally synchronized free-running rhythms, *Sleep* (1984) **7**, 27–51.

26. Wirz-Justice, A. Uncoupling of circadian rhythms in hamsters and man. In: Koella, W.P. (ed.) *Sleep 1980*, Basel: S. Karger (1981) 64–72.
27. Wirz-Justice, A. Sleep disturbances in relation to circadian rhythms. In: Komphuisen, H.A.C., Bruyn, G.W. & Visser, P. (eds.) *Sleep – Normal and Deranged Function*, Boerhaave Course State University Leiden (1981) 64–71.
28. Wirz-Justice, A., Wehr, T.A., Goodwin, F.K., Kafka, M.S., Naber, D., Marangos, P.J. & Campbell, I.C. Antidepressant drugs slow circadian rhythms in behaviour and brain neurotransmitter receptors, *Psychopharmacol. Bull.* (1980) **16**, 45–47.

THE SUPRACHIASMATIC NUCLEUS

29. Aschoff, J. Features of circadian rhythms relevant for the design of shift schedules, *Ergonomics* (1978) **21**, 739–754.
30. Borbély, A.A. Circadian rest–activity and sleep–wake rhythms. In: Koella, W.P. (ed.) *Sleep 1980* Basel: S. Karger (1981) 40–42.
31. Borbély, A.A., Baumann, F., Brandeis, D., Strauch, I. & Lehmann, D. Sleep deprivation effects on sleep stages and EEG power density in man, *Electroenceph. Clin. Neurophysiol.* (1981) **51**, 483–495.
32. Enright, J.T. *The Timing of Sleep and Wakefulness*, New York: Springer Verlag (1980).
33. Favrod, P. & Kučera, P. Suprachiasmatic nucleus projection to mesencephalic central grey in the woodmouse *(Apodemus sylvaticus)*, *Neuroscience* (1979) **4**, 1705–1716.
34. Fuller, C.A., Sulzman, F.M. & Moore-Ede, M.C. The effect of suprachiasmatic lesions on circadian rhythms in the squirrel monkey *(Saimiri sciureus)*, *Soc. Neurosci. Abstr.* (1977) **3**, 162.
35. Green, D.J. & Gillette, R. Circadian rhythm of firing rate recorded from single cells in the rat suprachiasmatic brain slice, *Brain Res.* (1982) **245**, 198–200.
36. Groos, G. Regulation of the circadian sleep–wake cycle. In: Koella, W. (ed.) *Sleep 1982*, Basel: Karger (1983) 19–29.
37. Groos, G.A. & van der Kooy, D. Functional absence of brain photoreceptors mediating entrainment of circadian rhythms in the adult rat, *Experientia* (1981) **37**, 71–72.
38. Groos, G.A. & Mason, R. The visual properties of rat and cat suprachiasmatic neurones, *J. Comp. Physiol.* (1980) **135**, 349–356.
39. Hauri, P. *The Sleep Disorders*, Kalamazoo, Michigan: Upjohn (1977) 10–12.
40. Inouye, S.T. & Kawamura, H. Persistence of circadian rhythmicity in a mammalian hypothalamic 'island' containing the suprachiasmatic nucleus. *Proc. Nat. Acad. Sci. USA* (1979) **76**, 5962–5966.
41. Lydic, R., Schoene, W.C., Czeisler, C. & Moore-Ede, M.C. Suprachiasmatic region of the human hypothalamus: homolog to the primate circadian pacemaker? *Sleep* (1980) **2**, 355–361.
42. Mai, J.K. The accessory optic system and the retino-hypothalamic system: a review, *J. Hirnforsch.* (1978) **19**, 213–288.
43. Miles, L.E.M., Raynal, D.M. & Wilson, M.A. Blind man living in normal society has circadian rhythms of 24.9 hours, *Science* (1977) **198**, 421–423.
44. Moore, R.Y. & Eichler, V.B. Loss of a circadian adrenal corticosterone rhythm following suprachiasmatic lesion in the rat, *Brain Res.* (1972) **42**, 201–206.
45. Moore, R.Y., Hellar, A., Bhatnager, R.R., Wartman, R.J. & Axelrod, J. Central control of the pineal gland: visual pathways, *Arch. Neurol.* (1968) **18**, 208–218.
46. Moore, R.Y. & Len, N.J. A retinohypothalamic projection in the rat, *J. Comp. Neurol.* (1972) **146**, 1–14.
47. Moore-Ede, M.C., Czeisler, C.A. & Richardson, G.S. Circadian time keeping in health and disease. 1. Basic properties of circadian pacemakers, *New Engl. J. Med.* (1983) **309**, 469–476.
48. Richter, C.P. *Biological Clocks in Medicine and Psychiatry*, Springfield Illinois: Charles C. Thomas (1965).
49. Richter, C.P. Sleep and activity: their relation to the 24-hour clock, *Res. Publ. Assoc. Rec. Nerv. Ment. Dis.* (1967) **45**, 8–27.
50. Rietveld, W.J. & Groos, G. In: Schevering, L.E. & Halberg, F. (eds.) *Chronobiology: Principles and Applications to Shifts in Schedules*, Alphen aan de Rijn: Sijthoff and Noordhof (1980) 189.
51. Rusak, B. & Zucker, I. Neural regulation of circadian rhythms, *Physiol. Rev.* (1979) **59**, 449–526.
52. Sawaki, Y. Suprachiasmatic nucleus neurones: excitation and inhibition mediated by the direct retino-hypothalamic projection, *Exp. Brain Res.* (1979) **37**, 127–138.

53. Schwartz, W.J., Smith, C.B. & Davidsen, L.C. *In vivo* glucose utilization of the suprachiasmatic nucleus. In: Suda, M., Hayaishi, O. & Nakagawa, H. (eds.) *Biological Rhythms and their Central Mechanism*, New York: Elsevier (1979).
54. Sofroniew, M.Y. & Windl, A. Neuroanatomical organization and connections of the suprachiasmatic nucleus. In: Aschoff, J., Daan, S. & Groos, G. (eds.) *Vertebrate Circadian Systems*, Berlin/Heidelberg: Springer Verlag (1982) 75–86.
55. Stephan, F.K. & Zucker, J. Circadian rhythms in drinking behaviour and locomotor activity of rats are eliminated by hypothalamic lesions, *Proc. Nat. Acad. Sci. USA* (1972) **69**, 1583–1586.
56. Winfree, A.T. The tides of human consciousness: descriptions and questions, *Am. J. Physiol.* (1982) **242**, R163–166.
57. Winfree, A.T. Circadian timing of sleepiness in men and women, *Am. J. Physiol.* (1982) **243**, R193–204.
58. Zatz, M. & Brownstein, M.J. Intraventricular carbachol mimics the effects of light on the circadian rhythm in the rat pineal gland, *Science* (1979) **203**, 358–360.

HOW MANY CLOCKS?

59. Aschoff, J. Circadian rhythms: influences of internal and external factors on the period measured in constant conditions, *Z. Tierpsychol.* (1979) **49**, 225–249.
60. Aschoff, J. & Wever, R. Spontanperiodik des Menschen bei Ausschluss aller Zeitgeber, *Naturwissenschaften* (1962) **49**, 337–342.
61. Czeisler, C.A., Weitzman, E.D., Moore-Ede, M.C., Zimmerman, J.C. & Knauer, R.S. Human sleep: its duration and organization depend on its circadian phase, *Science* (1980) **210**, 1264–1267.
62. Eastman, C. Spontaneous internal desynchronization of human circadian rhythms: two oscillators or one? In: Czeisler, C.A. & Moore-Ede, M.C. (eds.) *Mathematical Modelling of Circadian Systems*, New York: Raven Press (1982).
63. Fuller, C.A., Lydic, R., Sulzman, F.M., Albers, H.E., Tepper, B. & Moore-Ede, M.C. Circadian rhythm of body temperature persists after suprachiasmatic lesions in the squirrel monkey, *Am. J. Physiol.* (1981) **241**, R385–391.
64. Gibbs, F.P. Temperature dependence of rat circadian pacemaker, *Am. J. Physiol.* (1981) **241**, R17–20.
65. Kronauer, R.E., Czeisler, C.A., Pilato, S.F., Moore-Ede, M.C. & Weitzman, E.D. Mathematical model of the human circadian system with two interacting oscillators, *Am. J. Physiol.* (1982) **242**, R3–16.
66. Lewy, A.J., Wehr, T.A., Goodwin, F.K., Newsome, D.A. & Markey, S.P. Light suppresses melatonin secretion in humans, *Science* (1980) **210**, 1267–1269.
67. Lydic, R., Schoene, W.C., Czeisler, C. & Moore-Ede, M.C. Suprachiasmatic region of the human hypothalamus: homolog to the primate circadian pacemaker? *Sleep* (1980) **2**, 355–361.
68. Moore-Ede, M.C. The circadian timing system in mammals: two pacemakers preside over many secondary oscillators, *Fed. Proc.* (1983) **42**, 2802–2808.
69. Moore-Ede, M.C., Czeisler, C.A. & Richardson, G.S. Circadian timekeeping in health and disease. I. Basic properties of circadian pacemakers, *New Engl. J. Med.* (1983) **309**, 469–476.
70. Pickard, G.E. & Turek, F.W. The suprachiasmatic nuclei: two circadian clocks? *Brain Res.* (1983) **268**, 201–210.
71. Reppert, S.M., Perlow, M.J. & Ungerleider, L.G. Effects of damage to the suprachiasmatic area of the anterior hypothalamus on the daily melatonin and cortisol rhythms in the rhesus monkey, *J. Neurosci.* (1981) **1**, 1414–1425.
72. Richter, C.P. Deep hypothermia and its effects on the 24-hour clock of rats and hamsters, *Johns Hopkins Med. J.* (1975) **136**, 1–10.
73. Weitzman, E.D., Czeisler, C.A., Zimmerman, J.C. & Moore-Ede, M.C. Biological rhythms in man: relationship of sleep–wake, cortisol, growth hormone and temperature during temporal isolation. In: Martin, J.B., Reichlin, S. & Bick, K. (eds.) *Advances in Neurology*, New York: Raven Press (1980).
74. Wever, R. The circadian multi-oscillator system of man, *Int. J. Chronobiol.* (1975) **3**, 19–55.
75. Wever, R.A. *The Circadian System of Man: Results of Experiments under Temporal Isolation*, New York: Springer Verlag (1979) 218.

76. Winfree, A.T. The tides of human consciousness: descriptions and questions, *Am. J. Physiol.* (1982) **242**, R163–166.
77. Winfree, A.T. Impact of a circadian clock on the timing of human sleep, *Am. J. Physiol.* (1983) 245, R497–504.
78. Winfree, A.T. Circadian timing of sleepiness in man and woman, *Am. J. Physiol.* (1982) **243**, R193–204.
79. Zulley, J. Distribution of REM sleep in entrained 24-hour and free-running sleep–wake cycles, *Sleep* (1980) **2**, 377–389.

CAVES AND CELLARS

80. Aschoff, J. Circadian rhythms in man: a self-sustained oscillation with an inherent frequency underlies human 24-hour periodicity, *Science* (1965) **148**, 1427–1432.
81. Aschoff, J. Human circadian rhythms in activity, body temperature and other functions, *Life Sci. Space Res.* (1967) **V**, 159–173.
82. Aschoff, J. Desynchronization and resynchronization of human circadian rhythms, *Aerospace Med.* (1969) **40**, 44–49.
83. Aschoff, J. In: Hardy, J.D., Gagg, A.P. & Stolwijk, J.A. (eds.) *Physiological and Behaviour Temperature Regulation,* Springfield, Illinois: Charles C. Thomas (1970) 905–919.
84. Aschoff, J. Circadian rhythms: influences of internal and external factors on the period measured in constant conditions, *Z. Tierpsychol.* (1979) **49**, 225–249.
85. Aschoff, J., Gerecke, U., Jureck, A., Pohl, H., Reiger, P., Saint Paul, U. & Wever, R. In: Menaker, M. (ed.) *Biochronometry,* Washington: National Academy of Science (1971) 3–29.
86. Aschoff, J., Gerecke, U. & Wever, R. Phase relations between circadian activity periods and body temperature in man, *Eur. J. Physiol.* (1967) **295**, 173–183.
87. Aschoff, J., Gerecke, U. & Wever, R. Desynchronization of human circadian rhythms, *Jap. J. Physiol.* (1967) **17**, 450.
88. Aschoff, J. & Wever, R. Spontanperiodik des Menschen bei Ausschluss aller Zeitgeber, *Naturwissenschaften* (1962) **49**, 337–342.
89. Aschoff, J. & Wever, R. Human circadian rhythms: a multi-oscillatory system, *Fed. Proc.* (1976) **35**, 2326–2332.
90. Chouvet, G., Mouret, J., Coindet, J., Siffre, M. & Jouvet, M. Périodicité bicircadienne de cycle veillesommeil dans des conditions hors du temps étude, *Electroenceph. Clin. Neurophysiol.* (1974) **37**, 367–380.
91. Jouvet, M., Mouret, J., Chouvet, G. & Siffre, M. Experimental bicircadian rhythms in man. In: Schmitt, F. & Worden, F. (eds.) *The Neurosciences: Third Study Programme,* Cambridge, Massachusetts, MIT Press (1974) 491–497.
92. Kronauer, R.E., Czeisler, C.A., Pilator, S.F., Moore-Ede, M.C. & Weitzman, E.D. Mathematical model of the human circadian system with two interacting oscillators, *Am. J. Physiol.* (1982) **243**, R3–16.
93. Mills, J.N. Human circadian rhythms, *Physiol. Rev.* (1966) **46**, 128–171.
94. Mills, J.N., Minors, D.S. & Waterhouse, J.M. The circadian rhythms of human subjects without timepieces or indication of the alteration of day and night, *J. Physiol.* (1974) **240**, 567–594.
95. Siffre, M., Reinberg, A., Halberg, F., Chata, J., Perdriel, G. & Slind, R. L'isolement souterrain prolongé. Etude de deux sujets adultes sains avant, pendant et après cet isolement, *Presse Méd.* (1966) **74**, 915–920.
96. Webb, W.B. & Agnew, H.W. Regularity in the control of the free-running sleep–wakefulness rhythm, *Aerospace Med.* (1974) **45**, 701–704.
97. Weitzman, E.D., Czeisler, C.A. & Moore-Ede, M.C. In: Suda, M., Hayaishi, O. & Nakagawa, H. (eds.) *Biological Rhythms and their Central Mechanisms,* Amsterdam: Elsevier/North-Holland (1979).
98. Weitzman, E.D., Czeisler, C.A., Zimmerman, J.C. & Ronda, J.M. Timing of REM and stages 3 and 4 sleep during temporal isolation in man, *Sleep* (1980) **2**, 391–407.
99. Wever, R. Internal phase angle difference in human circadian rhythms: causes for changes and problems of determinations, *Int. J. Chronobiol.* (1973) **1**, 371–390.
100. Wever, R. Bedeutung der circadianen Periodik für das Alter, *Naturw. Rdsch. Stuttg.* (1974) **27**, 475–479.

101. Wever, R.A. Commentary on the mathematical model of the human circadian system by Kronauer *et al.*, *Am. J. Physiol.* (1982) **242,** R17–21.

ZEITGEBERS

102. Mills, J.N. Circadian rhythms during and after three months in solitude underground, *J. Physiol.* (1964) **174,** 217–231.
103. Moore-Ede, M.C. The circadian timing system in mammals: two pacemakers preside over many secondary oscillators, *Fed. Proc.* (1983) **42,** 2802–2808.
104. Moore-Ede, M.C., Czeisler, C.A. & Richardson, G.S. Circadian time keeping in health and disease. 1. Basic properties of circadian pacemakers, *New Engl. J. Med.* (1983) **309,** 469–476.
105. Sulzman, F.M., Fuller, C.A. & Moore-Ede, M.C. Feeding time synchronizes primate circadian rhythms, *Physiol. Behav.* (1977) **18,** 775–779.
106. Vernikos-Danellis, J. & Winget, C.M. The importance of light postural and social cues in the regulation of the plasma cortisol rhythms in man. In: Reinberg, A. & Hallberg, F. (eds.) *Chronopharmacology,* New York: Pergamon (1979) 101–106.
107. Webb, W.B. & Agnew, H.W. Regularity in the control of the free-running sleep–wakefulness rhythm, *Aerospace Med.* (1974) **45,** 701–704.
108. Weitzman, E.D., Czeisler, C.A., Zimmerman, J.C., Moore-Ede, M.C. & Ronda, J.M. Biological rhythms in man. In: Chase, M.H. & Weitzman, E.D. (eds.) *Sleep Disorders: Basic and Clinical Research,* New York: Spectrum (1983) 153–171.
109. Wever, R. Behavioural aspects of circadian rhythmicity. In: Brown, F.M. & Graeber, R.C. (eds.) *Rhythmical Aspects of Behaviour,* Hillsdale, New Jersey: Erlbaum (1982) 105–171.
110. Winfree, A.T. The tides of human consciousness; description and questions, *Am. J. Physiol.* (1982) **242,** R163–166.

PHASE–RESPONSE CURVES

111. Arendt, J. & Marks, V. Can melatonin alleviate jet-lag? *Brit. Med. J. (Clin. Res.)* (1983) **287,** 426.
112. de Coursey, P.J. Daily light sensitivity rhythm in a rodent, *Science* (1960) **131,** 33–35.
113. Hastings, J.W. & Sweeney, B.M. A persistent diurnal rhythm of luminescence in *Gonyaulax polyedra, Biol. Bull.* (1958) **115,** 440–458.
114. Mills, J.N., Minors, D.S. & Waterhouse, J.M. Adaptation to abrupt time shifts of the oscillator(s) controlling human circadian rhythms, *J. Physiol. (Lond.)* (1978) **285,** 455–470.
115. Moore-Ede, M.C., Czeisler, C.A. & Richardson, G.S. Circadian timekeeping in health and disease. 1. Properties of circadian pacemakers, *New Engl. J. Med.* (1983) **309,** 469–476.
116. Pittendrigh, C.S. Circadian rhythms and the circadian organization of living systems, *Cold Spring Harbor Symp. Quant. Biol.* (1960) **25,** 159–182.
117. Redman, J., Armstrong, S. & Ng, K.T. Free-running activity rhythms in the rat: entrainment by melatonin, *Science* (1983) **219,** 1089–1091.
118. Rusak, B. & Groos, G. Suprachiasmatic stimulation phase shifts rodent circadian rhythms, *Science* (1982) **215,** 1407–1409.
119. Taylor, W. & Hastings, J.W. Minute-long pulses of anisomycin phase-shift the biological clock in *Gonyaulax* by hours, *Naturwissenschaften* (1982) **69,** 94–96.

DEPRESSION AND CIRCADIAN TIMEKEEPING

120. Ceresa, F., Agneli, A., Boccuzzi, G. & Molino, G. Once-a-day neurally stimulated and basal ACTH secretion phases in man and their response to corticoid inhibition, *J. Clin. Endocrinol.* (1969) **29,** 1074–1082.
121. Coursey, R., Frankel, B. & Gaarder, K. EMG biofeedback and autogenic training as relaxation technique for chronic sleep-onset insomnia, *Biofeedback Self-Regulation* (1976) **1,** 353–354.
122. Doig, R.J., Mummery, R.V., Wills, M.R. & Elkes, A. Plasma cortisol levels in depression, *Brit. J. Psychiat.* (1966) **112,** 1263–1267.

123. Goodwin, F.K., Wirz-Justice, A. & Wehr T.A. Evidence that the pathophysiology of depression and the mechanism of action of antidepressant drugs both involve alterations in circadian rhythms, *Adv. Biochem. Psychopharmacol.* (1982) **32**, 1–11.
124. Gresham, S.C., Agnew, W.R. & Williams, R.L. The sleep of depressed patients, *Arch. Gen. Psychiat.* (1965) **13**, 503–507.
125. Haider, I. Patterns of insomnia in depressive illness: a subjective evaluation, *Brit. J. Psychiat.* (1968) **114**, 1127–1132.
126. Hartmann, E. Longitudinal studies of sleep and dream patterns in manic-depressive patients, *Arch. Gen. Psychiat.* (1968) **19**, 312–329.
127. Hauri, P. & Hawkins, D.R. Alpha-delta sleep, *Electroenceph. Clin. Neurophysiol.* (1973) **34**, 233–237.
128. Johnsson, A. & Engelman, W. Effect of lithium ions on human circadian rhythms, *Z. Naturforsch. (C)* (1980) **35**, 503–507.
129. Kupfer, D.J. REM latency: a psychobiologic marker for primary depressive disease, *Biol. Psychiat.* (1976) **11**, 159–174.
130. Kupfer, D.J. & Foster, G.F. Interval between onset of sleep and rapid-eye-movement sleep as an indicator of depression, *Lancet* (1972) **2**, 684–686.
131. Kupfer, D.J., Foster, F.G., Reich, L., Thompson, K.S. & Weiss, B. EEG sleep changes as predictors in depression, *Am. J. Psychiat.* (1976) **133**, 622–626.
132. Michaelis, R. & Hofmann, E. Zur phenomenologie und atiopathogenese der hypersomnie bei endogenphasischen depressionen. In: Jovanovic, U.J. (ed.) *The Nature of Sleep*, Stuttgart: Gustav Fischer (1973) 190–193.
133. Rudolf, G.A.E., Schilgen, B. & Tolle, R. Anti-depressive Behandlung mittels Schlafentzug, *Nervenarzt* (1977) **48**, 1–11.
134. Sachar, E.J., Hellman, L., Roffwarg, H.P., Halpern, F.S., Fukushima, D.K. & Gallagher, T.F. Disrupted 24 hour patterns of cortisol secretion in psychotic depression, *Arch. Gen. Psychiat.* (1973) **28**, 19–24.
135. Vogel, G.W. REM sleep deprivation and depression. In: Chase, M. & Weitzman, E.D. (eds.) *Sleep Disorders. Basic and Clinical Research*, Lancaster: MTP (1983) 393–400.
136. Vogel. G., McAbee, R. & Barker, K. REM pressure and improvement of endogenous depression. In: Chase, M.H., Mitler, M.M. & Walter P.L. (eds.) *Sleep Research, Vol 5*, Los Angeles: BIS/BRI UCLA (1976) 151.
137. Vogel, G.W., Thurmond, A., Gibbons, P., Sloan, K., Boyd, M. & Walker, M. REM sleep reduction effects on depression syndromes, *Arch. Gen. Psychiat.* (1975) **32**, 765–777.
138. Wehr, T.A., Gillin, J.C. & Goodwin, F.K. Sleep and circadian rhythms in depression. In: Chase, M.H. & Weitzman, E.D. *Sleep Disorders, Basic and Clinical Research*, New York: Spectrum (1983) 195–225.
139. Wehr, T.A., Goodwin, K.F., Wirz-Justice, A. & Lewy, A.J. Uncoupling of circadian oscillators in manic-depressive illness. Cited by Wirz-Justice, A. Uncoupling of circadian rhythms in hamsters and man. In: Koella, W.P. (ed) *Sleep 1980*, Basel: S. Karger (1981) 71.
140. Wehr, T., Wirz-Justice, A., Goodwin, R.K., Duncan, W. & Gillin, J.C. Phase advance of the circadian sleep–wake cycle as an antidepressant, *Science* (1979) **206**, 710–711.
141. Weitzman, E.D., Goldmacher, D., Kripke, D., MacGregor P., Kream, J. & Hellman, L. Reversal of sleep–waking cycle: Effect of sleep stage pattern and certain neuroendocrine rhythms, *Trans. Am. Neurol. Assoc.* (1968) **93**, 153–157.
142. Wirz-Justice, A., Wehr, T.A., Kafka, M.S., Naber, D., Marangos, P.J. & Campbell, I.C. Antidepressant drugs slow circadian rhythms in behaviour and brain neurotransmitter receptors, *Psychopharmacol. Bull.* (1980) **16**, 45–47.

SLEEP-ONSET RAPID EYE MOVEMENTS (SOREMS)

143. Carskadon, M.A. & Dement, W.C. Sleep studies on a 90-minute day, *Electroenceph. Clin. Neurophysiol.* (1975) **39**, 145–155.
144. Czeisler, C.A. Human circadian physiology: internal organization of temperature, sleep–wake and neuroendocrine rhythms monitored in an environment free of time cues, Ph.D. dissertation, Stanford (1978).
145. Endo. S., Yamamoto, T. & Sasaki, M. Effects of time zone changes on sleep: west–east flight and east–west flight, *Jikeikai Med. J.* (1978) **25**, 249–268.
146. Hume, K.I. & Mills, J.N. Rhythms of REM and slow-wave sleep in subjects living on

abnormal time schedules, *Waking Sleeping* (1977) **1**, 291–296.

147. Karacan, I., Finley, W.W., Williams, R.L. & Hursch. C.J. Changes in Stage 1 REM and stage 4 sleep during naps, *Biol. Psychiat.* (1970) **2**, 261–265.

148. Meddis, R. Human circadian rhythms and the 48 hour day, *Nature* (1968) **218**, 964–965.

149. Montplaisir, J., Billiard, M., Takahashi, S., Bell, I.R., Guilleminault, C. & Dement, W.C. Twenty-four hour recording in REM-narcoleptics with special reference to nocturnal sleep disruption, *Biol. Psychiat.* (1978) **13**, 73–89.

150. Paul, K. & Dittrichova, J. The process of falling asleep in infancy, *Activitas Nerv.* (1977) Suppl. 19, 272–273.

151. Rechtschaffen, A., Wolpert, E.A., Dement, W.C., Mitchell, S.A. & Fisher, C. Nocturnal sleep of narcoleptics, *Electroenceph. Clin. Neurophysiol.* (1963) **15**, 599–609.

152. Salzarulo, P., Fagioli, I., Salomon, F., Ricour, C., Raimbault, G., Ambrosi, S., Cicchi, O., Duhamel, J.F. & Rigoard, M.T. Sleep patterns in infants under continuous feeding from birth, *Electroenceph. Clin. Neurophysiol.* (1980) **49**, 330–336.

153. Schultz, H. Sleep onset REM episodes in depression. In: Koella, W.P. (ed.) *Sleep 1980*, Basel: S. Karger (1981) 72–79.

154. Sitaram, N., Mendelson, W.B., Wyatt, R.J. & Gillin, J.C. The time-dependent induction of REM sleep and arousal by physostigmine infusions during normal human sleep, *Brain Res.* (1977) **122**, 562–567.

155. Snyder, F. NIH studies of sleep in affective illness. In: Williams, I.A., Katz, M.M. & Shields, J. (eds.) *Recent Advances in the Psychobiology of the Depressive Illnesses*, Washington: US Government Printing Office (1972) 171–192.

156. Spielman, A.J., Pressman, M., Pollak, C.P., Rubinstein, M., Lamstein, S., Roffwarg, H.P. & Weitzman, E.D. REM deprivation of narcoleptics, *Sleep Res.* (1979) **8**, 216.

157. Webb, W.B., Agnew, H.W., Jr. & Williams, K.L. Effect on sleep of a sleep period time displacement, *Aerospace Med.* (1971) **42**, 152–155.

158. Weitzman, E.D., Nogeire, C., Perlow, M., Fukushima, D., Sassin, G., McGregor, P., Gallagher, T.F. & Hellman, L. Effect of a prolonged 3-hour sleep–wake cycle on sleep stages, plasma cortisol, growth hormone, and body temperature in men, *J. Clin. Endocrinol. Metab.* (1974) **38**, 1018–1030.

159. Zulley, J. *Der Einfluss von Zeitgebern auf den Schlaf des Menschen*, Frankfurt: Fischer (1979).

160. Zulley, J. Duration and frequency of bedrest episodes in internally desynchronised subjects, *Sleep* (1980) **2**, 344–346.

161. Zulley, J. & Schulz, H. Sleep and body temperature in free-running sleep–wake cycles. In: Popoviciu, L., Asgian, B. & Badine, J. (eds.) *Sleep 1978* Basel: S. Karger (1980) 341–344.

SLEEP DISORDERS DUE TO CIRCADIAN RHYTHM DISTURBANCES

162. Elliott, A.L. (Mills, J.N. & Waterhouse, J.M. A man with too long a day, *J. Physiol.* (1971) **212**, 30–31.

163. Fulton, J.F. & Bailey, P. Tumors in the region of the third ventricle: their diagnosis and relation to pathological sleep, *J. Nerv. Ment. Dis.* (1929) **69**, 1–25, 145–164, 261–277.

164. Gillespie, R.D. *Sleep and the Treatment of its Disorders*, New York: William Wood (1930).

165. Hauri, P. *The Sleep Disorders*, Kalamazoo, Michigan: Upjohn (1977) 1–76.

166. Krieger, D.T. & Krieger, H.P. Circadian patterns of urinary electrolyte excretion in central nervous system disease, *Metabolism* (1967) **16**, 815–823.

167. Lewis, H.E. & Masterton, J.P. British North Greenland expedition 1952–1954; medical and physiological aspects, *Lancet* (1955) **2**, 494–500, 549–556.

168. Lobban, M.C. The entrainment of circadian rhythms in man, *Cold Spring Harbour Symp. Quant. Biol.* (1960) **25**, 325–332.

169. Lobban, M.C. Seasonal variation in daily patterns of urinary excretion by Eskimo subjects. In: Shephard, R.J. & Itoh, S. (eds.) *Circumpolar Health*, Toronto: University of Toronto Press (1976) 17–23.

170. Miles, L.E.M., Raynal, D.M. & Wilson, M.A. Blind man living in normal society has circadian rhythms of 24.9 hours, *Science* (1977) **198**, 421–423.

171. Moore-Ede, M.C., Czeisler, C.A. & Richardson, G.S. Circadian timekeeping in health and disease. 2. Clinical implications of circadian rhythmicity, *New Engl. J. Med.* (1983) **309**, 530–536.

172. Page, R.B., Galicich, J.H. & Grunt, J.A. Alteration of circadian temperature rhythms with

third ventricular obstruction, *J. Neurosurg.* (1973) **38**, 309–319.

173.   Roffwarg, H., Clark, R.W. *et al.* Association of Sleep Disorders Centers. Diagnostic classification of sleep and arousal disorders, *Sleep* (1979) **2**, 1–137.

174.   Weber, A.L., Cary, M.S., Connor, N. & Keyes, P. Human non-24-hour sleep–wake cycles in an everyday environment, *Sleep* (1980) **2**, 347–354.

175.   Weitzman, E.D., Czeisler, C., Coleman, R., Dement, W., Richardson, G. & Pollak, C.P. Delayed sleep phase syndrome; a biological rhythm disorder, *Sleep* (1980) **2**, 221.

176.   Weitzman, E.D., Czeisler, C.A., Coleman, R.M., Spielman, A.J., Zimmerman, J.C., Dement, W., Richardson, G. & Pollak, C.P. Delayed sleep phase syndrome: a chronobiologic disorder with sleep onset insomnia, *Arch. Gen. Psychiat.* (1981) **38**, 737–746.

177.   Wirz-Justice, A. Sleep disturbances in relation to circadian rhythms. In: Kamphuisen, H.A.C., Bruyn, G.W. & Visser, P. (eds.) *Sleep. Normal and Deranged Function.* Boorhaave Course, State University Leiden (1981) 64–71.

178.   Yoshimura, H. Review of medical researches at the Japanese station (Syowa base) in the Antarctic. In: Edholm, O.G. & Gunderson, E.K.E. (eds.) *Polar Human Biology*, London: Heinemann (1973) 54–65.

SHIFTWORK AND SLEEP

179.   Akerstedt, T. & Torvall, L. Age, sleep, and adjustment to shift work. In: Koella, W.P. (ed.) *Sleep 1980*, Basel: S. Karger (1981) 190–195.

180.   Bilwise, D., Seidel, W., Greenblatt, D.J. & Dement, W. Night time and day time efficacy of flurazepam and oxazepam in chronic insomnia, *Am. J. Psychiat.* (1984) **141**, 191–195.

181.   Blake, M.J.F. & Corcoran, D.W.J. Introversion–extraversion and circadian rhythms. In: Colquhoun, W.P. (ed.) *Aspects of Human Efficiency*, London: English Universities Press (1972) 261–272.

182.   Colquhoun, W.P. & Folkard, S. Personality differences in body temperature rhythm and their relation to its adjustment to night work, *Ergonomics* (1978) **21**, 811–817.

183.   Czeisler, C.A., Moore-Ede, M.C. & Coleman, R.M. Rotating shift work schedules that disrupt sleep are improved by applying circadian principles, *Science* (1982) **217**, 460–463.

184.   Dahlgren, K. Adjustment of circadian rhythms and EEG sleep functions to day and night sleep amongst permanent nightworkers and rotating shiftworkers, *Psychophysiology* (1981) **18**, 381–391.

185.   Danchik, K.M., Schoenborn, C.A. & Elinson, J., Jr. (eds.) *Basic Data from Wave 1 of the National Survey of Personal Health Practices and Consequences: United States 1979*, Hyattsville, Maryland: Public Health Service (1981) DHSS publication No. (PHS) 81–1162.

186.   Foret, J. & Benoit, O. Predictable effects on individual sleep patterns during a rapidly rotating shift system, *Int. Arch. Occup. Environ. Health* (1980) **45**, 49–56.

187.   Foret, J. & Benoit, O. Individual factors, sleep characteristics, and circadian evolution of body temperature. In: Koella, W.P. (ed.) *Sleep 1980*, Basel: S. Karger (1981) 195–197.

188.   Foret, J., Bensimon, G., Benoit, O. & Vieux, N. Quality of sleep as a function of age and shift work. In: Reinberg, A. (ed.) *Studies on Night and Shift Work: a Multidisciplinary Approach*, New York: Pergamon (1981).

189.   Friedman, R.C., Bigger, J.T. & Kornfeld, D.S. The intern and sleep loss, *New Engl. J. Med.* (1971) **285**, 201–203.

190.   Guilleminault, C., Czeisler, C., Coleman, R. & Miles, L. Circadian rhythm disturbances and sleep disorders in shift workers, *Electroenceph. Clin. Neurophysiol. (Suppl.)* (1982) **36**, 709–714.

191.   Hartmann, E., Baekeland, F., Zwilling, G. & Hoy, P. Sleep need: how much sleep and what kind? *Am. J. Psychiat.* (1971) **127**, 1001–1008.

192.   Hauri, P. *The Sleep Disorders* Kalamazoo, Michigan: Upjohn (1977) 1–76.

193.   Horne, J.A. & Ostberg, O. A self assessment questionnaire to determine morningness–eveningness in human circadian rhythm, *Int. J. Chronobiol.* (1976) **4**, 97–110.

194.   Knauth, P. & Rutenfranz, J. Experimental shift work studies of permanent night and rapidly rotating shift systems. I. Circadian rhythms of body temperature and re-entrainment at shift change, *Int. Arch. Occup. Environ. Health* (1976) **37**, 125–137.

195.   Lund, R. Personality factors and desynchronization of circadian rhythms, *Psychosom. Med.* (1974) **36**, 224–228.

196.   Nicholson, A.N. & Stone, B.M. Hypnotic activity during the day of diazepam and its hydroxylated metabolites, 3-hydroxydiazepam (temazepam) and 3-hydroxy, *N*-desmethyl-

diazepam (oxazepam). In: Reinberg, A. & Halberg, F. (eds.) *Chronopharmacology*, Oxford: Pergamon (1979) 159–169.

197. Poulton, E.C., Hunt, G.M., Carpenter, A. & Edwards, R.S. The performance of junior hospital doctors following reduced sleep and long hours of work, *Ergonomics* (1978) **21**, 279–295.

198. Schaefer, K.E., Kerr, C.M., Buss, D. & Haus, E. Effect of 18-h watch schedules on circadian cycles of physiological functions during submarine patrols, *Undersea Biomed. Res.* (1979) **6**, 581–590.

199. Taub, J.M. Behavioural and psychophysiological correlates of irregularity in chronic sleep routines, *Biol. Psychol.* (1978) **7**, 37–53.

200. Webb, W.B. & Bonnet, M. The sleep of 'morning' and 'evening' types, *Biol. Psychol.* (1978) **7**, 29–35.

201. Weitzman, E.D., Nogeire, C., Perlow, M., Fukushima, D., Sassin, J., McGregor, P., Gallagher, T.F. & Hellman, L. Effects of a prolonged 3-hour sleep–wake cycle on sleep stages, plasma cortisol, growth hormone and body temperature in man, *J. Clin. Endocrinol.* (1974) **38**, 1018–1022.

JET LAG

202. Anton-Tay, F. & Wurtman, R.J. Regional uptake of ^{3}H melatonin from blood or cerebrospinal fluid by rat brain, *Nature* (1969) **221**, 474–475.

203. Conroy, R.T.W.L. Time zone transitions and business executives, *Trans. Soc. Occup. Med.* (1971) **21**, 69–72.

204. Golstein, J., van Cauter, E., Desir, D., Noel, P., Spire, J.P., Refetoff, S. & Copinschi, G. Effects of jet lag on hormonal patterns. IV. Time shifts increase growth hormone release, *J. Clin. Endocrinol. Metab.* (1983) **56**, 433–440.

205. Klein, K.E., Hermann, H., Kuklinski, P. & Wegmann, H.M. Circadian performance rhythms. Experimental studies in air operation. In: Mackie, J.R. (ed.) *Vigilance, Theory, Operational Performance and Physiological Correlates*, New York/London: Plenum Press (1977) 117–132.

206. McFarland, R.A. *Human Factors in Air Transportation: Occupational Health and Safety*, New York: McGraw-Hill (1953).

207. McFarland, R.A. Air travel across time zones, *Am. Sci.* (1975) **63**, 23–30.

208. Weitzman, E.D., Czeisler, C.A., Zimmerman, J.C., Moore-Ede, M.C. & Ronda, J.M. Biological rhythms in man: internal organization of the physiology during non-entrained (free-running) conditions and application to delayed sleep-phase syndrome. In: Chase, M.H. & Weitzman, E.D. (eds.) *Sleep Disorders. Basic and Clinical Research*, Lancaster: MTP (1983) 153–172.

209. Wirz-Justice, A. Sleep disturbances in relation to circadian rhythms. In: Kamphuisen, H.A.C., Bruyn, G.W. & Visser, P. (eds.) *Sleep. Normal and Deranged Function*, Boorhaave Course, State University Leiden (1981) 64–71.

HORMONES AND SLEEP

210. Chase, T.N. & Murphy, D.L. Serotonin and central nervous system function, *Ann. Rev. Pharmacol.* (1973) **13**, 181–197.

211. Danguir, J. Sleep deficits in rats with hereditary diabetes insipidus, *Nature* (1983) **304**, 163–164.

212. Gillin, J.C., Jacobs, L.S., Snyder, F. & Henkin, R.I. Effects of ACTH on the sleep of normal subjects and patients with Addison's disease, *Neuroendocrinology* (1974) **15**, 21–31.

213. Hjemdahl, P., Åkerstedt, T., Pollare, T. & Gillberg, M. Influence of ß-adrenoceptor blockade by metoprolol and propranolol on plasma concentrations and effects of noradrenaline and adrenaline during iv infusion, *Acta Physiol. Scand. (Suppl.)* (1983) **515**, 45–53.

214. Kalin, N.H., Insel, T.R., Cohen, R.M., Risch, S.C. & Murphy D.L. Diurnal variation in cerebrospinal fluid prolactin concentration of the rhesus monkey, *J. Clin. Endocrinol. Metab.* (1981) **52**, 857–858.

215. Krieger, D.T. & Gewitz, G.P. Recovery of hypothalamic-pituitary-adrenal function, growth hormone responsiveness and sleep EEG pattern in patient following removal of an adrenal

cortical adenoma, *J. Clin. Endocrinol. Metab.* (1974) **38**, 1075–1082.

216. Mendelson, W.B., Jacobs, L.S. & Gillin, J.C. Negative feedback suppression of sleep-related growth hormone secretion, *J. Clin. Endocrinol. Metab.* (1983) **56**, 486–488.

217. Milcu, S.M. & Nocolescu-Catargi, A. Deep-sleep phase alterations in patients with loss of the adrenal secretory rhythm and in hypophysectomized patients, *Electroenceph. Clin. Neurophysiol.* (1967) **22**, 574.

218. Quabbe, H.J., Kroll, M. & Thomsen, P. Dissociation of light onset and wake onset: effect on rhesus monkey growth hormone secretion, *Endocrinology* (1983) **112**, 1828–1831.

219. Ratge, D., Knoll, E., Diener, U., Hadjidimos, A. & Wisser, H. Circadian rhythm of catecholamines, cortisol and prolactin is altered in patients with apallic syndrome in comparison with normal volunteers, *Acta Endocrinol. (Copenh.)* (1982) **101**, 428–435.

220. Taylor, P.L., Garrick, N.A., Burns, R.S., Tamarkin, L., Murphy, D.L. & Markey, S.P. Diurnal rhythms of serotonin in monkey cerebrospinal fluid, *Life Sci.* (1982) **31**, 1993–1999.

221. Terry, L.C., Crowley, W.R. & Johnson, M.D. Regulation of episodic growth hormone secretion by the central epinephrine system; studies in the chronic cannulated cat, *J. Clin. Invest.* (1982) **69**, 104–112.

222. Turton, M.B. & Deegan, T. Circadian variations of plasma catecholamine, cortisol and immunoreactive insulin concentrations in supine subjects, *Clin. Chim. Acta* (1974) **55**, 389–397.

223. Wisser, H. & Knoll, E. Ergebnisse einer Kurtzeitsstudie über die circadiane Rhythmik bei normaler und erhöter Katecholaminausscheidung im Urin, *Clin. Chim. Acta* (1957) **59**, 1–7.

GROWTH HORMONE

224. Bansal, S.A., Lee, L.A. & Woolf, P.D. Dopaminergic stimulation and inhibition of growth hormone secretion in normal man: studies of the pharmacological specificity, *J. Clin. Endocrinol. Metab.* (1981) **53**, 1273–1277.

225. Carlson, H.E., Gillin, J.C., Gorden, P. & Snyder, F. Absence of sleep-related growth hormone peaks in aged normal subjects and in acromegaly, *J. Clin. Endocrinol. Metab.* (1972) **34**, 1102–1105.

226. Chambers, J.W. & Brown, S.M. Neurotransmitter regulation of growth hormone and ACTH in the rhesus monkey: effects of biogenic amines, *Endocrinology* (1976) **98**, 420–428.

227. Farthing, M.J., Campbell, C.A., Walker-Smith, J., Edwards, C.R., Rees, L.H. & Dawson, A.M. Nocturnal growth hormone and gonadotrophin secretion in growth retarded children with Crohn's disease, *Gut* (1981) **22**, 933–938.

228. Finkelstein, J.W., Roffwarg, H.P., Boyar, R.M., Kream, J. & Hellman, L. Age-related change in the twenty-four hour spontaneous secretion of growth hormone, *J. Clin. Endocrinol. Metab.* (1972) **35**, 665–670.

229. Horne, J.A. Human sleep and tissue restitution: some qualifications and doubts, *Clin. Sci.* (1983) **65**, 569–578.

230. Howse, P.M., Rayner, P.H.W., Williams, J.W. & Rudd, B.T. Growth hormone secretion during sleep in short children: a continuous sampling study, *Arch. Dis. Child.* (1974) **49**, 246.

231. Jacoby, J.H., Greenstein, M., Sassin, J.F. & Weitzman, E.D. The effect of monoamine precursors on the release of growth hormone in the rhesus monkey, *Neuroendocrinology* (1974) **14**, 95–102.

232. Kárteszi, M., Fiók, J. & Makara, G.B. Lack of episodic growth hormone secretion in rats with anterolateral deafferentation of the medial-basal hypothalamus, *J. Endocrinol.* (1982) **94**, 77–81.

233. Krieger, D.T., Albin, J., Paget, S. & Glick, S.M. Failure of suppression of nocturnal growth hormone rise by acute corticosteroid administration, *Hormone Metab. Res.* (1972) **4**, 463–466.

234. Krieger, D.T. & Glick, S. Absent sleep peak of growth hormone release in blind subjects: correlation with sleep EEG stages, *J. Clin. Endocrinol. Metab.* (1971) **33**, 847–850.

235. Lipman, R.L., Taylor, A.L., Schenk, A. & Mintz, D.H. Inhibition of sleep-related growth hormone release by elevated free fatty acids, *J. Clin. Endocrinol. Metab.* (1972) **35**, 592–594.

236. Lucke, C., Adelman, N. & Glick, S.M. The effect of elevated free fatty acids (FFA) on the sleep-induced human growth hormone (HGH) peak, *J. Clin. Endocrinol. Metab.* (1972) **35**, 407–412.

237. Lucke, C. & Glick, S.M. Effect of medroxyprogesterone acetate on the sleep-induced peak of growth hormone secretion, *J. Clin. Endocrinol. Metab.* (1971) **33**, 851–853.

238. Martinez-Campos, A., Giovanni, P., Cocchi, D., Zanardi, P., Parati, E.A., Caraceni, T. & Müller, E.E. Growth hormone secretion in neurological disorders, *Adv. Biochem. Psychopharmacol.* (1981) **28**, 521–540.

239. Mendelson, W.B., Jacobs, L.S. & Gillin, J.C. Negative feedback suppression of sleep-related growth hormone secretion, *J. Clin. Endocrinol. Metab.* (1983) **56**, 486–488.

240. Mendelson, W.B., Jacobs, L.S., Reichman, J.D., Othmer, E., Cryer, P.E., Trivedi, B. & Daughaday, W.H. Methysergide: suppression of sleep-related prolactin secretion and enhancement of sleep-related growth hormone secretion, *J. Clin. Invest.* (1975) **56**, 690–697.

241. Mendelson, W.B., Jacobs, L.S., Sitaram, N., Wyatt, R.J. & Gillin, J.C. Methscopolamine inhibition of sleep-related growth hormone secretion, *J. Clin. Invest.* (1978) **61**, 1683–1690.

242. Mendelson, W.B., Lantigua, R.A., Wyatt, R.J., Gillin, J.C. & Jacobs, L.S. Piperidine enhances sleep-related and insulin-induced growth hormone secretion: further evidence for a cholinergic secretory mechanism, *J. Clin. Endocrinol. Metab.* (1981) **52**, 409–415.

243. Minuto, F., Underwood, L.E., Grimaldi, P., Furlanetto, R.W., Van Wyk, J.J. & Giordino, G. Decreased serum somatomedin C concentrations during sleep: temporal relationship to the nocturnal surges of growth hormone and prolactin, *J. Clin. Endocrinol. Metab.* (1981) **52**, 399–403.

244. Pantelakis, S.N., Sinaniotis, C.A., Sbirakis, S., Ikkos, D. & Doxiadis, S.A. Night and day growth hormone levels during treatment with corticosteroids and corticotrophin, *Arch. Dis. Child.* (1973) **47**, 605–608.

245. Parker, D.C., Rossman, L.G. & Van der Laan, E.F. Persistence of rhythmic human growth hormone release during sleep in fasted and noniscocalorically fed normal subjects, *Metabolism* (1972) **21**, 241–252.

246. Parker, D.C., Rossman, L.G. & Van der Laan, E.F. Sleep-related nyctohumeral and briefly episodic variation in human plasma prolactin concentration, *J. Clin. Endocrinol. Metab.* (1973) **36**, 1119–1124.

247. Pimstone, B.L., Wittman, W., Hansen, J.D.L. & Murray, P. Growth hormone and kwashiorkor, *Lancet* (1966) **2**, 779–780.

248. Powell, G.F., Hopwood, N.J. & Barrett, E.S. Growth hormone studies before and during catch-up growth in a child with emotional deprivation and short stature, *J. Clin. Endocrinol. Metab.* (1973) **37**, 674–679.

249. Prinz, P.N., Halter, J., Raskind, M., Cunningham, G. & Karacan, I. Diurnal variation of plasma catecholamines and sleep-related hormones in man: relation to age and sleep pattern. In: Finch, C.A. (ed.) *Biological Mechanisms of Aging*, Conference Proceedings, Washington: USGPO (1981) 618–628.

250. Prinz, P.N., Roehrs, T.A., Vitaliano, P., Linnoila, M. & Weitzman, E.D. Effect of alcohol on sleep and night time plasma growth hormone and cortisol concentrations, *J. Clin. Endocrinol. Metab.* (1980) **51**, 759–764.

251. Quabbe, H.J. & Helge, H. *Verhandlungen der Deutschen Gesellschaft fur Innere Medizin 73 Kongress* (1967) 389.

252. Quabbe, H.J., Schilling, E. & Helge, H. Pattern of growth hormone secretion during a 24-hour fast in normal adults, *J. Clin. Endocrinol.* (1966) **26**, 1173–1175.

253. Rubin, R.T., Gouin, P.R., Arenander, A.T. & Poland, R.E. Human growth hormone release during sleep following prolonged flurazepam administration, *Res. Comm. Chem. Path. Pharmacol.* (1973) **6**, 331–334.

254. Sassin, J.F., Parker, D.C., Mace, J.W., Gotlin, R.W., Johnson, L.C. & Rossman, L.G. Human growth hormone release: Relation to slow-wave sleep and sleep–waking cycles, *Science* (1969) **165**, 513–515.

255. Schofield, J.G. The effects of neuroactive peptides on growth hormone release, *Proc. Nut. Soc.* (1981) **40**, 365–366.

256. Takahashi, Y., Kipnis, D.M. & Daughaday, W.H. Growth hormone secretion during sleep, *J. Clin. Invest.* (1968) **47**, 2079–2090.

257. Takahashi, K., Takahashi, S., Asumi, K., Honda, Y. & Utena, H. Changes of plasma growth hormone level in normal and hypersomnic patients during nocturnal sleep, *Adv. Neurol. Sci. (Tokyo)* (1971) **14**, 743–754.

258. Tanner, J.M. Human growth hormone, *Nature* (1972) **237**, 433–439.

259. Terry, L.C. & Martin, J.B. The effect of lateral hypothalamic-medial forebrain stimulation and somatostatin antiserum on pulsatile growth hormone secretion in freely moving rats: evidence for a dual regulatory mechanism, *Endocrinology* (1981) **109**, 622–627.

260. Underwood, L.E., Azumi, K., Voina, S.J. & Van Wyk, J.J. Growth hormone levels during

sleep in normal and growth hormone deficient children, *Pediatrics* (1971) **48,** 946–954.

261. Vigneri, R. & D'Agata, R. Growth hormone release during the first year of life in relation to sleep-wake periods, *J. Clin. Endocrinol. Metab.* (1971) **33,** 561–563.

262. Vogel, G.W., Rudman, D., Thurmond, A., Barrowclough, B., Giesler, D. & Hickman, J. Human growth hormone and slow-wave sleep, *Psychophysiology* (1972) **9,** 102.

263. Weinberg, U., Weitzman, E.D., Horowitz, Z.D. & Burg, A.C. Lack of an effect of melatonin on the basal and L-dopa stimulated growth hormone secretion in man, *J. Neural Transm.* (1981) **52,** 117–121.

264. Weitzman, E.D., Czeisler, C.A., Zimmerman, J.C. & Moore-Ede, M.C. Biological rhythms in man: relationship of sleep–wake, cortisol, growth hormone and temperature during temporal isolation. In: Martin, J.B., Reichler, S. & Bick, K. (eds.) *Advances in Neurology,* New York: Raven Press (1980).

265. Weitzman, E.D., de Graaf, A.S., Sassin, J.F., Hansen, T., Gotlibsen, O.B., Perlow, M. & Hellman, L. Seasonal patterns of sleep stages and secretion of cortisol and growth hormone during 24 hour periods in northern Norway, *Acta Endocrinol.* (1975) **78,** 65–76.

PROLACTIN

266. Barreca, T., Perria, C., Franceschini, R., Siani, C., Messina, V., Francaviglia, N. & Rolandi, E. Diurnal prolactin changes in human cerebrospinal fluid, *Clin. Endocrinol.* (1984) **20,** 649–655.

267. Boyar, R., Finkelstein, J., Roffwarg, H., Kapen, S., Weitzman, E.D. & Hellman, L. Twenty-four hour luteinizing hormone and follicle-stimulating hormone secretory patterns in gonadal dysgenesis, *J. Clin. Endocrinol. Metab.* (1975) **40,** 234–239.

268. Mendelson, W.B., Jacobs, L.S., Sitaram, N., Wyatt, R.J. & Gillin, J.C. Methscopolamine inhibition of sleep-related growth hormone secretion, *J. Clin. Invest.* (1978) **61,** 1683–1690.

269. Mendelson, W.B., Lantigua, R.A., Wyatt, R.J., Gillin, J.C. & Jacobs, L.S. Piperidine enhances sleep-related and insulin-induced growth hormone secretion: further evidence for a cholinergic secretory mechanism, *J. Clin. Endicrinol. Metab.* (1981) **52,** 409–415.

270. Nokin, J., Vekemans, M., L'Hermitte, M. & Robyn, C. Circadian periodicity of serum prolactin concentration in man, *Brit. Med. J.* (1972) **3,** 561–562.

271. Parker, D.C., Rossman, L.G. & Van der Laan, E.F. Relation of sleep-entrained human prolactin release to REM and non-REM cycles, *J. Clin. Endocrinol. Metab.* (1973) **36,** 1119–1124.

272. Parker, D.C., Rossman, L.G. & Van der Laan, E.F. Relation of sleep-entrained human prolactin release to REM–non REM cycles, *J. Clin. Endocrinol. Metab.* (1974) **38,** 646–651.

273. Sassin, J.F., Frantz, A.G., Kapen, S. & Weitzman, E.D. The nocturnal rise of human prolactin is dependent on sleep, *J. Clin. Endocrinol. Metab.* (1973) **37,** 436–440.

274. Sassin, J.F., Franz, A.G., Weitzman, E.D. & Kapen, S. Human prolactin 24-hour pattern with increased release during sleep, *Science* (1972) **177,** 1205–1206.

CORTISOL AND ACTH

275. Boyar, R.M., Wittan, M., Carruth, A. & Ramsey, J. Circadian cortisol secretory rhythms in Cushing's disease, *J. Clin. Endocrinol. Metab.* (1979) **48,** 760.

276. Dent, R.R., Guilleminault, C., Albert, L.H., Posner, B.I., Cox, B.M. & Goldstein, A. Diurnal rhythm of plasma immunoreactive ß-endorphin and its relationship to sleep stages and plasma rhythms of cortisol and prolactin, *J. Clin. Endocrinol. Metab.* (1981) **52,** 942–947.

277. Gallagher, T.F., Yoshida, K., Roffwarg, H.D., Fukushima, D.K., Weitzman, E.D. & Hellman, L. ACTH and cortisol secretory patterns in man, *J. Clin. Endocrinol. Metab.* (1973) **36,** 1058–1068.

278. Hellman, L., Nakada, F., Curti, J., Weitzman, E.D., Kream, J., Roffwarg, H., Ellman, S., Fukushima, D.K. & Gallagher, T.F. Cortisol is secreted episodically by normal man, *J. Clin. Endocrinol. Metab.* (1970) **30,** 411–422.

279. Jordan, R.M., Ramos-Garatin, A., Kendall, J.W., Gaudette, D. & Walls, R.C. Dynamics of adrenocorticotropin (ACTH) secretion in cyclic Cushing's syndrome: evidence for more than one abnormal ACTH biorhythm, *J. Clin. Endocrinol. Metab.* (1982) **55,** 531–537.

280. Katz, F.H., Romfh, P. & Smith, J.A. Episodic secretion of aldosterone in supine man: relationship to cortisol, *J. Clin. Endocrinol. Metab.* (1972) **35**, 178–181.
281. Katz, F.H., Romfh, P. & Smith, J.A. Diurnal variation of plasma aldosterone, cortisol and renin activity in supine man, *J. Clin. Endocrinol. Metab.* (1975) **40**, 125–134.
282. Kem, D.C., Weinberger, M.H., Gomez-Sanchez, C., Kramer, N.J., Lerman, R., Furuyama, S. & Nugent, C.A. Circadian rhythm of plasma aldosterone concentration in patients with primary aldosteronism, *J. Clin. Invest.* (1973) **52**, 2272–2277.
283. Krieger, D.T. & Gewirtz, G.P. The nature of the circadian periodicity and suppressibility of immunoreactive ACTH levels in Addison's disease, *J. Clin. Endocrinol. Metab.* (1974) **39**, 46–52.
284. Lacerda, L. de, Kowarski, A. & Migeon, C.J. Integrated concentration of plasma cortisol in normal subjects, *J. Clin. Endocrinol. Metab.* (1973) **36**, 227–228.
285. Mandell, A.J. & Mandell, M.P. Peripheral hormonal and metabolic correlates of rapid eye movement sleep, *Exp. Med. Surg.* (1969) **27**, 224–236.
286. Sederberg-Olsen, P., Binder, C., Kehlet, H., Neville, A.M. & Nielson, L.M. Variation in plasma corticosteroids in subjects with Cushing's syndrome of differing etiology, *J. Clin. Endocrinol. Metab.* (1973) **36**, 906–910.
287. Weitzman, E.D. Circadian rhythms and episodic hormone secretion in man, *Ann. Rev. Med.* (1976) **27**, 225–243.
288. Weitzman, E.D., Czeisler, C.A., Zimmerman, J.C., Moore-Ede, M.C. & Ronda, J.M. Biological rhythms in man: internal physiological organization during non-entrained (free-running) conditions and application to delayed sleep-phase syndrome. In: Chase, M.H. & Weitzman, E.D. (eds.) *Sleep Disorders: Basic and Clinical Research*, Lancaster: MTP (1983) 153–171.
289. Weitzman, E.D., Fukushima, D., Nogeire, C., Roffwarg, H., Gallagher, T.F. & Hellman, L. Twenty-four hour pattern of the episodic secretion of cortisol in normal subjects, *J. Clin. Endocrinol. Metab.* (1971) **33**, 14–22.
290. Weitzman, E.D., Goldmacher, D., Kripke, D., MacGregor, P., Kream, J. & Hellman, L. Reversal of sleep–waking cycle: Effect of sleep stage pattern and certain neuroendocrine rhythms, *Trans. Am. Neurol. Assoc.* (1968) **93**, 153–157.
291. Weitzman, E.D., Nogeire, C., Perlow, M., Fukushima, D., Sassin, J., McGregor, P., Gallagher, T.F. & Hellman, L. Effects of a prolonged 3-hour sleep–wake cycle on sleep stages, plasma cortisol growth hormone and body temperature in man, *J. Clin. Endocrinol. Metab.* (1974) **38**, 1018–1030.
292. Weitzman, E.D., Perlow, M., Sassin, F.J., Fukushima, D., Burack, B. & Hellman, L. Persistence of the 24-hour pattern of episodic cortisol secretion and growth hormone release in blind subjects, *Trans. Am. Neurol. Assoc.* (1972) **97**, 197–199.
293. Weitzman, E.D., Zimmerman, J.C., Czeisler, C.A. & Ronda, J. Cortisol secretion is inhibited during sleep in normal man, *J. Clin. Endocrinol. Metab.* (1983) **56**, 352–358.

MELATONIN

294. Arendt, J., Hampton, S., English, J., Kwasowski, P. & Marks, V. 24-hour profiles of melatonin, cortisol, insulin, C-peptide and GIP following a meal and subsequent fasting, *Clin. Endocrinol. (Oxf.)* (1982) **16**, 89–95.
295. Arendt, J. & Marks, V. Can melatonin alleviate jet-lag? *Brit. Med. J. (Clin. Res.)* (1983) **287**, 426.
296. Arendt, J., Symons, A.M., Laud, C.A. & Pryde, S. Abstract 58, *Social Study of Fertility, Conference, Nottingham, 1982.* Cited in: Lincoln, G. Melatonin as a seasonal time cue, *Nature* (1983) **302**, 755.
297. Arendt, J., Wirz-Justice, A., Bradtke, J. & Kornemark, M. Long-term studies on immunoreactive human melatonin, *Ann. Clin. Biochem.* (1979) **16**, 307.
298. Barber, S.G., Smith, J.A. & Hughes, R.C. Melatonin as a tumour marker in a patient with pineal tumour, *Brit. Med. J.* (1978) **2**, 328.
299. Beck, O., Borg, S. & Lundman, A. Concentration of 5-methoxyindoles in the human pineal gland, *J. Neural. Trans.* (1982) **54**, 111–116.
300. Braestrup, C., Nielson, M. & Olsen, C.E. Urinary and brain ß-carbolene-3-carboxylates as potent inhibitors of brain benzodiazepine receptors, *Proc. Nat. Acad. Sci. USA* (1980) **77**, 2288–2292.

301. Brown, G.M., Young, S.N., Gauthier, S., Tsui, H. & Grota, L.J. Melatonin in human cerebrospinal fluid in daytime: its origin and variation with age, *Life Sci.* (1979) **25**, 929–936.
302. Bubenik, G. Shift of seasonal cycle in white-tailed deer by oral administration of melatonin, *J. Exp. Zool.* (1983) **225**, 155–156.
303. Cheung, P.W. & McCormack, C.E. Failure of pinealectomy or melatonin to alter circadian rhythm of the rat, *Am. J. Physiol.* (1982) **242**, R261–264.
304. Cohen, H.N., Hay, I.D., Annesley, T.M., Beastall, G.H., Wallace, A.M., Spooner, R., Thomson, J.A., Eastwood, P. & Klee, G.G. Serum immunoreactive melatonin in boys with delayed puberty *Clin. Endocrinol. (Oxf.)* (1982) **17**, 517–521.
305. Cowen, P.J., Fraser, S., Sammons, R. & Green, A.R. Atenolol reduces plasma melatonin concentrations in man, *Brit. J. Clin. Pharmacol.* (1983) **15**, 579–581.
306. Cramer, H., Bohme, W., Kendel, K. & Donnadieu, M. Freisetzung von Wachstumsharmon und von melanozyten stimulierendem Hormon in durch Melatonin gebahnten Schlaf beim Menschen, *Arzneimittel-Forsch.* (1976) **26**, 1076–1078.
307. Cramer, H., Rudolph, J., Cornsbruch, U. & Kendel, K. On the effects of melatonin on sleep and behaviour in man, *Adv. Biochem. Psychopharmacol.* (1974) **11**, 187–191.
308. Ehrenkranz, J.R.L., Tamarkin, L., Comite, F., Johnsonbaugh, R.E., Bybee, D.E., Loriaux, D.L. & Cutler, G.B. Daily rhythm of plasma melatonin in normal and precocious puberty, *J. Clin. Endocrinol. Metab.* (1982) **55**, 307–310.
309. Fernandez-Guardiola, A.A. & Anton-Tay, F. Modulation of subcortical inhibitory mechanisms by melatonin, *Adv. Behav. Biol.* (1974) **10**, 273–287.
310. Ferrier, I.N., Arendt, J., Johnstone, E.C. & Crow, T.J. Reduced nocturnal melatonin secretion in chronic schizophrenia: relationship to body weight, *Clin. Endocrinol. (Oxf.)* (1982) **17**, 181–187.
311. Fevre, M., Segel, T., Marks, J.F. & Boyar, R.M. LH and melatonin secretion pattern in pubertal boys, *J. Clin. Endocrinol. Metab.* (1978) **47**, 1383–1386.
312. Fèvre-Montange, M., Cauter, E.V., Refetoff, S., Désir, D., Tourniaire, J. & Copinschi, G. Effects of jet lag on hormonal patterns: adaptation of melatonin circadian periodicity, *J. Clin. Endocrinol. Metab.* (1981) **52**, 642–649.
313. Garrick, N.A., Tamarkin, P.L., Markey, S.P. & Murphy, D.L. Light and propranolol suppress the nocturnal elevation of serotonin in the cerebrospinal fluid of rhesus monkeys, *Science* (1983) **221**, 474–476.
314. Harlow, H.J., Phillips, J.A. & Ralph, C.L. Day–night rhythm in plasma melatonin in a mammal lacking a distinct pineal gland, the nine-banded armadillo, *Gen. Comp. Endocrinol.* (1981) **45**, 212–218.
315. Harlow, H.J., Phillips, J.A. & Ralph, C.L. Circadian rhythms and the effects of exogenous melatonin in the nine-banded armadillo, *Dasypus novencintus:* a mammal lacking a distinct pineal gland, *Physiol. Behav.* (1982) **29**, 307–313.
316. Ho, A.K. & Smith, J.A. Effect of benserazide on the levels of pineal 5-hydroxytryptamine, melatonin synthesising enzymes and serum melatonin, *Biochem. Pharmacol.* (1982) **31**, 2251–2255.
317. Holmes, S.W. & Sugden, D. Effects of melatonin on sleep and neurochemistry in the rat, *Brit. J. Pharmacol.* (1982) **76**, 95–101.
318. Illnerova, H. & Vanecek, J. Extension of the rat pineal N-acetyltransferase rhythm in continuous darkness and on short photoperiod, *Brain Res.* (1983) **26**, 176–179.
319. Jimerson, D.C., Lynch, H.J., Post, R.M., Wurtman, R.J. & Bunney, Jr., W.E. Urinary melatonin rhythms during sleep deprivation in depressed patients and normals, *Life Sci.* (1977) **20**, 1501–1508.
320. Kennaway, D.J., Gilmore, T.A. & Seamark, R.F. Effect of melatonin feeding on serum prolactin and gonadotropin levels and the onset of seasonal estrous cyclicity in sheep, *Endocrinology* (1982) **110**, 1766–1772.
321. Kennaway, D.J., Gilmore, T.A. & Seamark, R.F. Effects of melatonin implants on the circadian rhythm of plasma melatonin and prolactin in sheep, *Endocrinology* (1982) **110**, 2186–2188.
322. Klein, D.C. & Moore, R.Y. Pineal N-acetyltransferase and hydroxy indole-O-methyl-transferase; control by the retinohypothalamic tract and the suprachiasmatic nucleus, *Brain Res.* (1979) **174**, 245–262.
323. Lang, U., Kornemark, M., Aubert, M.L., Paunier, L. & Sizonko, P.C. Radioimmunological determination of urinary melatonin in humans; correlation with plasma levels and typical 24-hour rhythmicity, *J. Clin. Endocrinol. Metab.* (1981) **53**, 645–650.

324. Lerner, A.B. & Norlund, J.J. Comment: administration of melatonin to human subjects. In: Altschule, M.D. (ed.) *Frontiers of Pineal Physiology*, Cambridge, Massachusetts: MIT Press (1975) 42–43.

325. Lewy, A.J. & Newsome, D.A. Different types of melatonin circadian secretory rhythms in some blind subjects, *J. Clin. Endocrinol. Metab.* (1983) **56**, 1103–1107.

326. Lewy, A.J., Wehr, T.A., Goodwin, F.K., Newsome, D.A. & Markey, S.P. Light suppresses melatonin secretion in humans, *Science* (1980) **210**, 1267–1268.

327. Lincoln, G. Melatonin as a seasonal time-cue: a commercial story, *Nature* (1983) **302**, 755.

328. Lynch, H.J., Ozaki, Y. & Wurtman, R.J. The measurement of melatonin in mammalian tissues and body fluids, *J. Neural. Transm. (Suppl.)* (1978) **13**, 251–264.

329. Marangos, P.J., Patel, J., Hirata, F., Sondheim, D., Paul, S.M., Skolnick, P. & Goodwin, F.K. Inhibition of diazepam binding by tryptophan derivatives including melatonin and its brain metabolite N-acetyl-5-methoxy kynurenamine, *Life Sci.* (1981) **29**, 259–267.

330. Moore, R.Y. & Lenn, N.J. A retinohypothalamic projection in the rat, *J. Comp. Neurol.* (1972) **146**, 1–14.

331. Namboodiri, M.A., Sugden, D. & Klein, D.C. 5-hydroxytryptophan elevates serum melatonin, *Science* (1983) **221**, 659–661.

332. Pavel, S., Goldstein, R. & Petrescu, M. Vasotocin, melatonin and narcolepsy: possible involvement of the pineal gland in its patho-physiological mechanism, *Peptides (Fayetteville)* (1980) **1**, 281–284.

333. Penny, R. Melatonin excretion in normal males and females: increase during puberty, *Metabolism* (1982) **31**, 816–823.

334. Redman, J., Armstrong, S. & Ng, K.T. Free-running activity rhythms in the rat: entrainment by melatonin, *Science* (1983) **219**, 1089–1091.

335. Reiter, R.J., Craft, C.M., Johnson, J.E., King, T.S., Richardson, B.A., Vaughan, G.M. & Vaughan, M.K. Age-associated reduction in nocturnal pineal melatonin levels in female rats, *Endocrinology* (1981) **109**, 1295–1297.

336. Reiter, R.J. The pineal gland: an intermediary between the environment and the endocrine system, *Psychoneuroendocrinology* (1983) **8**, 31–40.

337. Reppert, S.M. & Klein, D.C. Mammalian pineal gland: basic and clinical aspects. In: Motta, M. (ed.) *The Endocrine Functions of the Brain*, New York: Raven Press (1980) 327.

338. Reppert, S.M., Perlow, M.J., Ungerleider, L.G., Mishkin, M., Tamarkin, L., Orloff, D.G., Hoffman, H.J. & Klein, D.C. Effect of damage to the suprachiasmatic area of the anterior hypothalamus on the daily melatonin and cortisol rhythms in the rhesus monkey, *J. Neurosci.* (1981) **1**, 1414–1425.

339. Sallanon, M., Claustrat, B. & Touret, M. Presence of melatonin in various cat brainstem nuclei, *Acta Endocrinol. (Copenh.)* (1982) **101**, 161–165.

340. Sugden, D. *Actions of Melatonin on the Central Nervous System*, Ph.D. thesis (1980) London: Council for National Academic Awards.

341. Tamarkin, L., Abastillas, P., Chen, H.-C., McNemar, A. & Sidbury, J.B. The daily profile of plasma melatonin in obese and Prader–Willi syndrome children, *J. Clin. Endocrinol. Metab.* (1982) **55**, 491–495.

342. Tan, C.H. & Khoo, J.C.M. Melatonin concentrations in human serum, ventricular and lumbar cerebrospinal fluids as an index of the secretory pathways of the pineal gland, *Horm. Res.* (1981) **14**, 224–233.

343. Vaughan, G.M., Allen, J.P., Tullis, W., Siler-Khodr, T.M., Pena, A. & Sackman, J.W. Overnight plasma profiles of melatonin and certain adenohypophyseal hormones in man, *J. Clin. Endocrinol. Metab.* (1978) **47**, 566–571.

344. Vaughan, G.M., Bell, R. & de la Pena, A. Nocturnal plasma melatonin in humans: episodic pattern and influence of light, *Neurosci. Lett.* (1979) **14**, 81–84.

345. Vaughan, G.M., Pelham, R.W., Pang, S.F., Loughlin, L.L., Wilson, K.M., Sandock, K.L., Vaughan, M.K., Koslow, S.H. & Reiter, R.J. Nocturnal elevation of plasma melatonin and urinary 5-hydroxyindoleacetic acid in young men: attempts at modification by brief changes in environmental lighting and by sleep and by autonomic drugs, *J. Clin. Endocrinol. Metab.* (1976) **42**, 752–764.

346. Waldhauser, F., Weiszenbacher, G., Frisch, H., Zeitlhuber, U., Waldhauser, M. & Wurtman, R.J. Fall in nocturnal serum melatonin during prepuberty and pudescence, *Lancet* (1984) **1**, 362–365.

347. Wetterberg, L., Aperia, B., Beck-Friis J., Kjellman, B.F., Ljunggren, J.-G., Nilsonne, A.,

Petterson, U., Tham, A. & Unden, F. Melatonin and cortisol levels in psychiatric illness, *Lancet* (1982) **2**, 100.

348. Wurtman, R.J., Axelrod, J. & Barchas, J.D. Age and enzyme activity in the human pineal, *J. Clin. Endocrinol. Metab.* (1964) **24**, 299.
349. Wurtman, R.J. & Moskowitz, M.A. The pineal organ, *New Engl. J. Med.* (1977) **296**, 1329–1333.
350. Yu, H.S., Pang, S.F. & Tang, P.L. Increase in the level of retinal melatonin and persistence of its daily rhythm in rats after pinealectomy, *J. Endocrinol.* (1981) **91**, 477–481.

SLEEP AND THE KIDNEY: ADH

351. Danguir, J. Sleep deficits in rats with hereditary diabetes insipidus, *Nature* (1983) **304**, 163–164.
352. Leaf, A. & Liddle, G.W. Summarization of the effects of hormones on water and electrolyte metabolism. In: Williams, R.H. (ed.) *Textbook of Endocrinology*, Philadelphia: W.B. Saunders (1974) 938–947.
353. Mandell, A.J., Chaffey, B., Brill, P., Mandell, M.P., Rodnick, J., Rubin, R.T. & Sheff, R. Dreaming sleep in man: changes in urine volume and osmolarity, *Science* (1966) **151**, 1558–1560.
354. Mullen, P.E., James, V.H., Lightman, S.L., Linsell, C. & Peart, W.S. A relationship between plasma renin activity and the rapid eye movement phase of sleep in man, *J. Clin. Endocrinol. Metab.* (1980) **50**, 466–469.
355. Rubin, R.T., Poland, R.E., Gouin, R.R. & Tower, B.B. Secretion of hormones influencing water and electrolyte balance (antidiuretic hormone, aldosterone, prolactin) during sleep in normal adult men, *Psychosom. Med.* (1978) **40**, 44–52.
356. Rubin, R.T., Poland, R.E., Ravessoud, F., Gouin, P.R. & Tower, B.B. Antidiuretic hormone: episodic nocturnal secretion in adult man, *Endocr. Res. Comm.* (1975) **2**, 459–469.
357. Vitiello, M.V., Prinz, P.N. & Halter, J.B. Sodium restricted diet increases night time plasma norepinephrine and impairs sleep patterns in man, *J. Clin. Endocrinol. Metab.* (1983) **56**, 553–556.

THYROID HORMONE AND SLEEP

358. Alford, F.P., Baker, H.W.G., Patel, Y.C., Rennie, G.C., Youatt, G., Burger, H.G. & Hudson, B. Temporal patterns of circulatory hormones as assessed by continuous blood sampling, *J. Clin. Endocrinol. Metab.* (1973) **36**, 108–116.
359. Bellastella, A., Criscuolo, T., Mango, A., Perrone, L., Sinisi, A.A. & Faggiano, M. Circannual rhythms of plasma growth hormone, thyrotropin and thyroid hormones in prepuberty, *Clin. Endocrinol.* (1984) **20**, 531–537.
360. Lucke, C., Hehrmann, R., von Mayersbach, K. & von Zur Muhlen, A. Studies on circadian variations of plasma TSH, thyroxine and triiodothyronine in man, *Acta Endrocrinol. (Copenh.)* (1976) **86**, 81–86.
361. Opstad, P.K., Falch, D., Øktedalen, O., Fonnum, F. & Wergeland, R. The thyroid function in young men during prolonged exercises and the effect of energy and sleep deprivation, *Clin. Endocrinol.* (1984) **20**, 657–669.
362. Vanhaelst, L., Cauter, E. van, Degaute, J.P. & Goldstein, J. Circadian variations of serum thyrotropin levels in man, *J. Clin. Endocrinol. Metab.* (1972) **35**, 479–482.
363. Webster, B.R., Guansing, A.R. & Paice, J.C. Absence of diurnal variation of serum TSH, *J. Clin. Endocrinol. Metab.* (1972) **34**, 899–901.
364. Weeke, J. Circadian variation of the serum thyrotropin level in normal subjects, *Scand. J. Clin. Lab. Invest.* (1973) **31**, 337–342.

GONADOTROPHINS AND SLEEP

365. Boyar, R., Finkelstein, J., Roffwarg, H., Kapen, S., Weitzman, E. & Hellman, L. Synchronization of augmented luteinizing hormone secretion in normal man with sleep stage recording, *New Engl. J. Med.* (1972) **287**, 582–586.

366. Boyar, R., Finkelstein, J. Roffwarg, H., Kapen, S., Weitzman, E.D. & Hellman, L. Twenty-four hour luteinizing hormone and follicle-stimulating hormone secretory patterns in gonadal dysgenesis, *J. Clin. Endocrinol. Metab.* (1975) **40,** 234–239.
367. Cumming, D.C., Reid, R.L., Quigley, M.E., Rebar, R.W. & Yen, S.S.C. Evidence for decreased endogenous dopamine and opioid inhibitory influences on LH secretion in polycystic ovary syndrome, *Clin. Endocrinol.* (1984) **20,** 643–648.
368. Evans, J.I., MacLean, A.W., Ismail, A.A.A. & Love, D. Concentration of plasma testosterone in normal man during sleep, *Nature* (1971) **229,** 261–262.
369. Jung, R. Infantile precocious puberty, *Update* (1983) **9,** 1355–1362.
370. Kapen, S., Boyar, R.M., Finkelstein, J.W., Hellman, L. & Weitzman, E.D. Effect of sleep–wake cycle reversal on luteinizing hormone secretory pattern in puberty, *J. Clin. Endocrinol. Metab.* (1974) **39,** 293–299.
371. Kapen, S., Boyar, R., Hellman, L. & Weitzman, E.D. Effect of sleep–wake cycle reversal on LH secretory pattern in puberty, *J. Clin. Endocrinol. Metab.* (1973) **36,** 724–729.
372. Kapen, S., Boyar, R., Hellman, L. & Weitzman, E.D. Inhibition of LH secretion during the night time hours: a subgroup of the amenorrhoea–galactorrhoea syndrome. Presented at the Second International Sleep Research Congress, Edinburgh 30 June–4 July 1975.
373. Kawano, N. & Miyao, M. Studies on the gonadotropin secretion during sleep in patients with abnormal sexual development – the role of the CNS in the onset of puberty, *Brain Dev.* (1982) **4,** 421–428.
374. Kulin, H.E. & Reiter, E.O. Gonadotropins during childhood and adolescence: a review, *Pediatrics* (1973) **51,** 260–271.
375. Piro, C., Fraioli, F., Sciarra, F. & Conti, C. Circadian rhythm of plasma testosterone, cortisol and gonadotropins in normal male subjects, *Steroid Biochem.* (1973) **4,** 321–329.
376. Rose, R.M., Kreuz, L.E., Holaday, J.W., Sulak, K.J. & Johnson, C.E. Diurnal variation of plasma testosterone and cortisol, *J. Endocrinol.* (1972) **54,** 177–178.
377. Rosenfeld, R.S., Hellman, L., Roffwarg, H., Weitzman, E.D. & Gallagher, T.F. Dehydro-androsterone is secreted episodically and synchronously with cortisol in normal man, *J. Clin. Endocrinol. Metab.* (1971) **33,** 87.
378. Rubin, R.T., Poland, R.E., Rubin. L.E. & Gouin, P.R. The neuroendocrinology of human sleep, *Life Sci.* (1974) **14,** 1041–1052.
379. Weitzman, E.D. Circadian rhythms and episodic hormone secretion in man, *Ann. Rev. Med.* (1976) **27,** 225–243.
380. Winter, J.S.D. & Fairman, C. Pituitary-gonadal relations in male children and adolescents, *Pediat. Res.* (1972) **6,** 126–135.
381. Zumoff, B., Freeman, R., Coupey, S., Saenger, P., Markowitz, M. & Kream, J. A chronobiological abnormality in luteinizing hormone secretion in teenage girls with the polycystic ovary syndrome, *New Engl. J. Med.* (1983) **309,** 1206–1209.

PART II

SLEEP DISORDERS

CHAPTER 4

PARASOMNIAS

INTRODUCTION

The American Edgar Allan Poe, author of *Buried Alive*, and the Swiss composer Othmar Schoeck, who wrote a song cycle on the same topic, must have known sleep paralysis from first-hand experience to describe it so vividly. Sleep paralysis is not uncommon, and the maid described by St. Matthew (9:24), who was not dead but sleeping, may have suffered from this condition. The incubus or evil spirit that visited Dante's lost souls in Purgatory was surely a terror-by-night, and Lady Macbeth was a sleep walker. It is perhaps a little disappointing to find that most of these dramatic occurrences are normal physiological events.

Parasomnias (events around sleep) are non-epileptic in origin and include common, if not *universal* conditions such as nightmares and hypnic jerks: *common* disturbances, with no known pathological basis, such as sleep myoclonus; and also a number of *rare* conditions, due to definite disease, such as paroxysmal nocturnal haemoglobinuria. All these parasomnias can be very alarming, but few are serious. Most result in abnormal motor activity during half-sleep, or excessive autonomic discharge persisting into partial wakefulness. It is rare for parasomnias to cause a severe nocturnal sleep disturbance, but very occasionally they result in either insomnia or daytime drowsiness.

Parasomnias occur more often in *children* than in adults. Why this should be so is uncertain. Perhaps the normally deep sleep of children predisposes to parasomnias, and lightening of sleep with age accounts for growing out of them.[2] In some cases parasomnias are *familial*, as with somnambulism and night terrors.[4] Here there may be a neurochemical defect, but this has not yet been identified. In addition to childhood and occasional familial cases, a high incidence of parasomnias is found in some disease states of uncertain aetiology, such as in Gilles de la Tourette's syndrome, which is characterized by frequent somnambulism, enuresis and awakenings from sleep, as well as by tics.[5] Specific parasomnias occur frequently in some *primary sleep disorders,* including narcolepsy.

Psychiatric illnesses do not cause parasomnias in either children or adults, although bruxism, sleep walking and night terrors are increased by emotional and perhaps by physical stress.[3] Thus treatment of anxiety will sometimes prevent these parasomnias. Very occasionally, *disturbance of circadian rhythms*, as in endogenous depression, with early sleep-onset REM activity, can result in vivid sleep-onset nightmares, and perhaps also sleep paralysis. Practically any disturbance of sleep, whether due to sleep deprivation on previous nights, sleep discomfort, hypnotic or stimulant drugs, may make some parasomnias worse. Benzodiazepines can sometimes make nocturnal enuresis worse, not better.

The *treatment* of parasomnias often requires little more than the explanation to the child's parents of the benign nature of their child's sleep disturbance, laying stress on the absence of any serious psychopathology. The buzzer and pad remains the most effective treatment by far for nocturnal enuresis. (Why this should be so is not at all clear, since enuresis usually precedes rather than follows arousal.) Benzodiazepines will prevent night terrors, but this action has not been explained.

The *cause* of most parasomnias is unknown. Broughton[1] considered that sleep walking, sleep terrors and sleep enuresis were all disorders of arousal mechanisms. According to this view, arousal from stage 3–4 NREM sleep is incomplete. There is confusion upon awakening, amnesia for the event, a poor response to efforts to produce wakefulness, failure to react to external stimuli, minimal or fragmentary recall of dreams, and sometimes automatic behaviour. However, in the case of bed wetting, this may occur in any sleep stage, and the idea that children with parasomnias are somehow 'deeper' sleepers than others has no firm experimental basis. A few parasomnias may have a neurochemical basis, but most are probably multifactorial. In most cases we simply do not know why they happen.

Many parasomnias are strongly linked to one specific sleep stage, and occur therefore at a specific time of night (Table 4.1).

NOCTURNAL BEHAVIOURAL DISTURBANCES IN CHILDREN

The highly organized pattern of sleep undergoes major maturational changes in the first year of life, and the development of normal adult sleep behaviour continues until the age of 18 years. The development of normal sleep patterns in childhood requires consistency and regularity. At the age of 6–9 months, children spend 14–15 h of each 24 h period in sleep. This declines to 10–14 h at the age of 5 and to 7–9 h at the age of 15. However, the range of individual variation is large. Studies between 1954 and 1980 by Largo[8] in Swiss children in Zurich show that practically all healthy infants under the age of one sleep for 2–3 h each day as well as by night, but by the age of five the percentage of day sleepers has fallen to 21%. Sleep behaviour in pre-school age children has been reported from Los Angeles, Switzerland and London.[6,7,9] Differences in sleep depend largely on different conditioned learning patterns and on the mother's expectations. As would be expected, the more children sleep by day, the less they sleep by night and vice versa. The adage 'early to bed, early to rise' is demonstrably true in children. There is a good correlation between bedtime and the time of morning waking.

Night terrors, nightmares, sleep walking and bed wetting are common causes of sleep disturbance in young children, although there are major unexplained differences in the occurrence of these parasomnias in different populations of Zurich, Stockholm and Boston children. However, the major problem of childhood sleep is not the parasomnias but resistance to going to bed, evening wakefulness and frequent night arousals. Night awakening in childhood is entirely normal and occurs at one time or other in 50–70% of all young children; regularly in about 10%. Development factors are not of major importance. 6% of pre-term children at 3 years of age wake every night, 4% wake 4–5 nights a week, 8% 2–3 nights, and 28% one night. 34% have occasional screaming at bed time.[9] This behaviour is very similar to that reported for full-term children.

What constitutes a sleep problem in childhood is determined by the parents, not the child. In normal children, cutting out daytime sleep and enforcement of a regular night sleep schedule, with reassurance of the parents, rather than sedative or hypnotic drugs, may help to solve night restlessness. So sometimes will putting a child who is a poor sleeper into the bed of a brother or sister who sleeps well. A few children have a cyclical sleep disturbance, going to sleep progressively later and with more arousals for a few days, until they are so tired that one good night's sleep follows. The problem is different in blind, mentally retarded, brain-damaged or hyperexcitable children, in which behavioural techniques do not usually overcome sleep disturbances, and in whom these disturbances, with or without waking hyperactivity, may be neurologically based. Sleep problems in childhood are often blamed on divergent parental attitudes, marriage problems or ambivalent attitudes of the mother, but the reverse situation is sometimes true. Finally, in the area of childhood sleep disorders, it is important not to overlook the childhood form of sleep apnoea.

SLEEP AND MOVEMENT

Frequent *body movements* occur throughout normal sleep and 8–15 short arousals are normal, even in subjects who sleep well and do not recall these on waking. A shift of posture usually occurs about every 15–20 min. Some have considered that too few body movements are as detrimental to sleep as too many.[16] Body movements usually accompany sleep stage shifts, and it has been claimed that major body movements precede or follow a dream or interrupt a dream sequence.[11]

Finger, hand and face twitches, leg jerks, semi-purposeful arm movements and changes in posture occur throughout sleep. In NREM sleep these movements are most frequent in stage 1–2 and decrease during stage 3–4. They are stable and reliable indicators of sleep stage.[21] During REM sleep, brief phasic movements of the arms and legs occur. These movements are irregular, unlike the rhythmic periodic leg movements of sleep myoclonus that may

Table 4.1 *The parasomnias*

Parasomnia	Polysomnogram findings	Clinical features and differential diagnosis	Possible treatment
Sleep onset			
Hypnic jerks	Generalized myoclonus	Generalized body jerks at sleep onset (Distinguish from epilepsy)	None needed
Sensory starts	Uncertain	As hypnic jerks, with sensory paroxysm accompanying jerk	None needed
Sleep paralysis	Sleep-onset REM	1. Familial 2. Isolated 3. REM narcolepsy	Clomipramine 25–50 mg nocte Clonazepam 1–2 mg nocte
Hypnagogic hallucinations	NREM 1–2	Incorporation of waking material into dreams	
Bruxism	NREM 1–2	Usual age 2–15; or elderly subjects	Dental review Teeth protection 'Bite-guard'
Head banging	NREM 1–2	Young children (differentiate from seizure disorder)	None usually needed
Early sleep (first third of night)			
Nocturnal enuresis	NREM 3–4 (However, may occur in any sleep phase)	Up to 15% normal children More common in males (Urological evaluation)	Ephedrine 15–30 mg at night Tricyclics (suppress slow-wave sleep with also anticholinergic and bladder anaesthetic effect) Benzodiazepines may cause deterioration. Buzzer and pad
Sleep walking	NREM 3–4	Up to 15% of normal children	Avoid injury Short-acting benzodiazepine, e.g. triazolam 0.125 mg
Pavor nocturnus (night terrors)	NREM 3–4	1–4% of children Males more than females Confusion Severe autonomic overactivity	Benzodiazepines Psychotherapy may have a role

Middle and late sleep (REM sleep)			
Nightmares	REM	Universal; Good waking recall; Wake patient	None required, or benzodiazepines
Cluster headache	Usually REM sleep	Severe retro-orbital pain; Sympathetic signs	Ergotamine or indomethacin
Nocturnal painful erections	REM sleep	Check Hb, clotting factors, BP, vascular disease	Suppress REM sleep; Treat hypertension
Late night (?REM sleep-related)			
Cardiovascular symptoms, e.g. nocturnal angina	REM sleep or non-specific	Differentiate from gastro-oesophageal reflux	Coronary dilators; anti-arrhythmic drugs
Asthma	Sleep-stage related?	Distinguish from sleep apnoea, paroxysmal nocturnal dyspnoea, and abnormal swallowing syndrome	Asthma therapy
No specific time			
Gastrointestinal symptoms			
Gastro-oesophageal reflux			
Abnormal swallowing		Distinguish from asthma; pharyngeal pouch	Appropriate surgery; raise bed head; medical treatment
Paroxysmal nocturnal haemoglobinuria		May be chronic, not paroxysmal; differentiate from haematuria, local pathology, porphyria, drug metabolites	Blood transfusion if severe anaemia
Sleep myoclonus	EMG diagnosis	Periodic; May cause insomnia or daytime drowsiness; Association with akathisia	Clonazepam 2–4 mg; Cyproheptadine 4–12 mg
Sleep epilepsy	REM or NREM	Usually generalized seizures or psychomotor attacks; Peak occurrence first 2 h of sleep, second peak at 0400–0600, sometimes for 1 h after waking; Differentiate from automatisms and night terrors	Anticonvulsant drugs

occur throughout NREM but not during REM sleep. Periodically during REM sleep, rapid upper and lower facial jerking and eye jerks occur. The eye movements are binocularly symmetrical, rapid, vertical, oblique and horizontal. REM sleep movements have been related to dream content by Wolpert,[22] but despite some recent evidence in favour of this view[14] the proposition seems unlikely.

The eyelids of a sleeping person can easily be gently opened by hand, and, according to Oswald,[20] healthy children, and even more commonly dehydrated or sick children, often sleep with their eyes half open and their pupils partly exposed. Fuchs and Wu,[12] who studied the sleep of 500 healthy Chinese students, concluded that the facial structure of the Chinaman is such as to make him particularly liable to sleep with only half-closed eyes.

SLEEP IN MOVEMENT DISORDERS

The waking *involuntary movements* of extrapyramidal disease may be apparent in any stage of nocturnal sleep, although their attitudes during sleep are different according to the type of involuntary movement. Overall, with the reduction in awareness, loss of voluntary motor control and atonia of sleep, *spasticity* and *rigidity* due to pyramidal and extrapyramidal disease are reduced or abolished during sleep. In *Parkinson's disease,* tremor may persist to some extent during stage 1–2 NREM sleep, but is usually abolished during stage 3–4 NREM sleep and also during REM sleep. Involuntary gross body movements during sleep continue, but at a reduced level, in Parkinson's disease. Non-rhythmic involuntary movements, as well as abnormal postures, of *choreoathetosis* and *dystonia* may partly disappear during deep sleep.[18] Abnormal EMG groupings, particularly in chorea but also in generalized dystonia, decrease remarkably during sleep, proportional to the sleep stage, and are minimal in stages 3–4 NREM sleep. Abnormal EMG groupings, and clinical characteristics of dystonia, briefly return in REM sleep. The multiple tics of *Gilles de la Tourette's syndrome* occur throughout sleep in all stages including REM as well as NREM sleep.[13]

Neocortical seizure phenomena such as *Jacksonian status epilepticus* and *epilepsia partialis continua* show constant discharge rates across all sleep stages, although the convulsive movements may diminish in intensity with the atonia of NREM and REM sleep. The different forms of *myoclonus* show varied changes during sleep. As with epilepsia partialis continua, myoclonus of spinal cord origin and hemifacial spasm persist unchanged for the entire duration of sleep, as do the fasciculations of motor neurone disease. Likewise, palatal myoclonus associated with lesions of the olivodentate system usually persists throughout sleep, although occasional instances of the disappearance of palatal myoclonus during sleep have been recorded. Myoclonus in the course of encephalitis or following cerebral anoxia usually disappears in the course of NREM stage 1–2 sleep.[17]

The structure of sleep itself is abnormal in many motor disorders with primary involvement of the motor system (as in dystonia musculorum deformans) or with damage to adjacent sleep-related structures (e.g. Ramsay Hunt syndrome). Abnormal characteristics of sleep spindles in *dystonia* may indicate thalamic involvement here,[15] whilst REM sleep 'on' neurones may be damaged in *spinocerebellar ataxias*.

HYPNIC JERKS

Body jerks at sleep onset are clearly distinguished from other types of focal or generalized, single or multiple jerks that occur during other periods of sleep. They are a normal phenomenon. Hypnic jerks[19] occur only during the early stages of sleep. Between 60 and 70% of all normal subjects describe these jerks from time to time, but they are probably universal. Perhaps only violent movements causing arousal may be remembered. A hypnic jerk usually takes the form of a single, asymmetric, proximal or distal body twitch. The normal head droop with drowsiness when in the sitting position is not a true hypnic jerk, but related to the onset of sleep atonia in the neck muscles. Hypnic jerks are sometimes accompanied by a perception of falling, a vivid dream or hallucination, a sharp cry, or a sensory flash. The jerks of one of Oswald's subjects, a 40-year-old Oxford don, were accompanied by visual hallucinations, and were severe enough to prevent sleep, but this is unusual. Hypnic jerks are increased by prior physical work, emotional stress and caffeine, and reduced by alcohol and hypnotics. Their apparent association with anxiety may result from more ready recall of hypnic jerks and greater difficulty in falling asleep when anxious. Hypnic jerks are not related to other forms of waking or sleep myoclonus and are not a form of epilepsy. No EEG or clinical abnormality has been associated with them. Oswald[19] concluded that hypnic jerks were probably part of an arousal response to minimal stimuli.

BENIGN NEONATAL SLEEP MYOCLONUS

Rhythmic jerking of the hands, arms and legs with occasional, bilateral, synchronous, repetitive jerking of the fingers, wrists, elbows and ankles may occur during sleep in early infancy, both at sleep onset, but also during later stages of sleep. These repetitive and fragmentary jerks are found in only a small minority of infants, and disappear by the age of 1–2 years. Despite concern that such children may have serious neonatal seizures or central nervous system disease, the condition appears to be entirely benign.[10] Benign neonatal sleep myoclonus can be distinguished from other forms of myoclonus in infants, myoclonic epilepsy, benign myoclonus of early infancy, benign familial neonatal seizures, and myoclonic jerks in opsoclonus–myoclonus, by its occurrence during sleep only, and by the absence of any EEG or neurological abnormality, as well as by continued normality on follow-up. Neonatal sleep myoclonus may be a benign disturbance of the brain stem reticular activating control mechanism involved with the initiation and synchronization of normal sleep, and, as with hypnic jerks in adults, is probably a form of partial arousal response to noise or other stimuli.

RESTLESS LEGS AND SLEEP MYOCLONUS

RESTLESS LEGS (Table 4.2)

> *Wherefore to some, on being abed, they be taken themselves to sleep, presently in the arms and legs leapings and contractions of the tendons, and so great a restlessness and tossings of their members ensue that the diseased are no more able to sleep than if they were in a place of the greatest torture.*
>
> (Willis, 1685;[64] see Coleman[34].)

Willis's account of restless legs was followed by many other similar descriptions, but the syndrome of severe leg discomfort, with the inability to keep still, was not clearly defined until Ekbom's thesis of 1945.[39] The condition is really a waking, not a sleeping, disorder, although the restlessness usually persists into light sleep or prevents sleep onset. Restless legs are often accompanied by nocturnal myoclonus.[39] The restless leg syndrome has close similarity to the whole body restlessness induced by neuroleptic drugs and the motor restlessness of some neurotic individuals (akathisia), although sensory discomfort and motor 'impatience' are seldom a prominent feature of akathisia, in which restlessness may involve the whole body, not just the legs.[29, 32, 33, 39] Very occasionally, the arms and not the legs are restless.[63]

Table 4.2 *Restless legs and sleep myoclonus*

	Restless legs	Sleep myoclonus (periodic movements during sleep, PMS)
Time of occurrence	Wakefulness, evening early sleep	Sleep
Sleep stage	NREM 1 and 2	NREM sleep (inhibited during REM sleep)
Sensory component	Present	Absent
Character	Restless, not myoclonic	Periodic jerks
Distribution	Generalized, both legs	Tibialis anterior
Association	Anaemia, gastrectomy, sensory neuropathy, nerve damage, uraemia	Occult, but occurs in narcolepsy, sleep apnoea
Concurrence	Usually associated with sleep myoclonus	A third of cases associated with restless legs
Presenting complaint	Extreme sensory discomfort	No symptoms; sometimes insomnia or daytime drowsiness
Treatment	None very effective: sedatives	Uncertain: clonazepam and other benzodiazepines may reduce awareness of jerking

Clinical features

The sensory complaint is usually uppermost with deep, creeping, unpleasant or unbearable dysaesthesiae, sensations of cold, discomfort or weakness, usually most pronounced in the calves and accompanied by the irresistible desire or need to move the legs, and the inability to keep them still. This restlessness is most common in the evening and may persist for many hours, but is usually most severe before sleep onset. Rapid exercise, walking, leg rubbing or kicking may improve matters, but at best the relief is only temporary.

The severity of restlessness of the legs increases with age, sleep deprivation and mental stress. The degree of discomfort can be so great as to cause severe emotional disturbance or even suicide. Curiously, symptoms may be abolished with fever.

Ekbom[39, 41] suggested that the prevalence of the restless leg syndrome in the general population was as great as 5%. This figure is surely too high, obtained only when patients are questioned intensively, and even then most reports are of mild rather than severe symptoms. Murray[57] indicated a much lower prevalence, less than 1%.

Cause of restless legs

The cause of restless leg syndrome is usually occult, but there is often a hint of sensory nerve or root damage. Many case reports indicate a possible sub-clinical sensory neuropathy,[43, 61] amyloidosis[49] or diabetes.[44] Despite these clues, muscle biopsies done on 10 subjects by Harriman et al.[48] were all normal, with no evidence of muscle or nerve damage.

Many different conditions have been associated with the restless leg syndrome. These include motor neurone disease,[24] acute poliomyelitis,[52] drug toxicity, amphetamines, other CNS stimulants, and verapamil.[50] Other examples of the restless leg syndrome have been described in association with anaemia and deficiency states, gastrectomy,[42] iron deficiency anaemia, folate deficiency and malnutrition in prisoners of war,[24, 30, 39, 58] carcinoma,[40] uraemia[31] and normal pregnancy.[39]

Familial incidence

The restless leg syndrome is familial in up to a third of cases.[23] The familial restless leg syndrome is transmitted as an autosomal dominant trait. The age of onset of the disturbance varies, but most usually this starts in the second decade of life. The course is often stationary or with very slowly progressive symptoms, with wide fluctuations in the degree of disturbance. Spontaneous recovery does not occur. Montagna et al.[55] observed a family affected with the restless leg syndrome and also nocturnal myoclonus which they followed closely for over 20 years. The propositus was a 68-year-old monk whose symptoms started at the age of 15 and gradually got worse, causing severe insomnia and peculiar sensory disturbances in the legs by the age of 48.

Electromyography revealed slight slowing in sensory conduction velocity along the median, peroneal and sural nerves with a marked decrease in the amplitude of the sensory potentials. There was thus evidence for a sensory polyneuropathy due to loss of axons in this case. This was borne out on *sural* nerve biopsy, which showed loss of myelinated fibres and segmental demyelination. The patient also had signs of pyramidal and posterior column involvement. These signs were not present, however, in other affected family members.

Both non-familial and familial forms of the restless leg syndrome are frequently associated with severe nocturnal myoclonus.[28]

Polygraphic recording in the restless leg syndrome

Lugaresi *et al.*[53] were the first to carry out polygraphic recordings in the restless leg syndrome and to emphasize that this was a fairly common cause of insomnia.[32] They stressed the characteristic pre-sleep time of occurrence, but showed that the leg restlessness was continued into light sleep and could also wake the patient, usually from stage 1–2 NREM sleep.

Restless legs and sleep disturbance

In a few subjects, the restless leg syndrome causes a marked interruption of sleep, with numerous arousals and a considerable reduction in total sleep time. In these patients the number of sleep cycles as well as the percentage of deep NREM and of REM sleep is reduced, and there may be even the occasional appearance of motor restlessness in REM sleep.

Treatment for restless legs

Many treatments for the restless leg syndrome have been suggested, but most are completely ineffective or at best provide mild sedation only. These include folic acid,[30] 5-HTP,[26] carbamazepine,[37] vitamin E[25] and caffeine withdrawal.[54] Propranolol may reduce the severity of neuroleptic-induced akathisia.[51] Antihistamines (e.g. cyproheptadine 4–8 mg nightly), sedative anticholinergic drugs (e.g. benztropine 1 mg) and short-acting benzodiazepines (e.g. triazolam 250 µg) sometimes give partial relief, probably due to their sedative effect; and likewise the effect of beta blockers[38] is probably non-specific.

SLEEP MYOCLONUS (PERIODIC MOVEMENTS IN SLEEP, PMS)

Nocturnal or *sleep myoclonus,* with rhythmic, repetitive, synchronous or asynchronous, stereotyped, sudden non-epileptiform leg movement throughout sleep, is more common than the restless leg syndrome. About a third of patients with sleep myoclonus also have restless legs, whereas patients with restless legs almost always have sleep myoclonus. Both conditions have been extensively investigated by Coleman.[33]

Sleep myoclonus is much more common in middle-aged or old people than in young adults and children. Muscle jerks with continued dorsiflexion of the foot, extension of the big toe, and sometimes knee and hip jerks during sleep, can be easily monitored by tibialis anterior electromyograms (see refs. 34 and 60 for technical details).

The jerking of sleep myoclonus is confined to NREM sleep and is inhibited during REM sleep. Unlike hypnic jerking, sleep myoclonus does not occur at sleep onset. The contractions are brief (0.5–5 s), and occur at regular 20–40 s intervals throughout the night. Jerking occurs with repetitive groups of contraction lasting several minutes to an hour or more. The frequency and severity of leg jerking varies widely on different nights. Physical and emotional stress make the condition worse. Jerks have to be differentiated from myoclonus with epilepsy as well as from restlessness and jerking in sleep apnoea (Table 4.3).

Table 4.3 *Myoclonus and sleep*

Sleep-related jerks	
Pre-sleep	Restless leg syndrome, akathisia
Sleep onset	Physiological hypnic jerks; restless legs
NREM sleep	1. 'Essential' myoclonus, e.g. familial, sporadic myoclonus or benign sleep myoclonus of infancy
	2. Myoclonus with sleep apnoea, narcolepsy Drug-induced myoclonus
	3. Sleep myoclonus (periodic movements in sleep, PMS, see Table 4.2)
	4. Myoclonus with epilepsy
REM sleep	Normal phasic muscle jerks (very pronounced in some species, e.g. dog, but less obvious in humans)
Waking and sleeping jerks	
	Myoclonus with e.g. basal ganglia disease, dementias, viral encephalopathy, metabolic illness may persist during stage 2 NREM sleep
	Palatal myoclonus may persist unchanged throughout sleep

Sleep myoclonus is independent of other body movements in sleep, and does not occur in waking. It is not associated with any other neurological pathology, despite the marked increase in incidence with age.

Estimates of the prevalence of sleep myoclonus vary widely. It is found in roughly 1–2% of a normal elderly population and in 1–15% of patients investigated for the complaint of insomnia. In one series of 409 patients with many different disorders seen at a sleep disorder clinic, 53 (13%) had sleep myoclonus.[35] Approximately 15% of patients with obstructive sleep apnoea, and a similar number of those with REM narcolepsy, also have sleep myoclonus.

Sleep myoclonus is usually asymptomatic, but it can lead to either excessive daytime drowsiness or, alternatively, insomnia.[36, 65] Symonds[62] was the first to describe the disorder and associate it with daytime drowsiness. This is probably due to sleep disturbance at night; in Coleman's[33] series of patients with nocturnal myoclonus, sleep disturbance was common, with increased awakenings, a major decrease in stage 4 NREM sleep, and reduced sleep efficiency. However, these findings are similar to those reported from sleep studies in otherwise normal elderly subjects.[47]

Aetiology of sleep myoclonus

Symonds[62] suggested that in some instances sleep myoclonus was a form of epilepsy, but in most subjects this is not so: EEG and clinical findings are normal. Coleman[34] considered but rejected a wide variety of possible mechanisms, including spinal cord pathology, metabolic abnormalities as in uraemic myoclonus, hyperactivity of the alpha motor neurone, disruption of inhibitory neurotransmitter mechanisms, and primary disorders of sleep itself. The observation that periodic changes in respiratory rhythm, heart rate, blood pressure and muscle tone, with a superficial similarity to the periodicity of muscle jerking in sleep myoclonus, occur during sleep and coma, has given rise to the idea that sleep myoclonus may result from a brain stem pacemaker abnormality. However, practically any disturbance of the sleep–wake cycle may lead to sleep myoclonus. There is no conclusive evidence for the idea that sleep myoclonus is due to sleep anoxia, despite the association with old age and sleep apnoea.

The careful drug histories obtained by Coleman[33] in 53 of his patients gave no indication that periodic movements in sleep resulted from any one particular drug. There are inconclusive reports that *levodopa, clomipramine* and other *tricyclic drugs* occasionally provoke nocturnal myoclonus in parkinsonian and other elderly subjects. Sleep myoclonus is sometimes associated with *anticonvulsant drug treatment* or *hypnotic drug withdrawal*.

Treatment of sleep myoclonus

Clonazepam is the most widely used drug, and may benefit some but not most patients.[33, 59] Subjective reports of reduced arousals with clonazepam suggest improvement in sleep myoclonus, but often the number of leg jerks does not greatly alter, and other hypnotics may be equally effective. *Baclofen, 5-hydroxytryptophan* and *methysergide* have all been tried but seem to be ineffective.[45, 46]

HEAD BANGING

Jactatio capitis nocturnus or head banging usually occurs in early childhood and disappears by adolescence. Rhythmic to-and-fro head rocking, or less commonly whole body rocking, occurs just before and during light stage 1–2 NREM sleep, and in most cases disappears during slow-wave sleep.[67, 68] There is no waking problem.

Head banging has been attributed to many different organic, social and psychiatric factors, including low IQ, understimulation, stress or maternal neglect,[66, 77] excessive physical restraint[73] or erotic gratification.[74] Behaviouralists have divided head banging into two types, *auto-erotic*, said to start at the age of 6–12 months, and *tantrum* head banging, due to frustration, and beginning when the child is able to walk.[76] Despite all these theories, the real cause of head banging remains unknown.

Friedin *et al.*[68] described a 2-year-old boy with automatic stereotyped head banging preceded by body rocking for 2 h after he fell asleep. Head banging occurred during stage 1–2 NREM sleep, but, unusually for this sleep stage, in this child head banging was associated with confusion on awakening, amnesia for the event, poor response to arousal, and non-reactivity to external stimuli. A more typical picture of head banging was given by Walsh *et al.*[79] who described an 8-year-old girl with no physical or psychological problem, no evidence of maternal deprivation, movement restraint, need for erotic gratification or excess anxiety. This girl was responsive to external stimuli during rocking episodes, and showed only minimal disorientation on arousal.

Head banging is not a form of epilepsy, and although anticonvulsants have been tried, phenytoin is not effective.[75, 78]

Treatment of head banging is unsatisfactory. Low doses of oxazepam (e.g. 10–20 mg nightly) or other benzodiazepines will reduce the number of body movements at night,[69, 70] but tolerance usually develops over 1–4 weeks.[71, 72]

BRUXISM

The wicked shall see it and be grieved; he shall gnash with his teeth and melt away; the desire of the wicked shall perish.

(Psalm 112, v. 10)

Conscious teeth grinding (bruxomania) or sleep tooth grinding (bruxism) is, according to some dentists, common or even universal at all ages.[81, 92, 94] However, the true prevalence of bruxism is probably less than 5–10% of all children, and declines with age. Bruxism may start from the time the teeth erupt, persist throughout adolescence into adulthood, and still occur in elderly people with artificial teeth, or be practised by edentulous subjects on gum pads. Bruxism, in addition to unpleasant grinding, causes tooth wear, pain and damage to soft tissues with periodontal disease.

Ideas as to the cause of bruxism are legion, and include malocclusion,[85, 88] psychosomatic factors[91, 93], or often a combination of both.[96] As with other parasomnias, there is no definite relationship between tooth grinding and any personality type or psychological disorder, although bruxism is often most severe or most apparent at times of anxiety.

Bruxism occurs equally in men and women, and is sometimes accompanied by frequent body movements in sleep. One report has associated increased teeth contact, as measured by intra-oral radiotelemetry, with increased heart rate.[82] Bruxism occurs mainly in stage 2 NREM sleep or after lightening of sleep in REM episodes.[95, 97] Satoh and Haroda[98] found that bruxism was accompanied by slow ocular movements, and was always followed by a lighter phase of sleep.

Bruxism is undoubtedly sometimes stress-related. During stress, the masticatory muscles are amongst the first to be affected by increase in muscle tone.[99] Yemm[101] showed that when a human subject was stressed the EMG activity of both the masseter and temporal muscle was increased. A high incidence of tooth wear in prison inmates, as compared with 20- to 30-year-old male controls, has been reported by Cotman,[84] and sleep EMG studies have shown that marked bruxism follows days that are mentally stressful or physically fatiguing.[100] Also, the urinary adrenaline and noradrenaline output is sometimes higher in bruxers than in non-bruxers.[83]

No drug has any specific effect on bruxism, although benzodiazepines are possibly of limited value.[90] Of other treatments, including autosuggestion, hypnosis, occlusal adjustment and muscle relaxation exercises, aversion therapy, hypnotics and biofeedback, perhaps teeth 'nite-guards' are of greatest value.[80, 81, 86, 89, 90, 96, 99, 100]

SLEEP PARALYSIS (Plate 4b)

The American neurologist Weir Mitchell first reported night paralysis in 1876 in two healthy white males.[123] The condition was associated with narcolepsy and cataplexy by Adie[102] and Wilson.[136] Hishikawa[115] in a historical review detailed the many descriptive but sometimes incorrect terms that have been used for sleep paralysis, including nocturnal hemiplegia, nocturnal paralysis, sleep numbness, cataplexy of awakening and postchalastic fits.[107, 109, 110, 118] The French terms *crise à l'état de veille* and *cataplexie du réveil* stress the time of occurrence of sleep paralysis and its similarity to cataplexy. The well known night nurse's paralysis is probably an example of sleep paralysis.

Sleep paralysis occurs in four main circumstances:

1. *isolated sleep paralysis,* a rare event in normal people;
2. *familial sleep paralysis,* occurring in several members of one family, unaccompanied by other symptoms;
3. *narcoleptic sleep paralysis,* occurring as an accessory symptom in narcolepsy–cataplexy;
4. *hypersomnia with sleep paralysis,* seen occasionally in the Pickwickian syndrome and in other forms of obstructive sleep apnoea.[106, 112, 120, 122]

Apart from minor differences in frequency, sex incidence, pre- and postdormital timing and accompanying features, the essential details of sleep paralysis are similar in all four circumstances.

CLINICAL FEATURES

During sleep paralysis, there is partial or complete flaccid paralysis of skeletal, but not extra-ocular muscles with areflexia, similar to the findings during REM sleep, although the patient is awake. Sometimes respiratory muscles are involved to a minor extent, causing dyspnoea or a sense of suffocation. Most attacks start suddenly, last a few minutes and end gradually, although Bowling and Richards[105] described episodes of sleep paralysis lasting over 1 h. Although full consciousness is usually preserved, there may be rapid alternation between sleep paralysis and dreaming, with distortion or absence of time sense. The attack may be terminated by the onset of sleep or if the patient is touched or shaken. Some individuals can prevent paralysis by moving the eyes or arms. Most episodes occur when the patient is lying comfortably on a bed, and discomfort due to a standing or sitting sleep posture may prevent sleep paralysis.

The first attack of sleep paralysis is often terrifying. Anxiety is intensified by hallucinations and by respiratory movement, together with the mental struggle to move. There may be a corresponding increase in heart rate, sweating and widely dilated pupils. Because of terror, some victims of sleep paralysis ask to have their wrists cut before burial to prevent the possibility of being buried alive. Certainly many patients feel as though they are dying in their initial attacks of sleep paralysis, but with continued experience the benign and brief nature of the episodes become obvious and the only sequel is an occasional relapse into paralysis if the patient does not move around. Frequent attacks, however, can lead to the development of ritualistic behaviour, sleeping with the light or wireless on, or keeping a dog in the bedroom.

VARIANTS OF SLEEP PARALYSIS

Isolated sleep paralysis
This occurs at least once in a lifetime in up to 40–50% of all normal subjects.[108, 111, 127] This is most common in young adults and may be slightly more frequent in males than females. Attacks of isolated sleep paralysis are usually infrequent and more are postdormital than predormital in timing. Goode[113] studied all the nurses, patients and students of Duke Medical School. He found that 10 of 163 medical students, and overall 13 of 379 hospital personnel, had experienced one or more attacks of sleep paralysis. In four subjects sleep paralysis occurred 5–15 times a year. Sleep walking (22 persons) and sleep talking (87 persons) were both more common than sleep paralysis.

Familial sleep paralysis
This is a rare disorder and only a few families in which sleep paralysis, but not narcolepsy or cataplexy, has affected several generations have been described. Roth et al.[130, 131] studied 10 subjects in two families in whom sleep paralysis was frequent and always accompanied or preceded by terrifying dreams. Unlike subjects with isolated sleep paralysis, those with familial sleep paralysis have more attacks at sleep onset or during the first REM period of the night than during subsequent awakenings or at the end of sleep. Also, familial sleep paralysis may affect more women than men.

In individual families with sleep paralysis affecting many generations, the condition is transmitted as a dominant trait linked to the X chromosome. There are no other accompaniments, but in one patient with familial sleep paralysis studied by Roth and Bruhova[130] the feeling of terror and despair from the episode persisted next morning in the form of severe depression.

Sleep paralysis in narcolepsy
In subjects with narcolepsy (see Chapter 6), sleep paralysis has been reported to occur in between 17 and 50% of all cases.[113, 115, 133] As in isolated and familial cases, hallucinations accompany sleep paralysis in narcoleptics in about 50% of attacks. 80% of narcoleptics with sleep paralysis also have cataplexy, but only 20–60% of narcoleptics with cataplexy also have sleep paralysis.[115, 133] The frequency of attacks of sleep paralysis in narcoleptics is very variable (from a single episode to several each night), although in most instances sleep paralysis is less common than cataplexy with an average of perhaps 1–2 attacks a week.

Sleep paralysis in hypersomnia
Sleep paralysis is an uncommon accompaniment of forms of hypersomnia other than narcolepsy, including obstructive sleep apnoea or structural brain stem disease[128] and possibly severe endogenous depression (Toone, personal communication). In some of these instances, sleep paralysis may be associated with circadian mistiming of REM sleep or, in the case of sleep apnoea, sleep fragmentation.

PATHOPHYSIOLOGY OF SLEEP PARALYSIS

Langworthy and Betz[119] thought that sleep paralysis was a hysterical reaction, together with narcolepsy and cataplexy, being a neurotic defence with 'symbolic significance against primary anxieties associated with difficulties in realistic adjustments in personal relationships with others'. Genetic and physiological evidence has totally disproved these views. However, sleep paralysis is sometimes associated with psychiatric disorders. Van der Heider and Weinberg[135] described sleep paralysis accompanying combat fatigue in three young World War II soldiers with no preceding psychopathology. Perhaps sleep deprivation followed by a severe rebound of REM sleep, accompanied by sleep atonia, was responsible here.

There is no support for the belief that sleep paralysis is a form of epilepsy.[103, 109, 125] EEG recordings in patients during sleep paralysis are normal, except for the pattern of light sleep during conscious awareness.

In narcolepsy, sleep paralysis is usually preceded, accompanied or followed by a typical REM sleep picture. Hishikawa[115] found that the majority of narcoleptics who were awoken from a sleep-onset REM period claim to have been in a state of sleep paralysis, or to have had hypnagogic hallucinations. The generalized reduction of muscle tone, preservation of eye movements, and depression or loss of spinal reflexes of sleep paralysis are mirrored during REM sleep. Sleep paralysis thus appears to be a form of dissociated REM sleep, similar in many ways to cataplexy. The antithesis of sleep paralysis and cataplexy, where the subject is mentally awake but physically asleep, is observed during automatic behaviour and somnambulism.

PRE- AND POSTDORMITAL SLEEP PARALYSIS

Sleep paralysis occurs at the start or the end of sleep. The time tends to be constant in any individual. In one of the large families with sleep paralysis described by Roth, all the affected members had attacks only at the beginning of sleep, whilst, in another family, 14 members had attacks not at sleep onset, but always in the middle of the night.[129] In narcolepsy, sleep paralysis is usually experienced in sleep-onset REM sleep periods, whereas isolated sleep paralysis is more common at the end than at the start of the night. Hishikawa[115] found that most narcoleptics do not experience sleep paralysis during REM sleep when this commences more than 1 h after sleep onset. He suggested that these differences in the timing of attacks of sleep paralysis might be due to differences in the level of arousal and the degree of motor inhibition that occur throughout the night. There is some evidence that the level of consciousness in narcoleptics is slightly higher and the degree of motor inhibition is greater in sleep-onset REM periods than in subsequent REM periods.[117, 124]

TREATMENT OF SLEEP PARALYSIS

Isolated, familial and narcoleptic sleep paralysis may be prevented by imipramine, despramine (desmethylimipramine) and clomipramine. In equal doses (e.g. 25 mg), clomipramine is the most effective of these drugs. As in the case of cataplexy, adequate control of sleep paralysis is established within 24–48 h of starting treatment with lower dosages of tricyclic drugs than those that are used for the treatment of depression. These results therefore are unlikely to be due to any change in mood.[104, 114, 116, 126, 132, 134] Improvement in sleep paralysis is unlikely to be due simply to REM sleep suppression or alteration in REM sleep timing caused by tricyclic drugs, since other drugs with these properties (e.g. amphetamine) do not usually prevent sleep paralysis.

SLEEP WALKING

Sleep walking (Fig. 4.1) is an automatism that occurs during deep NREM sleep, usually in the first third of the night. It is much more common in children than in adults, and may be slightly more common in boys than in girls,[167] although Cirignotta et al.[144] found that the male: female ratio was 3:4. The usual age at which children start to sleep walk is between 4 and 6, accounting for half of all cases. Estimates of the frequency of sleep walking vary widely, but approximately 15% of children aged 5–12 years walk in their sleep at least

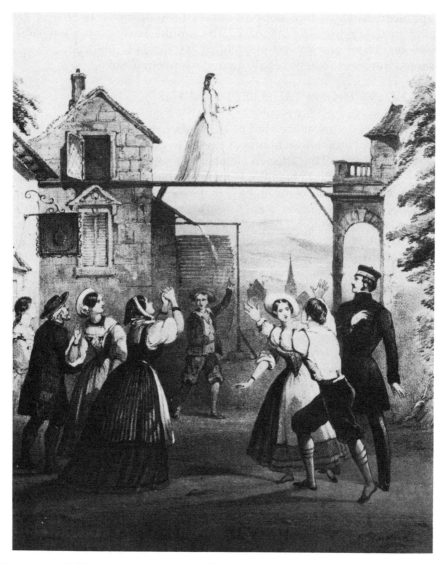

Figure 4.1 *Bellini:* La Sonnambula *Act II, Scene 2. The sleep walker Amina treads her way across a perilous bridge whilst her friends anxiously watch.*

once[138] and 3–6% do so more often. In contrast, less than 0.5% of adults are somnambulists.

Most children grow out of the condition between the ages of 7 and 14.[144]

FAMILIAL AND GENETIC FACTORS

Sleep walking is familial in 10–20% of all cases,[145] with an increased incidence of sleep walking in children when a parent has been a somnambulist. Bakwin[138] showed convincingly that monozygotic twins sleep walk much more often than dizygotic twins, and identical twins have a very similar sleep structure. Kales *et al.*[157] found that, in the families of children who sleep walk, other individuals tend to be deep sleepers with high thresholds for arousal from sleep.

CLINICAL CHARACTERISTICS

The pattern of sleep walking and the degree of responsiveness are very variable. Most children do not actually walk, but sit up in bed or on the edge of the bed, making repetitive, banal and purposeless movements. Less often, the child walks about the room, usually with the eyes wide open, avoiding familiar objects. At this time he or she may dress or undress, go to the toilet, rattle door handles, and sometimes repeat short phrases or incomprehensible sentences. Actual dialogue and complex behaviour such as cooking or eating food, playing the piano, or driving a car, are uncommon. If spoken to, the child usually does not respond, and avoids eye contact. He or she may have to be led back to bed. If awakened, the somnambulist is mildly disorientated for several minutes.

Dream reports during sleep walking lack clarity, with only fragmentary dream content. They differ qualitatively from reports of dreams occurring during REM sleep.

Most sleep walking episodes last a few seconds to a few minutes, rarely as long as an hour. Subsequent recall of events is uncommon, but a few children are aware that they have not slept very well.[152, 165] Contrary to general belief, the sleep walker may injure himself or others, and what appears to be purposeful behaviour can be dangerous when performed by an individual in the deep stages of sleep.

Factors which deepen night sleep (previous loss of sleep, anxiety, fever,[156] lithium, neuroleptic drugs[143] and some hypnotics[153]) increase the liability to sleep walk.

There is no evidence for any primary psychiatric abnormality in children who sleep walk.[154, 173]

Pierce and Lipcon[163] reported there was an association between sleep walking and enuresis, and the same was found in the sleep walking twins described by Bakwin.[138] However, this combination does not always occur; in families in the republic of San Marino, Cirignotta *et al.*[144] found that sleep walking, enuresis and also nightmares showed a family history positive for each specific disturbance, but not for the other two.

SLEEP WALKING IN ADULTS

Primary sleep walking is similar in nature in children and adults. In adults who present with sleep walking, and without any psychiatric illness, the problem usually dates from childhood without the normal adolescent remission.

Table 4.4 *Primary and secondary sleep walking*

Primary sleep walking	Automatic behaviour, fugue states during apparent 'sleep' in adults ('secondary' sleep walking)
Occurrence during sleep only	Occurrence both sleeping and waking
First third of the night	Usually no physiological evidence for sleep
	Any time of night
Simple repetitive behaviour	Sometimes complex and goal-directed behaviour
Short duration (minutes only)	Long duration (several hours)
Return to own bed	No return to own bed
Normal psychological background	Psychological background disturbed
Common in children, rare in adults	Uncommon in children
Family history of sleep walking	No family history

However, many psychiatric and other illnesses are accompanied by apparent sleep walking, although there may be clear differences in behaviour from that usually observed during primary somnambulism in childhood (Table 4.4).

The idea has arisen that sleep walking in adults is in some ways different from sleep walking in children. This confusion has been caused by the difficulty in distinguishing normal sleep walking behaviour from that seen in fugue states or automatic behaviour accompanying a psychiatric disorder, but without definite evidence of sleep. This is the likely explanation for the frequent association of so-called 'secondary' somnambulism in adults with severe psychopathology and precipitation by anxiety, emotional disturbances and severe traumatic psychological events.[148] The apparent sleep-walking episodes described by Sours et al.[173] which occurred in 14 young men from US Air Force bases who were thought to be schizophrenic or to have personality disorders, may thus have had a psychological basis. Many of these subjects had a disturbed family background, poor parental relationships, or a history of deliquency and theft, but in no case was there clear evidence that real sleep walking occurred.

The only factors that correlate well with primary sleep walking in children and adults are a family history of the condition, and an association of onset or exacerbation with extreme tiredness or stress.[152]

Here are two accounts of 'somnambulism' in adults. The first is a possible case of real sleep walking, but the second is clearly not.[151]

> *Marville quotes the case of a melancholic Italian of twenty who woke at midnight, brusquely tore the curtains of his bed aside, dressed himself, went to the stable, and mounted a horse. Soon he dismounted, went to the billiard room, and simulated all the movements of one playing. In another room, he struck with his hands a harpsichord, and finally retired to his bed. He was normally a deep sleeper, but did awake if a horn was blown in his ear.*
>
> *Mesnet speaks of a suicidal attempt made in his presence by a somnambulistic woman. She made a noose of her apron, fastened one end to a chair and the other to the top of a window. She then kneeled down in prayer, made the sign of the cross, mounted a stool and tried to hang herself. Mesnet, scientific to the utmost, allowed her to hang as long as he dared and then stopped the performance.*

CRIME WHILST ASLEEP?

Frenzy and aggression are sometimes reported during sleep walking and also during the related condition of sleep drunkenness. According to Broughton[140] and Roth,[171] a state similar to that of sleep walking or sleep drunkenness can occur from time to time in anyone who is awakened from inadequate sleep, in strange surroundings, or after taking a sedative or alcohol; in all these conditions it may be associated with aggressive behaviour. When aggression occurs whilst sleep walking, this may result from the terror and disorientation of partial arousal from stage 3–4 NREM sleep. Some of the adult cases referred as possible sleep walkers are adult men indicted for an offence carried out allegedly whilst asleep. However, it is very difficult to evaluate the evidence that a purposeful criminal act may be performed whilst sleep walking. Physiological evidence for a true state of sleep has never been presented.[137, 160, 164]

Roth[171] reported that quick-tempered subjects (especially aggressive psychopaths) are capable of murder in the state of sleep drunkenness, including killing the person who awakens them.[139, 141] Roth states that about 20 cases of manslaughter and 30 other crimes committed in a state of sleep drunkenness are known.[139-141, 168, 169] Also, some sleep walkers may be suggestible, as in hypnotic somnambulism. The problem in all these instances is to distinguish primary sleep walking episodes from states of altered automatic behaviour due to other causes. A defence to the charge of murder of diminished responsibility due to sleep walking carries little weight when we learn that a grave was dug the week before, again during an alleged somnambulistic episode (Millac, personal communication).

EEG CORRELATES

Sleep walking typically occurs during non-dream sleep, stage 3 and 4 NREM.[149] In sleep walkers the overall pattern of night sleep does not differ from normal. Episodes of sleep walking may commence with a paroxysmal burst of high-voltage slow-wave EEG activity. The nature of these bursts is in doubt, although brief similar EEG changes are seen in stage 3–4 NREM sleep in young children who do not sleep walk. They are uncommon in normal children after the age of 9.[150] Arousal may follow this high-amplitude slow-wave activity, with EEG flattening before walking or other movements occur.

At the time of the actual sleep walking episode, there is usually light stage 1 and 2 NREM sleep, with non-reactive alpha activity. Gibbs and Gibbs state that there is no difference in sleep pattern on nights with or without sleep walking.

SLEEP WALKING AND PSYCHOMOTOR ATTACKS

Sleep walking is not a form of epilepsy, but, since it is frequent, it can occur in children who also have unrelated psychomotor seizures. In any case, since

Table 4.5 *Sleep walking and psychomotor attacks*

Sleep walking	Psychomotor attacks during sleep
Nature of act	
Short, simple stereotyped behaviour but also longer periods of more complex behaviour	Short duration Totally unreactive If walking occurs, no return to own bed
Vocalization uncommon	Scream, vocalization may occur
Waking findings	
Attacks confined to sleep	In some instances, attacks both sleeping and waking
EEG correlates	
Stage 3–4 NREM sleep	Often REM sleep
Normal interictal EEG	Abnormal interictal EEG

psychomotor attacks occurring during sleep can result in a variety of repetitive automatic acts such as swallowing and hand rubbing, and which are exactly similar to somnambulistic activity, differentiation can be very difficult (Table 4.5).

Pedley and Guilleminault[161] described an unusual form of 'sleep walking' in six adult patients aged from 17 to 32 years. All had episodic screaming, vocalization, complex automatisms and walking during sleep. At least some of these episodes appear to have been epileptic in nature, since they stopped after anticonvulsant treatment, and epileptiform abnormalities were present in the EEG in four patients. However, polygraphic recording of two abortive attacks did not show any paroxysmal or other abnormal electrical activity at this time. A similar problem in diagnosis, but in children, is presented by patients described by Lugaresi and Cirignotti.[159] These children had periodic agitation during sleep – coarse, often violent trunk and limb movements lasting 15 – 40 s, occurring almost every night following arousal from NREM sleep. The clinical examination and EEG records during sleep and wakefulness were normal, but the occurrence of diurnal seizures and the response to carbamazepine suggests a possible epileptic basis of attack.

Differentiation between sleep walking and psychomotor attacks is made more difficult by the ocasional occurrence of benign epileptiform transients during sleep.[174] These are not associated with sleep walking, or with epilepsy, although Rowan and Protass[172] found independent medial temporal spike discharges in five of seven patients with periods of automatic behaviour and transient global amnesia.

CAUSE OF SLEEP WALKING

Ideas that sleep walking is due to dream acting or to any form of psychopathology can be discarded. Sleep studies have shown convincingly that the sleep walker is not acting out a dream, and there is no convincing evidence of any psychopathological basis. As evidence against the view that sleep walking is a symptom of neurosis, Kales *et al.*[155] pointed out that disappearance of the symptom did not lead to replacement by a substitute or equivalent syndrome.

The distinguishing feature of sleep walkers from normal children appears to be their inability to awaken into full contact with the environment. There is some apparent similarity between the automatic behaviour of sleep walking and that of hypnotic somnambulism, but sleep walkers, despite the preservation of normal reflex responses and the maintenance of some degree of sensory surveillance, lack the marked suggestibility of subjects under hypnosis. Also, EEG studies of hypnosis have shown that it differs very sharply from physiological sleep, and unlike sleep walking is not accompanied by any sign of sleep activity.[146, 170]

On the basis of the EEG changes in sleep walkers, and the clinical observation that children outgrow the habit, Kales *et al.*[155] concluded that sleep walking is due to physiological immaturity. Children who sleep walk, but not others, will sometimes reproduce this if stood on their feet during stage 3–4 NREM sleep. Broughton[142] considered that there was a general impairment of the mechanism for full awakening, with both a genetic and a neurochemical basis in sleep walkers. To what extent sleep walkers are simply very deep sleepers is unknown, and most evidence for this is anecdotal.

TREATMENT OF SLEEP WALKING

Sleep walkers need to be protected from injury, so that doors and windows should be locked, dangerous objects should be removed, and subjects should sleep on the ground floor if necessary. Behavioural therapy is occasionally successful in children,[162] probably due to reduction in anxiety and enforcement of a regular sleep schedule. Behavioural therapy is also sometimes successful in adults with psychopathology and perhaps fugue states rather than somnambulism.[152, 165] Most authors who have tried hypnosis report that it does not work.[147, 175] Hypnotics are by no means always successful, but 2–10 mg diazepam nightly will sometimes prevent sleep walking.[166]

BED WETTING

Bed wetting is due to involuntary micturition during sleep in individuals with normal waking bladder control. This should be established by the age of 3–4, but because of differences in gaining bladder mastery, bed wetting is only definitely abnormal over the age of 5. At the age of 5, about 15% of boys and 10% of girls are sometimes enuretic, and at about the age of 10, half these numbers. Overall, nocturnal enuresis occurs once a month, or more frequently, in 8% of school-age children. The condition usually improves at puberty, but still occurs in around 1–3% of late adolescents, and in a very small percentage of adults. Bed wetting is not associated with any psychopathology in children, but 35% of enuretic adults are said to be schizophrenic. Primary bed wetting must be differentiated from secondary enuresis, which is due to a high urinary output, small bladder, or disease of the urinary tract, spinal cord or cauda equina.

BED WETTING AND SLEEP STAGE

There is controversy as to whether bed wetting is most common in slow-wave sleep or not. Some attacks occur in the transition from deep slow-wave sleep to lighter stages, but bed wetting has been reported to occur in all sleep phases in proportion to the amount of sleep spent in them.[181, 182] Sphincter relaxation is preceded by body movements, accompanied by arousal, and followed by quiescence.

CAUSES OF BED WETTING

Enuresis is sometimes considered to be mainly functional, and perhaps associated with parent hostility, but it is unusual to find evidence of any severe emotional problem, particular kind of personality or abnormal psychological features in primary enuresis, unless these result from unusual methods of treatment, such as making older children launder their own soiled bed clothes.

The cystometric studies done in Marseilles by Gastaut and Broughton[180] have shown a peculiarity of bladder physiology in some children with nocturnal enuresis who have intravesicular pressures higher than normal, although the actual size of the bladder may be smaller than normal.[183] On the afferent side, any bladder sensory deficit will result in failure of perception of normal bladder stimuli. There is little evidence for the view that nocturnal enuresis is due to pathological deep sleep.[179] Broughton[177] concludes that nocturnal enuresis is probably multifactorial, with excessive bladder contractility, small bladder volume, possibly increased renal output, deep sleep, and failure of full arousal all contributing to the problem.

TREATMENT OF BED WETTING

Hypnotics, barbiturates and diazepam often increase rather than decrease the occurrence of enuresis. In contrast, tricyclic drugs (e.g. imipramine 10–25 mg nocte at 6–10 years) are of definite value. This result may be due in part to bladder-anaesthetizing effects. (It has also been claimed that imipramine is successful in some cases of childhood sleep walking and sleep terrors.[184])

Imipramine is easy to use and its effects are obvious within a few days of starting treatment. The likely explanation for the action of imipramine is not that this is an anticholinergic drug but that its sympathomimetic action produces an increase in pressure at the bladder outlet and in the urethra and a relaxation of the detrusor. Other anticholinergic drugs in general do not help nocturnal enuresis. The long-term results, including the treatment of relapses, are better with the alarm system than with imipramine. There have been no other important advances in the treatment of nocturnal enuresis, and current enthusiasms range from acupuncture to Zen Buddhism.

The sequence of development of bowel and bladder control is opposite. Bowel control is first gained at night whilst sleeping, bladder control by day whilst awake. Social factors have a considerable influence on the development of sphincter control whilst sleeping. Bladder mastery is delayed in children when the parents go out to work during the child's development from 6–12 months of age, and there is a marked social class gradient in bed wetting at 4–5 years of age (Table 4.6).

Table 4.6 *Bed wetting at 4–5 years of age*

Social class	Boys (%)	Girls (%)
I–II	22	10
III	16	0
IV–V	13	24

(Source: Stein, Z. & Susser, M. Social factors in the development of sphincter control, *Dev. Med. Child Neurol.* (1967) **9**, 692–706.)

Conditioning devices such as a buzzer that rings when the child wets the bed might be expected to be of no value, since arousal at this stage is too late. However, there is little doubt that the buzzer and pad alarm device is the most successful way of treating nocturnal enuresis.[176] One study has shown an inverse relationship between enuresis and nocturnal motor activity,[178] and the very fact of putting an appliance in the bed may lighten sleep. However, Sireling and Crisp[185] found that putting a buzzer-mesh device in the bed deepened, not lightened, sleep.

NIGHTMARES AND NIGHT TERRORS

A nightmare is an awakening from REM sleep, with detailed recall of a frightening dream. A night terror, in contrast, is an arousal in the first third of the night from NREM stage 3–4 sleep, almost always with a piercing scream or cry, and accompanied by signs of intense prolonged anxiety.[200] Nightmares and night terrors are associated with autonomic discharge, tachycardia, hypertension, sweating, pyelo-erection and mydriasis, but the response is much greater with sleep terrors than nightmares (Table 4.7).

Nightmares are rapidly followed by full alertness and a clear sensorium; waking often follows a dream motor reaction. Arousal from sleep terrors is usually incomplete.

Nightmares are universal, but they occur much more frequently in some individuals than in others. Any association with anxiety is probably due to easy arousal and good remembrance of dreams. Depression causes 'bad dreams'

Table 4.7 *Nightmares and night terrors*[189, 193–195, 199]

	Nightmares	Night terrors
Stage of sleep	REM (rarely stage 1–2 NREM)	Stage 3–4 NREM
Time of night	Mainly middle and late sleep	Most attacks (75%) occur in the first delta cycle, 60–90 min after sleep starts
Prevalence	Universal, all ages	Mainly children (1–4% have frequent attacks); sometimes associated with psychopathology in adults
Associated features	Hypnotic withdrawal, alcohol withdrawal, beta-blockers, previous sleep lack (usually less prominent than following hypnotic withdrawal)	Stress, previous sleep loss
Features of attack	Exact recall of frightening dream, with motor component, clear sensorium, rapid recovery, mild to moderate anxiety, some increase in pulse rate	Extreme terror, little or no dream recall, piercing cry, confusion, slow recovery (10–30 min), automatic behaviour, tachycardia (120 BPM), sweating, widely dilated pupils, hypertension
Other features	Also occur in day naps; some relationship to stress and anxiety	More common in deep than light sleepers, no consistent psychopathology, morning amnesia, familial, more common in males than females, associated with somnambulism and enuresis in some instances
Treatment	None required; check for alcoholism, hypnotic abuse	Benzodiazepines, behavioural therapy

rather than nightmares. Nightmares may result from drug treatment, or follow drug withdrawal. Reserpine, many different adrenergic blocking drugs and thiothixene[201] often produce nightmares. These are reported frequently following the withdrawal of alcohol and many drugs, such as amphetamine or hypnotics, at the time of REM rebound following REM suppression.

Night terrors (pavor nocturnus) are much less common events. They are sometimes familial, having been recorded as occurring in twins,[188] and in three generations of one family.[196] It is possible that upper airway obstruction may sometimes trigger night terrors in children, and Agrell and Axellson[186] reported 23 children with night terrors and very enlarged adenoids, in all but one of whom attacks ceased following adenoidectomy.

TREATMENT OF NIGHT TERRORS

Fisher *et al.*[194] introduced benzodiazepines to treat night terrors because of NREM stage 3–4 sleep suppression by these drugs. However, they found no correlation between the degree of stage 3–4 NREM sleep suppression and the clinical response, or, on drug withdrawal, between the timing of return of delta activity and reappearance of attacks. Various different benzodiazepines, bromazepam, and also imipramine, have been shown to be effective in preventing night terrors.[187, 191, 202] The cause of this effect of benzodiazepines remains unknown; Broughton[190] suggested that it might be simply due to reducing the intensity of arousal.

Kales *et al.*[198] reported that psychotherapy will prevent night terrors, and in children with severe anxiety this approach should be considered.

CAUSE OF NIGHT TERRORS

The extreme terror of pavor nocturnus is closely similar to the severe anxiety and panic that can be induced by some benzodiazepine antagonists. (These non-benzodiazepine agents act on brain benzodiazepine receptors.) Dorow *et al.*[192] reported that ethyl-ß-carboline-3-carboxylate (ß-CCE) caused severe agitation, tachycardia, muscle tension and heavy breathing, with a striking resemblance to the autonomic activity and panic of a night terror. Perhaps patients with night terrors produce such a compound, or alternatively lack endogenous benzodiazepine receptor ligands, thus accounting for the familial nature and neurochemical basis of night terrors.

Sleep disorders can sometimes kill. Narcolepsy may lead to a fatal automobile accident, and sleep apnoea to pulmonary hypertension, cor pulmonale and death. Even some parasomnias can be extremely dangerous. Hartmann[197] reported two patients with night terrors and sleep walking. In one case, an episode resulted in an automobile accident that killed three people, and in the other there was violence and a serious danger of loss of life. This was a young man with night terrors followed by episodes of violence. These occurred several times a week from the age of 5 or 6. A typical episode started with a yell, followed by muttering and cursing. During this state, the patient sometimes got out of bed, thrashed about, walked around, talked to people who were not present, and sometimes struck out violently and smashed things. Repetitive chewing movements sometimes occurred. There was complete amnesia for these episodes.

SLEEP, PAIN, PARALYSIS AND HEADACHE

Morning headache is common in any condition in which sleep is poor, particularly sleep apnoea. Night-time, *sleep-disturbing pains* are common in most, if not all, muscle and joint diseases. Nocturnal or waking *occipital and neck pain* is a characteristic feature of fibrositis and cervical spondylosis. Other pains may improve with sleep; the resolution of migraine not infrequently accompanies sleep.[203]

Two specific forms of headaches that occur during sleep and wake the patient are recognized; *cluster headache* and the related but more chronic condition of *paroxysmal hemicrania* (Table 4.8). Cluster headaches, so called because of the periodicity of bouts of attack which occur every two or three

Table 4.8 *Sleep-related headache*[205-207]

Cluster headache	Chronic paroxysmal hemicrania
Duration 1–5 h	Duration 20–30 min
Few attacks every 24 h	Up to 10–20 attacks every 24 h
Periodic bouts lasting 2–3 months	Chronic without remission
Slightly more frequent in females than males	Mainly men; adults, not children
Severe retro-orbital pain, lachrymation, nose blockage, Horner's syndrome, facial flushing, and sometimes aura of nausea, mood swings, and gastro-intestinal disturbance	Severe paroxysmal hemicrania
REM sleep-locked (but also attacks by day)	Both day and night – common during REM sleep
Occasionally familial	
Good response to ergotamine and indomethacin	Good response to indomethacin

months, are strongly linked to REM sleep, and cause frequent morning arousals at the time when REM sleep is most intense. The explanation for this timing may lie in the two-fold increase in regional blood flow that occurs during REM sleep,[208] changes in arterial dilatation being followed by oedema and severe pain. There are also changes in trigeminal motor neurone activity during sleep and wakefulness.[204.]

Pain and discomfort due to median nerve compression may cause arousal from any stage of sleep. Immobility, venostasis and pressure seem to be the main factors resulting in sleep dysaesthesiae.

SLEEP AND SEIZURES

Epilepsy has a predilection for sleep. In many instances, seizures occur mainly or entirely at a particular time of day or night. Langdon-Down and Brain,[227] Patry[236] and Janz,[223, 224] studied in detail the relationship between sleeping and waking and epilepsy. These studies in over 2000 patients established three different patterns of seizure occurrence. In individual patients, generalized convulsive seizures occur only or mainly during sleep (*nocturnal sleep epilepsy*); only during waking (*waking epilepsy*); or with a random distribution independent of the sleep–waking cycle (*diffuse or random epilepsy*). Of all the patients studied by Janz,[224] 45% had seizures mainly during sleep, 34% during wakefulness, and only 21% had seizures both sleeping and waking. Overall, between 0.5 and 24% of epileptics have seizures exclusively during sleep.[221, 227, 236]

NATURE OF SLEEP EPILEPSY

Sleep-related epileptic seizures usually have a fairly specific form and timing. Most of the epileptic events that occur during sleep are generalized seizures or focal psychomotor attacks. Generalized tonic–clonic seizures are similar in nature by day and by night, although incontinence of bladder or bowel is more common sleeping than waking. Likewise, the nature of psychomotor attacks is similar during sleep and wakefulness, but since sleep attacks may result in recurrent and stereotyped dreams, simple automatisms and periods of half-waking confusion, they need to be differentiated from non-epileptic parasomnias, dreams, nightmares, sleep walking, sleep talking and a variety of normal body movements. Occasionally, night terrors disappear after temporal lobectomy, suggesting that in these cases pavor nocturnus is an ictal manifestation of hippocampal epilepsy.[231]

Sleep epilepsy is more common in children than in adults, and in some children with severe epileptic encephalopathy up to 100 seizures may occur each night.

CAUSES OF SLEEP EPILEPSY

The causes of waking and sleeping epilepsy are a little different, although the borderland between the two conditions is far from distinct, and one form may change to the other, or random epilepsy occur over the years. Meldrum[229] suggested that this transition was sometimes due to progression of brain damage related to the seizures.

In patients with sleep epilepsy, the overall genetic factor is lower than for waking and random epilepsy.[239] Evidence of organic brain disease can be uncovered in approximately 10% of waking epilepsies, 25% of sleeping epilepsies, and the majority of random epilepsies.

SEIZURES AND SLEEP PHASE

Seizures tend to occur at specific times during the night. Tonic–clonic seizures mainly occur in the first 2 h after sleep onset or at 0400–0600.[239] In addition, both tonic–clonic seizures and myoclonic jerking are particularly common on awakening and during the first hour after arousal.

The overall activating effect of sleep on epileptic phenomena is seen in many ways. There is a particularly marked facilitation of generalized, as opposed to partial, seizures in NREM sleep, and in some but not all subjects with limbic seizures; these are activated during REM sleep.

Tonic–clonic seizures, generalized from the start, when occurring in sleep occur more frequently in NREM sleep than in REM sleep, and are especially common during stage 1–2 NREM sleep. Many studies have shown that generalized epileptic discharges increase in NREM sleep and decrease in REM sleep.[220] With other forms of generalized epilepsy, an opposite pattern is seen. In *petit mal*, the typical 3 per second spike and wave discharges are replaced by irregular polyspike and wave discharges in NREM sleep. If these episodes occur in REM sleep, the waveforms more resemble those of wakefulness. Isolated spike and wave episodes, or polyspike and wave discharges in generalized epilepsies usually become more 'spiky' in NREM sleep and are suppressed in REM sleep.

Tonic generalized seizures, seen most often in children, occur more or less exclusively in NREM sleep. This may markedly facilitate brief 1–3 s tonic attacks as well as more or less prolonged tonic seizures, sometimes terminated by several myoclonic jerks. In contrast, *clonic generalized seizures* are infrequent during sleep.

Focal attacks and *focal EEG abnormalities* may occur at random during both NREM and REM sleep. With partial epileptic phenomena, clear activation of waking discharges occurs in light NREM sleep in 76% of patients with anterior temporal discharges, and discharges occur exclusively in sleep in about a third of all such patients.[233] In some instances of partial epileptic seizures, these are activated in NREM sleep and deactivated in REM sleep relative to NREM sleep. However, there are many exceptions and some types of partial epileptic phenomena are selectively and markedly increased with REM sleep. This is seen particularly in *frontal lobe seizures, supplementary motor area seizures* and limbic, especially *amygdaloid attacks.* Broughton[214] has shown that REM sleep studies in epileptics are particularly useful in defining the presence and localization of an occult waking focus with secondary bilateral synchrony during wakefulness, since the generalized discharges are usually suppressed during REM sleep, thereby revealing the causal focus. In addition to activation during REM sleep, Weiser[245] has shown that activation of inter-ictal partial epileptic discharges varies with the time of night. Discharges arising in deep temporal lobe structures are mainly activated in the first NREM–REM cycle of the night, whilst frontal and parietal discharges show a relatively even activation for equivalent NREM stages across the night.

Psychomotor seizures that are largely if not entirely confined to REM sleep have been reported often. Epstein and Hill[219] reported a patient with recurrent dreams, with rhythmic continuous right temporal spiking during REM sleep. When the subject was aroused from these episodes he reported an unpleasant dream with an epigastric aura. Arguner *et al.*[210] recorded that of 40 seizures in 20 patients occurring during sleep, 23 started during REM sleep. A slightly lower REM seizure frequency was reported by Kikuchi,[226] who found that three out of nine nocturnal seizures in seven patients with psychomotor epilepsy started in REM sleep. In some subjects the association between psychomotor attacks and REM sleep may be near absolute. A 6-year-old girl described by Passouant[234] had six nocturnal seizures all during REM sleep, whilst a 12-year-old patient with nocturnal seizures and night terrors studied by Passouant and Cadilhac[235] had six nocturnal seizures during one night of sleep, five of which occurred during REM sleep and one at sleep onset. Montplaisir *et al.*[231] studied a patient with random hippocampal epilepsy who had frequent seizures both awake and asleep. Although focal seizure discharges were of shorter duration in REM than in NREM sleep, awakening, especially from REM sleep or shortly after a REM period, facilitated the occurrence of a generalized seizure (see below).

EFFECT OF SLEEP ON SPECIFIC EPILEPTIC CONDITIONS

In *hypsarrhythmia,* the waking EEG discharges fragment during sleep although sleep-related discharges are the last to disappear with steroid treatment of infantile spasms. Likewise, abnormal paroxysmal EEG discharges and myoclonus induced by photic stimulation decrease markedly in NREM sleep. An inverse pattern to that of hypsarrhythmia and absence seizures is seen in the condition of *epileptic encephalopathy* during slow-wave sleep with subclinical epileptic status described by Patry *et al.*[237] and Tassinari *et al.*[243] A diagnostic feature here is the particular activation of abnormal EEG features in NREM sleep, which disappears during REM sleep. The cause of the syndrome is unknown although it is associated with some degree of mental impairment, possibly aphasia or speech arrest, with daytime absence-type seizures and nocturnal orofacial seizures. The usual age of onset is 4–10, with a tendency to remit at puberty.

Marked activation of waking discharges during sleep, particularly REM sleep, occurs in other *benign partial epilepsies of childhood.* Some 50–60% of these subjects with benign forms of epilepsy in childhood, often mainly involving the mouth and face, no obvious organic disease and recovery at puberty, have seizures only whilst sleeping.[215] Waking EEGs show high-amplitude negative rolandic spikes with near-normal background activity. These waveforms show a marked increase in drowsiness and sleep. Sleep activation is greatest for children aged 5–9, when the nocturnal seizures are most common.

AROUSAL AND EPILEPSY

Arousal from sleep may precipitate both generalized and partial epileptic phenomena. Niedermeyer[232] described the most common form of awakening epilepsy. This is usually seen in young epileptics with no known CNS pathology, who on waking have recurrent episodes of generalized myoclonus terminating with a grand mal seizure. Meier-Ewart and Broughton[228] described a different variety of waking epilepsy in photic-sensitive epileptic patients. Transient changes in cortical activity on arousal may partly explain how arousal activates epileptic events.[215]

BIOLOGICAL RHYTHMS AND EPILEPSY

Psychomotor attacks sometimes show an ultradian rhythm, with a periodicity similar to the 90–110 min NREM–REM cycle, and here changes in arousal level with changes in sleep stage may activate the attack.[217, 231, 234, 242] Seizures sometimes show other striking patterns of ultradian or circadian rhythmicity, and changes in hormonal level may explain seizures related to menstruation, season or cyclical changes in mood.

SLEEP PATTERNS IN EPILEPSY

Many patients with epilepsy have abnormal sleep patterns but whether these are due to epilepsy, brain damage associated with the seizures, or anticonvulsant drugs is often uncertain. Jovanović[225] and Sterman[241] reported that some patients with sleep epilepsy taking anticonvulsant drugs had an excess of slow sleep, particularly in those with seizures starting in the temporal lobe, in contrast to an excess of light sleep in patients with waking epilepsy. As might be expected, more EEG abnormalities are found during sleep in patients with predominant sleep epilepsy than in patients with waking or random epilepsy;[246] whilst, in subjects with waking epilepsy, Christian[216] found that background slowing and dysrhythmias were more common in records taken during wakefulness than in similar recordings from subjects with sleep epilepsy. The effect of anti-epileptic drugs on sleep in epilepsy is largely unknown. Baldy-Moulinier *et al.*[211] suggested that anticonvulsant drugs might be responsible in part for disturbed sleep in epilepsy.

SLEEP DEPRIVATION AND SEIZURES

Seizures are known to be precipitated by prolonged sleeplessness in persons who have no previous history of epilepsy[212, 213, 222] Rodin *et al.*[238] were amongst the first to show that epileptogenic discharges occurred in the electro-encephalogram of normal subjects after sleep deprivation. One subject showed marked photosensitivity with EEG discharges elicited by intermittent light stimulation although subsequent studies have not shown such frequent EEG activation after sleep deprivation. Christian[216] and Bennett[212] suggested that sleep deprivation increases in particular the frequency of tonic–clonic seizures and brief absences. Bennett[212] reported four supposedly normal US aviators with well documented generalized tonic–clonic seizures during extensive stress and sleep deprivation. Light-sensitive epilepsies appear to be particularly prone to the effect of sleep deprivation. Broughton[215] suggested that this may be part of the reason that jazz players, and others living with frequent occupational curtailment of sleep, are apt to be bothered subjectively by lights and may even wear sunglasses indoors to reduce such discomfort.

Jazz (but not pop) players traditionally perform in ill-lit nightclubs and are not usually subject to flashing lights. In the bop era (late 1940s) jazz musicians wore dark glasses to look mysterious, not to prevent photic seizures. Sleep deprivation, hyperventilation, dehydration and alteration of circadian rhythms may be more potent precipitants of seizures in jazz players and other night artists than photic stimulation.

It is not clear whether sleep deprivation has a specific effect in provoking epilepsy or whether the procedure renders sleep and hence sleep epilepsy more likely to occur. Upwards of 25 different published studies of EEG recordings after sleep deprivation in people with epilepsy are unanimous in claiming that this procedure increases the yield of epileptiform activity and is therefore by implication of diagnostic value.[244] Although the literature is vast and the number of patients studied over 500, the evidence for EEG activation by sleep deprivation, other than simply as a means of sleep induction, is not good, and sleep deprivation may have no advantage over barbiturate-induced sleep as an EEG activating procedure. Because of the multiple effects of sleep, and sleep deprivation on epilepsy, it is essential in some patients to try and improve sleep, avoid unnecessary sleep loss, keep regular hours for sleeping and waking and avoid causes of late evening stress. The deleterious effect of alcohol on epilepsy is possibly due to subsequent poor sleep and sleep fragmentation following heavy alcohol consumption.

Why does seizure frequency depend on the sleep–waking cycle? Based on the experimental evidence linking changes in seizure threshold to changes in activity in brain amine systems,[230] Meldrum[229] has stressed the importance of changes between sleep and wakefulness in brain monoamine systems. Other sleep-related changes in cerebral blood flow, body temperature, water and electrolyte excretion, cortisol level and growth hormone level[218, 240] must be important. Anticonvulsant drug effectiveness may be lower sleeping than waking, although any major difference is unlikely. However, the practice of late evening rather than early morning phenytoin dosage has something to recommend it in sleep epilepsy, and anticonvulsant drug plasma levels should perhaps be monitored during sleep in these patients.

DIFFERENTIAL DIAGNOSIS OF EPILEPSY DURING SLEEP

Evidence for sleep epilepsy is sometimes difficult to evaluate, and both clinical observations and the EEG can be unreliable. The clinical feature of attack gives the best clue, but it is still sometimes impossible to classify attacks from the history alone, and both video recording and sleep monitoring can sometimes leave the diagnosis in doubt. A good response to anti-epileptic drugs is an insufficient criterion to judge the nature of attack. Clonazepam, for example, may improve sleep myoclonus, night terrors and bruxism, as well as tonic–clonic seizures and focal epilepsies, whilst phenytoin may improve migraine, trigeminal neuralgia, and even nocturnal enuresis. The existence of confirmed epileptic seizures in the same patient does not prove that sleep attacks are epileptic in nature, and the presence between attacks of epileptogenic EEG discharges can be very misleading since such 'abnormalities' can occur in entirely normal subjects. Thus it can be very difficult to distinguish between epileptic and non-epileptic attacks during sleep, and sometimes a definite diagnosis cannot be made (Table 4.9).

PAROXYSMAL NOCTURNAL HAEMOGLOBINURIA

This rare, acquired disorder of the bone marrow was first described by Gull[248] in the *Guy's Hospital Reports* for 1886, and by Strübing[257] in 1882. Classically it presents in young adults with weakness, pallor and iron deficiency anaemia,

Table 4.9 *Terminology of nocturnal cerebral 'attacks'*[215]

1. *Non-epileptic:* sleep walking, sleep terrors, terrifying dreams, nocturnal enuresis

2. *Partial epileptic seizures with automatisms*
   Nocturnal epileptic seizures with incontinence: proven epileptic variants which may simulate non-epileptic attacks

3. *Attacks of undetermined mechanism:* nature of attack uncertain as in paroxysmal nocturnal dystonia

together with the passing of dark red-brown urine after sleep in the morning, due to intravascular haemolysis with haemoglobinuria and haemoglobin-aemia. However, most cases are very different from this.[252] Usually the condition is chronic rather than paroxysmal, and presents with pancytopenia, abdominal, back or musculoskeletal pain (as a result of haemolysis or venous thrombosis), rather than with haemolytic anaemia. The most serious feature is sudden thrombosis of the cerebral, portal or other veins, leading occasionally to death.

Paroxysmal nocturnal haemoglobinuria is sometimes associated with aplastic anaemia, sideroblastic anaemia, myelofibrosis, or may evolve into acute leukaemia. Although the condition is usually chronic, acute haemolytic episodes can be precipitated by infection, vaccination, menstruation, transfusion, operation, ingestion of iron salts, and other unknown factors. The differential diagnosis includes other causes of intravascular haemolysis, as well as haematuria and acute porphyria.

Paroxysmal nocturnal haemoglobinuria has been shown to be due to a membrane defect of blood cells, not to any deficiency or abnormality of complement systems.[247, 256] However, red blood cells of monoclonal origin[255] may have a deficiency of the complement-regulating protein, decay-acceler-ating factor.[254] The diagnosis is based on the increased sensitivity of erythrocytes to complement-mediated haemolysis.[249]

The careful studies of Ham[250] suggested that the regular periods of increased haemolysis seen in some patients with paroxysmal nocturnal haemoglobinuria were related to sleep rather than to the night, as implied by the name of the disease. Ham studied the diurnal variations in plasma haemoglobin over several days and nights, and found increased concentrations of plasma haemoglobin during sleep, irrespective of whether the patient slept at night or during the day. Hansen[251] also attempted to relate plasma haemoglobin concentrations to sleep, and found that in some patients a rise in haemoglobin concentration did occur during sleep: he related sleep haemolysis to lowering of plasma cortisol levels. However, steroid treatment, with occasional exceptions, does not suppress sleep-related haemolysis.[253] When it occurs haemoglobinuria during sleep is probably due to the combined effect of mild respiratory acidosis, changes in acid–base balance and renal clearance or defective red blood cells.

NOCTURNAL PENILE TUMESCENCE (NPT)

With the development of an objective method of determining whether erection is physically possible,[262, 265, 277] it became apparent that there is more to the relationship between sleep and sexual function than the bed in which they both occur.[273] Sleep-related erections are entirely normal events.[259] All normal potent men have periodic penile erections during sleep, mainly concentrated at the start of REM sleep periods.[259] Their duration is, on average, 30 min per episode in young adults.[266] The period of total sleep time during which erection occurs declines with age from almost 200 min in the third decade to 100 min by the eighth decade.[261, 269, 270, 275]

Nocturnal penile tumescence (NPT) gives a fairly reliable index of physiological erectile capacity during waking.[271] Thus in most, if not all, cases where impotence is of *organic origin*, nocturnal tumescence is abnormal for age; and the degree of sleep-related erectile failure increases with the severity of patient disability. In contrast, impotence is likely to be of *psychogenic origin* if the patient has normal penile tumescence for age, and does not have any penile sensory deficit or penile pain. A history of the presence or absence of nocturnal erections is therefore of value in the diagnosis of male impotence.

However, there are some problems. The information may be misleading if variations in the degree of erection are disregarded, and also subjective accounts of morning erections may depend on whether the patient awakens from REM sleep or from another sleep stage in which erections are unlikely to occur. The absence of nocturnal emissions may be confused with the absence of nocturnal erections; the former suggests ejaculatory rather than erectile dysfunction.[273] Because of these difficulties, Karacan *et al.*[273] recommend nocturnal penile tumescence monitoring as a mandatory step in the diagnostic evaluation of every man who seeks medical or psychiatric treatment for impotence. With such detailed monitoring, the cause of impotence can be determined in up to 90% of patients who have impaired tumescence and no gross psychopathology.[260] This monitoring must include, however, a careful marital, medical, psychiatric and drug history, with full clinical and neurological examination, studies of gonadal function and urological examination, as well as assays of testosterone and prolactin levels.

NOCTURNAL PENILE TUMESCENCE MONITORING IN ORGANIC IMPOTENCE

Normal nocturnal penile tumescence in healthy males is not altered by the level or recency of sexual activity,[274] and also is not usually inhibited by general or acute psychological factors.[268] In contrast, patients with diabetes mellitus and other endocrine disorders, hyperprolactinaemia, penile diseases, priapism and Peyronie's disease, disorders of the central and autonomic nervous system, respiratory and haematological disorders, polycythaemia and lymphomas, have impaired penile tumescence.[258, 264, 267, 276] Excessive alcohol intake and many drugs, in particular adrenergic blocking agents and psychotropic drugs, cause both sexual dysfunction and NPT failure.[272] Vascular problems (arterial insufficiency is more common than venous pathology) have been discovered in more than 60% of patients presenting at special centres with impotence.[273] The demonstration of these requires photoelectric transducer measurements of dorsal penile artery blood flow, as well as Doppler tests, arteriograms and cavernosograms.

NOCTURNAL PENILE TUMESCENCE MONITORING IN PSYCHOGENIC IMPOTENCE

The diagnosis of psychogenic impotence is usually one of default. Although normal NPT findings largely exclude an organic basis for impotence, impaired sleep-related tumescence may possibly occur in some instances of psychogenic origin. For example, reversible loss of nocturnal penile tumescence during depression has been reported.[278] Unfortunately, there is no objective equivalent to NPT monitoring to assist the psychological and psychiatric evaluation of impotence, and the finding of psychopathology does not necessarily imply a cause for impotence. The majority of impotent men, of whatever cause, will show some reactionary emotional disturbance.

SLEEP-RELATED PAINFUL ERECTIONS

Physiological penile tumescence is non-painful. Very rarely, however, and often without any identifiable cause, prolonged, painful nocturnal erections may arouse the patient, followed, unlike priapism, by slow recovery, usually over a period of minutes. When severe, this may occur several times nightly, and frequent REM sleep-related arousals may cause insomnia. Waking sexual function is usually normal.[263] In some, but not all patients with this rare disorder, penile pathology, phymosis or Peyronie's disease is present.

SLEEP AND THE GUT

The gastrointestinal problems that present during sleep have been discussed by Orr and Robinson.[289]

Sleep-related reflux oesophagitis is often asymptomatic and is due more to change in posture than to sleep itself. Because of coughing and choking, it may produce arousal, with severe burning substernal pain, or a sour taste in the mouth. This is accompanied by heartburn, dysphagia, or laryngopharyngitis.[280] Because of the possibility of aspiration pneumonia, the diagnosis is important. This can be made by evidence of oesophagitis and by acid clearance studies during sleep.[288, 290, 291]

Sleep-related abnormal swallowing is a rare disorder. The patient, as in reflex oesophagitis, coughs, chokes and splutters, but in this case the problem is due to inadequate swallowing or pooling of saliva. The patient is usually aware of this and may also complain of restlessness and insomnia.[281] Occasionally a pharyngeal pouch is discovered.

Gastric acid secretion has been studied in normal subjects during sleep. There is a rise in gastric acidity and a decrease in the volume of gastric secretion during sleep, shown by Johnson and Washeim as early as 1924.[284] Even higher sleep acid secretion occurs with a duodenal ulcer.[286] No definite correlation has yet been described between acid secretion and sleep stage.[287] The increase in gastric acidity during sleep and lack of food in the stomach to buffer acid probably accounts for sleep arousal with ulcer symptoms.

Peristalsis is not greatly affected by sleep. The first studies on the small intestine during sleep were made by Hines and Mead,[283] who found that in a man with a congenital umbilical hernia and exteriorized intestine there were no sleep-related changes in intestinal movement. Unlike the small intestine, where movements continue throughout sleep, the normal external anal sphincter tone may be considerably suppressed during sleep and colonic motor activity may disappear.[292] It is perhaps therefore a little surprising that sleep incontinence is not more common. Loss of anal sphincter tone may account for the nocturnal rather than continuous faecal incontinence found in some diabetic patients with neuropathy,[293], as well as in gluten-sensitive enteropathy and cholera.[279, 285]

In 1917 in the *Glasgow Medical Journal* (**88**, 129) MacLennon gave the first account of *proctalgia fugax* when he reported two cases of rectal crises of non-tabetic origin. Proctalgia fugax most often occurs during sleep at night, and often wakes the patient, but may also occur whilst resting in bed at night and also after straining at stool, sudden explosive bowel action, or ejaculation.[282, 294] Intense levator ani spasm causes cramp-like and sometimes unbearable pain. This can cause fainting. The pain is situated in the rectum 5–10 cm above the anus and lasts a few minutes to half an hour, with spontaneous resolution, although very occasionally proctalgia is continuous, not intermittent. The pain usually recurs at regular intervals and there are no organic features. Proctalgia fugax is reputedly an occupational disease of young doctors and others suffering from anxiety or acute stress. The cause is quite unknown, although the condition is sometimes considered to be due to sigmoidorectal intussusception. The condition is incurable, very unpleasant, but harmless. Treatment is thoroughly unsatisfactory. Advice to inhale amyl nitrite, take a hot sitz bath, or put the finger in usually comes from those who have not suffered from the condition.

SLEEP AND THE CARDIOVASCULAR SYSTEM (Table 4.10)

Blood pressure, heart rate, cardiac output and peripheral resistance all fall in many species throughout sleep or in specific sleep stages, although it is not proven that cardiac output drops in human REM sleep. There is an overall

Table 4.10   *Effects of sleep on cardiovascular disease*[300, 305, 308, 310, 311, 313]

Cardiovascular symptoms	
Paroxysmal nocturnal dyspnoea	Posture-related rather than sleep-related symptoms
Orthopnoea	
Myocardial infarction	Peak occurrence at 0400–0600
Nocturnal angina	Coronary artery spasm is associated with restless sleep, dreaming and REM sleep, but also occurs during stage 3–4 NREM sleep
Cardiac dysrhythmias	Premature ventricular beats are more common in REM sleep than in other sleep stages
	Bradycardia followed by abrupt tachycardia with resumption of air exchange and arousal in sleep apnoea
Blood pressure	Slight hypotension (2–5 mmHg) during stage 3–4 NREM sleep, minimal increase in blood pressure during REM sleep

increase in visceral blood flow and decrease in muscle blood flow. The depressor action of sleep on the heart is mediated through the vagus nerve, whilst the effect of sleep on peripheral muscle blood flow is largely mediated by changes in sympathetic tone.

Changes in *blood pressure* during sleep are minor in man. In normal subjects blood pressure is usually somewhat lowered in stage 1–2 NREM sleep, more so in stage 3–4 NREM sleep and for brief periods during REM sleep. However, during REM sleep, blood pressure is very variable, and this phase usually includes both the highest and the lowest pressures of the night.

Sleep does not usually greatly alter blood pressure in hypertensive subjects and the basic pattern of minor changes with NREM-REM sleep is unaltered although, in a few hypertensive patients that have been studied, blood pressure occasionally falls during sleep to near normal values.[301] Lowered blood pressure during NREM sleep, or early congestive heart failure, may precipitate angina during sleep.[304]

Kleitman[303] noticed a pronounced 3–4 h rhythm in the heart rate during sleep. Nocturnal heart rate is usually slightly slower than daytime rate.

The most marked changes in *heart rate* during sleep are found in obstructive sleep apnoea syndromes. Here, airway obstruction with lowering of the diaphragm leads to a large venous return to the heart, a rise in blood pressure with baroceptor response and subsequent cardiac slowing.

Cardiac dysrhythmias may increase or decrease during sleep. Ventricular premature beats are sometimes more common during sleep than during waking. In 30 nights of records from ten cardiac patients, Rosenblatt *et al.*[310] found that ventricular premature beats were increased during REM sleep; but in another group of coronary patients, Smith *et al.*[311] found no differences in the occurrence of ventricular premature beats sleeping and waking, although these occurred a little more frequently during wake–sleep transitions than during NREM–REM sleep transitions. In individual patients, there is a great variability in the effect of sleep on ventricular premature beats, which in some instances are reduced more by sleep than by anti-arrhythmic drugs.[305]

Overall, the decreased sympathetic activity of sleep may decrease the vulnerability of the heart to ventricular premature beats, and possibly to fibrillation. In normal subjects, not coronary patients, ventricular or atrial premature beats are unusual both sleeping and waking, but in a study of 50 medical students, Brodsky et al.[295] found that A–V nodal blocks and sinus bradycardia were fairly common, and more marked sleeping than waking. Conduction block may be a normal occurrence during REM sleep.[297]

A group of individuals with ventricular arrhythmias who increase the frequency and complexity of premature ventricular beats during sleep was described by Rosenberg et al.[309] Such subjects comprise 3–36% of all those investigated. A high prevalence of neurological diseases, in particular cerebrovascular disease, is present in these individuals. The most frequent explanation given for the occasional increase in ventricular premature beats during sleep is that this unmasks a ventricular focus owing to the slower nocturnal heart rate, with overdrive suppression by the more rapid daytime rate.

Although the heart rate typically falls during sleep, pauses longer than 2–3 s are unusual and probably abnormal. Guilleminault et al.[299] have described four apparently normal young persons with prolonged periods of asystole, some as long as 9 s, mainly whilst asleep and during REM sleep. REM sleep-related sinus arrest occurred without any evident cardiac abnormality, although with vague chest-related symptoms. Perhaps asystole related to REM sleep may underlie some cases of unexpected death, although these appear to be rare medical curiosities, and not in need of urgent pacemaker implantation. However, unexpected nocturnal cardiac arrest and death may in some instances be the result of ventricular fibrillation, not asystole, in conditions long recognized in Asia: in the Philippines as *bangungut* ('to arise and moan'), in Laos as *non-laitai* ('sleep death') and in Japan as *pokkuri* ('sudden death').

Heart attacks and *strokes* are common during sleep, but surprisingly little is known about the mechanisms involved. Traditionally, cardiac deaths and angina occur in the early morning, at a sleep time associated with high REM activity, but there is no definite evidence that ECG changes of ischaemia, or nocturnal angina, are specifically associated with REM sleep, despite the relationship by MacWilliam[306] of dreaming to angina, sudden death and cerebral haemorrhage. However, it is not infrequent for angina to occur during REM sleep. In four patients studied by Nowlin et al.,[307] nocturnal angina with ST segment depression was associated in 32 of 39 episodes with REM periods, but did occur in other sleep phases; and in 25 patients studied by Chierchia[298] ST segment depression was most common in REM sleep and in stage 1–2 NREM sleep, and least common in stage 3–4 NREM sleep. Overall, ECG abnormalities may decrease, increase or remain unaltered during sleep.[312] King et al.[302] reported a patient with Prinzmetal variant angina in which ST segment changes and anginal attacks were confined to REM sleep. Broughton and Baron[296], in their study of sleep following myocardial infarction showed that sleep was fragmented and REM sleep reduced for 1–2 weeks after the acute episode.

REFERENCES

INTRODUCTION

1. Broughton, R.J. Sleep disorders: disorders of arousal, *Science* (1968) **159**, 1070–1078.
2. Broughton, R. Childhood sleep walking, sleep terrors and enuresis nocturna: their pathophysiology and differentiation from nocturnal epileptic seizures, *Sleep 1978*, Basel: S. Karger (1980) 103–111.
3. Gutnick, B.D. & Reid, W.H. Adult somnambulism: two treatment approaches, *Nebr. Med. J.* (1982) **67**, 309–312.
4. Hällström T. Night terror in adults through three generations, *Acta Psychiat. Scand.* (1972) **48**, 350–352.
5. Nee, L.E., Caine, E.D., Polinsky, R.J., Eldridge, R. & Ebert, M.H. Gilles de la Tourette syndrome: clinical and family study of 50 cases, *Ann. Neurol.* (1980) **7**, 41–49.

NOCTURNAL BEHAVIOURAL DISTURBANCES IN CHILDREN

6. Basler, K., Largo, R.H. & Molinari, L. Die Entwicklung des Schlafverhaltens in den ersten fünf Lebensjahren, *Helv. Paed. Acta* (1980) **35**, 211–223.
7. Jenkins, S., Bax, M. & Hart, H. Behaviour problems in pre-school children, *J. Child Psychol. Psychiat.* (1980) **21**, 5–17.
8. Largo, R. Nocturnal behavioural disturbances of the child. In: *Proceedings International Conference on Sleep in Relation to Respiratory Disease, 10–13 July 1983, Oxford,* 60.
9. Ungerer, J.A., Sigman, M., Beckwith, L., Cohen, S.E. & Parmelee, A.H. Sleep behaviour of pre-term children at three years of age, *Dev. Med. Child Neurol.* (1983) **25**, 297–304.

SLEEP AND MOVEMENT

10. Coulter, D.L. & Allen, R.J. Benign neonatal sleep myoclonus, *Arch. Neurol.* (1982) **39**, 191–192.
11. Dement, W.C. & Wolpert, E.A. The relation of eye movements, body movement and external stimuli to dream content, *J. Exp. Psychol.* (1958) **55**, 543–553.
12. Fuchs, A. & Wu, F.C. Sleep with half-open eyes, *Am. J. Opthal.* (1948) **31**, 717.
13. Glaze, D.G., Frost, J.D., Jr. & Jankovic, J. Sleep in Gilles de la Tourette's syndrome: disorder of arousal, *Neurology (Cleveland)* (1983) **33**, 586–592.
14. Herman, J.H., Erman, M., Boys, R., Peiser, L., Taylor, M.E. & Roffwarg, H.P. Evidence for a directional correspondence between eye movements and dream imagery in REM sleep, *Sleep* (1984) **7**, 52–63.
15. Jankel, W.R., Allen, R.P., Niedermeyer, E. & Kalsher, M.J. Polysomnographic findings in dystonic musculorum, *Sleep* (1983) **6**, 281–285.
16. Jovanovic, U.J. *Der Schlaf. Neurophysiologische Aspekte,* Munich: J.A. Barth (1969) 223–232.
17. Lugaresi, E., Coccagna, G. & Mantovani, M. The evolution of different types of myoclonus during sleep, *Eur. Neurol. Basel* (1970) **4**, 321–333.
18. Mano, T., Shiozawa, Z. & Sobue, I. Polygraphic study of extrapyramidal involuntary movements in man during sleep, *Sleep Res.* (1979) **8**, 234.
19. Oswald, I. Sudden bodily jerks on falling asleep, *Brain* (1959) **82**, 92–103.
20. Oswald, I. *Sleeping and Waking. Physiology and Psychology,* Amsterdam: Elsevier (1962) pp. 58, 232.
21. Suzuki, Y., Hosaka, S., Shinomiya, N., Muraki, N., Nomura, Y., Hachimori, K., Iwakawa, Y., Niwa, T. & Segawa, M. Body movements during sleep. Their significance in childhood dystonia, *Sleep Res.* (1979) **8**, 245.
22. Wolpert, E.A. Studies in psychophysiology of dreams. II: An electromyographic study of dreaming, *Arch. Gen. Psychiat.* (1960) **2**, 231–241.

RESTLESS LEGS AND SLEEP MYOCLONUS

23. Ambrosetto, C., Lugaresi, E., Coccagna, G. & Tassinari, C.A. Clinical and polygraphic remarks in the restless legs syndrome, *Riv. Patol. Nerv. Ment.* (1965) **86,** 244–251.
24. Ask-Upmark, E. & Meurling, S. On the presence of a deficiency factor in the pathogenesis of amyotrophic lateral sclerosis, *Acta Med. Scand.* (1955) **52,** 217.
25. Ayres, S. & Mihan, R. Nocturnal leg cramps (*systremma*): a progress report on response to vitamin E, *South. Med. J.* (1974) **67,** 1308–1312.
26. Billiard, M., Besset, A. & Passouant, P. Treatment of chronic insomnia: long term follow up, *Sleep Res.* (1978) **7,** 210.
27. Bixler, E.O. Nocturnal myoclonus and nocturnal myoclonic activity in the normal population, *Res. Comm. Chem. Pathol. Pharmacol.* (1982) **36,** 129–140.
28. Boghen, D. & Peyronnard, J.-M. Myoclonus in familial restless legs syndrome, *Arch. Neurol.* (1976) **33,** 368–370.
29. Bornstein, B., Restless legs, *Psychiat. Neurol.* (1961) **141,** 165–201.
30. Botez, M.I., Cadotte, M., Beaulieu, R., Pichette, L.P. & Pison, C. Neurological disorders responsive to folic acid therapy, *Med. Hypotheses* (1976) **2,** 135–140.
31. Callaghan, N. Restless legs syndrome in uremic neuropathy, *Neurology (Minn.)* (1966) **16,** 359–361.
32. Coccagna, G., Lugaresi, E., Tassinari, A. & Ambrosetto, C. La sindrome delle gamba senza riposo, *Omni. Med. Ther.* (1966) **44,** 619–667.
33. Coleman, R.M. *Periodic Nocturnal Myoclonus in Disorders of Sleep and Wakefulness,* Ph.D.thesis, Yeshiva University; Ann Arbor, Michigan: University Microfilms (1979).
34. Coleman, R.M. Periodic movements in sleep (nocturnal myoclonus) and restless leg syndrome. In: Guilleminault, C. (ed.) *Sleeping and Waking Disorders: Indications and Techniques,* Menlo Park, California: Addison-Wesley (1982) 265–296.
35. Coleman, R.M., Pollak, C.P., Kokkoris, C.P., McGregor, P.A. & Weitzman, E.D. Periodic nocturnal myoclonus in patients with sleep–wake disorders. A case series analysis. In: Chase, M.H., Mitler, M. & Walker, P.L. (eds.) *Sleep Research,* Vol. 8, Los Angeles: Brain Information Service/Brain Research Institute, UCLA (1979) 175.
36. Coleman, R.M., Pollak, C.P. & Weitzman, E.D. Periodic movements in sleep (nocturnal myoclonus): relation to sleep disorders, *Ann. Neurol.* (1980) **8,** 416–421.
37. Dement, W., Guilleminault, C. & Zarcone, V. *Progress in Clinical Sleep Research,* Scientific exhibit at the American Medical Association meeting, Atlantic City, New Jersey, 14–18 June 1975.
38. Derom, E., Elinck, W., Buylaert, W. & van der Straeten, M. Which beta-blocker for the restless leg? *Lancet* (1984) **1,** 857.
39. Ekbom, K. Restless legs, *Acta Med. Scand. (Suppl.)* (1945) **158,** 4–122.
40. Ekbom, K. Restless legs som tidigsymptom vid cancer, *Sv. Lakastidn.* (1955) **52,** 1875–1883.
41. Ekbom, K.A. Restless legs syndrome, *Neurology* (1960) **10,** 868–873.
42. Ekbom, K. Restless legs syndrome after partial gastrectomy, *Acta Neurol. Scand.* (1966) **2,** 79–89.
43. Frankel, B.L., Patten, B.N. & Gillin, J.C. Restless legs syndrome. Sleep electroencephalographic and neurologic findings, *J. Am. Med. Assoc.* (1974) **230,** 1302–1303.
44. Gorman, C., Dyck, P. & Pearson, J. Symptoms of restless legs, *Arch. Int. Med.* (1965) **115,** 155–160.
45. Guilleminault, C., Raynal, D., Phillips, R. & Dement, W. Action of GABA derivative (BA-3467) on sleep of patients with nocturnal myoclonus and idiopathic insomnia, *Sleep Res.* (1975) **4,** 219.
46. Guilleminault, C., Raynal, D., Weitzman, E.D. & Dement, W.C. Sleep-related periodic myoclonus in patients complaining of insomnia, *Trans. Am. Neurol. Assoc.* (1975) **100,** 19–21.
47. Hammond, E. Some preliminary findings on physical complaints from a prospective study of 1 064 004 men and women, *Am. J. Public Health* (1964) **54,** 11–12.
48. Harriman, D., Taverner, D. & Woolf, A. Ekbom's syndrome and burning paraesthesiae, *Brain* (1970) **93,** 393–406.
49. Heinze, F., Frame, B. & Fine, C. Restless legs and orthostatic hypotension in primary amyloidosis, *Arch. Neurol.* (1967) **16,** 497–500.
50. Kumana, C.R. & Mahon, W.A. Bizarre perceptual disorders of extremities in patients taking verapramil, *Lancet* (1980) **1,** 1324.

51. Lipinski, J.F., Zubenko, G.S., Berreira, P. & Cohen, B.M. Propranolol in the treatment of neuroleptic-induced akathisia, *Lancet* (1983) **2**, 685.
52. Luft, R. & Muller, R. 'Crampi, och 'restless legs' vid akut poliomyelit, *Nord. Med.* (1947) **33**, 748–750.
53. Lugaresi, E., Tassinari, C.A., Coccagna, G. & Ambrosetto, C. Particularités cliniques et polygraphiques du syndrome d'impatience des membres inférieurs, *Rev. Neurol. (Paris)* (1965) **113**, 545–555.
54. Lutz, E. Restless legs, anxiety and caffeinism, *J. Clin. Psychiat.* (1978) **39**, 693–698.
55. Montagna, P., Coccagna, G., Cirignotta, F. & Lugaresi, E. Familial restless leg syndrome. In: Guilleminault, C. & Lugaresi, E. (eds.) *Sleep/Wake Disorders: Natural History, Epidemiology and Long-term Evolution*, New York: Raven Press (1983) 231–235.
56. Murphy, T. The restless legs syndrome, *Can. Med. Assoc. J.* (1959) **17**, 201.
57. Murray, T. The restless legs syndrome, *Can. Med. Assoc. J.* (1967) **96**, 1571–1574.
58. Norlander, N.B. Therapy in restless legs, *Acta Med. Scand.* (1953) **145**, 453.
59. Oshtory, M. & Vijayan, N. Clonazepam treatment of insomnia due to sleep myoclonus, *Arch. Neurol.* (1980) **37**, 119–120.
60. Pollak, C., Coleman, R., Kokkoris, C., Marmarou, A. & Weitzman, E. New technique for recording and displaying long-term EMG data: application to ambulatory patients with nocturnal myoclonus, *Sleep Res.* (1979) **8**, 271.
61. Roth, B., van Thanh, L. & Vacek, J. Syndrom neklidnych nohov. Klinicka a polygraficka studie, *Cask. Neurol. Neurochir.* (1974) **37**, 374–379.
62. Symonds, C.P. Nocturnal myoclonus, *J. Neurol. Neurosurg. Psychiat.* (1953) **16**, 166–171.
63. Webb, A.T. Restless arms syndrome, *J. Am. Med. Assoc.* (1976) **236**, 822.
64. Willis, T. *The London Practice of Physick*, 1st edn., London: Bassett and Crooke (1685) 404.
65. Zorick, F., Roth, T., Salis, P., Kramer, M. & Lutz, T. Insomnia and excessive daytime sleepiness as presenting symptoms in nocturnal myoclonus. In: Chase, M.H., Mitler, M. & Walter, P.L. (eds.) *Sleep Research*, Vol. 7, Los Angeles: Brain Information Service/Brain Research Institute, UCLA (1978) 256.

HEAD BANGING

66. Brody, S. Self-rocking in infancy, *J. Am. Psychoanal. Assoc.* (1960) **8**, 464–491.
67. Evans, J. Rocking at night, *J. Child Psychol. Psychiat.* (1961) **2**, 71–85.
68. Freidin, M.R., Jankowski, J.J. & Singer, W.D. Nocturnal head banging as a sleep disorder: a case report, *Am. J. Psychiat.* (1979) **136**, 1469–1470.
69. Glick, B.S., Schulman, D. & Turecki, S. Diazepam (Valium) treatment in childhood sleep disorders, *Dis. Nerv. Syst.* (1971) **32**, 565–566.
70. Kales, A. & Kales, J. Evaluation diagnosis and treatment of clinical conditions related to sleep, *J. Am. Med. Assoc.* (1970) **213**, 2229–2235.
71. Kales, A. & Scharf, M.B. Sleep laboratory and clinical studies of the effects of benzodiazepines on sleep: flurazepam, diazepam, chlordiazepoxide and R05-4200. In: Garattini, S., Mussini, E. & Randall, L.O. (eds.) *The Benzodiazepines*, New York: Raven Press (1973).
72. Kay, D.C., Blackburn, A.B., Buckingham, J.A. & Karacen, I. Human pharmacology of sleep. In: Williams, R.L. & Karacan, I. (eds.) *Pharmacology of Sleep*, New York: Wiley (1976) 83–210.
73. Lewy, D.M. On the problem of movement restraint (tics, stereotyped movements, hyperactivity), *Am. J. Orthopsychiat.* (1944) **14**, 651–669.
74. Lourie, R.S. The role of rhythmic patterns in childhood, *Am. J. Psychiat.* (1956) **105**, 653–660.
75. Pedley, T.A. & Guilleminault, C. Episodic nocturnal wanderings responsive to anticonvulsant drug therapy, *Ann. Neurol.* (1977) **2**, 30–35.
76. Silberstein, R.M., Blackman, S. & Mandell, W. Autoerotic head banging: a reflection on the opportunism of infants, *J. Am. Acad. Child Psychiat.* (1966) **5**, 235–242.
77. Spitz, R.A. & Wolf, K.M. Autoeroticism: some empirical findings and hypotheses on three of its manifestations in the first year of life. In: *Psychoanalytical Study of the Child*, Vol. 3/4, New York: International Universities Press (1949).
78. Tassinari, C.A. & Monica, D. Pavor nocturnus of non-epileptic nature in epileptic children, *Clin. Neurol.* (1972) **33**, 603–607.
79. Walsh, J.K., Kramer, M. & Skinner, J.E. A case report of jactatio capitis nocturna, *Am. J. Psychiat.* (1981) **138**, 524–526.

BRUXISM

80. Berlin, R. & Dessner, L. Bruxism and chronic headache, *Odontol. Tidskr.* (1960) **68**, 261–262.
81. Boyens, P.J. Value of autosuggestion in the therapy of 'bruxism' and other biting habits, *J. Am. Dent. Assoc.* (1940) **27**, 1773–1774.
82. Butler, J.H. Occlusal adjustment, *Dent. Dig.* (1970) **76**, 442–446.
83. Clark, G.T., Rugh, J.D. & Handelman, S.L. Nocturnal masseter muscle activity and urinary catecholamine levels in bruxers, *J. Dent. Res.* (1980) **59**, 1571–1576.
84. Cotman, L. Bruxism amongst prison inmates, *Dent. Survey* (1970) **46**, 31–34.
85. Dawson, P.E. *Evaluation, Diagnosis and Treatment of Occlusal Problems,* St. Louis: C.V. Mosby (1974) 101.
86. Glebred, M.B. Treatment of bruxism: a case report, *J. Hypnos. Psychol. Dent.* (1958) **1**, 18–20.
87. Heller, R.F. & Strang, H.R. Controlling bruxism through automated adversive conditioning, *Behav. Res. Ther.* (1973) **11**, 327–329.
88. Jankelson, B. Physiology of human dental occlusion, *J. Am. Dent. Assoc.* (1955) **50**, 665–680.
89. Kardachi, B.J. & Clarke, N.G. The use of biofeedback to control bruxism, J. Periodontol. (1977) **48**, 639–642.
90. Kutscher, A.H., Zegarell, E.V. & Lamont-Havers, R.W. Pharmacological methods. In: Schwartz, L. & Chayes, C.M. (eds.) *Facial Pain and Mandibular Dysfunction,* Philadelphia/London/Toronto: W.B. Saunders (1968) 300.
91. Laskin, D.M. Etiology of the pain–dysfunction syndrome, *J. Am. Dent. Assoc.* (1969) **79**, 147–153.
92. Leof, M. Clamping and grinding habits: their relation to periodontal disease, *J. Am. Dent. Assoc.* (1944) **31**, 184–190.
93. Moulton, R.E. Psychological consideration in the treatment of occlusion, *J. Prosthet. Dent.* (1957) **7**, 148–157.
94. Nadler, S.C. Bruxism: A classification, critical review, *J. Am. Dent. Assoc.* (1957) **54**, 615–622.
95. Powell, R.N. Tooth contact during sleep: association with other events, *J. Dent. Res.* (1965) **44**, 959–967.
96. Ramfjord, S. Bruxism: a clinical and electromyographic study, *J. Am. Dent. Assoc.* (1961) **62**, 21–44.
97. Reding, G.R., Zepelin, H., Robinson, J.E., Zimmerman, S.O. & Smith, V.H. Nocturnal teeth grinding: all night psychophysiological studies, *J. Dent. Res.* (1968) **47**, 786–797.
98. Satoh, Y. & Haroda, Y. Electrophysiological study on tooth grinding during sleep, *Electroenceph. Clin. Neurophysiol.* (1973) **35**, 267.
99. Schwartz, L. & Chayes, C.M. *Facial Pain and Mandibular Dysfunction,* Philadelphia/London/Toronto: W.B. Saunders (1968) 152.
100. Solberg, W.K. & Rugh, J.D. The use of biofeedback devices in the treatment of bruxism, *J. Sci. Dent. Assoc.* (1972) **40**, 825.
101. Yemm, R. Variations in the electrical activity of the human masseter muscle occurring in association with emotional stress, *Arch. Oral Biol.* (1969) **14**, 873.

SLEEP PARALYSIS

102. Adie, W.J. Idiopathic narcolepsy: a disease sui generis, with remarks on the mechanism of sleep, *Brain* (1926) **49**, 257–306.
103. Aird, R.B. Use of phenacemide (Phenurone) in the treatment of narcolepsy and cataplexy, *Arch. Neurol. Psychiat.* (1953) **70**, 510.
104. Akimoto, H., Honda, Y. & Takahashi, Y. Pharmacotherapy in narcolepsy, *Dis. Nerv. Syst.* (1960) **21**, 704–706.
105. Bowling, G. & Richards, N.G. Diagnosis and treatment of the narcolepsy syndrome, *Cleveland Clin. Quart.* (1961) **28**, 38–45.
106. Chodoff, P. Sleep paralysis, *J. Nerv. Ment. Dis.* (1944) **100**, 278.
107. Daniels, L.E. Narcolepsy, *Medicine* (1934) **13**, 1–122.
108. Dement, W. In: Hishikawa, Y.[115], p. 123.
109. Ethelberg, S. Symptomatic cataplexy or chalastic fits in cortical lesions of the frontal lobe, *Brain* (1950) **73**, 499–512.

110. Ethelberg, S. Sleep paralysis or postdormital chalastic fits in cortical lesions of the frontal lobe, *Acta Psychiat. Scand. (Suppl.)* (1956) **108,** 121–130.
111. Felci, L.L., Caliskan, A. & Nazilli, R. Sleep paralysis, *Nord-Psikiyat. Ass.* (1970) **7,** 108.
112. Gooddy, W. Sensation and volition, *Brain* (1949) **72,** 312–339.
113. Goode, G.B. Sleep paralysis, *Arch. Neurol.* (1962) **6,** 228–234.
114. Guilleminault, C., Carskadon, M. & Dement, W.C. On the treatment of rapid eye movement in narcolepsy, *Arch. Neurol.* (1974) **30,** 90–93.
115. Hishikawa, Y. Sleep paralysis. In: Guilleminault, C., Dement, W.C., & Passouant, P. (eds.) *Narcolepsy,* New York: Spectrum (1976) 97–124.
116. Hishikawa, Y., Ida, H., Nakai, K. & Kaneko, Z. Treatment of narcolepsy with imipramine (Tofranil) and desmethylimipramine (Pertofran), *J. Neurol. Sci.* (1966) **3,** 453–461.
117. Hishikawa, Y. & Kaneko, Z. Electroencephalographic study on narcolepsy, *Electroenceph. Clin. Neurophysiol.* (1965) **18,** 249–259.
118. Kleitman, N. *Sleep and Wakefulness,* Chicago: University of Chicago Press (1963) 233–242.
119. Langworthy, O.R. & Betz, B.J. Narcolepsy as a response to emotional conflicts, *Psychosom. Med.* (1944) **6,** 211–226.
120. Levin, M. The pathogenesis of narcolepsy with consideration of sleep paralysis and localized sleep, *J. Neurol. Psychiat.* (1933) **14,** 1–14.
121. Lhermitte, J. & Gauthier, A. La cataplexie et ses composants somatiques et psychiques; l'onirisme hallucinatoire cataplectique, *Ann. Med.* (1937) **42,** 50–68.
122. Lichtenstein, B.W. & Rosenblum, A.H. Sleep paralysis, *J. Nerv. Ment. Dis.* (1945) **95,** 153–155.
123. Mitchell, S.W. Some disorders of sleep, *Am. J. Med. Sci.* (1890) **C,** 109–127.
124. Nan'no, H., Hishikawa, Y., Koida, H., Takahashi, H. & Kaneko, Z. A neurophysiological study of sleep paralysis in narcoleptic patients, *Electroenceph. Clin. Neurophysiol.* (1970) **28,** 382–390.
125. Notkin, J. & Jeliffe, S.E. The narcolepsies, *Arch. Neurol. Psychiat.* (1934) **31,** 615–634.
126. Passouant, P., Baldy-Moulinier, M. & Aussiloux, C. Etat de mal cataplectique au cours d'une maladie de Gélineau: influence de la clomipramine, *Rev. Neurol.* (1970) **123,** 56–60.
127. Penn, N.E., Kripke, D.F. & Scharff, J. Sleep paralysis among medical students, *J. Psychol.* (1981) **107** (2), 247–252.
128. Rosa, R., Kramer, M. & Ebright, P. Central sleep apnoea associated with sleep paralysis: a case report, *Sleep Res.* (1979) **8,** 212.
129. Roth, B., see Hishikawa[115], p. 123.
130. Roth, B. & Bruhova, S. Dreams in narcolepsy, hypersomnia and dissociated sleep disorders, *Exp. Med. Surg.* (1969) **27,** 187–209.
131. Roth, B., Bruhova, S. & Berková, L. Familial sleep paralysis, *Arch. Suisse Neurol. Neurochir. Psychiat.* (1968) **102,** 321–330.
132. Roth, B., Faber, J., Nervsimalova, S. & Tosovsky, J. The influence of imipramine, dexphenmetrazine and amphetamine sulphate upon the clinical and polygraphic picture of narcolepsy–cataplexy, *Arch. Suisse Neurol. Neurochir. Psychiat.* (1971) **108,** 251–260.
133. Sours, J.A. Narcolepsy and other disturbances in the sleep–waking rhythm: a study of 115 cases with review of the literature, *J. Nerv. Ment. Dis.* (1963) **137,** 525–542.
134. Takahashi, Y. & Honda, Y. Pharmacotherapy in narcolepsy, *Clin. Psychiat.* (1964) **6,** 673–682, 775–784.
135. Van der Heide, C. & Weinberg, J. Sleep paralysis and combat fatigue, *Psychosom. Med.* (1945) **7,** 330–334.
136. Wilson, S.A.K. The narcolepsies, *Brain* (1928) **51,** 63–109.

SLEEP WALKING

137. Anonymous editorial, Sleep walking and guilt, *Brit. Med. J.* (1970) **2,** 186.
138. Bakwin, H. Sleep-walking in twins, *Lancet* (1970) **2,** 446–447.
139. Bonkalo, A. Impulsive acts and confusional states during incomplete arousal from sleep: criminologic and forensic implications, *Psychiat. Quart.* (1974) **48,** 400–409.
140. Broughton, R. Sleep disorders: disorders of arousal? *Science* (1968) **159,** 1070–1078.
141. Broughton, R. Confusional sleep disorders: interrelationship with memory consolidation and retrieval in sleep. In: Boag, J.W. & Cambell, T. (eds.) *A Triune Concept of the Brain and Behaviour,* Toronto: University of Toronto Press (1972) 115–127.

142. Broughton, R. Childhood sleep walking, sleep terrors and enuresis nocturna: their pathophysiology and differentiation from nocturnal epileptic seizures, *Sleep 1978*, Basel: S. Karger (1980) 103–111.
143. Charney, D.S., Kales, A., Soldatos, C.R. & Nelson, J.C. Somnambulistic-like episodes secondary to combined lithium-neuroleptic treatment, *Brit. J. Psychiat.* (1979) **135**, 418–424.
144. Cirignotta, F., Zucconi, M., Mondini, S., Lenzi, P.L. & Lugaresi, E. Enuresis, sleep walking and nightmares: an epidemiological survey in the republic of San Marino. In: Guilleminault, C. & Lugaresi, E. (eds.) *Sleep/Wake Disorders. Natural History, Epidemiology and Long-Term Evolution*, New York: Raven Press (1983) 237–241.
145. Davies, E., Hayes, M. & Kirman, B.H. Somnambulism, *Lancet* (1942) **1**, 186.
146. Diamant, J., Dufek, M., Hoskovec, J., Krištof, M., Pekárek, V., Roth, B. & Velek, M. An EEG study of the waking state and hypnosis with particular reference to subclinical manifestations of sleep activity, *J. Clin. Exp. Hypnos.* (1960) **8**, 199–212.
147. Eliseo, T.S. The hypnotic treatment of sleep walking in an adult, *Am. J. Clin. Hypnos.* (1975) **17**, 272–276.
148. Fenichel. O. The psychoanalytic theory of neurosis, New York: W.W. Norton (1945).
149. Gastaut, H. & Broughton, R. A clinical and polygraphic study of episodic phenomena during sleep, *Rec. Adv. Biol. Psychiat.* (1965) **7**, 197–221.
150. Gibbs, F.A. & Gibbs, E.L. *Atlas of Electroencephalography*, Cambridge, Massachusetts: Addison-Wesley (1950).
151. Gould, G.M. & Pyle, W.L. *Anomalies and Curiosities of Medicine*, London: Rebman (1898) 864–865.
152. Gutnik, B.D. & Reid, W.H. Adult somnambulism: two treatment approaches, *Neb. Med. J.* (1982) **67**, 309–312.
153. Huapaya, L.V.M. Seven cases of somnambulism induced by drugs, *Am. J. Psychiat.* (1979) **136**, 985–986.
154. Kales, A., Jacobson, A., Paulson, M.J., Kales, J.D. & Walter, R.D. Somnambulism; Psychophysiological correlates. I. All-night EEG studies, *Arch. Gen. Psychiat.* (1966) **14**, 586–594.
155. Kales, A., Jacobson, A., Kales, J.D., Kun, T. & Weissbuch, R. All-night EEG sleep measurements in young adults, *Psychon. Sci.* (1967) **7**, 67–68.
156. Kales, J.D., Kales, A., Soldatos, C.R., Chamberlin, K. & Martin, E.D. Sleep walking and night terrors related to febrile illness, *Am. J. Psychiat.* (1979) **136**, 1214–1215.
157. Kales, A., Soldatos, C.R., Bixler, E.O., Ladda, R.L., Charney, D.S., Weber, G. & Schweitzer, P.K. Hereditary factors in sleepwalking and night terrors, *Brit. J. Psychiat.* (1980) **137**, 111–118.
158. Lishman, A. *Organic Psychiatry: The Psychological Consequences of Cerebral Disorder*, Oxford: Blackwell Scientific (1978).
159. Lugaresi, E. & Cirignotti, F. Hypnogenic paroxysmal dystonia: epileptic seizure or a new syndrome? *Sleep* (1981) **4**, 129–138.
160. Mick, B.A. Headaches and sleepwalking, (1974) **229**, 393.
161. Pedley, T.A. & Guilleminault, C. Episodic nocturnal wanderings responsive to anticonvulsant drug therapy, *Ann. Neurol.* (1977) **2**, 30–35.
162. Persikoff, R.B. & David, P.C. Treatment of pavor nocturnus and somnambulism in children, *Am. J. Psychiat.* (1971) **128**, 778–781.
163. Pierce, C.M. & Lipcon, H.H. Somnambulism psychiatric interview studies, *US Armed Forces Med. J.* (1956) **7**, 1143–1153.
164. Reid, W.H. Sleepwalking, *West. J. Med.* (1975) **122**, 417–420.
165. Reid, W.H., Ahmed, I. & Levie, C.A. Treatment of sleepwalking: a controlled study, *Am.J. Psychother.* (1981) **35**, 27–37.
166. Reid, W.H. & Gutnik, B. Treatment of intractable sleepwalking, *Psychiat. J. Univ. Ottawa* (1980) **5**, 86–88.
167. Roffwarg, H.P., Clark, R.W. *et al.* Association of Sleep Disorders Centers. Diagnostic Classification of Sleep and Arousal Disorders, 1st edn, prepared by the Sleep Disorders Classification Committee, *Sleep* (1979) **2**, 1–137.
168. Roth, B. *Narcolepsy and Hypersomnia from the Aspect of Physiology of Sleep*, Prague (1957) 331.
169. Roth, B. *Narkolepsie und Hypersomnie vom Standpunkt der Physiologie des Schlafes*, Berlin: VEB Verlag Volk Gesundheit (1962) 428.
170. Roth. B. EEG in narcolepsy and hypersomnia. In: Passouant, P. (ed.) *EEG and Sleep: Handbook of Electroencephalography*, Vol. 7A, Amsterdam: Elsevier (1975) 43–56.

171. Roth, B. *Narcolepsy and Hypersomnia*, Basel: S. Karger (1980) 226.
172. Rowan, A.J. & Protass, L.M. Transient global amnesia: clinical and electroencephalographic findings in 10 cases, *Neurology* (1979) **29**, 869–872.
173. Sours, J.A., Frumkin, P. & Indermill, R.R. Somnambulism: its clinical significance and dynamic meaning in late adolescence and adulthood, *Arch. Gen. Psychiat.* (1963) **9**, 400–413.
174. White, J.C., Langston, J.W. & Pedley, T.A. Benign epileptiform transients of sleep, *Neurology (Minneap.)* (1977) **27**, 1061–1068.
175. Wolberg, L.R. Hypnotherapy. In: Arietti, S. (ed.) *American Handbook of Psychiatry*. Vol. 2, New York: Basic Books (1959).

BED WETTING

176. Berg, I. Child psychiatry and enuresis, *Brit. J. Psychiat.* (1981) **139**, 247–248.
177. Broughton, R. Childhood sleep walking, sleep terrors and enuresis nocturna: their pathophysiology and differentiation from nocturnal epileptic seizures, *Sleep 1978*, Basel: S. Karger (1980) 103–111.
178. Crisp, A.H. & Hafner, J. Nocturnal activity and enuresis, *J. Neurol. Neurosurg. Psychiat.* (1974) **37**, 610–613.
179. Gambi, D., Pinto, F., Forrioli, M.G. & Bertolini, R. Night sleep in enuretic children. In: Levin, P. & Koella, W.P. (eds.) *Sleep*, Basel: S. Karger (1975) 92–97.
180. Gastaut, H. & Broughton, R. A clinical and polygraphic study of episodic phenomena during sleep, *Rec. Adv. Biol. Psychiat.* (1965) **7**, 197–221.
181. Kales, A., Kales, J.D., Jacobson, A., Humphrey, F.J. & Soldatos, C.R. Effects of imipramine on enuretic frequency and sleep stages, *Pediatrics* (1977) **60**, 431–436.
182. Mikkelsen, E.J. & Rapoport, J.L. Enuresis: psychopathology, sleep stage and drug response, *Urol. Clin. North Am.* (1980) **7**, 361–377.
183. Muellner, S.R. Development of urinary control in children: a new concept in cause, prevention and treatment of primary enuresis, *J. Urol.* (1960) **84**, 714–716.
184. Pesikoff, R.B. & Davis, P.C. Treatment of pavor nocturnus and somnambulism in children, *Am. J. Psychiat.* (1971) **128**, 778–781.
185. Sireling, L.I. & Crisp. A.H. Sleep and the enuresis alarm device, *J. Roy. Soc. Med.* (1983) **76**, 131–133.

NIGHTMARES AND NIGHT TERRORS

186. Agrell, I.-G. & Axellson, A. The relationship between pavor nocturnus and adenoids, *Acta Paedopsychiat.* (1972) **39**, 46–53.
187. Allen, R.M. Attenuation of drug-induced anxiety dreams and pavor nocturnus by benzodiazepines, *J. Clin. Psychiat.* (1983) **44**, 106–108.
188. Bakwin, H. Sleep walking in twins, *Lancet* (1970) **2**, 446–447.
189. Broughton, R. Sleep disorders: disorders of arousal? *Science* (1968) **159**, 1070–1078.
190. Broughton, R. Confusional sleep disorders: interrelationship with memory consolidation and retrieval in sleep. In: Boag, J.W. & Campbell, T. (eds.) *A Triune Concept of the Brain and Behaviour*, Toronto: University of Toronto Press (1972) 115–127.
191. Burstein, A. & Burstein, A. Treatment of night terrors with imipramine (letter), *J. Clin. Psychiat.* (1983) **44**, 82.
192. Dorow, R., Howowski, R., Paschelke, G., Amin, M. & Braestrup, C. Severe anxiety induced by FG 7142, a ß-carboline ligand for benzodiazepine receptors, *Lancet* (1983) **2**, 98–99.
193. Fisher, C.J., Byrne, J., Edwards, R. & Kahn, E. A psychophysiological study of nightmares, *J. Am. Med. Assoc.* (1970) **18**, 747–782.
194. Fisher, C., Kahn, E., Edwards, A. & Davis, D. A psychophysiological study of nightmares and night terrors. Physiological aspects of the stage 4 night terror, *J. Nerv. Ment. Dis.* (1973) **157**, 75–98.
195. Gastaut, H. & Broughton, R. Paroxysmal psychological events and certain phases of sleep, *Percept. Mot. Skills* (1963) **17**, 362.
196. Hällström, T. Night terror in adults through three generations, *Acta Psychiat. Scand.* (1972) **48**, 350–352.

197. Hartmann, E. Two case reports: night terrors with sleep-walking – a potentially lethal disorder, *J. Nerv. Ment. Dis.* (1983) **171**, 503–505.
198. Kales, J.C., Cadieux, R.J., Soldatos, C.R. & Kales, A. Psychotherapy with night-terror patients, *Am.J. Psychother.* (1982) **36**, 399–407.
199. Kales, J.D., Kales, A., Soldatos, C.R., Caldwell, A.B., Charney, D.S. & Martin, E.D. Night terrors. Clinical characteristics and personality patterns, *Arch. Gen. Psychiat.* (1980) **37**, 1413–1417.
200. Roffwarg, H.P., Clark, R.W. *et al.* Association of Sleep Disorders Centers. Diagnostic Classification of Sleep and Arousal Disorders, 1st edn, prepared by the Sleep Disorders Classification Committee, *Sleep* (1979) **2**, 1–137.
201. Solomon, K. Thiothixene and bizarre nightmares: an association? *J. Clin. Psychiat.* (1983) **44**, 77–78.
202. Vela, A., Dobladez, B. & Rubio, M.E. Action of bromazepam on sleep of children with night terrors. 1. Sleep organization and heart rate, *Pharmatherapeutica* (1982) **3**, 247–258.

SLEEP, PAIN, PARALYSIS AND HEADACHE

203. Blau, J.N. Resolution of migraine attacks – sleep and the recovery phase, *J. Neurol. Neurosurg. Psychiat.* (1982) **45**, 223–226.
204. Chandler, S.H., Chase, M.H. & Nakamura, Y. Intracellular analysis of synaptic mechanisms controlling trigeminal motoneuron activity during sleep and wakefulness, *J. Neurophysiol.* (1980) **44**, 359–371.
205. Dexter, J.D. The relationship between stage III and IV and REM sleep and arousals with migraine, *Headache* (1979) **19**, 364–369.
206. Dexter, J.D. & Weitzman, E.D. The relationship of nocturnal headaches to sleep stage patterns, *Neurology (Minneap.)* (1970) **20**, 513–516.
207. Kayed, K., Godtlibsen, O.B. & Sjaastad, O. Chronic paroxysmal hemicrania IV: 'REM sleep locked' nocturnal headache attacks, *Sleep* (1978) **1**, 91–95.
208. Sakai, F., Meyer, J.S., Karacan, I., Yamaguchi, F. & Yamamoto, M. Narcolepsy: regional cerebral bloodflow during sleep and wakefulness, *Neurology* (1979) **29**, 61–67.
209. Treadwell, B.L. Fibromyalgia or the fibrositis syndrome: a new look, *N.Z. Med. J.* (1981) **94**, 457–459.

SLEEP AND SEIZURES

210. Arguner, A., Billiard, M., Besset, M. & Passouant, P. Psychomotor seizures during sleep, *Sleep Res.* (1975) **4**, 206.
211. Baldy-Moulinier, M., Touchon, J., Besset, A., Billiard, M., Cadilhac, J. & Passouant, P. Sleep architecture and epileptic seizures. In: Degen, R. & Niedermeyer, E. (eds.) *Epilepsy, Sleep and Sleep Deprivation*, Amsterdam: Elsevier (1984) 109–118.
212. Bennett, D.R. Sleep deprivation and major motor seizures, *Neurology (Minneap.)* (1963) **13**, 953–959.
213. Bennett, D.R., Mattson, R.H, Ziter, F.A., Calverley, J.R., Liske, E.A. & Pratt, K.L. Sleep deprivation: neurological and electroencephalographic effects, *Aerospace Med.* (1964) **35**, 888–890.
214. Broughton, R.J. Sleep and epilepsy. In: *Epilepsy 1978*, London: British Epilepsy Association (1978) 57–62.
215. Broughton, R.J. Epilepsy and sleep: a synopsis and prospectus. In: Degen, R. & Niedermeyer, E. (eds.) *Epilepsy, Sleep and Sleep Deprivation*, Amsterdam: Elsevier (1984) 317–356.
216. Christian, W. Biolektrische Characteristik tages-periodisch gebundener Verlaufsformen epileptischer Erkrankungen, *Deutsch. Z. Nervenheilk.* (1960) **181**, 413–444.
217. Daly, D.D. Circadian cycles and seizures. In: Brazier, M.A.B. (ed.) *Epilepsy, its Phenomena in Man*, UCLA Forum in Medical Sciences, Vol. 7, New York: Academic Press (1973) 215–232.
218. Dixon, P.F., Booth, M. & Butler, J. The corticosteroids. In: Gray, C.H. & Basarach, A.L. (eds.) *Hormones in Blood, Vol 2* London/New York: Academic Press (1974) 305.
219. Epstein, A.W. & Hill, W. Ictal phenomena during REM sleep of the temporal lobe epileptic, *Arch. Neurol.* (1966) **15**, 367–375.

220. Gastaut, H., Batini, C., Fressy, J., Broughton, R., Tassinari, C.A. & Vittini, F. Étude électroencéphalographique des phénomènes épisodiques épileptiques au cours du sommeil. In: *Le Sommeil de Nuit Normal et Pathologique*, Paris: Masson (1965).

221. Gibbard, F. & Bateson, M. Sleep epilepsy: its patterns and prognosis, *Brit. Med. J.* (1974) **2**, 403–405.

222. Gunderson, C.H., Dunne, P.B. & Feher, T.L. Sleep deprivation seizures, *Neurology (Minneap.)* (1973) **23**, 678–686.

223. Janz, D. The grand mal epilepsies and the sleeping–waking cycle, *Epilepsia* (1962) **3**, 69–109.

224. Janz, D. Epilepsy and the sleep–waking cycle. In: Vinken, P.J. & Bruyn, G.W. (eds.) *Handbook of Clinical Neurology 15, The Epilepsies*, Amsterdam: North-Holland (1974) 311.

225. Jovanovič, U.J. Das Schlafverhalten der Epileptiker. 1. Schlafdauer, Schlaftiefe und Besonderheiten der Schlafperiodik, *Deutsch. Z. Nervenheilk.* (1967) **190**, 159–172.

226. Kikuchi, S. An electroencephalographic study of nocturnal sleep in temporal lobe epilepsy, *Folia Psychiat. Neurol. Jap.* (1969) **23**, 59–81.

227. Langdon-Down, M. & Brain, W. Time of day in relation to convulsions in epilepsy, *Lancet* (1929) **2**, 1029–1032.

228. Meier-Ewart, K.-H. & Broughton, R. Photomyoclonic response of epileptic and non-epileptic subjects during wakefulness, sleep and arousal, *Electroenceph. Clin. Neurophysiol.* (1967) **23**, 142–151.

229. Meldrum, B.S. In: Laidlaw, J. & Richens, A. (eds.) *A Textbook of Epilepsy*, Edinburgh: Churchill Livingstone (1982) 456–487.

230. Meldrum, B.S., Anlezark, G. & Trimble, M. Drugs modifying dopaminergic activity and behaviour, the EEG and epilepsy in *Papio papio*, *Eur. J. Pharmacol.* (1975) **32**, 203–213.

231. Montplaisir, J., Laverdière, M., Saint-Hilaire, J.M., Walsh, J. & Bouvier, G. Sleep and temporal lobe epilepsy: a case study with depth electrodes, *Neurology (NY)* (1981) **31**, 1352–1356.

232. Niedermeyer, E. Awakening epilepsy ('Aufwachepilepsie') revisited 30 years later. In: Degen, R. & Niedermeyer, E. (eds.) *Epilepsy, Sleep and Sleep Deprivation*, Amsterdam: Elsevier (1984) 85–96.

233. Niedermeyer, E. & Rocca, U. The diagnostic significance of sleep electroencephalograms in temporal lobe epilepsy: a comparison of scalp and depth tracings, *Eur. Neurol.* (1972) **7**, 119–129.

234. Passouant, P. Influence des états de vigilance sur les épilepsies. In: Koella, W.P. & Levin, P. (eds.) *Sleep, Vol. 3*, Basel: S. Karger (1977) 57–65.

235. Passouant, P. & Cadilhac, J. Décharges épileptiques et sommeil. In: Thieme, G. (ed.) *Epilepsy: Modern Problems in Pharmacopsychiatry, Vol. 4*, Basel: S. Karger (1980) 87–104.

236. Patry, F. The relation of time of day, sleep and other factors to the incidence of epileptic seizures, *Am. J. Psychiat.* (1931) **87**, 789–813.

237. Patry, G., Lyagoubi, S. & Tassinari, C.A. Subclinical 'electrical status epilepticus' induced by sleep in children, *Arch. Neurol.* (1971) **24**, 242–252.

238. Rodin, E., Luby, E.D. & Gottlieb, J.S. The electroencephalogram during prolonged experimental sleep deprivation, *Electroenceph. Clin. Neurophysiol.* (1962) **14**, 544–551.

239. Roffwarg, H.P., Clark, R.W. *et al.* Association of Sleep Disorders Centers. Diagnostic Classification of Sleep and Arousal Disorders, 1st edn, prepared by the Sleep Disorders Classification Committee, *Sleep* (1979) **2**, 1–137.

240. Sassin, J.F., Parker, D.C., Mace, J.W., Gerlin, R.W., Johnson, L.C. & Roseman, L.G. Human growth hormone release: relation to slow-wave sleep–waking cycles, *Science* (1969) **165**, 513–515.

241. Sterman, M.B. Power spectral analysis of EEG characteristics during sleep in epileptics, *Sleep* (1981) **22**, 95–106.

242. Stevens, J.R., Kodama, H., Lonsbury, B. & Mills, L. Ultradian characteristics of spontaneous seizure discharges recorded by radio-telemetry in man, *Electroenceph. Clin. Neurophysiol.* (1971) **31**, 313–325.

243. Tassinari, C.A., Dravet, C. & Roger, J. Encephalopathy related to electrical status epilepticus during slow sleep, *Electroenceph. Clin. Neurophysiol.* (1977) **43**, 529–530.

244. Veidhuizen, R., Binnie, C.D. & Beintema, D.J. The effect of sleep deprivation on the EEG in epilepsy, *Electroenceph. Clin. Neurophysiol.* (1983) **55**, 505–512.

245. Wieser, H.G. Temporal lobe epilepsy, sleep and arousal: stereo-EEG findings. In: Degen, R. & Niedermeyer, E. (eds.) *Epilepsy, Sleep and Sleep Deprivation*, Amsterdam: Elsevier (1984) 137–167.

246. White, P., Dyken, M., Grant, P. & Jackson, L. Electroencephalographic abnormalities during sleep as related to the temporal distribution of seizures, *Epilepsia* (1962) **3**, 167–174.

PAROXYSMAL NOCTURNAL HAEMOGLOBINURIA

247. Dessypris, E.N., Clark, D.A., McKee, L.C., Jr. & Krantz, S.B. Increased sensitivity to complement of erythroid and myeloid progenitors in paroxysmal nocturnal hemoglobinuria, *New Engl.J. Med.* (1983) **309**, 690–693.
248. Gull, W.W. A case of intermittent haematuria, with remarks, *Guy's Hosp. Rep.* (1866) **12**, 381–392.
249. Ham, T.H. Chronic hemolytic anemia with paroxysmal nocturnal hemoglobinuria: study of the mechanism of hemolysis in relation to acid–base equilibrium, *New Engl. J. Med.* (1937) **217**, 915–917.
250. Ham, T.H. Studies on destruction of red blood cells; chronic haemolytic anaemia with paroxysmal nocturnal haemoglobinuria: investigation of mechanism of haemolysis with observations on 5 cases, *Arch. Int. Med.* (1939) **64**, 1271–1305.
251. Hansen, N.E. Sleep related plasma haemoglobin levels in paroxysmal nocturnal haemoglobinuria, *Acta Med. Scand.* (1968) **184**, 547–549.
252. Hansen, N.E. & Killmann, S.-A. Paroxysmal nocturnal haemoglobinuria, *Acta Med. Scand.* (1968) **184**, 525–541.
253. Morley, A.A., Baker, L.R.J., Beardwell, C.G. & Burke, C.W. Adrenal steroids and haemolysis in paroxysmal nocturnal haemoglobinuria, *Lancet* (1967) **2**, 448–450.
254. Nicholson-Weller, A., March, J.P., Rosenfeld, S.I. & Austen, K.F. Affected erythrocytes of patients with paroxysmal nocturnal hemoglobinuria are deficient in the complement regulatory protein, decay-accelerating factor, *Proc. Nat. Acad. Sci.* (1983) **80**, 5066–5070.
255. Oni, S.B., Osunkoya, B.O. & Luzzatto, L. Paroxysmal nocturnal hemoglobinuria: evidence for monoclonal origin of abnormal red cells, *Blood* (1970) **36**, 145–152.
256. Schreiber, A.D. Paroxysmal nocturnal hemoglobinuria revisited, *New Engl. J. Med.* (1983) **309**, 723–725.
257. Strübing, P. Paroxysmale Hemoglobinurie, *Deutsch. Med. Wockenschr.* (1882) **8**, 1–14.

NOCTURNAL PENILE TUMESCENCE

258. Cooper, A.J. The causes and management of impotence, *Postgrad. Med. J.* (1972) **48**, 548–552.
259. Fisher, C., Gross, J. & Zuch, J. Cycle of penile erection synchronous with dreaming (REM) sleep – Preliminary report, *Arch. Gen. Psychiat.* (1965) **12**, 29–45.
260. Fisher, C., Shiavi, R.C., Edwards, A., Davis, D.M., Reitman, M. & Fine, J. Evaluation of nocturnal penile tumescence in the differential diagnosis of sexual impotence. A quantitative study, *Arch. Gen. Psychiat.* (1979) **36**, 431–437.
261. Hursch, C.J., Karacan, I. & Williams, R.L. Some characteristics of nocturnal penile tumescence in early middle-aged males, *Comp. Psychiat.* (1972) **13**, 539–548.
262. Karacan, I. A simple and inexpensive transducer for quantitative measurements of penile erection during sleep, *Behav. Res. Meth. Instr.* (1969) **1**, 251–252.
263. Karacan, I. Painful nocturnal penile erections, *J. Am. Med. Assoc.* (1971) **215**, 1831.
264. Karacan, I. Diagnosis of erectile impotence in diabetes mellitus. An objective and specific method, *Ann. Int. Med.* (1980) **92**, 334–337.
265. Karacan, I. Evaluation of nocturnal penile tumescence and impotence. In: Guilleminault, C. (ed.) *Sleeping and Waking Disorders: Indications and Techniques*, Menlo Park, California: Addison-Wesley (1982) 343–372.
266. Karacan, I., Asian, C. & Hirschkowitz, M. Erectile mechanisms in man, *Science* (1983) **220**, 1080–1082.
267. Karacan, I., Dervent, A., Salis, P.J., Ware J.C., Scott, F.B., Dervent, B. & Williams, R.L. Spinal cord injuries and NPT, *Sleep Res.* (1978) **7**, 261.
268. Karacan, I., Goodenough, D.R., Shapiro, A. & Starker, S. Erection cycle during sleep in relation to dream anxiety, *Arch. Gen. Psychiat.* (1966) **15**, 183–189.
269. Karacan, I., Hursch, C.J., & Williams, R.L. Some characteristics of nocturnal penile tumescence in elderly males, *J. Gerontol.* (1972) **27**, 39–45.

270. Karacan, I., Hursch, C.J., Williams, R.L. & Thornby, J.I. Some characteristics of nocturnal penile tumescence in young adults, *Arch. Gen. Psychiat.* (1972) **26**, 351–356.

271. Karacan, I., Salis, P.J. & Williams, R.L. The role of the sleep laboratory in the diagnosis and treatment of impotence. In: Williams, R.L. & Karacan, I. (eds.) *Sleep Disorders: Diagnosis and Treatment,* New York: Wiley (1978) 353–382.

272. Karacan, I., Snyder, S., Salis, P.J., Williams, R.L. & Derman, S. Sexual dysfunction in male alcoholics and its objective evaluation. In: Fann, W.E., Karacan, I., Pokorny, A.D. & Williams, R.L. (eds.) *Phenomenology and Treatment of Alcoholism,* New York: Spectrum Publications (1980) 259–268.

273. Karacan, I., Williams, R.L., Derman, S. & Aslan, C. Impaired sleep-related penile tumescence in the diagnosis of impotence. In: Zales, M.R. (ed.) *Eating, Sleeping and Sexuality,* New York: Brunner-Mazel (1982) 186–199.

274. Karacan, I., Williams, R.L. & Salis, P.J. The effect of sexual intercourse on sleep patterns and nocturnal penile erections, *Psychophysiology* (1970) **7**, 338–339.

275. Karacan, I., Williams, R.L., Thornby, J.I. & Salis, P.J. Sleep-related penile tumescence as a function of age, *Am. J. Psychiat.* (1975) **132**, 932–937.

276. Moore, C., Karacan, I. & Taylor, A. Erectile dysfunction in Shy–Drager syndrome, *Sleep Res.* (1979) **8**, 240.

277. Moraise, A., Marshall, P.G., Surridge, D.H. & Fenemore, J. A new device for diagnostic screening of nocturnal penile tumescence, *J. Urol.* (1983) **129**, 288–290.

278. Roose, S.P., Glassman, A.H., Walsh, B.T. & Cullen, K. Reversible loss of nocturnal penile tumescence during depression: a preliminary report, *Neuropsychobiology* (1982) **8**, 284–288.

SLEEP AND THE GUT

279. Cooper, B.T., Holmes, G.K.T. & Ferguson, R. Gluten-sensitive diarrhoea without evidence of celiac disease, *Gastroenterology* (1980) **79**, 801–806.

280. Dent, J., Dodd, W.J. & Friedman, R.H. Mechanism of gastro-oesophageal reflux in recumbent asymptomatic human subjects, *J. Clin. Invest.* (1980) **65**, 256–257.

281. Guilleminault, C., Eldridge, F.L., Phillips, J.R. & Dement, W.C. Two occult causes of insomnia and their therapeutic problems, *Arch. Gen. Psychiat.* (1976) **33**, 1241–1245.

282. Harvey, R.F. Colonic motility in proctalgia fugax, *Lancet* (1979) **2**, 713–714.

283. Hines, L.F. & Mead, H.C.A. Peristalsis in a loop of small intestine, *Arch. Int. Med.* (1926) **38**, 539.

284. Johnson, R.L. & Washeim, H. Studies in gastric secretion, *Am. J. Physiol.* (1924) **70**, 247–253.

285. Khan, M. Hour of onset of cholera and diarrhoea, *Lancet* (1979) **1**, 834–835.

286. Levin, E., Kirsner, J.B. & Palmer, W.L. A comparison of the normal gastric secretion in patients with duodenal ulcer and in normal individuals, *Gastroenterology* (1948) **10**, 952–964.

287. Orr, W.C., Hall, W.H., Stahl, M.L., Durkin, M.G. & Whitsett, T.L. Sleep patterns and gastric acid secretion in duodenal ulcer disease, *Arch. Int. Med.* (1976) **136**, 655–660.

288. Orr, W.C., Martin, R.J., Imes, N.K., Rogers, R.M. & Stahl, M.L. Hypersomnolent and nonhypersomnolent patients with upper airway obstruction during sleep, *Chest* (1979) **75**, 418–422.

289. Orr, W.C. & Robinson, M.G. The sleeping gut, *Med. Clin. N. Am.* (1981) **65**, 1359–1376.

290. Orr, W.C., Robinson, M.G. & Johnson, L.F. Acid clearing during sleep in patients with oesophagitis and controls, *Gastroenterology* (1979) **76**, 1213.

291. Orr, W.C., Robinson, M.G. & Johnson, L.F. Acid clearance during sleep in the pathogenesis of reflux oesophagitis, *Dig. Dis. Sci.* (1981) **26**, 423–427.

292. Schuster, M.M., Hookman, P. & Hendrix, T.S. Simultaneous manometric recording of internal and external and sphincteric reflexes, *Bull. Johns Hopkins Hosp.* (1965) **116**, 79–88.

293. Sleisinger, M.H. & Fordtran, J.S. Gastrointestinal disease: pathophysiology, diagnosis and management, 2nd edn., Philadelphia: W.B. Saunders (1978).

294. Spiro, H. *Clinical Gastroenterology,* New York: MacMillan (1977).

SLEEP AND THE CARDIOVASCULAR SYSTEM

295. Brodsky, M., Wu, D., Denes, P., Kanakis, C. & Rosen, K.M. Arrhythmias documented by 24 hour continuous electrocardiographic monitoring in 50 male medical students without apparent heart disease, *Am. J. Cardiol.* (1977) **39**, 390–395.

296. Broughton, R. & Baron, R. Sleep patterns in the intensive care unit and on the ward after acute myocardial infarction, *Electroenceph. Clin. Neurophysiol.* (1978) **45**, 348–352.
297. Buguet, A., Roussel, B., Canicave, J.-C., Grippari, J.-L. & Viola, P. Heart blocks during sleep: a case report in a healthy subject, *Sleep* (1981) **4**, 99.
298. Chierchia, S. Pathogenetic mechanisms of coronary vasospasm, *Acta Med. Scand.* (1982) Suppl. **660**, 49–56.
299. Guilleminault, C., Pool, P., Motta, J. & Gillis, A.M. Sinus arrest during REM sleep in young adults, *New Engl. J. Med.* (1984) **311**, 1006–1010.
300. Karacan, I., Williams, R.L. & Taylor, W.J. Sleep characteristics of patients with angina pectoris, *Psychometrics* (1969) **10**, 280–284.
301. Khatri, J.M. & Freis, E.D. Hemodynamic changes during sleep in hypertensive patients, *Circulation* (1969) **39**, 785–790.
302. King, M.J., Zir, L., Kaltman, A.J. & Fox, A.C. Case report. Variant angina associated with angiographically demonstrated coronary artery spasm and REM sleep, *Am. J. Med. Sci.* (1973) **265**, 419.
303. Kleitman, N. *Sleep and Wakefulness*, Chicago: University of Chicago Press (1963) 552.
304. Lichstein, E., Alosilla, C., Chadda, K.D. & Gupta, P.K. Significance and treatment of nocturnal angina preceding myocardial infarction, *Am. Heart J.* (1977) **93**, 723–728.
305. Lown, B., Tykocinski, M., Garfein, A. & Brooks, P. Sleep and ventricular premature beats, *Circulation* (1973) **48**, 691–701.
306. MacWilliam, J.A. Blood pressure and heart action in sleep and dreams: their relation to haemorrhages, angina and sudden death, *Brit. Med. J.* (1923) **2**, 1196–1197.
307. Nowlin, J.B., Troyer, W.G., Collins, W.S., Silverman, G., Nichols, C.R., McIntosh, H.D., Estes, E.H. & Bogdonoff, M.D. The association of nocturnal angina pectoris with dreaming, *Ann. Int. Med. (Chicago)* (1965) **63**, 1040–1046.
308. Roffwarg, H.P., Clark, R.W. *et al* Association of Sleep Disorders Centers. Diagnostic Classification of Sleep and Arousal Disorders, 1st edn, prepared by the Sleep Disorders Classification Committee, *Sleep* (1979) **2**, 1–137.
309. Rosenberg, M.J., Uretz, E. & Denes, P. Sleep and ventricular arrhythmias, *Am. Heart J.* (1983) **106**, 703–709.
310. Rosenblatt, G., Hartmann, E. & Zwilling, G.R. Cardiac irritability during sleep and dreaming, *J. Psychosom. Res.* (1973) **17**, 129–134.
311. Smith, R., Johnson, L., Rothfield, D., Zir, L. & Tharp, B. Sleep and cardiac arrhythmias, *Arch. Int. Med.* (1972) **130**, 342–349.
312. Stern, S. & Tzivoni, D. Dynamic changes in the S–T segment during sleep in ischemic heart disease, *Am. J. Cardiol.* (1973) **22**, 17–20.
313. Williams, R.L. Sleep disturbances in various medical and surgical conditions. In: Williams, R.L. & Karacan, I. (eds.) *Sleep Disorders: Diagnosis and Treatment*, New York: Wiley (1978) 285–301.

CHAPTER 5

INSOMNIA

THE COMPLAINT

My first contact with a real insomniac was a lady who was referred to me in 1959 by a New York physician; she stated that she never slept. We thought perhaps she was the unique individual for whom we all had been searching, i.e. someone who did not need sleep. In fact she was dependent on barbiturates, and was taking more than 2000 mg of Seconal and Amytal at bedtime. Naturally, when she did not take the medication, she did not sleep. Nonetheless I decided to record her once with her medication and once without. I was slightly startled to find that she weighed nearly 300 pounds; however, my prior experience did not prepare me for what followed when she took her medication. She downed some 20 capsules and oozed onto the floor in a coma. Because I was alone, I could not move her into bed that night.

(Dement, W.C.[34])

James Thurber stayed up nights playing word games and wrote 'Insomnia, it comes to us all'.

Insomnia is a subjective phenomenon, a complaint of disordered sleep. Insomnia causes difficulty in falling asleep, repeated waking and early morning arousal. Some insomniacs have round-the-clock 24 h insomnia, and are unable to sleep by day as well as by night. As well as sleepless nights, the major result is a feeling of not being refreshed by sleep, but as far as we know no one ever died from insomnia. Records for staying awake have been set by a man from San Diego who stayed awake for eleven days and did not suffer any ill effects[67] and by a patient with *chorée fibrillaire de Morvan* who went four months without sleep.[39]

Morvan's article, published in 1890, was founded on a study of five cases of which only the first was described in detail. After 8 days of weakness and fatigue the patient, a man, showed continuous fibrillation of the calves and hamstrings, but the face, tongue, hands and feet were not affected. There was profuse sweating with fever, and the illness took a downward course with delirium, coma, and death by the twenty-seventh day. The other four cases were trivial and none fatal. What was this illness?

Insomnia is difficult to verify objectively. There is often little correspondence between sleeplessness as reported by a person and sleeplessness as determined by a machine wired up to him to measure sleep. Nevertheless, people who do complain of insomnia mostly sleep worse than controls, sleep less and wake in the night more often.[41] Sleep laboratory investigation rarely reveals a hidden cause. Kales *et al.*, in a comparison of 200 insomniac patients and 100 normal controls, found no examples of sleep apnoea and about the

Table 5.1   *Causes of insomnia*

Physiological factors: environmental factors, noise, discomfort, time-zone changes, shiftwork, old age, naturally short sleep
Psychological factors: normal life stress, anxiety with e.g. bereavement, sickness, exams
Psychiatric illness: endogenous depression, anorexia nervosa, obsessive–compulsive neurosis, anxiety neurosis
Physical causes, painful and distressing conditions: cardiorespiratory distress, arthritis, terminal cancer, nocturia, gastrointestinal disease, renal failure, thyrotoxicosis, Parkinson's disease
Pharmacological causes: alcohol, coffee, anorectic and stimulant drugs
Parasomnias: sleep apnoea, sleep myoclonus, 'non-restorative' sleep
Primary sleep disorders: 'primary' insomnia, delayed sleep phase syndrome
'Pseudo'-insomnia: hypochondriasis, misinterpretation, misattribution of fatigue

same number of individuals (5%) with nocturnal leg jerks among the controls as among the insomniacs (Table 5.1).[72]

PREVALENCE OF INSOMNIA

The complaint of insomnia is far more common than any other complaint about sleep. A number of questionnaire surveys in different countries have suggested that the prevalence of sleep problems (mainly insomnia) in the general adult population is about 15% in Scotland,[97] 25% in Florida[79] and 42.5% in Los Angeles.[13] In the Los Angeles metropolitan area one-third of those questioned about their sleep complained of insomnia, difficulty in falling asleep, difficulty in staying asleep or too-early final waking.[13] Although the magnitude of these figures invites disbelief, they have been repeatedly confirmed. At least a quarter of adults and a higher percentage of old people complain of insomnia at some time or other each year.[86] As with population studies, surveys by physicians of their patients indicate that a high percentage of the adult population complain of insomnia,[12] although a few reports are not representative of the whole population. Clift,[24] a GP in Manchester, wrote a report based chiefly on hypnotic drug users and their sleep characteristics, and Gnirrs[45] described sleep disturbances in a psychiatric department. Some indication of the size of the problem of chronic insomnia in the general adult

Table 5.2   *Frequency of different causes of insomnia*

Cause	Percentage of cases
Psychiatric causes	
depression	17
personality disorder	18
'Psychophysiological' insomnia	15
Alcoholism, drug abuse	12
Sleep myoclonus	12
Sleep apnoea	6
Other insomnias – alpha–delta sleep, REM awakenings	6
Medical and toxic conditions	4
'Pseudo'-insomnia – normal EEG findings	9

Data from Coleman *et al.*[26] based on findings in patients with insomnia seen at sleep disorder clinics.

population is given by the fact that in 1979 it was reported that 4% of people in the United States used prescription drugs from time to time to help them sleep,[132] and a similar number of Londoners in a 1977 survey had taken a hypnotic in the preceding two weeks.[105]

Family practice surveys show that far fewer patients complain to their doctors about insomnia than experience sleeplessness from time to time. In Holland, de Graaf and Pluymen[33] showed that only about 3% of patients attending a general practice surgery had a sleep problem of any importance, whilst in a family practice in Canada, only one in 500 of patients listed insomnia as a complaint (See Table 5.2).[22, 23]

WHO COMPLAINS?

The complaint of poor sleep is made especially by patients who are female, old, neurotic, thin, and who smoke and drink alcohol. Overall, women complain twice as often about their sleep as men,[13, 79, 97] and housewives in particular are often bad sleepers.[33] Poor sleep is sometimes accepted as an inevitable consequence of old age. The normal elderly person lies awake for one-fifth of the night, and the complaint of insomnia is much more common amongst old people than the young.[13, 65, 97, 139] Psychiatric problems often lead to insomnia and patients who believe they sleep poorly are, as a group, more anxious than controls.[13, 65, 97] Anxious subjects may greatly overestimate the time taken to fall asleep and underestimate their total sleep duration.[20] Insomnia is frequently associated with psychiatric difficulties, whilst hypersomnia more often results from organic disease.

The higher the educational level, the better the sleep. Kales and Kales[75] showed that the complaint of insomnia was most common in subjects from lower socioeconomic groups and of poor education.

The nature of insomnia carries with it a high risk of self-medication, hypnotic drug abuse and alcoholism. Both heavy drinkers and heavy smokers describe themselves as sleeping less than non-drinkers or non-smokers.[111]

In young adults the difference between good and poor sleepers has been associated with differences in body temperature, skin resistance and frequency of vasoconstriction during sleep.[104] Total 24 h corticosteroid excretion[66] and body core temperature[104] may be higher in poor than in good sleepers. Oversleeping, sleeping for very long periods, or merely staying in bed, can lead to a feeling of poor sleep and sometimes to the complaint of insomnia.

THE EFFECTS OF INSOMNIA

If sleep is the major restorative process which overcomes the wear and tear of wakefulness, or if it is important for memory, chronic insomnia would be expected to have dire results. However, all studies have shown that short periods of sleep lack do not greatly impair any aspect of waking performance. We all seem to get much more sleep than we need. Following sleep loss, only about one third of the total amount of sleep that is lost is regained. In people who are naturally very short sleepers, all but the essential core of deep sleep may have been eliminated (see Chapter 1: Sleep deprivation; Good and poor sleepers).

Common observation shows that the more deeply one sleeps the more alert one is when awake, but this is surprisingly difficult to quantify. After a good night's sleep, daytime tests of most performance tasks rise to peak or plateau levels between 1200 and 2100, and the rhythm of body temperature follows a similar pattern. More complex performance tests, however, requiring memory or logical reasoning, may fall steadily throughout the day and be completely out of phase with temperature rhythms.[107] Initiation and motivation may suffer after a poor night's sleep, although there may be little or no deterioration in simple motor and memory tasks. The major effect of insomnia in patients is to cause sleepiness, fatigue, lack of concentration and sometimes muscle aching and mild depression, similar to the results of sleep deprivation experiments in healthy young volunteers.

Two studies have shown that, in those who regularly sleep for only short periods, the mortality rate is surprisingly high.[85, 86]

Medical conditions inducing insomnia and leading to the taking of sleeping pills would be expected to produce a high death rate. Wingard and Berkman[152] demonstrated a high mortality rate amongst those who sleep only 6 h or less, with a high death rate for ischaemic heart disease, stroke, cancer and all causes combined. The relative mortality rate of short sleepers was 1.3 times greater than that of normal sleepers when correction was made for age, sex, race, socioeconomic status, physical health, weight, smoking, alcohol consumption and so on (see Chapter 1: 'Death at night', ref. 8).

Why does a poor night's sleep cause muscle aching? Chronic alpha intrusion into the normal sleep pattern was reported by Hauri and Hawkins[57] to be associated with feelings of general fatigue, malaise and muscle aching. Many patients with fibrositis and sleep discomfort show alpha intrusion into NREM sleep.[103] However, not everyone with non-restorative sleep and morning fatigue has alpha intrusion into sleep, and 'alpha–delta' sleep may accompany the chronic use of either hypnotics or stimulants, with no relationship to muscle aching. Fibrositis is very unlikely to originate in poor sleep.

SLEEP AND AGE

Sleep gradually changes in quality throughout life (see Chapter 1) and both sexes complain more about their sleep as they get older. The number of insomniacs and the severity of insomnia both increase with age.[85]

As the years pass, total sleep time decreases from 8 h daily in young adulthood to about 6 h daily at age 90. There is much less stage 4 sleep, or the deepest phase of sleep may disappear altogether. Changes in REM sleep are unimpressive if we consider only the averages, which remain at about 22% of total sleep time from age 16 to age 79, although REM sleep time becomes a little shorter with age.[63] More nocturnal waking periods disrupt sleep. Sleep is less refreshing in the elderly than in young people and cat-naps occur frequently during daytime. The normal sleep pattern of an old man can be very similar to that of a young adult with maintenance insomnia.[151]

These changes do not affect only the very elderly.[119] The 30-year-old gets only half the amount of stage 4 NREM sleep that the 20-year-old gets, and shows twice the amount of intervening wakefulness over the night.[43] The time spent in bed awake, not asleep, each night increases from 5% at the age of 20 to 15% at age 70 and over 20% at age 85.[37] The sleep of old people is much more easily disrupted by noise than that of young people[122] and the sleep-disrupting effect of coffee greatly increases with age.[78] However, at all ages there is an enormous variability in sleep patterns and some 90-year-olds sleep just like young adults.[117]

Do old people need as much sleep as young adults? Of the 2466 people questioned in Scotland by McGhie and Russell,[97] only the young, not the old, complained of being tired in the morning, despite better sleep in the young. However, the usual nature of morning activity is very different in young and old people.

The results of McGhie and Russell's survey showed a regular rise in the incidence of complaints of disturbed sleep with each succeeding decade so that by the age of 75 disturbed sleep occurred in one-third of all the people surveyed.[97] Likewise Tune[139] found that many healthy English people over the age of 70 often reported irregular sleep.

Insomnia in the elderly is due to a mixture of medical, psychological and social factors, medical disorders, pain, depression, loneliness, absence of regular activities and interests, long daytime naps, worry about financial problems or health; but in addition Regelstein[119] suggested that much of the insomnia in the elderly is related to the evolution of sleep patterns with age itself.

The total number of neurones in the brain declines by about 20% between birth and old age[18] but this involves the cortex much more than the brain stem nuclei that are involved in the control of sleep. Hazeman et al.[60] did all-day monitoring in 22 old people aged from 82 to 97 and found that the amount of wakefulness, somnolence and naps, as behaviourally measured, correlated both with age and with the waking frequencies of the EEG. The preservation of REM sleep in the elderly correlates with the preservation of intelligence, as measured by WAIS subscales[114] and there is much less REM sleep time amongst the elderly demented.[37]

Circadian disturbances have been held responsible for the poor sleep of the elderly, but will not explain the whole problem. Circadian regulatory mechanisms do break down in old people,[128] and Wever[150] showed that in subjects living in temporal isolation, internal desynchronization between sleep and temperature rhythms occurred in 21% of young subjects aged 17–33, but 100% of older people aged 44–69. Regelstein[119] suggested that loss of social contacts, important for the synchronization of the normal sleep–wake cycle, may explain partly the fitful sleep of old people.

As many as one-third to one-half of all people over 60 have sleep apnoea and sleep myoclonus[85] and both of these may sometimes account for poor sleep in the elderly. However, in most of these instances, sleep apnoea or myoclonus is only of minor severity and do not cause symptoms. In a group of elderly people with no sleep problems investigated by Carskadon and Dement[19] 37.5% had sleep apnoea. The definition of sleep apnoea in the elderly requires reappraisal.

Inside and outside hospital, the elderly are saturated with hypnotics. Such treatment is ubiquitous. In women of 75, McGhie and Russell[97] found that 45% regularly used sleeping pills. In old people's homes for healthy old people in Edinburgh, Oswald[110] reported that the nightly hypnotic intake varied from 15% for inmates in one home to 50% in another. There is much evidence that this practice is harmful. There is no doubt that daytime sedation as a result of night hypnotics will impair the already diminished cortical function of the elderly and impair patterns of mood and daytime performance.[125] Agitation and confusion are increased in the elderly by hypnotics.[47] Learoyd[94] showed that one sixth of elderly patients admitted to mental hospitals showed a disappearance of behavioural disturbances when sedatives were stopped. Sleep apnoea, which is present in up to 50% of people aged over 65, is increased in severity by hypnotics.

Demented patients may show an exaggeration of the normal age-related changes in sleep (reduction in total sleep time, absence of delta sleep and frequent awakenings). Dementia is an important cause of chronic insomnia. In addition to normal age-related changes, demented subjects often show loss of REM sleep, confusion and restlessness at night, and displacement of sleep from night to day.[37] Loss of REM sleep is particularly marked in *progressive supranuclear palsy*, with involvement of brain stem nuclei, and sleep myoclonus may contribute to insomnia in *Jakob–Creutzfeldt disease*. Sleep fragmentation, sleep reversal, and sleep apnoea are found with increased frequency in *Alzheimer's disease*. The response to sedatives in demented subjects, particularly those who are most disturbed, is often irregular, and paroxysmal rage reactions and further disturbances in behaviour are not unusual.

STRUCTURE OF INSOMNIA (Table 5.3)

Two kinds of information are necessary to assess insomnia; the history of the sleep problem (transient or chronic) and the pattern of insomnia (e.g. change in sleep onset, sleep interruption, alteration in circadian rhythm).

Table 5.3   *Patterns of insomnia*

1. Sleep-onset insomnia
      anxiety, tension, phobia of insomnia
      drugs
2. Sleep-maintenance insomnia
      drugs, hypnotic withdrawal, alcohol, daytime stimulants
      medical diseases
      neurological and psychiatric disorders
      parasomnias
      restless legs, sleep myoclonus
3. Early morning waking
      affective disorders
4. Phase-shift disorders
5. Cyclical insomnia

TRANSIENT AND CHRONIC INSOMNIA

Most authorities divide insomnia into *transient* (less than 3–4 weeks) or *chronic* (more than 3–4 weeks) varieties. *Transient insomnia* is due to many different causes, including life stress, brief illness, hypnotic withdrawal, time-zone travel or temporary sleep deprivation. Recovery is usually rapid after a period of maximum sleep disruption of 2–3 weeks. Transient insomnia as a result of change in environment, emotional crisis, a new baby, illness or bereavement, and so on, is experienced by everyone several times during their lives. The sleep disruption can take any form (difficulty in falling asleep, intermittent awakenings or premature morning arousal), dependent on age, previous sleep habit and personality. Transient situational insomnia is sometimes multifactorial, as occurs before, during and after surgery, with apprehension, physical discomfort and pain, a change in environment from familiar surroundings to an often noisy ward, premedication and general anaesthetic, analgesics and sedatives all interfering with normal sleep habits. Despite this multifactorial aetiology, psychological factors have been shown to play a role in as many as 80% of all insomniacs.[107]

Chronic insomnia may be life-long. It is usually the consequence of old age, medical, behavioural or psychiatric problems.

PATTERNS OF INSOMNIA

Difficulty in falling asleep (prolonged sleep latency, *sleep-onset insomnia*; i.e. longer than 30 min before sleep supervenes) is usually related to sudden anxiety, bereavement, accident, noise, environmental changes or stimulant drugs. This pattern of insomnia is also an early presenting feature in some instances of depressive illness. The high level of arousal that prevents sleep is probably due to both psychological and physiological factors[42] and in some cases is associated with high plasma noradrenaline levels.[116] High noradrenaline levels may also explain the insomnia of people on a diet who go to bed in a state of physiological starvation.

Sleep maintenance insomnia, with frequent nocturnal arousals, has many different causes. The interruptions in sleep may occur at specific times, or be entirely random. Frequent arousals at 90 min intervals are almost always due to REM sleep nightmares, and awakenings from REM sleep are characteristic of night terrors and cluster headache. In contrast, sleep acroparaesthesiae, sleep apnoea and also neurotic anxiety cause random multiple awakenings with full arousal from both NREM and REM sleep.

Early morning awakening without further sleep, although seen with any kind of excitement, is a specific feature of major depressive illness, in particular endogenous bipolar depression and hypomania.

Phase-shift disorders can masquerade as insomnia, when the patient is unable to go to sleep at the expected time. However, despite late sleep onset, sleep itself is normal in duration in the delayed sleep phase syndrome.

Cyclical insomnia may conceal drug abuse, alcoholism, or cyclical medical and psychiatric disorders.

CHRONIC INSOMNIA

Three classes of insomnia can be recognized in people with prolonged difficulty in sleeping:

1. *primary* or *idiopathic* chronic insomnia, occurring without unambiguous cause;
2. *secondary* chronic insomnia associated with:
   (a) medical problems,
   (b) physiological problems,
   (c) psychological problems,
   (d) psychiatric problems,
   (e) drugs,
   (f) cyclical causes;
3. a class where sleep difficulty is part of *a sleep disorder.*

The frequency of these three different classes of insomnia is approximately as follows: *primary chronic insomnia* accounts for about 10–25% of all cases of chronic insomnia; *secondary chronic insomnia* for most examples; whilst a *sleep disorder* (e.g. alteration in sleep architecture *per se* or the delayed sleep phase syndrome) is rarely associated with the presenting complaint of chronic insomnia.

These three classes of chronic insomnia are considered in detail below.

PRIMARY CHRONIC INSOMNIA

Primary insomnia of infancy and childhood

Hauri and Olmstead[58] established the clinical features of a disorder characterized by unexplained, life-long, fragmented, short sleep. A remarkable lack of sleep commences in infancy, with in adult life fitful sleep for 3–4 h each night, very early arousals and insomnia by day as well as by night. Unlike short sleepers, subjects with primary insomnia complain about their sleep and also of daytime fatigue, irritability, tension and somatic depression. The diagnosis should be considered when insomnia goes back to childhood or adolescence, with no obvious internal or external environmental cause sufficient to produce the symptoms. This condition is sometimes familial. In others, a possible structural basis is suggested by the occasional finding of signs of minimal brain damage, dyslexia or hyperkinesis.[58] The pattern of this type of insomnia is very similar to that seen in secondary insomnia due to psychophysiological causes, at least at a descriptive level, and it may be impossible to distinguish the two conditions in adult life.

Minor abnormalities of sleep structure have been demonstrated in some cases of primary insomnia. There may be diffuse EEG abnormalities, atypical EEG findings such as lack of sleep spindles or frequent intrusion of alpha bursts into sleep,[113] or a poverty of eye movements during REM sleep. One patient described by Hauri had almost no delta sleep.[55]

Hypnotics are usually unsuccessful in primary insomnia. Biofeedback and conditioning techniques may cause minimal improvement. Feinstein et al.[38] and Jordan et al.[70] attempted to improve sleep structure in primary insomnia by sensory–motor rhythm biofeedback, based on the observation that this may increase sleep spindles during the night in animals.[135] This treatment may be no less successful than any other.

Chronic 'pseudo'-insomnia of adults

In primary chronic insomnia, the complaint dates from childhood with short sleep and an abnormal sleep structure. However, some subjects complain of insomnia starting in adult life, sometimes associated with daytime sleepiness, impaired mood or wellbeing, but detailed investigation does not reveal any major abnormality in the duration or structure of their sleep or any obvious cause for insomnia.[121] The term 'pseudo'-insomnia is a product of sleep laboratory investigation of such patients.[20] This term may be inappropriate, and Nicholson and Marks[107] point out that some of these patients may need more sleep, or sleep of a different pattern, from that they habitually obtain. Perhaps the sleep of patients with 'pseudo'-insomnia may involve abnormalities that are not yet appreciated.

The group of 'pseudo'-insomnias is very heterogeneous. It probably includes subjects who: (1) are natural short sleepers; (2) complain of insomnia due to abnormal expectation about sleep; (3) have delayed (or, less often, advanced) sleep phase syndromes; and (4) are old and do not sleep at night but function normally by day. And what are we to make of subjects who have very disturbed sleep whilst in the laboratory, but no complaint about either sleeping or waking?

SECONDARY CHRONIC INSOMNIA

Most chronic insomnias are associated with obvious medical, psychiatric or behavioural problems. Almost any medical condition may disturb sleep by discomfort, pain, cough, breathlessness, nocturia, angina or other symptom, and the structure of sleep is altered by many metabolic diseases.[121]

Medical causes of chronic insomnia
Many *neurological disorders* cause insomnia, including head injury, infection, parkinsonism, encephalitis, psychomotor and generalized seizures, cortical and subcortical lesions, damage to the spinal cord, cerebrovascular disease and dementia. Insomnia in neurological disorders can result from primary involvement of sleep mechanisms (e.g. progressive supranuclear palsy), be due to alteration in sensory mechanisms (e.g. spinal cord lesions) or occur as a consequence of stress, discomfort and pain, sometimes with nerve or root compression as in nerve entrapment, lumbar disc lesions, night cramps,[129] the 'tired arm' syndrome[40] or fibrositis.[102]

Any *medical condition* causing night pain or discomfort will disturb sleep.[25] Common causes of night waking due to pain or discomfort include ulcer pain,[6, 35] nocturnal angina,[108, 130] nocturnal asthma[118] and chronic as well as intermittent airflow obstruction. Here hypnotics can be dangerous, although some pink puffers who retain normal nocturnal oxygen saturation benefit from sedatives.[21, 101]

Chronic renal insufficiency causes short, fragmented and disorganized sleep patterns.[112] Following dialysis or transplantation, sleep may improve, but it rarely achieves a normal pattern.[82] Poor sleep in uraemia has been attributed to irreversible neuronal changes, but is more likely to result from the severe metabolic disturbance.

Several endocrine disorders may produce insomnia. *Hyperthyroidism* can cause fragmented, short sleep with excessive amounts of delta activity, and *hypothyroidism* causes excessive sleepiness with lack of delta activity as well as obstructive sleep apnoea. Following return to the euthyroid condition, return to normal sleep patterns can be very slow, taking up to one year.[36] The sleep of between 5% and 25% of all *acromegalics* may be disturbed by obstructive sleep apnoea. Insomnia is occasionally secondary to *hypogonadism,* or anxiety associated with this. Insomnia in menopausal women may improve with conjugated oestrogen 0.625 mg daily.[127]

Physiological causes of chronic insomnia
Physiological factors resulting in poor sleep are usually easy to identify; these include change in environment, time change, shiftwork or old age. In addition to the physiological effect of aging on sleep, insomnia in old people is often multifactorial, with increase in general medical illness, psychological problems, decline of physical health, concern about approaching death and age-related changes in sleep mechanisms, nocturnal myoclonus and pathological (i.e. frequent episodes) sleep apnoea.

Psychological causes of chronic insomnia

Sleep is to some extent a learned habit and is easily upset by increased arousal, excitement and anxiety in some people in whom conditioned arousal responses prevent sleep and cause transient or chronic insomnia. Several studies have shown that people who are vulnerable to worry by reason of a nervous temperament regard themselves as habitual poor sleepers.[75, 97, 131]

The personality pattern of up to 70–80% of patients attending sleep disorder clinics complaining of insomnia is abnormal, with elevated Minnesota Multiphasic Personality Inventory scales for depression, conversion hysteria and psychoaesthenia.[74, 75] Retrospective studies in these patients show a high frequency of emotional and health problems going back to childhood, and sometimes severe stress in the period leading up to the development of insomnia.[61] Psychophysiological factors perpetuate insomnia, with emotional arousal preventing sleep, and also producing the fear of sleeplessness. This can lead to a vicious circle of physiological activation, sleeplessness, more fear of sleeplessness, further emotional arousal, and still further sleeplessness.[75] Several studies have established a diagnostic entity of *persistent psychophysiological insomnia*. However, this includes a very heterogeneous group of patients who cannot sleep, have a sense of not being refreshed by sleep, or merely visit sleep disorder clinics.

Psychiatric causes of chronic insomnia

Sleep may be severely disturbed in depression, anxiety, rumination, obsessive–compulsive disorders, psychosis and hypochondriasis.

Psychiatric problems lie at the roots of many sleep problems and in particular insomnia. Psychiatric disorders frequently cause a greater degree of sleep disturbance than any other cause of insomnia. In a study by Zorick et al.,[156] the total sleep of a group of psychiatric patients was much reduced as compared to both normal controls and other insomniacs. Hauri[55] has estimated that psychiatric problems lie at the root of 80% of all insomniacs seen by a psychiatrist, but only 30% seen by a neurologist. A sleepless night itself looks bad, and causes hopelessness with depression – this is of course normal, not a sign of depressive illness.

Depression. (See also Chapter 1: Sleep deprivation and mood; Chapter 3: Depression and circadian timekeeping.)

> In the true endogenous depressive we see a shift in the 24 h rhythm . . . the night becomes day . . . anyone knowing the material would look for the CNS origin in the midbrain, where the entire vegetative nervous system is controlled by a central clock whose rhythmicity . . . regulates and balances the biological system.
> (Georgi, 1947; in Wehr et al.[143])

The traditional idea that depression as a result of difficult life circumstances is associated with difficulty in falling asleep and that endogenous depression unrelated to external events is accompanied by frequent awakenings and early morning insomnia is not always borne out by sleep laboratory studies.[55, 91]

Some severely depressed patients sleep for excessively long, and not short, periods[99] or have normal sleep.[57] However, fragmented sleep is common in depression, and the subjective complaint of early morning waking is statistically associated with endogenous depression.[51]

Sleep changes in depression have been carefully documented over the last decade. Severe endogenous depression is accompanied by difficulty in staying asleep and early morning arousal, but without necessary delay in sleep onset; whilst in mania and hypomania the onset of sleep is delayed and sleep is short. Most patients with bipolar illness sleep more when they are depressed and less when they are manic.[53] Occasionally during the switch from depression to mania, 48 h may pass without sleep. Sleep is always shortened in the milder forms of mania and gravely disturbed during severe mania.

Sleep disturbance is one of the most important bodily symptoms of depression. Insomnia may precede all other psychological symptoms of depression, and restoration of sleep may be the first sign of recovery. Sleep is unrefreshing and sometimes with horrible dreams.

Anxiety. Neurotic anxiety and tension cause sleep-onset insomnia. This is more common in young people than in the elderly. A variety of physical symptoms are usually present. Rumination is common, which by itself impairs the ability to get to sleep. Coursey[28] suggested that rumination maintained arousal at too high a level, thus preventing sleep.

Sleep phobia. Many patients who have experienced frequent insomnia, or labelled themselves as insomniac, dread a further bad night's sleep. This in itself may cause fear and panic in the poor sleeper, leading to a self-fulfilling prophecy, and a phobia of sleepless nights develops. This can sometimes be improved by behavioural therapy, with relaxation and support to help the patient face the thought of another sleepless night without fear and arousal.

Schizophrenia. Most chronic schizophrenics sleep surprisingly well[93] with fairly normal sleep patterns and a normal amount of REM sleep. Minor changes are described in REM sleep in schizophrenics, but these may be due to neuroleptic drug treatment. Zarcone[153] found that when acutely ill schizophrenics are sleep-deprived they have little or no REM rebound, whilst sleep deprivation after recovery can result in an excessive rebound in REM sleep.[154]

Obsessive–compulsive disorders. In obsessive–compulsive disorders, patient with classic symptoms such as washing and checking rituals often complain o poor sleep and frequent awakenings, although a few suffer from hypersomnia with over 12 h of sleep per day. Most have short sleep times, frequen awakenings, short REM latency, and little stage 4 NREM sleep. This pattern i very similar to that found in endogenous depression.[64]

Drug and alcohol-induced chronic insomnia. Coffee, tea, cola, nicotine beta-blockers, α-methyldopa, phenytoin, bronchodilators, monamine oxidase inhibitors, amphetamine and other central nervous system stimulants, anoretic drugs, thiazides and other diuretics all interfere with sleep. A caffeine dose equivalent to four cups of coffee just before bedtime markedly increases arousals in normal subjects[77] and coffee disturbs sleep even in those who claim to be unaffected by it.[81] Alcohol is even more disruptive to sleep than coffee. Cigarette smoking close to bedtime, starvation, and possibly some food allergies, may also cause insomnia.

The acute administration of a short half-life *benzodiazepine* may produce early morning rebound insomnia and anxiety, not sedation, the morning after. With chronic treatment, withdrawal of short-acting hypnotic drugs can lead to a temporary insomnia of greater severity than that prior to drug administration. The severity of rebound insomnia is related to the dose, the period of administration and the benzodiazepine used. With short-acting benzodiazepines (e.g. triazolam) the rapid disappearance of drug from the receptors to which they are bound can result in severe rebound insomnia, accompanied by considerable anxiety, which can last for a few days and nights after a short period of drug administration[27] whilst, after more prolonged use, rebound insomnia may last as long as 2–3 weeks.[109] Severe rebound insomnia is usually more prominent in old than young people.

Alcohol shortens sleep latency, but causes subsequent sleep disruption. There is a dose-dependent depression of REM sleep with a compensatory increase on withdrawal and an increase in delta sleep with intoxication, a decrease with withdrawal.[50, 68, 84] Depending on the alcohol dose, compensatory REM sleep rebound on withdrawal may occur on the same night or on the following night.[124] Gross *et al.*[49] suggested that the degree of general excitement in delirium tremens was related to the disruption of REM sleep after alcohol withdrawal, with REM breakthrough into wakefulness. Several studies have shown that delirium tremens is closely correlated with a high REM time.[7, 46] There is marked but variable decrease in slow-wave sleep following alcohol withdrawal, perhaps related to different levels of tolerance.[4] Sleep may be totally abolished during heavy binges.

Chronic alcoholics have fragmented sleep, little or no delta sleep, decreased REM sleep and many arousals.[68] The sleep–wake cycle becomes blurred, with excessive daytime sleepiness and a lot of naps.[98] Normal motor inhibition during REM sleep may be lost, and EMG activity during REM sleep in the recovering alcoholic may be increased, not decreased.[136] The sleep of many alcoholic patients can remain disturbed for as long as 1–2 years after alcohol withdrawal, with continuous difficulty in falling asleep, fragmented sleep and low delta sleep.[3] Sleep changes, particularly loss of REM sleep and alcohol-provoked sleep apnoea, may contribute to memory impairment in chronic alcoholics.[9]

Periodic causes of chronic insomnia. Insomnia is occasionally cyclical. In many instances, cyclical insomnia is due to recurrent depressive episodes, or to severe manic–depressive psychosis. Occasionally, however, cyclical insomnia is related to menstruation or endocrine disorders.[10, 11]

CHRONIC INSOMNIA DUE TO ABNORMAL SLEEP CONTROL OR CIRCADIAN RHYTHM DISORDERS

Alterations in sleep architecture

The occasional brief arousal due to *parasomnias* rarely produces insomnia. Obstructive *sleep apnoea* causes a complaint of daytime drowsiness much more often than a complaint of insomnia, although the reverse is true in central sleep apnoea. Between 70% and 80% of *narcoleptics* complain of a poor night's sleep although here, as in obstructive sleep apnoea, the major complaint is usually one of daytime drowsiness, not one of nocturnal insomnia. *Sleep myoclonus* is a non-specific accompaniment of many different disorders, including narcolepsy, respiratory insufficiency and sleep apnoea, as well as chronic myelopathy and neuropathy;[95] and only the minority of cases are associated with the complaint of insomnia.

Delayed sleep phase syndrome

A small number of patients sleep quite normally, awaken spontaneously, and feel refreshed, but are unable to go to sleep at socially acceptable hours. These subjects have normal sleep itself, and normal somnographic recordings, but abnormal circadian sleep timing.[147] The condition, which is sometimes familial, often dates from childhood or early adolescence. If made to go to bed early, sleep does not follow (hence the classification of sleep-onset insomnia, or better, since insomnia is not a feature, delayed sleep phase syndrome). The clock times of sleep onset and of waking remain stable, but are unusual and antisocial. Most subjects with this rare syndrome go to bed and fall asleep readily at between 0300 and 0600 but are unable to fall asleep earlier. If undisturbed, they sleep well and thoroughly until 1000–1500. The major problems are arousal at a normal time and the maintenance of normal morning vigilance at work or at school. The syndrome causes considerable personal and social problems. All the patients with this problem described by Weitzman *et al.*[147] were 'evening' people or 'owls' on the 'owl' and 'lark' scale of Horne and Ostberg.[62]

Subjects often spend many years attempting to achieve conventional sleep and wake times, but this is usually not successful. Sedatives are ineffective but a rapid, progressive, fixed sleep phase delay of 2–3 h per night, until the clock is reset to an acceptable sleep onset and wake time, is sometimes successful.[32] Attempts at sleep phase alteration are much more successful in some individuals than others (it is perhaps relevant here that there are very large individual differences in phase shift responses after transmeridian flights).[83, 148] It is still not established whether melatonin, or exposure to a bright white light early in the morning, will act as a phase-setter in patients who cannot get to sleep until later than they wish.[22]

INSOMNIA IN CHILDREN (see also p. 191)

Insomnia is one of the most common disorders reported in pre-school children by their parents. The usual problem is either difficulty in falling asleep or intermittent sleep.[120] As many as 14% of children have sleep difficulties at 3 years of age. At least some of these derive from early disturbances in sleep–waking rhythms.[126] Bax has drawn attention to the frequent association of insomnia with child abuse.[8]

Rocking, the constant stimulation of sound, light, a comfortable temperature and swaddling help sleep in babies, and constant bedtime rituals, reduced attention on waking and 'star' charts will reinforce good sleep habits in older children. Very high success rates are claimed for behavioural treatment of childhood sleep problems.[69] Behavioural techniques are effective in the management of many childhood psychological problems associated with insomnia and may also help in the treatment of parasomnias, when, as in night terrors, waking anxiety increases the problem.[73] Behavioural treatment is usually unsuccessful, however, when insomnia is associated with brain damage, blindness or mental retardation.

INSOMNIA IN PREGNANCY AND THE PUERPERIUM

The safety of benzodiazepines with respect to the fetus has not been established, and hypnotics should not be prescribed in pregnancy, especially in the first trimester. Diazepam crosses the placenta and enters breast milk, and drowsiness in children has been attributed to drug intake via maternal milk.[96] Insomnia in pregnancy should be treated by non-pharmacological methods where possible, although, when insomnia is associated with severe psychiatric illness, depression or psychosis, treatment will depend on the severity of the primary condition.

THE HEALTHY LIFE APPROACH TO INSOMNIA (Table 5.4)

Oswald[110] gives simple rules for better sleep:

> The patient should avoid worry and forgive those who anger him ('impossible' he may cry). Learning to relax through meditation, yoga, or music, or after sex (or whatever takes your fancy) is recommended . . . Those who get up regularly to milk the cows or go for a cross-country run at 6 every morning are always sleepy by 11 at night.

Since regularity is associated with feeling happier and being more efficient in the day,[137] there is a lot to recommend a regular time for going to bed and for getting up.

Can patients be taught to control sleep onset and prevent arousal? Cleghorn et al.[22] suggested that the expectation of the experience of not going to sleep (and the belief that the onset of sleep cannot be controlled) can be altered, and

Table 5.4 *Sleep hygiene rules*[55, 110]

1. Sleep as much as you feel you need for refreshment, but not too much. If awake, get out of bed. An excess of bed time, rather than sleep time, may be related to shallow fragmented sleep.
2. Keep to regular sleep and arousal times. This may strengthen circadian rhythms.
3. Regular morning or afternoon exercise, not too near sleep time, may deepen sleep.
4. Try to avoid excessive sudden noise. If necessary, use earplugs.
5. Very warm (but not cold) rooms will interfere with sleep.
6. Hunger may prevent sleep. Have regular evening food and a bedtime milk drink.
7. Caffeine in the evening disturbs sleep even in people who think it does not.
8. Alcohol is much more disruptive than caffeine. It may improve sleep onset, but later causes sleep fragmentation.
9. Occasional, but not regular, sleeping pills may help some insomniacs.
10. During a poor night, rather than trying harder and harder to fall asleep by counting sheep, get out of bed, switch on the light and read, write or eat until tired.

sleep-preventing stimuli abolished. Relaxation exercises and avoiding inappropriate stimuli ('stimulus control') with or without EMG feedback will sometimes promote sleep, and the slow lengthening of sleep by around 1–2 h per week may eventually establish a normal sleep habit in chronic insomniacs.[59] Nicassio *et al.*[106] have used relaxation techniques in chronically sleep-disturbed adults to reduce sleep onset latency and to improve the subjective and objective quality of sleep. If rumination prevents sleep onset, the active switching of thoughts from a problem to a pleasant memory can be taught.[100]

REFERENCES

1. Adam, K. Brain rhythm that correlates with obesity, *Brit. Med. J.* (1977) **ii**, 234.
2. Adam, K. Dietary habits and sleep after bedtime food drinks, *Sleep* (1980) **3**, 47–58.
3. Adamson, J. & Burdick, J.A. Sleep of dry alcoholics, *Arch. Gen. Psychiat.* (1973) **28**, 146–149.
4. Allen, R.P., Wagman, A.M.I., Funderburk, F.R. & Wells, D.T. Slow-wave sleep: a predictor of individual differences in response to drinking? *Biol. Psychiat.* (1980) **15**, 345–348.
5. Anders, T.F., Carskadon, M.A. & Dement, W.C. Sleep and sleepiness in children and adolescents, *Pediat. Clin. N. Am.* (1980) **27**, 923–948.
6. Armstrong, R.H., Burnap, D., Jacobson, A., Kales, A., Ward, S. & Golden, J. Dreams and gastric secretion in duodenal ulcer patients, *New Physician* (1965) **14**, 241–243.
7. Bates, R.C. Delirium tremens and sleep deprivation, *Mich. Med.* (1972) **71**, 941–944.
8. Bax, M.C.O. Sleep disturbances in the young child, *Brit. Med. J.* (1980) **280**, 1177–1179.
9. Benson, K., Cohen, M. & Zarcone, V. REM sleep time and digit span impairment in alcoholics, *J. Stud. Alcohol* (1978) **39**, 1488–1498.
10. Billiard, M., Guilleminault, C. & Dement, W.C. A menstruation-linked periodic hypersomnia, *Neurology* (1975) **25**, 436–443.
11. Billiard, M. & Passouant, P. Sleep study in women. In: Koella, W.P. & Levin, P. (eds.) *Sleep, First European Congress on Sleep Research 1972*, Basel: S. Karger (1973) 395–399.
12. Bixler, E.O., Kales, A. & Soldatos, C.R. Sleep disorders encountered in medical practice: a national survey of physicians, *Behav. Med.* (1979) **6**, 1–6.
13. Bixler, E., Kales, A., Soldatos, C., Kales, J.D. & Healey, S. Prevalence of sleep disorders in the Los Angeles Metropolitan area, *Am. J. Psychiat.* (1979) **136**, 1257–1262.
14. Borbély, A.A., Baumann, F., Brandeis, D., Strauch, L. & Lehmann, D. Sleep-deprivation effect on sleep stages and EEG power density in man, *Electroenceph. Clin. Neurophysiol.* (1981) **51**, 483–493.
15. Borbély, A.A., Huston, J.P. & Waser, P.G. Physiological and behavioural effects of parachlorphenylalanine in the rat, *Psychopharmacology* (1973) **31**, 131–142.
16. Borbély, A.A., Tobler, I. & Groos, G. Sleep homeostasis and the circadian sleep–wak

rhythm. In: Chase, M.H. & Weitzman, E.D. (eds.) *Sleep Disorders: Basic and Clinical Research* New York: Spectrum (1983) 227–243.

17. Brezinova, V. & Oswald, I. Sleep after a bedtime beverage, *Brit. Med. J.* (1972) **2**, 431–433.
18. Brody, H. & Vijayashankar, N. Anatomical changes in the nervous system. In: Finch, C.E. & Hayflick, I. (eds.) *Handbook of the Biology of Aging*, New York: Van Nostrand Reinhold (1977) 241–261.
19. Carskadon, M.A. & Dement, W.C. Respiration during sleep in the aged human, *J. Gerontol.* (1981) **36**, 420–423.
20. Carskadon, M., Dement, W., Mitler, M., Guilleminault, C., Zarcone, V. & Spiegel, R. Self-reports versus sleep laboratory findings in 122 drug-free subjects with complaints of chronic insomnia, *Am. J. Psychiat.* (1976) **133**, 1382–1388.
21. Clark, T., Collins, J. & Tong, D. Respiratory depression caused by nitrazepam in patients with respiratory failure, *Lancet* (1971) **2**, 737–738.
22. Cleghorn, J.M., Bellissimo, A., Kaplan, R.D. & Szatmari, P. Insomnia: II. Assessment and treatment of chronic insomnia, *Can. J. Psychiat.* (1983) **28**, 347–353.
23. Cleghorn, J.M., Kaplan, R.D., Bellissimo, A. & Szatmari, P. Insomnia: I. Classification, assessment and pharmaceutical treatment, *Can. J. Psychiat.* (1983) **28**, 339–346.
24. Clift, A.D. *Sleep Disturbance and Hypnotic Drug Dependence*, Amsterdam: Excerpta Medica (1975).
25. Coccagna, G. & Lugaresi, E. All-night polygraph in patients with painful disease, *EEG EMG* (1982) **13**, 149–153.
26. Coleman, R.M., Roffwarg, H.P., Kennedy, S.J., Guillaminault, C., Cinque, J., Cohn, M.A. & Karacan, I. Sleep wake disorders based on a polysomnographic study: a national cooperative study, *J. Am. Med. Assoc.* (1982) **247**, 997–1003.
27. Committee on the Review of Medicines. Systematic review of the benzodiazepines, *Brit. Med. J.* (1980) **280**, 910, 1053, 1085.
28. Coursey, R.D. Personality measures and evoked responses in chronic insomnia, *J. Abnorm. Psychol.* (1975) **84**, 239–249.
29. Coursey, R., Frankel, B. & Gaarder, K. EMG biofeedback and autogenic training as relaxation technique for chronic sleep-onset insomnia, *Biofeedback Self-Regulation* (1976) **1**, 353–354.
30. Crisp, A.H. & McGuiness, B. Jolly fat: relation between obesity and psychoneurosis in general population, *Brit. Med. J.* (1976) **i**, 7–9.
31. Crisp, A.H. & Stonehill, E. Aspects of the relationship between sleep and nutrition: a study of 375 psychiatric out-patients, *Brit. J. Psychiat.* (1973) **122**, 379–394.
32. Czeisler, C.A., Richardson, G.S., Coleman, R.M., Zimmerman, J.C., Moore-Ede, M.C., Dement, W.C. & Weitzman, E.D. Chronotherapy: resetting the circadian clocks of patients with delayed sleep phase insomnia, *Sleep* (1981) **4**, 1–21.
33. de Graaf, W. & Pluymen, J. Sleep disturbances in a general practice. In: Kamphuisen, H.A.C., Bruyn, G.W. & Visser, P. *Sleep, Normal and Deranged Function*, Leiden: Mefar (1981) 72–75.
34. Dement, W.C. A life in sleep research. In: Chase, M.T. & Weitzman, E.D. (eds.) *Sleep Disorders, Basic and Clinical Research*, New York: Spectrum (1983) 540–541.
35. Dragstedt, L.L. Causes of peptic ulcer, *J. Am. Med. Assoc.* (1959) **169**, 203–209.
36. Dunleavy, D.L.F., Oswald, I., Brown, P. & Strong, J.A. Hyperthyroidism, sleep and growth hormone, *Electroenceph. Clin. Neurophysiol.* (1974) 259–263.
37. Feinberg, I. & Carlson, V.R. Sleep variables as a function of age in man, *Arch. Gen. Psychiat.* (1968) **18**, 239–250.
38. Feinstein, B., Sterman, M.B. & MacDonald, L.R. Effects of sensorimotor rhythm biofeedback training on sleep. In: Chase, M.H., Stern, W.C. & Walter, P.L. (eds.) *Sleep Research, Vol. 3*, Los Angeles: BIS/BRI UCLA (1974) 134.
39. Fischer-Perroudon, C., Mouret, J. & Jouvet, M. Four months without sleep (agrypnia) in a case of 'chorée fibrillaire de Morvan' – improvement after 5HTP. In: Chase, M.H., Stern, W.C. & Walter, P.L. (eds.) *Sleep Research*, Los Angeles: BIS UCLA (1973) 148.
40. Ford, F.R. The tired arm syndrome. A common condition manifest by nocturnal pain in the arm and numbness of the hand, *Bull. Johns Hopkins Hosp.* (1956) **98**, 464–466.
41. Frankel, B.L., Coursey, R.D., Buchbinder, R. & Snyder, F. Recorded and reported sleep in chronic primary insomnia, *Arch. Gen. Psychiat.* (1976) **33**, 615–623.
42. Freedman, R.R. & Sattler, H.L. Physiological and psychological factors in sleep-onset insomnia, *J. Abnorm. Psychol.* (1982) **91**, 308–309.

43. Gaillard, J.-M. Chronic primary insomnia: possible physiopathological involvement of slow wave sleep deficiency, *Sleep* (1978) **1**, 133–147.
44. Gillin, J.C., Sitaram, N., Duncan, W.C., Gershon, E.S., Nurnberger, J., Post, R.E.M., Murphy, D.L., Wehr, T., Goodwin, F.K. & Bunney, W.E., Jr. Sleep abnormalities in depression: diagnostic potential and pathophysiology, *Psychopharmacol. Bull.* (1980) **16**, 40–42.
45. Gnirrs, F. Schlafstörungen bei psychisch Kranken, *Nervenarzt*. (1978) **48**, 394–401.
46. Greenberg, R. & Pearlman, C. Delirium tremens and dreaming, *Am.J. Psychiat.* (1967) **124**, 37–46.
47. Greenblatt, D.J., Allen, M.D. & Shader, R.I. Toxicity of high-dose flurazepam in the elderly, *Clin. Pharmacol. Ther.* (1977) **21**, 355–361.
48. Gresham, S.C., Agnew, W.R. & Williams, R.L. The sleep of depressed patients, *Arch. Gen. Psychiat.* (1965) **13**, 503–507.
49. Gross, M., Goodenough, D., Hasty, J., Rosenblatt, S. & Lewis, E. Sleep disturbances in alcoholic intoxication and withdrawal. In: Mello, N. & Mendelson, J. (eds.) *Recent Advances in Study of Alcoholism. An Interdisciplinary Symposium*, Rockville Maryland: NIMH (1971) 317–397.
50. Gross, M.M. & Hastey, J.M. A note on REM rebound during experimental alcohol withdrawal in alcoholics. In: Gross, M.M. (ed.) *Advances in Experimental Medicine and Biology, Vol. 59*, New York: Plenum Press (1975) 509–513.
51. Haider, I. Patterns of insomnia in depressive illness: a subjective evaluation, *Brit. J. Psychiat.* (1968) **114**, 1127–1132.
52. Hallstrom, C. Which hypnotic – if any? *Brit. J. Hosp. Med.* (1983) **30**, 188–192.
53. Hartmann, E. Longitudinal studies of sleep and dream patterns in depressive patients, *Arch. Gen. Psychiat.* (1968) **19**, 312–329.
54. Hauri, P. A case series analysis of 141 consecutive insomniacs evaluated at the Dartmouth Sleep Laboratory, *Sleep Res.* (1976) **5**, 173.
55. Hauri, P. *Current Concepts – The Sleep Disorders*, Kalamazoo, Michigan: Upjohn (1977) 54.
56. Hauri, P., Chernik, D., Hawkins, D. & Mendels, J. Sleep of depressed patients in remission, *Arch. Gen.Psychiat.* (1974) **31**, 386–391.
57. Hauri, P. & Hawkins, D.R. Individual differences in the sleep of depression. In: Jovanovic, U.J. (ed.) *The Nature of Sleep*, Stuttgart: Gustav Fisher (1973) 193–197.
58. Hauri, P. & Olmstead, E. Childhood-onset insomnia, *Sleep* (1980) **3**, 59–66.
59. Hauri, P., Percy, L., Hellekson, C., Harmann, E. & Russ, D. The treatment of psychophysiological insomnia with biofeedback: a replication study, *Biofeedback and Self-Regulation* (1982) **7**, 223–235.
60. Hazeman, P., Laffort, F. & Lille, F. Elucidation of vigilance level in aged persons, *Rev. Electroenceph. Neurophysiol.* (1977) **7**, 203–209.
61. Healey, E.S., Kales, A., Monroe, L.J., Bixler, E.O., Chamberlin, K. & Soldatos, C.R. Onset of insomnia: role of life-stress events, *Psychosom. Med.* (1981) **43**, 439–451.
62. Horne, J.A. & Ostberg, O. A self-assessment questionnaire to determine morningness–eveningness in human circadian rhythms, *Int. J. Chronobiol.* (1976) **4**, 97–110.
63. Hursch, C.J., Karacan, I. & Williams, R.L. Stage 1-REM from infancy to old age, *Sleep Res.* (1972) **1**, 87.
64. Insel, T.R., Gillin, J.C., Moore, A., Mendelson, W.B., Loewenstein, R.J. & Murphy, D.L. The sleep of patients with obsessive–compulsive disorder, *Arch. Gen. Psychiat.* (1982) **39**, 1372–1377.
65. Johns, M.W., Egan, P., Gay, T.J.A. & Masterton, J.P. Sleep habits and symptoms in male medical and surgical patients, *Brit. Med. J.* (1970) **2**, 509–512.
66. Johns, M.W., Gay, T.J.A., Masterton, J.P. & Bruce, D.W. Relationship between sleep habits, adrenocortical activity and personality, *Psychosom. Med.* (1971) **33**, 499–508.
67. Johnson, L.C. Psychological and physiological changes following total sleep deprivation. In: Kales, A. (ed.) *Sleep Physiology and Pathology, a Symposium*, Philadelphia: Lippincott (1969) 206–207.
68. Johnson, L.C., Burdick, J.A. & Smith, J. Sleep during alcohol intake and withdrawal in the chronic alcoholic, *Arch. Gen. Psychiat.* (1970) **22**, 406–418.
69. Jones, D.P.H. & Verduyn, C.M. Behavioural management of sleep problems, *Arch. Dis. Child.* (1983) **58**, 442–444.
70. Jordan, J.B., Hauri, P. & Phelps, P.J. The sensorimotor rhythm (SMR) in insomnia. In: Chase, M.H., Mitler, M.M. & Walter, P.L. (eds.) *Sleep Research, Vol. 5*, Los Angeles: BIS/BRI UCLA (1976) 175.

71. Kales, A., Allen, C., Scharf, M.B. & Kales, J. All night EEG studies of insomniac subjects, *Arch. Gen. Psychiat.* (1970) **23**, 226–232.
72. Kales, A., Bixler, E.O., Soldatos, C.R., Vela-Bueno, A., Caldwell, A.B. & Cadieux, R.J. Biopsychobehavioural correlates of insomnia. Part 1: Role of sleep apnoea and nocturnal myoclonus, *Psychosomatics* (1982) **23**, 589–600.
73. Kales, J.C., Cadieux, R.J., Soldatos, C.R. & Kales, A. Psychotherapy with night-terror patients, *Am.J. Psychother.* (1982) **36**, 399–407.
74. Kales, A., Caldwell, A.B., Preston, T.A., Healey, S. & Kales, J.D. Personality patterns in insomnia, *Arch. Gen. Psychiat.* (1976) **33**, 1128–1134.
75. Kales, A. & Kales, J. Sleep laboratory studies of hypnotic drugs: efficacy and withdrawal effects, *J. Clin. Psychopharmacol.* (1983) **3**, 140–150.
76. Kales, A., Soldatos, C.R., Bixler, E.O. & Kales, J.D. Rebound insomnia and rebound anxiety. A review, *Psychopharmacology* (1983) **26**, 121–137.
77. Karacan, I., Booth, G.H. & Thornby, J.I. The effect of caffeinated and decaffeinated coffee on nocturnal sleep in young adult males. Paper presented at Annual Meeting of Association for the Psychophysiological Study of Sleep, San Diego, California (1973).
78. Karacan, I., Thornby, J.I. & Anch, A.M. Dose–response effects of coffee on the sleep of normal middle-aged man, *Sleep Res.* (1976) **5**, 71.
79. Karacan, I., Thornby, J.I., Anch, M., Holzer, C.E., Warheit, G.J., Schwabb, J.J. & Williams, R.L. Prevalence of sleep disorders in a primarily urban Florida county, *Soc. Sci. Med.* (1976) **10**, 239–244.
80. Karacan, I., Thornby, J.I., Booth, G.H., Salis, P.J., Anch, A.M., Okawa, M. & Williams, R.L. Dose–response effects of natural and decaffeinated coffee and caffeine on the sleep of normal young adult males (abstract). In: Chase, M.H., Stein, W.C. & Walter, P.L. (eds.) *Sleep Research, Vol. 3*, Los Angeles: BIS/BRI UCLA (1974) 56.
81. Karacan, I., Thornby, J.I., Booth, G.H., Salis, P.J., Anch, A.M., Okawa, M. & Williams, R.L. Dose-response effects of coffee on objective (EEG) and subjective measures of sleep. In: Levin, P. & Koella, W.P. (eds.) *Sleep 1974. Second European Congress on Sleep Research, Rome, 1974*, Basel: S. Karger (1975) 504–509.
82. Karacan, I., Williams, R.L., Bose, J., Hursch, C.J. & Warson, S.R. Insomnia in haemodyalitic and kidney transplant patients, *Psychophysiology* (1972) **9**, 137.
83. Klein, K.E., Hermann, H., Kuklinski, P. & Wegmann, H.-M. Circadian performance rhythms: experimental studies in air operation. In: Mackie, R.R. (ed.) *Vigilance, Theory, Operational Performances and Physiological Correlates*, New York/London: Plenum Press (1977) 117–132.
84. Knowles, J., Laverty, S. & Kuechler, H. The effects of alcohol on REM sleep, *J. Stud. Alcohol* (1968) **29**, 342–349.
85. Kripke, D.F., Ancoli-Israel, S., Mason, M. & Messin, S. Sleep related mortality and morbidity in the aged. In: Chase, M.H. & Weitzman, E.D. (eds.) *Sleep Disorders: Basic and Clinical Research*, New York: Spectrum (1983) 415–444.
86. Kripke, D.F., Simons, R.M., Garfinkel, L. & Hammond, E.C. Short and long sleep and sleeping pills, *Arch. Gen. Psychiat.* (1979) **36**, 103–116.
87. Kupfer, D.J. REM latency: a psychobiological marker for primary depressive disease, *Biol. Psychiat.* (1976) **11**, 159–174.
88. Kupfer, D.J. Sleep and affective disorders, quoted in Wheatley, D. (ed.) *Psychopharmacology of Sleep*, New York: Raven Press (1981), p. 172.
89. Kupfer, D.J., Broudy, D., Coble, P.A. & Spiker, D.G. EEG sleep and affective psychosis, *J. Affective Disord.* (1980) **2**, 17–25.
90. Kupfer, D.J. & Foster, G.F. Interval between onset of sleep and rapid-eye-movement sleep as an indicator of depression, *Lancet* (1972) **2**, 684–686.
91. Kupfer, D.J., Foster, F.G. & Detre, T.P. Sleep continuity changes in depression, *Dis. Nerv. Syst.* (1973) **34**, 192–195.
92. Kupfer, D.J., Foster, F.G., Reich, L., Thompson, K.S. & Weiss, B. EEG sleep changes as predictors in depression, *Am. J. Psychiat.* (1976) **133**, 622–626.
93. Kupfer, D.J., Wyatt, R.J., Scott, J. & Snyder, F. Sleep disturbance in acute schizophrenic patients, *Am.J. Psychiat.* (1970) **126**, 1213–1223.
94. Learoyd, B.M. Psychotropic drugs and the elderly patient, *Med. J. Australia* (1972) **1**, 1131–1133.
95. Lugaresi, E., Cirignotta, F., Montagna, P. & Coccagna, G. Myoclonus and related phenomena during sleep. In: Chase, M.H. & Weitzman, E.D. (eds.) *Sleep Disorders, Basic and Clinical Research*, New York: Spectrum (1983) 123–127.
96. McEwan, H. Drugs in pregnancy, *Brit. J. Hosp. Med.* (1982) **28**, 559–565.

97. McGhie, A. & Russell, S.M. The subjective assessment of normal sleep patterns, *J. Ment. Sci.* (1962) **8**, 642–654.

98. Mello, N.K. & Mendelson, J.H. Behavioural studies of sleep patterns in alcoholics during intoxication and withdrawal, *J. Pharmacol. Exp. Ther.* (1970) **175**, 94–112.

99. Michaelis, R. & Hofmann, E. Zur Phenomenologie und Atiopathogenese der Hypersomnie bei endogenphasischen Depressionen. In: Jovanović, U.J. (ed.) *The Nature of Sleep*, Stuttgart: Gustav Fischer (1973) 190–193.

100. Mitchell, K. & White, R. Self-management of severe predormital insomnia, *J. Behav. Ther. Exp. Psychiat.* (1977) **8**, 57–63.

101. Mitchell-Heggs, P., Murphy, K., Minty, K., Guz, A., Patterson, S.C., Minty, P.S.B. & Rosser, R.M. Diazepam in the treatment of dyspnoea in the 'pink puffer' syndrome, *Quart. J. Med.* (1980) **49**, 9–20.

102. Moldofsky, H. & Scarisbrick, P. Induction of neurasthenic musculoskeletal pain syndrome by selective sleep-stage deprivation, *Psychosom. Med.* (1976) **38**, 35–44.

103. Moldofsky, H., Scarisbrik, P., England, R. & Smythe, H. Musculoskeletal symptoms and non-REM sleep disturbance in patients with 'fibrositis syndrome' and healthy subjects, *Psychosom. Med.* (1975) **37**, 341–351.

104. Monroe, L.J. Psychological and physiological differences between good and poor sleepers, *J. Abnorm. Psychol.* (1967) **72**, 255–264.

105. Murray, J., Dunn, G., Williams, P. & Tarnopolsky, A. Factors affecting the consumption of psychotropic drugs, *Psychol. Med.* (1981) **11**, 551–560.

106. Nicassio, P.M., Boylan, M.B. & McCabe, T.G. Progressive relaxation, EMG biofeedback, and biofeedback placebo in the treatment of sleep-onset insomnia, *Brit. J. Med. Psychol.* (1982) **55**, 159–166.

107. Nicholson, A. & Marks, J. *Insomnia. A Guide for Medical Practitioners*, Lancaster: MTP (1983) 1–124.

108. Nowlin, J.B., Troyer, W.G., Collins, W.S., Silverman, G., Nichols, C.R., McIntosh, H.D., Estes, E.H., Jr. & Bogdonoff, M.D. The association of nocturnal angina pectoris with dreaming, *Am. Intern. Med.* (1965) **63**, 1040–1046.

109. Oswald, I. Drug research and human sleep. In: Tucker, E. (ed.) *Progress in Drug Research*, Basel: Birkhauser Verlag (1978).

110. Oswald, I. Symptoms that depress the doctor: insomnia, *Brit. J. Hosp. Med.* (1984) **31**, 219–224.

111. Palmer, C.D., Harrison, G.A. & Hiorns, R.W. Association between smoking and drinking and sleep duration, *Ann. Human Biol.* (1980) **7**, 103–107.

112. Passouant, P., Cadillhac, J., Baldy-Moulinier, M. & Mion, C. Etude du sommeil nocturne chez des urémiques chroniques soumis à une épuration extrarénale, *Electroenceph. Clin. Neurophysiol.* (1970) **29**, 441–449.

113. Phillips, R.L., Spiegel, R. & Clayton, D. A study of short arousals in insomnia and normals. In: Chase, M.H., Stern, W.C. & Walter, P.L. (eds.) *Sleep Research, Vol. 4*, Los Angeles: BIS/BRI UCLA (1975) 231.

114. Prinz, P.N. Sleep patterns in the healthy aged: relationship with intellectual function, *J. Gerontol.* (1977) **2**, 179–186.

115. Prinz, P.N. & Halter, J.B. Sleep disturbance in the elderly: neurohormonal correlates. In: Chase, M.H. & Weitzman, E.D. (eds.) *Sleep Disorders: Basic and Clinical Research*, Lancaster: MTP (1983) 463–488.

116. Prinz, P.N., Halter, J., Benedetti, C. & Raskind, M. Circadian variation of plasma catecholamines in young and old men: relation to rapid eye movement and slow wave sleep, *J. Clin. Endocrinol. Metab.* (1979) **49**, 300–304.

117. Prinz, P.N., Obrist, W.D. & Wang, H.S. Sleep patterns in healthy elderly subjects. Individual differences as related to other neurobiological variables, *Sleep Res.* (1975) **4**, 132.

118. Ravenscroft, K., Jr. & Hartmann, E.L. The temporal correlation of nocturnal asthmatic attacks and the D-state, *Psychophysiology* (1968) **4**, 396–397.

119. Regelstein, Q.R. Insomnia and sleep disturbances in the aged. Sleep and insomnia in the elderly. *J. Geriat. Psychiat.* (1980) **13**, 153–171.

120. Richman, N. Sleep problems in young children, *Arch. Dis. Child.* (1981) **56**, 491–493.

121. Roffwarg, H.P. & Clark, W. *et al.* Diagnostic classification of sleep and arousal disorders, *Sleep* (1979) **2**, 1–137.

122. Roth, T., Kramer, M. & Trinder, J. The effect of noise during sleep on the sleep patterns of different age groups, *Can. Psychiat. Assoc. J.* (1972) **17**, Suppl. 2, 197–201.

123. Rudolf, G.A.E., Schilgen, B. & Tolle, R. Anti-depressive Behandlung mittels Schlafenzug, *Nervenarzt.* (1977) **48**, 1–11.
124. Rundell, O.H., Lester, B.K., Griffiths, W.J. & Williams, H.L. Alcohol and sleep in young adults, *Psychopharmacologia* (1972) **26**, 201–218.
125. Saario, I. & Linnoila, M. Effect of subacute treatment with hypnotics alone or in combination with alcohol, on psychomotor skills related to driving, *Acta Pharmacol. Toxicol.* (1976) **38**, 382–392.
126. Salzarulo, P. & Chevalier, A. Sleep problems in children and their relationship with early disturbances of the waking–sleeping rhythms, *Sleep* (1983) **6**, 47–51.
127. Schiff, I., Regelstein, Q., Talchinsky, D. & Ryan, K.J. Effects of oestrogens on sleep and psychological states of hypogonadal women, *J. Am. Med. Assoc.* (1979) **242**, 2405–2407.
128. Shock, N.W. Systems integration. In: Finch, C.E. & Hayflick, I. (eds.) *Handbook of the Biology of Aging*, New York: Van Nostrand Reinhold (1977) 639–665.
129. Simpson, R.G. Nocturnal disorders of medical interest, *Practitioner* (1969) **202**, 259–269.
130. Snyder, F. Autonomic nervous system manifestations during sleep and dreaming. Sleep and altered states of consciousness, *Res. Pub. Assoc. Res. Nerv. Ment. Dis.* (1967) **45**, 469–487.
131. Soldatos, C.R., Kales, A. & Kales, J. Management of insomnia, *Ann. Rev. Med.* (1979) **30**, 301–312.
132. Solomon, F., White, C.C., Parron, D.L. & Mendelson, W.B. Sleeping pills, insomnia and medical practice, *New Engl. J. Med.* (1979) **300**, 803–808.
133. Southwell, P., Evans, C. & Hunt, J. Effect of a hot milk drink on movements during sleep. *Brit. Med. J.* (1972) **2**, 429–431.
134. Sterman, M.B. Sleep. In: Di Cara, K.V. (ed.) *Limbic and Autonomic Nervous Systems Research*, New York: Plenum Press (1974) 395–417.
135. Sterman, M.B., Howe, R.C. & MacDonald, L.R. Facilitation of spindle-burst sleep by conditioning of electroencephalographic activity whilst awake, *Science* (1970) **167**, 1146–1148.
136. Tachibana, M., Tanaka, K., Hishikawa, Y. & Kaneko, Z. A sleep study of acute psychotic states due to alcohol and meprobimite addiction. In: Weitzman, E.D. (ed.) *Advances in sleep research, Vol. 2*, New York: Spectrum Publications (1975) 177–205.
137. Taub, J.M. Behavioural and psychophysiological correlates of irregularity in chronic sleep routines, *Biol. Psychol.* (1978) **7**, 37.
138. Taub, J.M., Globus, G.G., Phoebus, E. & Drury, R. Extended sleep and performance, *Nature* (1971) **233**, 142–143.
139. Tune, G.S. Sleep and wakefulness in normal human adults, *Brit. Med. J.* (1968) **2**, 269–271.
140. Vogel, G.W. REM sleep deprivation and depression. In: Chase, M. & Weitzman, E.D. (eds.) *Sleep Disorders: Basic and Clinical Research*, Lancaster: MTP (1983) 393–400.
141. Vogel, G., McAbee, R. & Barker, K. REM pressure and improvement of endogenous depression. In: Chase, M.H., Mitler, M.M. & Walter, P.L. (eds.) *Sleep Research, Vol. 5*, Los Angeles: BIS/BRI UCLA (1976) 151.
142. Vogel, G.W., Thurmond, A., Gibbons, P., Sloan, K., Boyd, M. & Walker, M. REM sleep reduction effects on depression syndromes, *Arch. Gen. Psychiat.* (1975) **32**, 765–777.
143. Wehr, T.A., Gillin, J.C. & Goodwin, F.K. Sleep and circadian rhythms in depression. In: Chase, M.H. & Weitzman, E.D. (eds.) *Sleep Disorders: Basic and Clinical Research*, New York: Spectrum (1983) 195–225.
144. Wehr, T.A. & Goodwin, F.K. Biological rhythms and psychiatry. In: Arieti, S. & Brodie, H.K.H. (eds.) *American Handbook of Psychiatry, Vol. 6*, New York: Basic Books (1981).
145. Wehr, T., Wirz-Justice, A., Goodwin, R.K., Duncan, W. & Gillin, J.C. Phase advance of the circadian sleep–wake cycle as an antidepressant, *Science* (1979) **206**, 710–711.
146. Weiss, H.R., Kasinoff, B.H. & Bailey, M.A. An exploration of reported sleep disturbance, *J. Nerv. Ment. Dis.* (1962) **134**, 528–534.
147. Weitzman, E.D., Czeisler, C.A., Coleman, R.M., Spielman, A.J., Zimmerman, J.C., Dement, W., Richardson, G. & Pollak, C.P. Delayed sleep-phase syndrome: a chronobiologic disorder with sleep onset insomnia, *Arch. Gen. Psychiat.* (1981) **38**, 737–746.
148. Weitzman, E.D., Czeisler, C.A., Zimmerman, J.C., Moore-Ede, M.C. & Ronda, J.M. Biological rhythm in man: internal physiological organisation during non-entrained (free-running) conditions and application to delayed sleep-phase syndrome. In: Chase, M.H. & Weitzman, E.D. (eds.) *Sleep Disorders: Basic and Clinical Research*, New York: Spectrum Publications (1983) 153–171.
149. Weitzman, E.D., Goldmacher, D., Kripke, D., MacGregor, P., Kream, J. & Hellman, L.

Reversal of sleep–waking cycle: effect on sleep-stage pattern and certain neuroendocrine rhythms, *Trans. Am. Neurol. Assoc.* (1968) **93,** 153–157.

150. Wever, R. The meaning of circadian periodicity for old people, *Verhand. Deutsch. Gesell. Path.* (1975) **59,** 160–180.

151. Williams, R.L., Karacan, I. & Hursch, C.J. *Electroencephalography (EEG) of Human Sleep: Clinical Implications,* New York: J Wiley (1974).

152. Wingard, D.L. & Berkman, L.F. Mortality risk associated with sleeping pattern among adults, *Sleep* (1983) **6,** 102–107.

153. Zarcone, V. REM phase deprivation and schizophrenia. II. *Arch. Gen. Psychiat.* (1975) **32,** 1431–1436.

154. Zarcone, V., Gulevich, G., Pivik, T. & Dement, W. Partial REM phase deprivation and schizophrenia, *Arch. Gen. Psychiat.* (1968) **18,** 194–202.

155. Zarcone, V. & Hoddes, E. Effects of 5-hydroxytryptophan on fragmentation of REM sleep in alcoholics, *Am. J. Psychiat.* (1975) **132,** 74–76.

156. Zorick, F., Roth, T., Hartse, K., Piccione, P. & Stepanski, E. Evaluation and diagnosis of persistent insomnia, *Am.J. Psychiat.* (1981) **138,** 769–773.

157. Zucker, I., Rusak, B. & King, R.C., Jr. Neural bases for circadian rhythms in rodent behaviour. In: Riesen, A.H. & Thompson, R.F. (eds.) *Advances in Psychobiology, Vol. 3,* New York: Wiley (1976) 35–74.

CHAPTER 6

DAYTIME DROWSINESS

DAYTIME DROWSINESS

TERMINOLOGY

The terms used to describe daytime drowsiness by doctors (narcolepsy, hypersomnolence and sub-wakefulness) are as difficult to define as the terms used to describe sleep by patients (good, bad, light, deep – see p. 12). *Narcolepsy* was defined at a conference in Montpellier in 1976 as 'an illness with excessive sleep, sleep episodes and cataplexy, with or without sleep paralysis, hypnagogic hallucinations and disturbed nocturnal sleep'. Although night sleep is disturbed in narcolepsy, it is not usually prolonged. The term 'narcolepsy' is used both to describe short sleep attacks during wakefulness and the syndrome itself. *Hypersomnolence* is more difficult to define. In the day, there are prolonged sleep periods and night sleep is often prolonged. Thus, hypersomnia (like occasional instances of insomnia) is sometimes a 24 h disorder. In addition to prolonged day-sleep periods, the term hypersomnia includes dozing and sub-wakefulness. *Sub-wakefulness* is the most difficult of all these terms to define exactly. It implies a reduction in normal levels of waking alertness and not short or long day-sleep attacks. Narcolepsy and hypersomnolence are sometimes but not always accompanied by sub-wakefulness. In all instances, it is of great importance to separate daytime sleepiness from less specific symptoms such as tiredness or excess fatigue.

DAYTIME DROWSINESS IN NARCOLEPSY AND HYPERSOMNOLENCE

There is no absolute boundary between short sleep attacks and more prolonged daytime sleep periods. Both short and long sleep episodes occur in the daytime in patients with the narcoleptic syndrome as well as in patients with daytime drowsiness from other causes such as sleep apnoea. Although two different patterns of symptomatology can be distinguished (Table 6.1) the reality of any major distinction between the two symptoms (narcolepsy and periods of hypersomnolence in the daytime) is sometimes doubtful.

Table 6.1. *Distinction between narcolepsy and hypersomnolence*

Narcolepsy	Hypersomnolence
Short (less than 1 h) day-sleep attacks	Long (over 1–2 h) day-sleep attacks
Sub-wakefulness mild	Sub-wakefulness severe
Day-sleep onset sudden	Day-sleep onset gradual
Day-sleep attacks irresistible	Day-sleep attacks resistible
Sleep attacks under unusual circumstances	Sleep with monotony but not in unusual circumstances
Daytime drowsiness most severe in the evening	Daytime drowsiness most severe in the morning
CNS stimulants partially effective	CNS stimulants are sometimes reported to be ineffective: this is doubtful
Night sleep often interrupted	Prolonged, deep night sleep
Conceptual disorder of REM sleep	Conceptual disorder of NREM sleep

PREVALENCE OF DAYTIME DROWSINESS

The prevalence of excessive daytime sleepiness revealed by questionnaire surveys or reported from the sleep laboratory is between 0.3% and 4% of the adult population.[2, 8, 17] These figures suggest that daytime drowsiness is less common than insomnia, which has been estimated to occur in between 14% and 35% of all adults.[1, 3, 17] However, looking at subjects with sleep–wake disorders, Coleman[6] found in a sample of 8000 patients that hypersomnia was a more common complaint than insomnia. Some surveys probably overestimate the frequency of serious daytime drowsiness. Results are derived from non-representative sleep laboratory populations, the use of questionnaire or telephone surveys, and the inclusion of transient as well as chronic problems. Headache, epilepsy, dizziness, fatigue and muscle weakness are all more common complaints in general neurological practice than daytime drowsiness.

PROBLEMS ASSOCIATED WITH DAYTIME DROWSINESS

Daytime drowsiness, although less common, is as severe a medical problem to the patient as the other chronic neurological illnesses listed above. Many hypersomniacs are considered to be dull, lazy, work-shy or stupid and, if they need treatment, to be amphetamine addicts. Fortunately, recent publicity about sleep disorders, particularly in the United States, has led to a wider knowledge of them by both patients and physicians, although long gaps between presentation and diagnosis, sometimes up to 10 years in narcolepsy, remain common, and up to a half of all narcoleptics may never be recognized. This situation should be reversed. With good investigative facilities, Guilleminault and Dement[12] showed that the diagnosis of the cause of persistent daytime drowsiness could be established in over 90% of subjects.

CAUSES OF DAYTIME DROWSINESS

The main causes of persistent daytime drowsiness (Table 6.2) are narcolepsy

Table 6.2. *Clinical and polysomnographic criteria for the diagnosis of different types of daytime drowsiness*

Condition	Main clinical features	Polysomnogram findings
Narcolepsy–cataplexy	Brief (1–30 min) irresistible day naps under unusual circumstances	SOREM (may need multiple recordings to demonstrate)
Hypersomnolence	1. Wrong diagnosis; should be monosymptomatic narcolepsy	SOREM
	2. Diagnostic entity, with daytime tiredness and sleepiness, prolonged deep night sleep and difficulty in arousal (see text: idiopathic hypersomnolence)	SO NREM
'Secondary' hypersomnolence	Daytime sleepiness with structural (e.g. head injury or encephalitis) or metabolic cause (e.g. uraemia)	Often diffuse slowing of EEG dominant frequencies
'Neurotic' hypersomnolence	1. Hysterical manifestation 2. Idiopathic hypersomnolence occurring in neurotic individuals. 3. Hypersomnia occurring as a prominent feature of depressive illness	No specific findings throughout this group
Nocturnal hyperkinesis with daytime hypersomnolence	Severe sleep myoclonus, akathisia, bruxism and frequent arousal (unnoticed) from sleep	Abnormal sleep EMG
Sleep apnoea	Snoring, restlessness, apnoea Hypersomnia, automatic behaviour Cor pulmonale	Obstructive, central, mixed apnoeic episodes, sleep fragmentation
Long-cycle hypersomnia	Recurrent hypersomnia at intervals of more than a day (e.g. Kleine–Levin syndrome)	Variable; usually EEG slowing during attacks
Drug- or alcohol-associated hypersomnia (often both)	Chronic hypnotic intake, alcoholism	Sleep fragmentation, nocturnal insomnia, REM rebound on drug withdrawal

SOREM: Sleep onset with REM periods.
SO NREM: Sleep onset with NREM periods.

and sleep apnoea. *Narcolepsy* occurs with an approximate prevalence of between 0.01% and 0.09% of the adult population.[5, 9] *Sleep apnoea* is equally or more common than narcolepsy in American sleep laboratory series,[7] although not in United Kingdom experience. Lavie[21] recently established the prevalence of sleep apnoea as 1.1% of all Israeli industrial workers. *Parasomnias* sometimes cause daytime drowsiness and may be more frequent than one would expect, at least as shown by questionnaire surveys.[2, 27] With the exception of endogenous depression[20] it is uncommon for *psychiatric disorders* to produce daytime drowsiness. Other causes of persistent daytime drowsiness include any type of persistent insomnia, and, particularly in children, long-term treatment with anticonvulsants in high dosages. Finally, the syndrome (or syndromes) of 'essential' hypersomnolence described below accounts for perhaps 10–15% of all adult cases of severe daytime drowsiness.[29, 35, 39]

MEASUREMENT OF DAYTIME DROWSINESS

The Multiple Sleep Latency Test (MSLT) and the Stamford Sleepiness Scale (SSS) are very useful objective and subjective measures of daytime sleepiness. The MSLT, developed by Richardson et al.[31] is a practical means of investigating excessive daytime somnolence. The time taken to fall asleep on 4–5 successive occasions is measured at 2 h intervals from 1000. A repeated latency of less than 5–10 min is abnormal. Also, this test will show that sleep-onset REM periods occur within 10 min of going to sleep on at least two occasions in most narcoleptics. The SSS[14] is a very long and comprehensive subjective rating scale designed to determine levels of sleepiness in subjects with daytime drowsiness.

CATEGORIES OF HYPERSOMNOLENCE

Hypersomnolence, not due to narcolepsy or sleep apnoea, can be divided into the following three broad diagnostic categories:

1. *Essential hypersomnolence* is defined as chronic persistent daytime drowsiness without obvious organic cause. The diagnosis covers several different syndromes – and misdiagnoses – described below.
2. *Secondary hypersomnolence.* In contrast to essential hypersomnolence, the cause is apparent, with daytime drowsiness or 24 h sleepiness the result of many different organic disorders.
3. *Neurotic hypersomnolence.* A poorly defined group of patients complain of chronic fatigue and sub-wakefulness, sometimes attributed to personality problems, anxiety or conversion symptomatology.

Criteria for clinical and polysomnographic diagnosis of different types of daytime drowsiness are shown in Table 6.2. In addition to the above categories of persistent hypersomnolence, in rare instances (e.g. the Kleine–Levin syndrome) hypersomnolence is *cyclical.*

HYPERSOMNOLENCE SYNDROMES ('ESSENTIAL' HYPERSOMNOLENCE)

Daytime sleepiness, with the pattern of hypersomnolence rather than narcolepsy (Table 6.1) may be the presenting feature of a number of different illnesses, in addition to occurring in narcolepsy, sleep apnoea and many different structural and metabolic diseases. In some of these conditions, fatigue, not daytime sleepiness, is the most prominent symptom.

1. In a few instances, daytime drowsiness is the presenting feature of a *depressive illness*.
2. The complaint of hypersomnolence may be due to one extreme of *the normal distribution of sleepiness*.
3. Some hypersomniacs seem to have a specific illness, *'idiopathic hypersomnolence'*.
4. A few patients with a typical presentation of hypersomnia develop, after many years, cataplexy and other typical features of *the narcoleptic syndrome*.

These four presentations of hypersomnia are considered in greater detail below.

Depression and hypersomnia

Although much less common than insomnia, the association of hypersomnia with depression is well documented.[11, 22–24, 28] Sometimes hypersomnia has a fluctuating course and is associated with mild cyclical mood changes. 79 of Roth's 167 patients with hypersomnia had psychological problems, excess fatigue, or a psychopathic personality, and 24 were depressed.[35] In 23 random patients with hypersomnia, Roth and Nevšímolová[37] found an even higher incidence of depression (26%). In hypersomnolence, sexual disturbances (diminished libido and potency in men, menstrual abnormalities in women) are common. In at least some of these subjects, hypersomnolence appears to be an early or predominant symptom of a depressive illness, although this may be denied by the patient,[12] and nocturnal sleep recordings commonly show multiple arousals in depressed subjects, unlike the picture of deep sleep with few awakenings associated by Rechtschaffen and Roth[30] with hypersomnolence. Nevertheless hypersomnia, as well as depression, sometimes responds to treatment with MAO inhibitors.[28] However, MAO inhibitors and tricyclic drugs are ineffective in the treatment of subjects with hypersomnia who are not depressed.

Normal sleep habits

The borderland between normal long sleepers, with normal daytime alertness, and others with essential hypersomnolence is sometimes uncertain, but only subjects in the second group usually complain of daytime drowsiness. Minor changes in lifestyle or occupation, or minor delays in the time of going to bed at night may be more disruptive to daytime alertness in a few poorly adapted individuals than in most subjects, leading to the complaint of excessive daytime tiredness, which is sometimes accompanied by sleepiness.

'Idiopathic' hypersomnolence

Does a syndrome of 'idiopathic' hypersomnolence (Table 6.3), distinct from hypersomnolence in depression or in narcolepsy, exist?

Roth[32–35] showed that many hypersomniacs have a somewhat similar clinical picture, with recurrent attacks of daytime sleepiness, lengthy non-refreshing naps, no sleep attacks, and no respiratory problems during sleep. This clinical

Table 6.3. *Idiopathic hypersomnolence and the narcoleptic syndrome*

	Idiopathic hypersomnolence	Narcolepsy-cataplexy
Estimated prevalence (UK)	4000	20 000
Sex distribution	M=F	M=F
Familial occurrence (% affected first degree relative)	35	50
Age at onset (years: mean and range)	22 (11–53)	24 (4–72)
Day sleep (% of subjects)		
short attack (under 1 h)	20	92
long attack (over 1 h)	84	28
sleep standing up	18	88
sub-wakefulness	Major problem	Variable
Night sleep (% of subjects)	Deep 80	Disturbed 72
morning waking	Difficult 60	No problem
sleep drunkenness	50–60	10–15
automatic behaviour	30	33
Associated features (% of subjects)		
migraine	16	6
fainting	8	2
cataplexy, sleep paralysis	0	100
EEG findings (% of subjects)		
sleep latency (min: mean and range)	6 (1–30)	6 (1–30)
SOREM on single day recording	0	40
SOREM on repeated day and night recordings	0	80
Treatment	Morning or evening stimulant drug	Morning stimulant drug
Pathophysiological mechanisms	Facilitation of NREM sleep	Facilitation of sleep; dissociation of REM sleep

Clinical characteristics of idiopathic hypersomnolence and narcolepsy. Data from Parkes.[29]

presentation is different from that of narcolepsy, and neither cataplexy nor sleep paralysis occurs (Table 6.1).

Night sleep in some of these patients is very different from that in narcolepsy. Sleep latency is usually short in both conditions, but some hypersomniacs have deep night sleep lasting longer than average (8–12 h or more) without waking or restlessness. Dreams may never be recalled. Morning arousal can be particularly difficult, despite loud alarms and buckets of cold water, and getting up can take half an hour or more. This pattern contrasts with the light sleep, frequent arousals and early waking of 70–80% of narcoleptics.

EEG sleep recordings in most subjects considered to have 'idiopathic' hypersomnia are normal, apart from the short sleep latency and prolonged sleep time. Sleep-onset REM periods do not occur; if present they indicate the definitive diagnosis of narcolepsy (Table 6.4).

It has been suggested that 'idiopathic' hypersomnolence represents a heredofamilial excess of stage 3–4 NREM sleep at night, with a high arousal threshold, daytime drowsiness and perhaps a low setting of the ascending reticular activating system.[36] This condition, however, may alternatively

Table 6.4.   *EEG findings in different forms of daytime drowsiness*

REM sleep onset (SOREM)
1. Monosymptomatic narcolepsy (e.g. narcolepsy alone, isolated cataplexy or sleep paralysis)
2. Polysymptomatic narcolepsy (e.g. narcolepsy plus one or more accessory symptom)
3. Rare examples of hypersomnia with:
   (a) depression
   (b) circadian rhythm disturbance
4. 'Secondary' narcolepsy, (clinical presentation usually atypical)

NREM sleep onset (SO NREM)
1. 'Idiopathic' hypersomnolence
2. Secondary hypersomnia
   (a) structural brain disease, head injury, encephalitis
   (b) situational or due to drug abuse
   (c) metabolic disease
   (d) sleep apnoea, sleep myoclonus, other parasomnias
3. Cyclical hypersomnia
   (a) Kleine–Levin syndrome (usually slow-wave EEG activity)
   (b) sleep-cycle shifts (may be SOREM)
   (c) menstrual hypersomnia (usually slow-wave EEG activity)

represent one extreme of the normal distribution of drowsiness (see Normal sleep habits, p. 271).

Roth[35] divides hypersomnolence into two levels of severity. Patients with minor symptoms have diurnal hypersomnia alone, whilst the more disabled have 24 h hypersomnia with prolonged nocturnal sleep and sleep drunkenness or morning arousal. Morning symptoms of sleep drunkenness, sub-wakefulness and automatic behaviour may contribute to the extraordinarily bad record of driving, household and occupational accidents uncovered in patients with daytime sleepiness by Broughton and Ghanem.[4]

Despite differences in presentation, the age of onset, sex distribution and familial occurrence of idiopathic hypersomnia and narcolepsy are closely similar. Both conditions often start at puberty or shortly after. Roth[35] has followed patients in whom idiopathic hypersomnolence remains stationary for up to 20 years. A clear distinction between the conditions is particularly difficult in families with narcolepsy, where a history of either 'narcolepsy' or 'hypersomnolence' may be found in first-degree relatives of subjects with definite narcolepsy, cataplexy and sleep-onset REM activity.[15, 18] Some 30–40% of patients with 'hypersomnolence' have a drowsy first-degree relative.[26]

Hypersomnolence and the narcoleptic syndrome
A few subjects considered to have idiopathic hypersomnolence at initial presentation eventually develop cataplexy or sleep paralysis, have REM sleep onset, or, as described above, a relative with the narcoleptic syndrome. Recent studies of patients presenting with the clinical diagnosis of idiopathic hypersomnolence have shown that 60% of these, like all narcoleptics, have the human leucocyte antigen DR$_2$.[16] Most of these subjects probably have monosymptomatic narcolepsy.

TREATMENT FOR HYPERSOMNIA

This depends on the cause. Thus, for example, hypersomnia with depression responds to antidepressant drugs, and daytime fatigue due to an abnormal lifestyle may improve with change of occupation or regularity of habit. The idea has arisen that the response to central stimulant drugs is not as good in hypersomnia as in narcolepsy. This is almost certainly incorrect, but due to difficulty in clinical distinction between different forms of hypersomnolence. Overall, central stimulant drugs are as effective in preventing daytime drowsiness in idiopathic hypersomnolence as in narcolepsy.

Dextroamphetamine 10 mg, phenbutrazate 20 mg, methylphenidate 20 mg, levoamphetamine 30 mg, phentermine 30 mg or pemoline 40 mg, all improve daytime drowsiness in hypersomniacs. Higher oral doses are usually not much more effective. Late evening rather than morning CNS stimulant drug treatment is sometimes necessary in subjects with 24 h hypersomnolence. Dexamphetamine 10–20 mg (or the longer-acting fencamfamin 20–40 mg) taken at bedtime will facilitate morning arousal and improve subsequent alertness without preventing night sleep in many of these subjects. Wyler *et al.*[40] reported that methysergide (2–6 mg daily) improved hypersomnia and narcolepsy, but this has not been confirmed.

The similar drug response in some patients with hypersomnia and narcolepsy may indicate, as already suggested (see p. 273), that the two conditions are in reality similar or identical.

SUB-WAKEFULNESS SYNDROMES

Several different sub-wakefulness syndromes have been described in otherwise normal subjects with normal physical and mental findings, no history of drug intake, sleep apnoea, sleep myoclonus or other recognized cause of daytime hypersomnolence. The diagnostic status of most of these is uncertain. A *neutral state syndrome* was associated by Guilleminault *et al.*[13] with daytime hypersomnia and automatic behaviour, normal 24 h total sleep time, but abnormal sleep structure, lack of stages 2–4 NREM sleep, and the occurrence of frequent microsleep episodes. These possibly accounted for the many periods of automatic behaviour reported by the patient. Cerebrospinal fluid homovanillic acid and 5-HIAA levels were normal. Amphetamine, methylphenidate and levodopa had no effect.

A somewhat similar *sub-wakefulness syndrome* with constant irresistible fatigue and sleepiness was described by Klimková-Deutschová *et al.*[19] EEG recordings showed frequent stage 1 NREM sleep episodes by day, but, unlike the neutral state syndrome, normal sleep patterns at night. This condition resembles that described by Mouret *et al.*,[25] who suggested a defect in the waking system as the cause. Normal variation in cerebrospinal fluid serotonin content in man with sleeping and waking is not established, although there is a 20-fold difference in level in the rhesus monkey.[38] This variation makes it difficult to assess the significance of elevated cerebrospinal fluid 5-HIAA levels found in a group of sleepy patients by Guilleminault and Dement.[12]

HYPERSOMNIA WITH CENTRAL STIMULANT DRUGS

Central stimulant drug dependency may result in hypersomnia, not insomnia, although the diagnosis is usually obvious. Dement and Guilleminault[10] described hypersomnia in patients who had taken stimulant drugs for an inadequate indication, or illicitly, and in whom drug withdrawal was followed by improvement in excess sleepiness.

NARCOLEPSY

In the past, the term 'narcolepsy' has often been applied mistakenly to any patient complaining of sleepiness.[95] However, Adie[41] confined the term to a specific syndrome with frequent day naps, but in addition cataplexy, sleep paralysis or both. These clinical features remain the criteria for diagnosis, to which may be added hypnagogic hallucinations, sleep-onset REM periods, a very short sleep latency, daytime sub-wakefulness, a heredofamilial incidence in up to 50% of cases, and a high if not absolute association with the HLA antigen DR_2. DR antigens are present in the brain.

Narcolepsy and cataplexy are due to a disturbance of the brain stem mechanisms for sleep but no anatomical lesion has ever been found. The cause may be either immunological or biochemical. A possible defect in brain amines, catecholamines or serotonin has been most studied, but other possibilities seem more likely. The condition is life-long, cures are extremely rare, and remissions are very uncommon.

HISTORY

Sleepy giants were recognized in the Bible, but definite narcoleptics were not described in English or American literature until the 18th century. Edgar Allan Poe, who may have suffered from sleep paralysis himself, depicted in *The Premature Burial* a character with 'a species of exaggerated lethargy . . . without ability to stir'; Melville described in *Moby Dick* a character with narcolepsy; and the hero of George Eliot's novel *Silas Marner* had paralysis with surprise.[212]

The first Europeans to observe sleeping sickness were probably sea captains involved in the slave trade in the Bay of Benin on the west coast of Africa. There was an endemic area of South African trypanosomiasis in Sierra Leone and from Senegal to the Congo. More cases were found inland than on the coast, with pathological sleep after prolonged and fatiguing work had exhausted the victim's strength. De Manacéine[130] described the first symptoms of sleeping sickness as enlarged lymph nodes followed by drooping of the eyelids.

> *Initially the subjects can be roused but periods of sleep become longer and more frequent until at last sleep is almost continuous, food is refused, and death ensues in the course of weeks or months.*

The brain was described as anaemic and usually firm with inflammation of the membranes.[80] It is now recognized that African sleeping sickness is the result of trypanosome colonization of the choroid plexus and the surrounding brain.

Many sleepy people in Europe were thought last century to have African sleeping sickness. However, in Africa this was a disease of blacks, not whites, and Professor Senelaigne, commenting on a case of Caffé,[62] rejected the diagnosis of 'the sleep sickness' in a French patient plagued by hallucinations and an overpowering need to sleep and concluded his argument by saying:

> I'm sure that you will be inclined to agree with me, my dear colleague, that we would be better off leaving sleep diseases to the blacks, at least temporarily anyway, since the whites have plenty of problems without that one too.

Many patients with narcolepsy were described in the 18th and 19th centuries. In 1704, Oliver in the *Philosophical Transactions*[153] related the history of 'an extraordinary sleepy person at Tinsburg, near Bath', and a century and a half later the Dublin physician, Graves,[91] described a gentleman who always

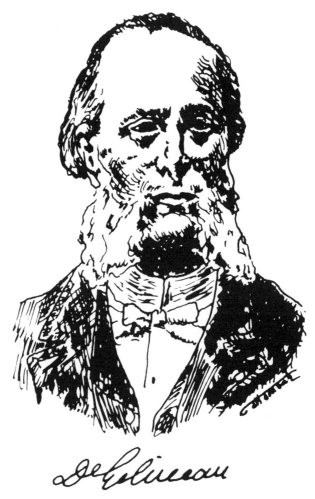

Figure 6.1.   *Dr. E. Gélineau (reprinted with permission from Passouant[158]).*

fell asleep in his soup, an early report of the striking association between eating and narcolepsy. Lasegue (see de Manacéine[130]) reported a young waiter who fell asleep whilst serving and de Manacéine recounts the case of a servant who dropped the baby on the floor and nearly killed him. The best description came, however, from Gélineau in 1880 (Fig. 6.1). Gélineau started his medical career as a French naval officer and then practised near Rochefort until ill-health obliged him to set up as a neuropsychiatrist in Paris. Eventually he became a leading authority on phobias as well as on narcolepsy before retiring in 1900 at the age of 72 to his castle of Sainte Luce La Tour and devoting his energies to viticulture. He was amply rewarded for his Bordeaux wine: a gold medal at the Anvers exhibition, a diploma of excellence in Amsterdam, and a great gold medal at the Paris Universal Exhibition of 1900.[158]

In the *Gazette des Hopitaux* for 1880 (Fig. 6.2) Gélineau described two patients, one a sleepy syphilitic and the other a Parisian hogshead seller, who attended his clinic on 15 February 1879. At the age of 36, and following an unhappy love affair, as many as 200 sudden sleep attacks a day commenced, lasting from a few minutes to half an hour or more. Attacks could be brought on in a number of ways; by walking or other muscular exertion, by emotion, by sexual excitement; and they were particularly common during thunderstorms. He once fell asleep near the monkey cage in the Jardin des Plantes. The patient had a lively sense of humour and the sight of a grotesque person or being dealt a good hand at cards made him weak with laughter and fall. Gélineau named this symptom astasia. For treatment, Gélineau gave amyl nitrite, apomorphine, picrotoxin, strychnine and caffeine, and advised bathing in the Seine. Gélineau distinguished narcolepsy from phobias which required a different treatment:

> The sufferer from agoraphobia takes five times daily at two hour intervals . . . iron, morphine, strychnine . . . viandes rouges et vin de Bordeaux.

(Gélineau[88])

In his monograph *De la Narcolepsie* published in 1881 (Fig. 6.3), Gélineau[87] analysed 14 cases, and differentiated two types of narcolepsy; an independent syndrome, and cases secondary to other illnesses.

DE LA NARCOLEPSIE

Par le docteur GÉLINEAU.

I

Je propose de donner le nom de narcolepsie (de νάρχωσις, somnolence, et λαμβάνειν, saisir, prendre) à une névrose rare ou du moins peu connue jusqu'à ce jour, caractérisée par un besoin de dormir impérieux, subit et de courte durée, se reproduisant à des intervalles plus ou moins rapprochés. Ce nom rappellera la double analogie de la narcolepsie avec la somnolence et la catalepsie.

Figure 6.2. *Definition of narcolepsy (from Gélineau[87]).*

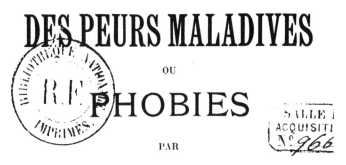

DES PEURS MALADIVES

OU

PHOBIES

PAR

le Docteur E. GÉLINEAU

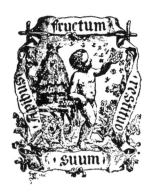

PARIS

SOCIÉTÉ D'ÉDITIONS SCIENTIFIQUES

PLACE DE L'ÉCOLE DE MÉDECINE

4, RUE ANTOINE-DUBOIS, 4

—

1894

NARCOLEPSY IN THE EARLY 20TH CENTURY

Despite the excellent descriptions of Graves,[91] Caffé,[62] Westphal[202] and Gélineau,[87] narcolepsy was little known and rarely recognized until the second decade of the 20th century. It was, and still sometimes is, wrongly considered to be due to encephalitis or hysteria. Gowers[90] stated that most attacks of narcolepsy occur in hysterical subjects, and that for every case of narcolepsy 2000 cases of epilepsy came under observation. However, the 1917–1927 epidemic of encephalitis lethargica focused attention on narcolepsy, although most cases of narcolepsy had no history of encephalitis. Wilson's report of 43 cases in 1928 was followed by reports of 45 cases at the Mayo Clinic,[64] then about 100[163] and subsequently more than 200.[123–125] By the time of Adie's classic paper in *Brain*[41] it was recognized, as Gélineau had originally suggested, that narcolepsy was a specific disease.

PRINCIPAUX OUVRAGES

DU MÊME AUTEUR

Des Névroses spasmodiques. Paris 1879.

Prix **3 fr.**

De la Kénophobie ou peur des espaces

Prix **3 fr.**

De la Narcolepsie   Prix **2 fr. 50**

Traité de l'angine de poitrine. Prix **8 fr.**

**Maladies et hygiène des gens
nerveux**   Prix **4 fr.**

N.-B. — Ces ouvrages se trouvent à la Société
d'Editions scientifiques, 4, rue Antoine-Dubois, Paris.

Figure 6.3. *Above and left: some of the principal works of Gélineau (Bibliothèque Nationale, Paris).*

CATALEPSY AND CATAPLEXY

In much of the early sleep literature, catalepsy is often confused with cataplexy.

Catalepsy is the term now used to describe increase in muscle tone resulting in fixed postures that can be maintained for long periods without fatigue accompanied by apparent paralysis of voluntary movement (Fig. 6.4). This state disappears with sleep, and is frequently associated with psychiatric disorders, epilepsy and hysteria.

A typical example of catalepsy last century was the outbreak which raged endemically for several years at Billinghausen, near Würzburg, and described by Vogt. Half the inhabitants suffered from catalepsy, often lasting for a few minutes, during which the face became intensely pale, the limbs motionless, speech embarrassed and consciousness, if not altogether abolished, much obscured. The attacks were liable to occur at any moment and fixed the patient in the position in which they caught him. All those who were attacked showed a very feeble physical and intellectual development. The disease was thought to be transmitted by heredity, not immediately by parents to children, but atavistically by skipping a generation, from grandparents to grandchildren. Those attacked by this disorder were commonly called die Starren (the rigid ones).

Gélineau observed somewhat similar behaviour due to acute anxiety in agoraphobic patients who were paralysed by the fear of mutilation and death, due to a possible carriage accident on crossing the streets and squares of Paris.

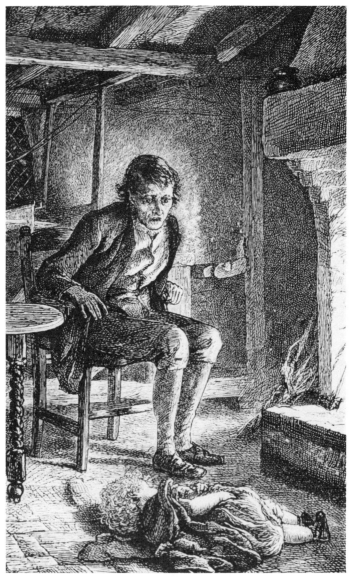

Figure 6.4. *In* Silas Marner, *by George Eliot (Mary Anne Evans), Victorian novelist 1819–1880, the weaver's lost gold is replaced by a strange child. The book has suffered unfairly from being forced on generations of school children. Here immobility is due to catalepsy, not cataplexy.*

Attempts were made to localize the lesions responsible for catalepsy when due to organic causes. This appeared to be anywhere between and including the mamillary bodies and the corpora striata. Ingram *et al.*[106] reported that lesions of a region between the mamillary bodies and the third nerve, thus involving the caudal hypothalamus, were followed by a state resembling catalepsy with a remarkable plastic hypertonus but also accompanied by somnolence or lethargy.

Catalepsy seems to have been a common occurrence during the last century and in many early accounts of narcolepsy the falling or astasic attacks of Gélineau were described as 'catalepsy'.

A motor inhibitory phenomenon with similarities to catalepsy occurs in laboratory animals, certain birds and some reptiles. A painful stimulus or holding the animal on its back for a few seconds causes a state of immobility with waxy flexibility lasting many minutes and possibly accompanied by analgesia.[115] There is no accompanying abnormality of sleep or REM sleep in such animals and the condition does not reliably occur in higher mammals or primates.

Cataplexy, unlike catalepsy, is characterized by loss of muscle tone as well as paralysis. A similar flaccid paralysis with areflexia occurs in sleep paralysis and during REM sleep. Loss of muscle tone and reflexes during sleep was first clearly described by Lombard[128] and by Rosenbach,[168] who made the observation that a dream of active movement was associated with a very violent knee kick.

THE NARCOLEPTIC SYNDROME

Prevalence
The exact frequency of narcolepsy is not known. It is probably slightly less common than multiple sclerosis or myasthenia gravis. All reports agree that about as many males as females are affected. Frequency estimates are often greatly biased by the method of search and thus general hospital records suggest that the condition is rare, whereas newspaper or television advertising produces many cases. Estimates of perhaps 20 000 narcoleptics in the United Kingdom and 100 000 in the United States are based on relatively small samples. A reasonable guess is that narcolepsy occurs at a rate of 4 cases per 10 000. Roth[169] found a prevalence of 2–3 cases per 10 000 in Czechoslovakia, whilst Dement and his colleagues estimated that the prevalence of narcolepsy in the San Francisco area was between 5 and 6.7 per 10 000. Relatives of index cases have a 60-fold greater risk of having the condition than individuals in the general population.[77]

Age of onset
The age of onset of narcolepsy (Fig. 6.5) varies from childhood to the mid-50s with a median around 25, although Sours[184] reported the mean age of onset as a little lower, 18 years (range 6–52).

Pre-pubertal cases of narcolepsy–cataplexy undoubtedly occur. Roth[171] reported that the disease was manifest in 23 of 360 cases before the age of 10, and Guilleminault and Anders[93] found that 20% of cases started before the age of 11.[147]

Onset over the age of 50 accounts for less than 5% of all cases.

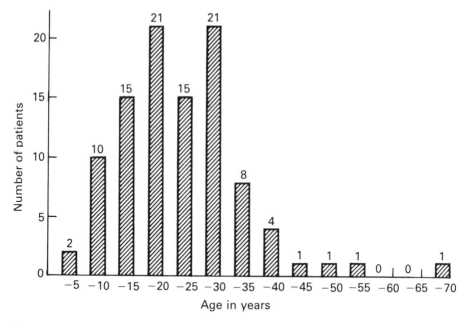

Figure 6.5. *Age at onset of narcolepsy as reported by 100 patients.*

Precipitating factors

In most instances, there are no definite precipitants to narcolepsy. A few patients give a history of sudden abrupt changes of the sleep–wake cycle, or psychological stress. Head injury is also frequently mentioned, but some of these cases are not genuine examples of narcolepsy. Menstruation and narcolepsy may start together or menstruation or pregnancy may intensify the symptoms. Wilson[204] stresses the frequency of epistaxis as a precipitating factor. In a series of 100 narcoleptics, possible antecedents were given as the menarche (4), pregnancy or childbirth (4), infectious diseases (2), emotional shock (4), operation (2), head injury (1) and anaesthetic (1), by Parkes *et al.*[155] Wilson[203] described cases after influenza, encephalitis and head injury, and Vein[194, 195] after typhoid, pneumonia, mumps, scarlet fever, malaria, infectious hepatitis and sinusitis.

Familial and genetic factors

The first report of *familial narcolepsy* (Table 6.5, Fig. 6.6) came from Westphal[202] who described a mother and a son who both had sleep paralysis and narcolepsy. Krabbe and Magnussen[118] described a family of 12 sibs, four of whom had narcolepsy. In a review of the literature they found 54 narcoleptics in 19 families with a distribution suggestive of a single dominant mode of inheritance, amongst a total of 200–300 people with excessive sleep. However, the diagnosis of narcolepsy was uncertain in many of these cases. More convincing descriptions came from Roth,[170] who found a heredofamilial

Table 6.5.   *Heredofamilial incidence of narcolepsy*[171]

Form of condition	Total no. of patients	Heredofamilial cases
Monosymptomatic narcolepsy	113	9(7.9%)
Monosymptomatic cataplexy	3	1(33.3%)
Monosymptomatic sleep paralysis	10	8(80%)
Polysymptomatic narcolepsy	234	37(15.8%)
Total	360	55(15.3%)

pattern of narcolepsy in 12 patients from two families, and Yoss and Daly[208] who initially found a hereditary occurrence of narcolepsy in 40 of 400 of their cases. On close questioning a much higher familial occurrence was revealed and up to 30% of subjects with the narcoleptic syndrome had an affected relative. Other estimates of the number of affected first-degree relatives of index cases of narcolepsy vary from 12%[184] to 50%[46] and 52%.[113]

Twin studies of narcolepsy have been too few to give a reliable estimate of the frequency of the condition in monozygotic and dizygotic pairs. Imlah[105] described identical twins who both developed narcolepsy and cataplexy at the age of 13, but in another pair of identical twins reported by Mitchell and Cummins[136] only one had narcolepsy (attributed in this instance to birth trauma).

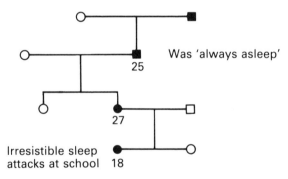

Figure 6.6.   *Inheritance of narcolepsy–cataplexy in the family of a schoolgirl with narcolepsy: narcolepsy in the schoolgirl; cataplexy, sleep paralysis and narcolepsy in her mother; cataplexy and narcolepsy in a grandfather; and narcolepsy in a great grandfather. The age of onset is given where known (the unaffected sister was 15 at the time of the study).*

Nevšímalová-Brühová and Roth[148] made the observation that in the families of subjects with monosymptomatic narcolepsy (narcolepsy or cataplexy alone) identical symptoms appear in each affected family member; whilst in families with polysymptomatic narcolepsy, it is rare to find identical symptom combinations among the affected relatives. Some of these have independent narcolepsy or hypersomnia without other symptoms.

There are several reports of different families in which several members, over several generations, have had only narcolepsy, cataplexy or sleep paralysis. Daly and Yoss[70] described a family with *narcolepsy* in 12 members over four generations, only three of whom had cataplexy. Gelardi and Brown[86] studied a family in which 15 members had *cataplexy*, but only three had sleep paralysis and three had possible narcolepsy. Rushton[176] described a family with isolated *sleep paralysis* without other symptoms.

Overall, between a quarter and a half of all narcoleptics have an affected close relative. A number of different patterns of inheritance of narcolepsy have been described. There is no evidence for consanguineous marriages in the parents of narcoleptics, as is likely to occur with autosomal recessive traits. Because of the findings on pupillography, Yoss and Daly[208] considered that narcolepsy represented one extreme of the normal distribution of drowsiness, and had a polygenic mode of inheritance. However, in family studies where relatives of narcoleptics were personally interviewed, Baraitser and Parkes[46] found a dominant mode of inheritance, although the degree of severity of this was variable, and occasionally 'skipped' generations occurred. Also, many subjects with narcolepsy do not have an affected parent. There is no clear maternal or paternal age effect. Although the effect of a dominant gene in the heterozygous state may result in narcolepsy, intermediate patterns of inheritance and also environmental factors may account for the disease in some instances.

There is no certain method of identifying which, if any, of the children of parents with narcolepsy will develop the condition, although it is helpful to know that, at the age of 25 years, nearly 85% of the risk has gone. Carskadon *et al.*[63] reported the development over 1–2 years of a short sleep latency and sleep-onset REM activity in an asymptomatic young adolescent daughter of a narcoleptic mother, and in some instances abnormal sleep structure may predict the onset of clinical symptoms of narcolepsy. HLA typing (Table 6.6), should the DR_2 grouping be absent, may help to exclude narcolepsy if the initial reports of an absolute linkage between narcolepsy and the DR_2 antigen are confirmed.[121]

Table 6.6. *HLA frequency in narcolepsy: percentage of subjects (42 narcoleptics, 200 controls) with each antigen*[121]

	Antigen			
	HLA A_3	HLA Cw7	HLA B_7	HLA DR_2
Narcoleptics	33	74	67	100
Control subjects	26	48	22	22

Narcoleptic dogs, like humans, show a variety of patterns of inheritance. In the Labrador and Doberman pinscher, narcolepsy is inherited in a pattern consistent with an autosomal recessive defect,[82] whilst in miniature poodles narcolepsy has a multifactorial aetiology.

The genetic basis for narcolepsy has recently been confirmed by studies of major histocompatibility complex (MHC) human leucocyte antigen (HLA) frequency in the disorder. HLA A, B and C antigens show some linkage with narcolepsy, but the strongest connection is with the D-related (DR) antigen

DR_2. This antigen, which also occurs in the brain, has been found in all of 37 narcoleptic subjects so far investigated, as compared with a frequency of approximately 20% in the general Caucasoid population. This is the strongest HLA–disease linkage so far discovered, and connects narcolepsy with the short arm of chromosone 6.[121] Linkage disequilibrium between the various HLA A, B, C and D antigens probably accounts for the finding of Billiard et al.[51] that the HLA B_7 antigen was present in 52.6% of 38 unrelated French Caucasoid subjects with narcolepsy as compared with the 14.6% of the general population.

Course, fluctuations, prognosis
Narcolepsy usually starts gradually and takes several years to develop. Once established, symptoms show minor fluctuations but almost always persist into old age. Roth[171] estimated that 88% of cases have a steady course and 12% have remissions and exacerbations. Fluctuations in the severity of symptoms depend on mood, psychological state, types of work, climatic conditions, and drug treatment.

A few cases commence abruptly, sometimes with very severe cataplexy,[171] whilst 10% of narcoleptics have a prodromal period of 1–20 years before the establishment of definite symptoms.[155] Clinical diagnosis during this period may be impossible.

Narcolepsy may improve with increasing age, although Prüll,[159] Yoss and Daly[207] and Billiard et al.[50] found no evidence of complete spontaneous remission in any patient. Ohta et al.[152] reported a slightly better prognosis in Japanese patients followed up over 10–20 years, some of whom had occasional prolonged symptom remission or slow improvement. Short remissions lasting 1–6 months occur in a minority of patients. A single severe narcoleptic for 20 years observed at King's College Hospital has had a complete remission for 2 years.

The prognosis for cataplexy and sleep paralysis is better than for narcolepsy, and in 10–20% of subjects cataplexy disappears spontaneously.

There is no evidence that long-term amphetamine–tricyclic treatment alters the eventual prognosis of narcolepsy or cataplexy in any way. Life-span in narcolepsy is normal.

Symptom combination
Yoss and Daly[207] found that in 241 patients with the narcoleptic syndrome seen at the Mayo clinic between 1950 and 1954 all patients had narcolepsy, 68% cataplexy, 24% sleep paralysis and 30% hypnagogic hallucinations. Comparable figures are reported in other series; e.g. Wolfenden[205] found that 70% of patients with the narcoleptic syndrome had cataplexy as well as narcolepsy, 24% sleep paralysis and 30% hypnagogic hallucinations. The most common association is narcolepsy– cataplexy alone, and the full tetrad occurs in only the minority of subjects. Of 190 patients described by Bowling and Richards[54] and Sours[184] only 10% had all four symptoms. Roth[171] reported that

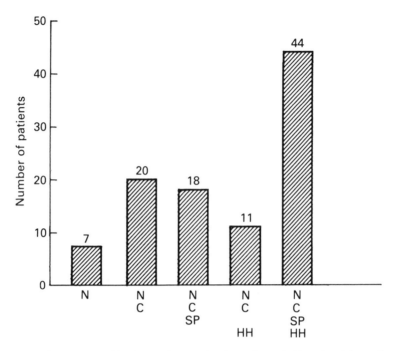

Figure 6.7.   *Symptom combination in the narcoleptic syndrome (100 patients) (reproduced with permission from Parkes et al.[155]).*

the four main symptoms of narcolepsy can be demonstrated in only about 10–15% of all subjects; Yoss and Daly[207] in 11%; and Wolfenden[205] in 30% (Fig. 6.7).

Symptom order
Symptoms usually appear in the order: (1) narcolepsy, (2) cataplexy, (3) sleep paralysis. It is difficult to document accurately the onset of hypnagogic hallucinations. In 70 narcoleptic patients described by Billiard et al.[50] the mean age of onset for these various symptoms was 22, 28, 29 and 27 years respectively.

Cataplexy is the first symptom of the narcoleptic syndrome on rare occasions. Guilleminault et al.[96] found, in 50 patients with narcolepsy, that cataplexy was the first symptom in three subjects (narcolepsy in 34, with simultaneous onset of narcolepsy and cataplexy in 13). This is very comparable to the finding of Roth[171] that, in 288 patients, cataplexy was the first symptom in 28 (sleep paralysis in 12 and narcolepsy in 221).

Very rarely the narcoleptic syndrome presents with headache, somnambulism, sleep drunkenness or nocturnal sleep disturbance.

'Monosymptomatic' narcolepsy
The marked variability of symptom presentation can cause diagnostic

confusion when a single symptom alone is present for many years. The term 'monosymptomatic' narcolepsy (i.e. narcolepsy, cataplexy or sleep paralysis alone) is purely descriptive and does not imply a separate disease entity. Monosymptomatic narcolepsy is common. Yoss and Daly[209, 210] reported that a single symptom alone was present in 110 of 390 subjects considered to have the narcoleptic syndrome; Janzen et al.[108] in 13 of 50 subjects; Rüther et al.[177] in 8 of 51; and Roth[171] in 113 of 360. Billiard et al.[50] described a narcoleptic who had his first sleep attack at the age of 63 after he had had cataplexy for 11 years; and an even more unusual example with the first appearance of cataplexy at 68 years of age, 47 years after the start of excessive daytime sleepiness.

A classification of the narcolepsies is given in Table 6.7.

Table 6.7. *Classification of the narcolepsies*

Monosymptomatic narcolepsy
Narcolepsy alone (or cataplexy or sleep paralysis alone)
Single symptom of narcolepsy–cataplexy:
   (a) sometimes family history of narcolepsy, cataplexy or both
   (b) subjects may later develop cataplexy (or other accessory symptoms)
The narcoleptic syndrome
Idiopathic or primary narcolepsy
Narcolepsy–cataplexy: sleep-onset REM activity, no structural lesion (sleep paralysis may replace
   cataplexy as a positive diagnostic feature)
   (a) familial
   (b) non-familial

*Narcolepsy–cataplexy associated with definite structural lesion**
(Clinical presentation usually highly atypical)
   (a) encephalitis lethargica and other forms of encephalitis
   (b) multiple sclerosis
   (c) infiltrating brain stem neoplasm
   (d) head injury

---

* 'Secondary' narcolepsy (see p. 308). Here: (1) environmental factors may precipitate narcolepsy
   in a genetically predisposed subject, or (2) two separate diseases may coexist, or (3) daytime
   drowsiness with structural or metabolic disease may be confused with true narcolepsy.

Clinical features of narcolepsy

Warmth, monotony, eating, travelling and tiredness predispose to narcolepsy. All narcoleptics go to sleep in trains, buses or cars, after meals and whilst reading or relaxing. Most nap during monotonous tasks at home or at work and some go to sleep on the toilet. Eating sweet foods and, in particular, a large carbohydrate meal is a common cause of narcolepsy.[199] Some narcoleptics cannot eat an apple, a bar of chocolate or a doughnut without falling asleep. However, an essential feature of narcolepsy is the tendency to go to sleep in unusual, as well as usual, circumstances; and there are many descriptions of sleep in odd surroundings – standing up, walking, cycling, horse riding, examining patients, skiing, during sexual intercourse or orgasm, and even whilst having a painful tooth drilled. Unusually, sleep may follow emotional crisis at a time of high arousal, rather than boredom. Most attacks come on gradually and occur with warning. They can be postponed to some extent, but

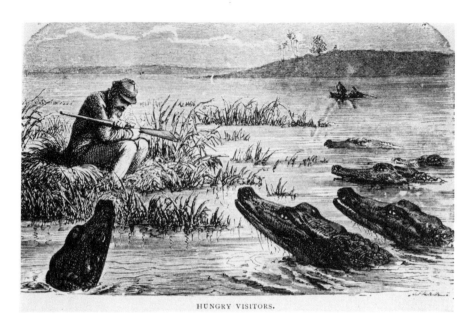

HUNGRY VISITORS.

PEANUTS

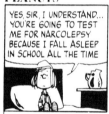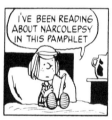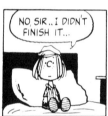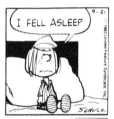

Figure 6.8. *Two views of narcolepsy. (a) David Livingstone.* Missionary Travels and Adventures in Africa, *London: Hodder and Stoughton (1880); (b) Charlie Brown.* International Herald Tribune, *21 September 1983.* © 1983 United Features Syndicate, Inc.

only at the expense of irritability. Sleep is often preceded by tiredness, heaviness of the limbs, drooping eyelids, loss of neck muscle tone, defocusing or double vision, limb paraesthesiae and hypnagogic hallucinations, but a few attacks are sudden or catastrophic and occur with no warning. On average, attacks last 10–30 min, with a range from 10–20 s to several hours. The mean duration of naps is longer in the evening than in the morning. Very long sleep periods, continuing over several days, are sometimes described in females at the start of narcolepsy, occasionally in relation to menstruation.

Nap frequency is very variable, and most patients claim to have 1–8 sleep periods per day. However, EEG studies show that these estimates are mostly false with a large number of short sleep periods as well as frequent microsleeps lasting a few seconds in most subjects. Loss of sleep, hypnotics, phenothiazines, sedatives, antihistamines and alcohol all make narcolepsy worse.

There is no constant pattern of arousal from attacks. Arousal may be spontaneous or result from environmental stimuli and be followed by feelings of either refreshment or tiredness.

Constant daytime sub-wakefulness, as well as sleep attacks, occurs in some but not all narcoleptics. In the EEG recordings of these subjects, states corresponding to full wakefulness may be absent altogether.[75, 169, 171, 209, 210]

Age does not greatly alter the pattern of narcolepsy, and the normal pattern of age-related night-sleep changes also occurs in narcoleptics.

Night sleep in narcoleptics

Disturbed nocturnal sleep develops in the majority of narcoleptics, either at the start or later in the illness. Between 60% and 80% of all established narcoleptics complain of poor night sleep; 68 out of 102 patients;[71] 17 of 30;[98] and 66 of 97.[169, 171] The usual complaints are of light sleep, frequent awakenings, non-refreshing sleep, morning headache and sometimes muscle aching. Sleep apnoea, sleep myoclonus and somnambulism are more frequent than in the normal population. Amongst 100 narcoleptics, 88 woke once or more nightly, 48 complained of muscle jerking at the start of day or night sleep, three of bruxism and three of generalized body vibration on sleep onset. Snoring, yawning and muscle aching occurred in 37 subjects and somnambulism in seven.[155] Jovanović[109] claimed that some narcoleptics wake over 300 times each night.

Narcoleptics usually wake up normally after night sleep, although morning headaches, sleep paralysis and sleep drunkenness may occur.[171] The morning is usually a good time and the evening a bad one.

CATAPLEXY (Fig. 6.9, Table 6.8)

The phrase 'weak with laughter' reflects the fact that hearty laughter, as well as fright, surprise or sudden noise, causes muscular hypotonia and partial paralysis in normal subjects. This affects in particular the face, jaw and neck muscles. Scollo-Lavizarri[181] attributed this phenomenon to an inhibitory brain stem reflex which can be demonstrated successively in the muscles of the jaw, trunk and limbs. This physiological event rarely if ever causes real incapacity, but in people with narcolepsy sudden attacks of paralysis with tonelessness (cataplexy) are frequent and disabling.

Cataplexy is conditioned by the presence of trigger factors. Over 95% of attacks are the result of sudden stimuli, and less than 5% appear to be spontaneous. Spontaneous episodes of cataplexy are usually identical with sleep paralysis.

Laughter is the commonest cause of cataplexy, but anger, fright, joy, surprise or other sudden emotion, intense concentration or motor effort during sport, coughing, sneezing and nose blowing, rage, or the fear of corporal punishment will trigger an attack. Many sporting activities, angling, hunting, table tennis, rugby or ice hockey, will produce cataplexy, with the combination

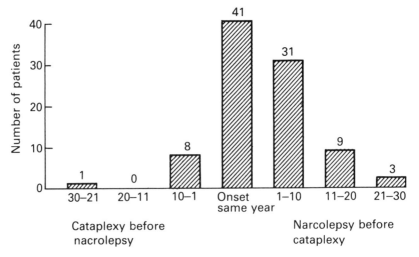

Figure 6.9. *Onset of cataplexy and narcolepsy: the horizontal axis shows the number of years by which the onset of one condition preceded the other.*

of excitement and the need for motor response. Occupational cataplexy is no uncommon; there are reports of a surgeon with attacks due to a spurt of blood a railway signalman paralysed on the approach of a train, and a priest unable to elevate the Host. A patient described by Roth[171] had cataplexy whilst reading Czechoslovak lyric poetry. The common feature in all these examples is th sudden increase in alertness. This may explain why cataplexy has bee confused with ethnically determined startle responses, including *myriach* (Siberia), *latah* (the Far East), *jumping Frenchmen* (Atlantic seaboard of the USA and *piblokto* (Arctic Eskimos). However, unlike cataplexy, none of thes conditions is associated with atonia.

The severity and frequency of cataplexy differ greatly in individual subjects Attack frequency varies from several episodes a day to a single attack ove many years. Attack duration varies from a second or two to 5–10 min Cataplexy is most frequent when background vigilance is low and subjects a tired, sleep-deprived or taking hypnotics. A few patients learn to contro cataplexy by avoiding laughter, or by increasing muscle tension in know trigger situations.

Partial and complete cataplexy
Partial episodes of cataplexy involve mainly bulbar-innervated muscles, wit loss of speech, jaw sagging, neck bending, rolling or vergence of the eye double vision and ptosis but not complete collapse. Voluntary eye movement sometimes preserved. *Generalized cataplexy* causes complete skeletal musc atonia and paralysis with falling, although respiration is not compromised ar sphincter disturbance, when it occurs, is due not to cataplexy, but to stre incontinence. Bad falls and self-injury are uncommon. Normal awarene persists throughout cataplexy unless there is a transition to sleep hallucinosi

Table 6.8. *Clinical characteristics of narcolepsy*

Symptom	Narcolepsy	Cataplexy	Sleep paralysis	Night sleep	Hypnagogic hallucinations
Usual age of onset	10–30	15–30	15–30	–	–
Average attack frequency	6–8 per day	Very variable	A few each year	–	Very variable
Average attack duration	5–30 min	Few seconds	Few minutes	–	–
Characteristic features	Tiredness, sub-wakefulness with sleep attacks in both usual and unusual circumstances	Paralysis with atonia; almost always triggered by sudden increase in alertness, startle or laughter	Sleep onset or termination Eye movements, respiration maintained; intense fear	70–80% have disturbed sleep, many awakenings, nocturnal myoclonus, sometimes sleep apnoea	Pre-sleep and sometimes waking hallucinatory experiences
Ultimate recovery	Life-long	Improves with age	May improve with age	Deterioration with age	Uncertain
Drug response	CNS stimulants	Clomipramine	Clomipramine	Benzodiazepines may reduce movement and arousal	CNS stimulants

Status cataplecticus

Status cataplecticus is usually confined to subjects with very severe narcolepsy–cataplexy, and occurs mainly at the onset of the illness or following tricyclic drug withdrawal. There may be severe generalized atonia, partial or complete paralysis, facial fasciculation, rolling and jerking eye movements, with frequent transition from sleep to waking and marked oscillations in motor control, lasting hours or days.

Unilateral cataplexy

Cataplexy is usually bilateral, but Wilson[203] described focal cataplexy, affecting only one arm or leg, in sportsmen making a difficult stroke at tennis or kicking a ball. Cataplexy is unilateral in 0.5–1% of all cases.[207] Lascelles et al.[122] described the occurrence of unilateral cataplexy in a patient with systemic lupus erythematosus, who also had narcolepsy and sleep paralysis. Laughter caused complete loss of use of the right arm and leg with ptosis and jaw sagging for 15 s to 3 min. The authors suggested that focal vasculitis in the pons and mesencephalon accounted for the cataplexy, which improved with corticosteroids.

The finding of unilateral cataplexy is very odd when one considers that sleep atonia is always bilateral, and that the EEG changes of sleep and wakefulness are also bilateral. The usual result of a unilateral stimulus to the reticular formation is EEG activation of the entire cortex. Perhaps isolated hemicerebrum experiments are relevant here; hemisection of the midbrain and pons has shown that the EEG may be synchronized ipsilateral to a chronic lesion of the midbrain tegmentum[117] whilst pontine sections have the opposite effect, hemisection at the pretrigeminal level causing episodes of synchronization contralateral to the lesion.[67, 68] However, there is a remarkably fast recovery of EEG symmetry with isolated hemicerebrum experiments. These may indicate that the ascending reticular formation of the level of the upper midbrain divides into two ascending channels, although there must be functional cross-connections; the clinical observation of unilateral cataplexy in man indicates that there must also be two descending reticulospinal motor inhibitory pathways that may be triggered independently. These findings argue against any circulating hypnotoxin theory of sleep atonia.[48]

Clinical examination during cataplexy

When Adie's paper was published (September 1926), he remarked that no patient had been examined by a competent neurologist during an attack of cataplexy. However, in the same year, Mankowski reported absence of reflexes, and Mussio Fournier described total electrical inexcitability of the facial muscles. (This has never been confirmed.)

Wilson gave his classic account of cataplexy in 1928:

> The clinical value of this striking case of narcoleptic and emotional attacks is enhanced by the fact that I was able to observe one of the latter from beginning to end and to examine the patient's neurological condition during it. Dr. Macdonald Critchley, the present registrar at the National Hospital, was with me at the time and helped materially in the examination, which was of necessity hurried. Description of attack of 'powerlessness' – while I was occupied with another patient, E.C. was sitting behind me and as afterwards appeared was endeavouring to keep himself from falling asleep. Suddenly I heard a slight groaning noise coming from him, and at once looking around, I saw his head nodding gently on his chest as he sank forward into a bent position and a moment or two later slid or 'slithered' off the chair to the floor. The

arms were by the side and the fingers semiflexed; the eyes were closed. Lifting the arms, I found him absolutely atonic and flaccid. When let go they fell like lumps of lead by his side. The legs similarly were absolutely atonic, sprawling out on the floor. Lifting the eyelids, I observed that the pupils reacted to light slightly but definitely, while the eyelid muscles were so toneless that little or no reflex contraction took place on my touching the cornea. Testing the knee jerks I found them completely abolished on both sides. In the meantime, Dr. Critchley had hurriedly taken off the patient's shoe and sock on the left side and testing the plantar reflex obtained a slight, but definite left extensor response which he demonstrated to me and I corroborated. Just as we were finishing this rapid examination, the patient suddenly said 'I am alright sir' in his ordinary voice and with a faint smile. Muscular power came back, he moved his limbs, got onto the chair, and told us that he had been conscious the whole time.

Examination of other patients during cataplexy has confirmed Wilson's account of loss of the tendon reflexes,[41] a mute, flexor[131] or sometimes extensor plantar response,[56, 203] and occasionally loss of pupillary light reaction, bradycardia or tachycardia. The pallor, pupillary dilatation, sweating and increase in pulse rate sometimes recorded during cataplexy are probably due to the shock that starts the attack and not to the attack itself (Table 6.9).

Table 6.9.   *Differential diagnosis of cataplexy*

1. Cataplexy
2. Ethnically determined startle responses (e.g. latah in Malaysians)
3. Myoclonic jerks causing falls
4. Tonic fits
5. Akinetic fits
6. Psychomotor attacks
7. Drop attacks in transient ischaemic episodes
8. Intermittent hydrocephalus producing drop attacks
9. Idiopathic drop attacks
10. Petit mal triad (Zellweger[213] described a case of 'narcolepsy' with spike and wave paroxysms in the EEG)

Polygraphic studies of cataplexy

During cataplexy, tonic muscular activity disappears with loss of the monosynaptic H reflex if attacks are prolonged.[56, 92, 101, 103] Wakefulness at the start of attack rapidly turns to sleep and REM episodes occur after 1–2 min.[92, 101, 180] Cataplexy is often followed by REM sleep, just as sleep paralysis is often followed by intense hypnagogic hallucinations.[99, 146] Sometimes the change from the descending inhibition of REM sleep with preserved alertness to full REM sleep can be seen clinically, when atonia and paralysis with preserved eye movements at the start of attack are followed by jerking eye movements, complete atonia, facial flickering and irregular respiration.

Emotional factors and cataplexy

To explain the role of emotional factors in the provocation of cataplexy, Vizioli[196, 197] considered that cataplexy was related to activation of an inhibitory bulbar-spinal motor system originating in limbic areas. This idea is perhaps given some support (see Roth,[171] p. 174) by the observation of hippocampal theta activity during cataplectic attacks and also during REM sleep in narcoleptic dogs.[139] However, many non-emotional stimuli that alter the activity of brain stem motor mechanisms also cause alteration of muscle tone, but do not provoke cataplexy.

Puizillout[160] demonstrated that stimulation of the aortic trunk of the vagus in cats causes reflex triggering of paradoxical sleep, an effect, like cataplexy, that is more obvious after sleep deprivation. Dell and Puizillout[74] found that vago-aortic stimulation in the cat, after sleep deprivation, produced sleep-onset REM periods and also reflex 'cataplexy', although stimulation without previous sleep deprivation usually caused manifestations of NREM sleep.[76] The sudden fall of anti-gravity tonus, the strong inhibition of motor neurones and the depression of spinal reflexes during paradoxical sleep are exactly similar during cataplexy, and the frequent transition of cataplexy to full REM sleep suggests that cataplexy is an isolated fragment of this sleep stage, but occurring during waking.

SLEEP PARALYSIS

Weir Mitchell in 1896 considered that sleep paralysis was a normal physiological event, the spell to be broken by the mental effort to move.[200]

Sleep paralysis in the narcoleptic syndrome is not as common an accompaniment of narcolepsy as cataplexy, and in most patients attacks are infrequent, at most one or two a week. A small minority of patients have more frequent attacks, sometimes several each night. Sleep paralysis occurs in between 10%[195] and 45%[171] of cases of polysymptomatic narcolepsy.

Lhermitte[127] described sleep paralysis as 'waking cataplexy' and Daniels[71] described it as 'hypnagogic cataplexy'. Sleep paralysis and cataplexy are almost identical, apart from the absence of trigger factors, longer duration of attack, and occasional sense of respiratory embarrassment in sleep paralysis as compared with cataplexy.[60]

Sleep paralysis is more common at sleep onset than at termination in narcoleptics, and in about half all subjects is accompanied by hypnagogic hallucinations. Recovery is either spontaneous or due to noise or other external stimulus. This is occasionally useful in the differential diagnosis from periodic paralysis in which weakness is not overcome by noise.

HYPNAGOGIC HALLUCINATIONS (Fig. 6.10)

Hypnagogic hallucinations were described by Maury[132] as the sensory errors of half sleep. Maury considered that hypnagogic hallucinations were a normal event. He described the whole range of visual imagery with luminous phenomena, flowers, landscapes, arabesques of geometrical figures and fragments of waking imagination incorporated into dreams that could be summoned but not controlled in the moments before falling asleep. Visual, auditory or somaesthetic hallucinations occur, and the patient may hear his name, sentences that do not make sense, other sounds or neologisms.[154]

The half-sleep sensory errors of narcoleptics may be more vivid and dream-like in quality than the above description. Hypnagogic episodes in

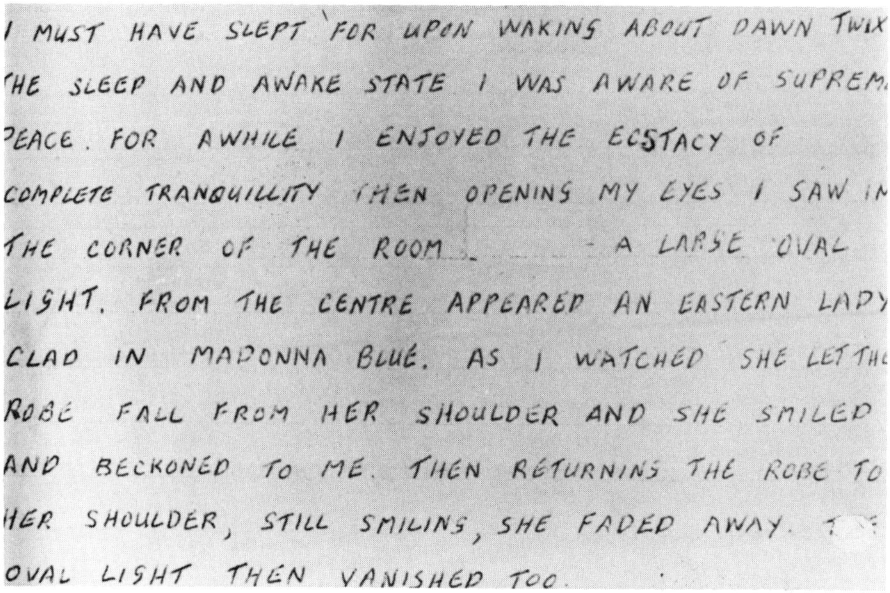

I MUST HAVE SLEPT FOR UPON WAKING ABOUT DAWN TWIX THE SLEEP AND AWAKE STATE I WAS AWARE OF SUPREM. PEACE. FOR AWHILE I ENJOYED THE ECSTACY OF COMPLETE TRANQUILLITY THEN OPENING MY EYES I SAW IN THE CORNER OF THE ROOM - A LARGE OVAL LIGHT. FROM THE CENTRE APPEARED AN EASTERN LADY CLAD IN MADONNA BLUE. AS I WATCHED SHE LET THE ROBE FALL FROM HER SHOULDER AND SHE SMILED AND BECKONED TO ME. THEN RETURNING THE ROBE TO HER SHOULDER, STILL SMILING, SHE FADED AWAY. T OVAL LIGHT THEN VANISHED TOO.

Figure 6.10.   *Hypnagogic hallucinations described by a subject with narcolepsy.*

normal subjects are accompanied by signs of stage 1 NREM sleep[85, 212] whilst those of narcoleptics are often accompanied by REM sleep. Hypnagogic hallucinations, like the episodes of sleep paralysis that they often accompany, last several minutes and may occur by day as well as night. Visual hallucinations can also occur independently of sleep in 10–15% of narcoleptics, sometimes leading to the mistaken diagnosis of schizophrenia. About 20–50% of narcoleptics have fairly frequent hypnagogic hallucinations, whereas a small number lack dream recall.

AUTOMATIC BEHAVIOUR (Fig. 6.11)

Many subjects with narcolepsy are constantly sub-alert, perform badly on tests requiring sustained attention, and have frequent lapses of vigilance.[192] States of automatic behaviour were described in detail in Maury,[132] Daniels[71] and Guilleminault et al.[94] These states occur in 20–40% of all narcoleptics but also in many other conditions associated with sub-wakefulness.

Maury[132] thought that this intermediate state between sleeping and waking, when motor function was largely preserved but consciousness was inert, was due to too short a natural sleep or one interrupted by force, and that it could be diminished by intellectual pursuits. As such, it was a normal state for the time when rest was insufficient – 'such half-awakening was particularly common in children belonging to the working class'. Automatic behaviour was also well known to le Manacéine, who observed that 27 of 84 people she saw with this condition came from Finland, explicable by the fact that amongst natives of that country it was nearly impossible to find a person of sanguine temperament'.

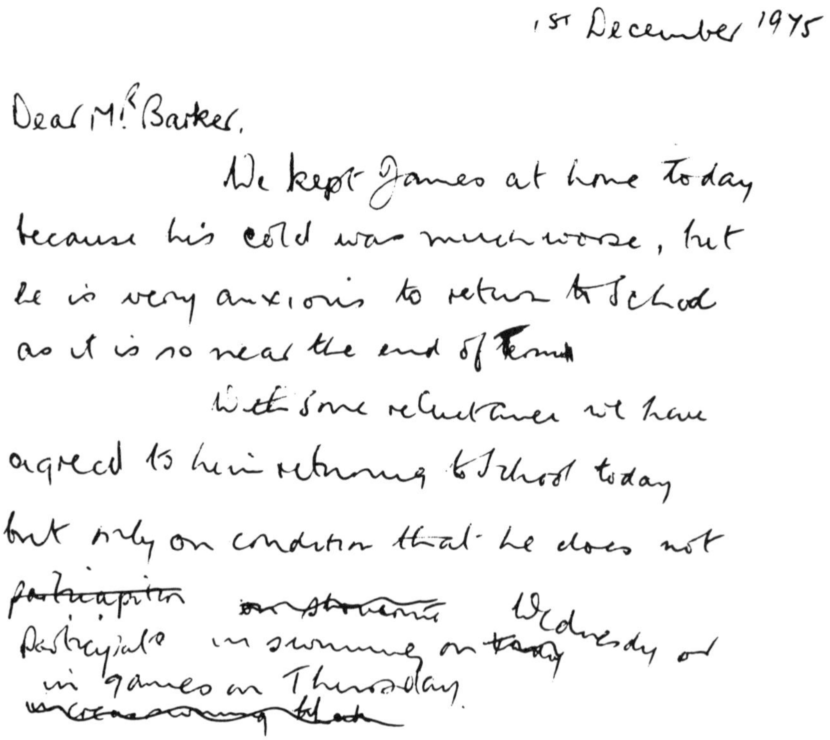

1st December 1975

Dear Mr Barker,

We kept James at home today because his cold was much worse, but he is very anxious to return to school as it is so near the end of term

With some reluctance we have agreed to him returning to school today but only on condition that he does not participate ~~on~~ Particularly in swimming on ~~t~~ Wednesday or in games on Thursday.

Figure 6.11. *Automatic behaviour whilst writing a letter to the patient's son's schoolmaster.*

A typical description of automatic behaviour is given by Guilleminault et al.[94]:

> The patient left Reno alone at 1000 to drive to Tahoe, a 70-mile distance. 'I remember perfectly what happened to Carson City (30 miles away). After that I had a complete blackout. I found myself at the reception desk of the hotel at Tahoe, knocking on the desk and the receptionist asked me what he could do to help. I suddenly "came back". I could not remember why I was in that hotel, where I had parked my car and what had happened in the past 90 minutes.'

The alteration in awareness is not perceived and complete or partial amnesia for the attack is usual.[214] Simple repetitive activity, sudden bursts of meaningless written or spoken language with no relationship to what has gone before, inability to perform complex tasks or learn new ones, and frequent automobile accidents, driving on the wrong side of the road, neglecting traffic signals, and loss of all sense of passage of time are typical features of these attacks. Identical symptoms occur during episodes of transient global amnesia in non-narcoleptics, although these are usually of longer duration. In contrast to automatic behaviour, somnambulism (which usually occurs from deep NREM sleep) is uncommon in narcoleptics, present in only 1.7% of Roth's cases.[171]

REM sleep periods, microsleeps and more prolonged attention lapses may all contribute to automatic behaviour in narcoleptics. Daytime REM episodes always impair performance. In addition to REM episodes, polygraphic recording in narcoleptics shows very frequent or continuous microsleep episodes. These periods of NREM microsleep are accompanied by interruption of performance of vigilance tests. As well as REM sleep periods and microsleep episodes, Iijima et al.[104] found that many narcoleptics dozed or fell into the light stages of NREM sleep very often during examination.

Sleep drunkenness, ataxia often accompanied by automatic behaviour, occurs in 11% of all cases of polysymptomatic narcolepsy.[171] Microsleeps have been observed during sleep drunkenness[94, 171] with incomplete arousal, impaired motor control, mental clouding and confusion lasting 30–60 min after waking.

Automatic behaviour and sleep drunkenness in narcoleptics have to be distinguished from drug-induced confusional states and metabolic disorders as well as disordered awareness related to seizure activity, automatisms with partial complex seizures of fronto-temporal origin, absence status and post-ictal confusional states.

OTHER SYMPTOMS IN THE NARCOLEPTIC SYNDROME

Pain in the neck (sometimes associated with frequent cataplexy), jumping of the facial or limb muscles before night-sleep onset, morning headache, mild anxiety or depression are not uncommon. Peptic ulcer, essential tremor and chorea, possibly as complications of stimulant drug treatment, are sometimes described. The association of narcolepsy with extreme obesity, kyphoscoliosis, hypothyroidism, severe sexual disturbance or hypopituitarism is usually because of failure to distinguish between idiopathic narcolepsy, obstructive sleep apnoea and other causes of daytime drowsiness.

EYE MOVEMENTS, SLEEP AND NARCOLEPSY

Most normal people when drowsy have blurring of vision or diplopia (Fig. 6.12). Similar disturbances of vision precede or accompany narcolepsy in many instances and ptosis, insufficiency of convergence, accompanied by subjective ocular fatigue, defocusing, diplopia and eyelid fasciculation are common findings.[65, 69, 111, 126, 171, 194, 195] These abnormalities may improve or disappear after a good night's rest or amphetamine treatment, and simply reflect the fairly constant vigilance defect in narcoleptics. Van Bogaert[193] suggested that there may be a sleep centre in relation to the oculomotor nuclei and commented that in most of the published cases of sleep problems there had also been an associated abnormality of eye movement. Anderson and Salmon[44] believed this indicated physiological, if not also anatomical, proximity of REM sleep centres to the oculomotor nuclei.

The following example (from Wilson[203]) illustrates visual problems in narcolepsy:

P.O.R. aged 24. Occupation, railway carpenter: unmarried.
History of present illness – *In April, 1924, the patient had his first attack of irresistible sleep when actually on the top of a signal post executing a repair. He managed to climb down and fell fast asleep at the foot of it, for perhaps half an hour. Ever since, he has suffered from continually recurring diurnal attacks of sleep, not a single day passing without them. About the same time as the original attack, or rather later, he noticed occasional double vision, independent of the sleep 'turns', the images being on the same horizontal level and a little way apart.*

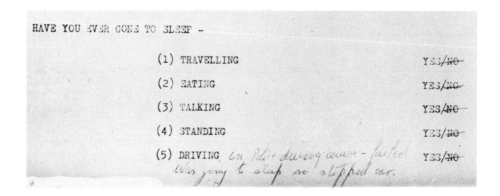

Figure 6.12. *Driving problems illustrated by response to narcolepsy questionnaire.*

There are several reports of other ocular abnormalities in narcolepsy. Roth[171] described congenital oculomotor paresis in three subjects with familial narcolepsy, one of whom also had bilateral sixth nerve palsies and cataracts. Van Bogaert[193] records the familial occurrence of congenital cataract with cataplexy, accompanied by narcolepsy in one member of the family, while Lösner and Zett[129] described narcolepsy associated with congenital bilateral sixth cranial nerve palsies.

THE PUPILLOGRAM AND NARCOLEPSY

The ability to remain alert in the dark can be measured by pupillography. An awake and alert person in total darkness has large pupils. In sleep the pupils are small, and, between the two extremes of vigilance, intermediate in size. Yoss *et al.*[206, 211] found that in patients with narcolepsy the pupillary responses to flashes of light were sluggish. However, non-narcoleptic subjects also sometimes had sluggish pupillary responses, and occasionally found it difficult to remain alert in the dark. Because of these findings, Yoss[206] suggested that the sleepiness of narcolepsy was comparable to other human traits such as stature and intelligence, representing one extreme of the normal distribution of vigilance in the general population.

PSYCHIATRIC ASPECTS OF NARCOLEPSY

The mean IQ of narcoleptics is within the normal range.[175] Personality traits are usually normal, although, as with epilepsy, a distorted self-image, social withdrawal, exclusion by peer groups, difficulty in maintaining employment and heterosexual contacts due to narcolepsy can lead to the development of a personality disorder.[156, 175] However, most narcoleptics adapt appropriately to their disability, and although discouragement is frequent real attacks of depression are not very common.[71] 20% of the narcoleptics reported by Parkes *et al.*[155] were mildly anxious or depressed and Roth and Nevšímalová[173] found a somewhat higher incidence of depression in narcolepsy than in the general population. Cave[64] and Daniels[71] observed three patients who suffered from narcolepsy only during periods of depression.

Chronic sexual disorder is not uncommon, with impotence in men and frigidity in women. Sexual problems, at least in males, may be due in part to tricyclic drug treatment of cataplexy. Up to a half of all patients with narcolepsy have symptom-related difficulties at work, in marriage or in their social lives.[175]

A psychogenic basis for narcolepsy using sleep as an escape from anger, guilt, resentment or sexual impulse is often considered in the psychoanalytic literature but there are no convincing psychotic features in these patients, despite hypnagogic hallucinations. Most reported examples of psychosis occurring in narcolepsy are due to amphetamine treatment and, with this exception, psychosis is no more frequent in patients with narcolepsy than would be expected by chance.[55]

DROWSINESS AND DRIVING

There is ample evidence that barbiturates, benzodiazepines, alcohol and other sedatives impair performance in driving tasks, although the driver may be unaware of any impairment (Anonymous; *Brit. Med. J.* (1978) 2 1415–1417). Sedatives and antihistamines increase the risk of fatal road traffic accidents at least five-fold, whilst following short general anaesthesia for minor surgical procedures, drowsiness may persist for up to 3 days.[174] The evidence that daytime drowsiness as a result of narcolepsy or any other disorder such as sleep apnoea is a common cause of road traffic accidents is a little less conclusive than in the case of alcohol or hypnotics, but there is no doubt that this is an increasing modern problem.

A considerable amount of research has been done to establish the part that day-sleep attacks in narcoleptics and daytime drowsiness in sleep apnoea may play in the causation of road accidents. Although some of these reports are anecdotal, there is no doubt that daytime drowsiness whilst driving is very dangerous.

Kennedy,[112] from the University of Wales, described a narcoleptic driver who had sleep attacks at the wheel occurring with no warning, or double vision lasting 5–10 min. Bartels and Kusakcioglu[47] reported that sleep attacks were a not uncommon cause of road accidents on the major highways of the eastern United States. These authors found that 40% of narcoleptics had fallen asleep whilst driving on New England turnpikes, compared with 7% of controls. Many subjects fall asleep when they have to stop at crossroads or wait until the lights change or the way is clear. Roth[171] reported that some drivers fall asleep whilst on the move, often with disastrous results, particularly rear-end collisions.

In addition to daytime sleep episodes, sub-wakefulness, automatic behaviour and sleep drunkenness in people with daytime drowsiness may all contribute to road traffic accidents, and, in rare instances of narcolepsy, cataplexy and sleep paralysis, if they occur whilst driving, can be dangerous.

Both the driving ability of patients with daytime drowsiness and the physician's responsibility to the sleepy driver are ill-defined in the United Kingdom. When the accused has no memory whatsoever of events prior to a car crash at a crossroads, Lord Chief Justice Goddard made this caveat: 'that drivers do fall asleep is a not uncommon cause of serious road accidents and it would be impossible, as well as disastrous, to hold that falling asleep at the wheel was any defence to a charge of dangerous driving. If a driver finds that he is getting sleepy he must stop' (Hill *v.* Baxter, 1958, 1 AER 193). A patient with daytime drowsiness may thus fail in his essential duty to stay awake.

Driving ability in anyone with daytime drowsiness or sleep attacks depends on the severity and frequency of attack, the degree of warning of impending sleep, the possibility that such attacks may occur whilst driving, and the degree of symptom control by treatment. With all these variables there can be no hard and fast rules as to the driving ability of patients with many different kinds of day-sleep disorders. Each individual subject needs separate consideration. General guidelines in narcolepsy, sleep apnoea and hypersomnolence may be as given in Table 6.10.

Table 6.10   *Guidelines on driving*

	Can drive?
Narcolepsy	
Off treatment	No
On treatment (control good)	Yes
On treatment (control poor)	No
Sudden attacks	No
Idiopathic hypersomnolence	As narcolepsy
Persistent sub-wakefulness	No
Obstructive sleep apnoea	No
With tracheostomy, on CPAP* or with other effective treatment	Yes
Kleine–Levin syndrome	Yes (between attacks)

* CPAP – continuous positive airway pressure, see p. 384.

If there is any doubt as to driving ability, and bearing in mind the high proportion of road traffic accidents shown in Table 6.11, it is often in the patients' best interest that they are advised not to drive. (Figures in respect of sleep apnoea, hypersomnolence syndromes and other causes of daytime drowsiness are probably similar to those shown for narcolepsy in Table 6.11.)

Table 6.11. *Reported frequency of road traffic accidents in narcoleptics who drive or have driven (64 narcoleptics)*

Gone to sleep whilst driving	48%
Had road traffic accident due to sleep whilst driving	25%
Stopped driving because of narcolepsy	4%

Source: Parkes, J.D. The sleepy driver. In: *Driving and Epilepsy and Other Causes of Impaired Consciousness.* Godwin-Austen, R.B. & Espir, M.L.E. (eds.) London: Royal Society of Medicine (1983) 25.

BIOCHEMICAL FINDINGS IN NARCOLEPSY

Blood
There are no constant abnormal findings in the blood. *Polycythaemia, low 17-ketosteroid levels,* decrease in circulating noradrenaline, lymphocytosis[169] and an increase in *blood sugar*[71, 166] are occasionally found. Blood gas changes with mild *hypoxia* and *hypercapnia*[53] may result from sleep apnoea, not narcolepsy. Isolated *thyrotropin* deficiency has been reported in a single patient.[151] Serum *melatonin* concentration during night sleep is unremarkable.[52] Frequent short sleep periods throughout the day and fragmented night sleep result in disturbance of the normal pattern of sleep-onset *GH release* over a 24 h period, but usually the total amount of GH released over 24 h is normal.[49, 186, 187, 201]

Urine
There is no constant abnormality in urinary catecholamine content. Gunne and Lidvall[97] found the urinary output of dopamine, adrenaline and catecholamine metabolites was normal, but the noradrenaline excretion was high (controls 18 µg/24 h, narcoleptic patients 31 µg/24 h) in six narcoleptics. Ishiguro *et al.*[107] likewise found high noradrenaline but also high dopamine with low homovanillic acid urinary excretion in narcoleptics.

Cerebrospinal fluid
Rennert[164] reported raised CSF pressure, and in 25% of cases found a mild lymphocytosis in the CSF. In a quarter of Roth's cases of idiopathic narcolepsy, a slight increase in lymphocyte count or protein content was present in the CSF.[171] In a small number of narcoleptics there is a rise in CSF immunoglobulin concentration and also oligoclonal bands.

Changes in the CSF monoamine content are inconstant or small.[89, 145, 155] Gunne and Lidvall[97] found normal CSF 5-HIAA levels, although other authors have found the concentration of this 5-HT metabolite raised. In normal subjects, CSF 5-HT levels are very low, sometimes below the detection limit of the assay, whilst dopamine, noradrenaline and adrenaline concentrations are very variable. Montplaisir *et al.*[142] reported that narcoleptics and other hypersomniac patients had low concentrations of dopamine and of the tryptamine metabolite indole acetic acid in the CSF, although the concentration of 5-HIAA was raised. Thal and Sharpless[189] have criticized many of the observations on the biogenic amine content of the CSF in narcolepsy. The results are influenced by very many factors; age, sex, presence of other clinical conditions, time of day, technique of lumbar puncture and position of the patient, degree of previous activity prior to puncture, sample manipulation, storage temperature, as well as the method used for chemical determination.

The basal metabolic rate has been reported to be normal in narcolepsy by Wilson[204] and Roth[171]. Hypertension was recorded by Redlich[163] in narcolepsy, but this is not usual in untreated patients or in those on conventional doses of central nervous system stimulant drugs.

CEREBRAL BLOOD FLOW IN NARCOLEPSY

Regional cerebral blood flow changes with sleep in normal subjects. There is a marked reduction of hemispheric grey matter blood flow during state 1–2 NREM sleep and a greater reduction of brain stem and cerebellar blood flow. In REM sleep these changes are reversed, with a two-fold increase in brain stem blood flow above normal values.[179] The pattern of cerebral blood flow throughout the night is altered in narcolepsy, with an increase rather than decrease in hemispheric grey matter blood flow in early night sleep. This may be due, at least in part, to the early onset of REM sleep, and also to the effect of previous treatment, since methylphenidate increases cerebral blood flow both sleeping and waking.[78, 179]

SLEEP STUDIES IN NARCOLEPTICS

The nocturnal sleep of narcoleptics shows: (1) a short sleep latency; (2) sleep onset REMs or short latency REMs; (3) increase in stage 1 and decrease in stage 3–4 NREM sleep; (4) a normal amount of REM sleep; (5) frequent movement; (6) poor periodicity of REM–NREM cycles; (7) numerous nightmares.[140, 141, 165]

The mean *24 h total sleep time* including day naps in narcoleptics is slightly higher than in age-matched control subjects. The total sleep time and the average REM episode length during the night slowly declines with advancing age in narcoleptics as in normal subjects.[50]

Laboratory studies confirm the clinical observation that 70–80% of subjects with narcolepsy–cataplexy have *restless fragmented night sleep*. Waking after the onset of night sleep is more common in narcoleptics than in controls and increases with the progression of the disease and in elderly subjects. Usually many short periods of wakefulness occur each night. However, total nocturnal sleep time is not usually greatly reduced.

Sleep myoclonus is found in up to half of all narcoleptics[167, 172] and obstructive central and mixed *sleep apnoeic episodes* are more common in narcoleptics than in non-narcoleptics.[42, 61, 75, 120, 157] Guilleminault and Dement[95] found unequivocal sleep apnoea in 10 subjects with narcolepsy and Rosa et al.[167] in six of 28 narcoleptics.

The number and duration of day sleep episodes is best assessed by continuous polygraphic recordings. Hishakawa *et al.*[100] showed that narcoleptics fall asleep in the daytime with a shorter latency and spend more time asleep than controls. The multiple sleep latency test (MSLT) used as an index of daytime drowsiness indicates that most narcoleptics fall asleep in under 5 min when lying down in a quietened room as compared with periods of 10–20 min in normal subjects. Likewise, many narcoleptics find it extremely difficult to stay awake and REM sleep episodes during attempts to maintain wakefulness are of value in diagnosis.[59]

SLEEP ONSET REM IN NARCOLEPSY

Documentation of sleep-onset REM episodes during nocturnal sleep is highly diagnostic of narcolepsy but only in the absence of sleep disturbance related to medication use or drug withdrawal, any other sleep disorder, or previous disruption of the sleep–wake schedule. Although most narcoleptics have REM periods within 10–15 min of nocturnal sleep onset, some do not. Mosko *et al.*[144] have noted that approximately one in five of all narcoleptics have an unusually long (over 150 min) REM sleep latency. This is sometimes related to the occurrence of other sleep disorders, particularly sleep-related leg movements, in narcolepsy.

Sleep onset REM (SOREM) periods in narcolepsy were first described by Vogel[198] and confirmed by Rechtschaffen *et al.*[162] and by Takahashi and Jimbo.[185] SOREM periods occur during day naps less commonly than at the start of night sleep, but the tendency for day sleep periods to begin with REM activity increases throughout the day. Overall in a single recording night at least one SOREM episode occurs in 50% or more of all subjects with narcolepsy and cataplexy. This figure rises to 75% and 85% with two and three recording nights respectively. With additional day nap recordings, SOREM periods can be found in over 95% of all subjects with narcolepsy.[167] In a study at Stanford, SOREM periods occurred 39 out of 48 times in 23 patients with narcolepsy–cataplexy and all patients had at least one positive recording.[212] However, others have found a somewhat lower frequency of SOREM periods in narcoleptics. These are most common with short sleep periods, in home circumstances before the first consolidated night sleep period begins, and if the patient is examined lying down rather than sitting up or in an uncomfortable posture.[58, 171] SOREM periods in narcoleptics are usually brief and are not accompanied by penile tumescence, although the total nocturnal penile tumescence time and amount of tumescence simultaneous with REM sleep across the night is normal.[188]

Most narcoleptics, because of frequent sleep attacks and sleep onset REM activity, have many more REM periods over 24 h than normal subjects during an 8 h sleep period, although there is not a large overall excess of total 24 h REM time.[137] The mistiming of REM sleep results in a bimodal, rather than the normal unimodal, distribution of REM peaks in the first third of night sleep in narcoleptics. However, the circadian peak of REM sleep at around 0300–0700 occurs at the same time in narcoleptics as in normal subjects.

DIAGNOSIS OF NARCOLEPSY

The diagnosis of narcolepsy depends on an accurate history more than on polygraphic studies. Narcolepsy can be separated from normal everyday variation in alertness by the repeated occurrence of sleep attacks and the unusual circumstances in which they occur. Not all patients are constantly sub-alert and the pattern of waking, tired or refreshed, is not of diagnostic value. Cataplexy and sleep paralysis must be distinguished from epilepsy, other causes of atonia and sometimes periodic paralysis. When, as occasionally occurs, automatic behaviour is the presenting symptom of narcolepsy, initial diagnosis is difficult. Minor symptoms, disturbed night sleep, muscle twitching, paraesthesiae as a prelude to sleep spells, loss of muscle tone, double vision accompanying cataplexy, or sweating and hypoglycaemia with amphetamine treatment may confuse the diagnosis. Dream timing, rather than dream frequency or nature, is important. The finding of a positive family history may help to confirm the diagnosis.

Polysomnographic studies will confirm the diagnosis of narcolepsy, but may need to be repeated several times before REM activity within 10 min of falling asleep is shown. A single negative EEG study by day or night does not exclude the diagnosis of narcolepsy. Also, the finding of a short sleep latency does not necessarily confirm the diagnosis of narcolepsy for there are many other causes of excessive daytime drowsiness.

A few patients feign a history of narcolepsy in order to obtain amphetamines. The history may sound convincing, but previous records or relative interview may reveal the truth. When in doubt, polysomnographic studies must be done and drug supplies should always be limited to one source.

ANIMAL NARCOLEPSY

Two breeds of dogs, Labrador retrievers and Doberman pinschers, have been identified at Stanford with a condition very similar, if not identical to narcolepsy–cataplexy in man. These animals transmit narcolepsy to their offspring through a presumed autosomal recessive mechanism.[82] Narcolepsy has also been found in other dog and animal species (the poodle, the corgi and the horse), although the genetic mechanism is not well defined in these animals.[72, 116] Cases in Siamese cats have little resemblance to the human condition.

Narcoleptic dogs have frequent drowsiness – light sleep on EEG recordings – and also have sleep-onset REM periods (possibly a normal characteristic in some animal species). They also have attacks of paralysis and loss of muscle tone. During these, dogs, like man, can blink and make following eye movements.

Foutz et al.[83] described a continuously sleepy Shetland–Welsh cross female pony with cataplexy caused by excitement and petting, but, unlike dogs, not by food. Cataplexy started 2–3 days after birth, with focal attacks involving forelimbs and generalized attacks when the pony lay on her side with flaccid limbs for a few seconds to over 10 min. The EEG at this stage showed a desynchronized pattern. Methylphenidate 20 mg i.v. abolished narcolepsy and cataplexy, and imipramine 100 mg i.v. abolished cataplexy but not narcolepsy. Physostigmine 10 mg i.v. made cataplexy worse.

Biochemical studies suggest a possible defect of serotonin and catecholamine turnover in the cerebrospinal fluid in narcoleptic poodles[79] but not in narcoleptic Doberman pinschers.[135] In the brain of genetically narcoleptic Doberman pinschers, an increase in dopamine and the dopamine metabolite 3,4-dihydroxyphenylacetic acid but not of homovanillic acid has been demonstrated. The ratio of homovanillic acid to dopamine in the caudate nucleus is reduced and the dopamine content in the amygdala and brain stem reticular formation nuclei is increased.[135] These results may indicate a focal depression of dopamine utilization, turnover, or both.

Narcolepsy and cataplexy respond to amphetamine and tricyclic drugs respectively in both animals and man, although there are species differences in the responses to some cholinergic and anticholinergic drugs, which in the doses investigated affect cataplexy in animals, but not in man. *Clomipramine* is successful in the prevention of cataplexy in dogs, horses and man. In dogs, increase in central cholinergic activation by *physostigmine* and *arecoline* increases the number of attacks of cataplexy by around 200–300%, whilst muscarinic blockade with *atropine* and *scopolamine* reduces the frequency of cataplexy. *Nicotine* and the nicotinic-blocking drug *mecamylamine* are ineffective in dogs.[73] Delashaw *et al.* showed that drugs that do not cross the blood-brain barrier (e.g. *atropine methylnitrite, neostigmine*) do not affect cataplexy in dogs. Anticholinergic drugs, in the comparatively low doses that have been investigated, do not prevent cataplexy in man.[191] However, the anticholinesterase drug physostigmine elicits early onset REM sleep in normal humans[182] and carbachol introduced directly into the pons elicits a state similar to cataplexy in cats.[139]

Blockade of noradrenaline re-uptake with the drug *nisoxetine* suppresses cataplexy in dogs.[81] This drug, like tricyclics,[110] will suppress REM sleep[183] but has not been investigated in human cataplexy.

THEORIES AS TO THE CAUSE OF NARCOLEPSY

In the past narcolepsy has been considered to be due to epilepsy;[66, 161, 190] to be associated with psychiatric disorders;[55] to be due to structural brain disease (here we have confusion with symptomatic narcolepsy); to be related to one normal extreme of vigilance level;[209] and to result from diabetes in lethargic American negroes.[166]

PHYSIOLOGICAL MECHANISMS

Is narcolepsy due to circadian mistiming?

The general consensus is that narcolepsy is a disorder of sleep, and despite disturbed REM sleep timing is not a primary disorder of circadian mechanisms. Temporal peaks and nadirs of REM sleep, temperature and hormonal rhythms are not greatly disturbed in narcolepsy[143] and the abnormal temporal pattern of growth hormone secretion over 24 h is likely to be the consequence of sleep attacks, and not due to a primary disorder of circadian timekeeping. It seems unlikely that day naps and lowered vigilance are simply the consequence of REM sleep mistiming, and neither the night sleep fragmentation nor the frequent nocturnal arousals that occur in narcoleptics will account entirely for daytime drowsiness or cataplexy.

Is narcolepsy a disorder of reticular activation?

Sours[184] considered that narcolepsy was due to a pathophysiological disorder of the reticular activating system resulting in lowered vigilance and microsleeps by day. In contrast, because of REM sleep mistiming and frequent REM sleep episodes, Mitchell and Dement[137] suggested that narcolepsy was due to overactivity of the REM system. Cataplexy and sleep paralysis occur largely, if not only, in relation to REM sleep periods.[99] Underactivity of the reticular activating system might result in overactivity of REM systems. The correct conclusion is surely that cataplexy, sleep paralysis and also hypnagogic hallucinations are manifestations of partial REM sleep in which only some of the physiological consequences of this sleep stage appear. The muscle atonia of cataplexy and sleep paralysis are probably mediated by the same brain stem mechanisms and the same descending pathways as mediate the generalized atonia of normal REM sleep.

What is the cause of cataplexy?

Mitler[138] considered three possible neurophysiological explanations for the motor inhibition of cataplexy: (1) that it resulted from loss of fusimotor fibre activity; (2) that it was due to abnormal high frequency PGO wave-like phasic presynaptic volleys; or (3) that it was due to tonic, REM-sleep-like, post-synaptic inhibition, mediated by a cortico-bulbar-spinal inhibitory pathway.

There are some experimental data which suggest that a shut-down of the fusimotor gamma fibre system occurs during REM sleep. Kubota and Tanaka,[119] recording from gamma motor neurones in the ventral horn, found evidence of deactivation of the gamma efferent system in REM sleep, and Gassel and Pompeiano[84] obtained evidence of depression of the gamma system during sleep by contrasting the electrically induced H tibial nerve reflex with the mechanically induced Achilles tendon reflex. They showed that the second was markedly more reduced than the first in REM sleep.

There is no support for the second idea, that PGO waves occur in train throughout cataplexy, in either animals or man.[138]

The third possibility, that of anterior horn cell inhibition mediated by a descending cortico-bulbar-spinal inhibitory pathway during cataplexy, seems likely and would account for the loss of H reflexes during cataplexy, due to increase in inhibition at the anterior horn cell.[56, 92, 101, 103] The latency of motor response to electrical cortical stimulation in humans during cataplexy is normal (Dick, personal communication), and by this criterion the pyramidal pathway remains functional.

PATHOLOGICAL MECHANISMS

Is narcolepsy a biochemical or immunological disorder?

The familial incidence of narcolepsy and the firm association with major histocompatibility antigens shows that narcolepsy must have a genetic and probably a neurochemical or immunological basis. If narcolepsy is due to a *biochemical error* affecting the reticular activating system and REM sleep mechanisms, real clues as to the nature of this are few.

The exaggeration of the normal association between a large carbohydrate meal and sleep in narcolepsy may indicate an error of *carbohydrate metabolism* or may result from a non-specific reduction in arousal threshold. Amphetamine increases cerebral glucose oxidative metabolism. Low glutamate and aspartate levels occur in the cerebrospinal fluid of narcoleptics.[155] Both these amino acids occur in high concentration in the cerebral enzyme glucose-6-phosphatase. This is one of the few enzymes so far characterized in which activity varies with sleep.[43]

The possibility that narcolepsy–cataplexy is due to a defect of *neurotransmitter monoamine systems* in the brain has been closely examined. Most of the evidence for this view is indirect, based on a study of neurotransmitter mechanisms involved in sleep in animals, and on a study of the mode of action of antinarcoleptic and anticataplectic drugs in animals and man. The initiation and maintenance of sleep and of REM sleep in animals is critically dependent on the balance between catecholamine, serotonin and acetylcholine neurone activity in the pontine areas of the brain stem,[102, 178] although other neurotransmitter systems have been little studied. The stimulant action of amphetamine and the anticataplectic action of tricyclic drugs has been attributed to enhancement of catecholamine mechanisms, and to anticholinergic (or 5-HT) effects respectively, but other possibilities have been neglected. Certainly direct amine precursors (levodopa, 1-DOPS and 5-HTP), as well as physostigmine and atropine, have at best only minor effects on sleep, narcolepsy and cataplexy in man. In contrast to the stimulant effect of amphetamines, the hypnotic effect of benzodiazepines may be entirely independent of catecholamine mechanisms. Benzodiazepine hypnosis is reversed by amphetamines, but also by the calcium re-entry antagonist nifedipine as well as by ß-carboline benzodiazepine antagonists, which have different pharmacological effects from the amphetamines.[45, 114, 133, 134]

The involvement of other neurotransmitter mechanisms in narcolepsy remains to be explored. There are at least 20 different amino acid and *peptide neurotransmitters* present within a very small area of the pontine tegmentum. The secret of narcolepsy may lie here.

Narcolepsy is associated with a major histocompatibility antigen DR_2 found otherwise in association with diseases considered to have an autoimmune component (multiple sclerosis and Goodpasture's syndrome). There is no definite pathological marker in the brain or firm disease association to suggest that any immune mechanism may be operant in narcolepsy, although the association with the antigen DR_2 is surprisingly tight. Cataract, glaucoma, familial tremor, multiple sclerosis, oculomotor palsies, lymphoma, polycythaemia, myotonic dystrophy, acromegaly and diabetes have all occasionally been described in association with apparent narcolepsy, but in some of these instances 'narcolepsy' is due to sleep apnoea, and both the HLA status and involvement of immune mechanisms in many of these disorders is uncertain. However, a more definite indication of possible immunological mechanisms in narcolepsy is given by the finding of Rennert[164] and Roth[171] of an increase in protein content and mild lymphocytosis in the CSF of up to a quarter of all subjects with idiopathic narcolepsy.

The HLA locus has consistently misled its investigators, but the antigen DR has a widespread distribution throughout the brain, and may be an important functional component of the sleep–wake system. If so, the presence of DR_2 within the brain may itself determine the occurrence of narcolepsy. Since only 1 in 500–1000 of all DR_2-positive subjects develops narcolepsy, an additional component is required. This may be specific antigenic determinant (epitope) on the DR_2 molecule itself or one in close linkage disequilibrium with DR. Alternatively, in those cases in which narcolepsy has a sudden onset, sometimes with a prodromal illness, environmental contact with a foreign DR_2-related molecule, or virus infection that results in the expression of normally absent brain antigens, may trigger the disease.

Both genetic and environmental factors are involved in narcolepsy. In cases of so-called 'primary' narcolepsy, and occurring without any obvious environmental cause, the genetic predisposition to the disease is probably the primary determinant factor. However, in so-called 'secondary' narcolepsy (see below: as, for example, when narcolepsy–cataplexy follows encephalitis lethargica, pp. 81, 311), the main determinant may be viral or other infection occurring in a genetically susceptible person. Although the distinction between 'primary' and 'secondary' narcolepsy is clinically important, as discussed below, the division is probably artificial, and in reality all cases of typical narcolepsy–cataplexy are examples of one illness.

SECONDARY NARCOLEPSY

The term 'narcolepsy' is used nowadays to denote quite unequivocally 'idiopathic' narcolepsy.[224] The case for 'secondary' narcolepsy (Table 6.12), i.e. narcolepsy with cataplexy or sleep paralysis, due to definite disease of the brain, has been poorly presented and its authenticity is doubtful.[265] In almost all instances the sleep disturbance is highly atypical or not the presenting feature, and the presence or nature of cataplexy is open to doubt. In all early cases there are no sleep studies and no information on sleep latency or the possible occurrence of sleep-onset REM activity. The usual clinical picture is very different from that of narcolepsy. A further problem is raised by the very long latency, often several years, between the initial illness and the subsequent development of narcolepsy.[259] Only a handful of post mortem reports on these cases are available.[219, 232, 252, 272] In a survey of 34 patients over 20 years Bonduelle and Degos[224] could only find two examples of what they considered to be authentic symptomatic narcolepsy.

Table 6.12. *Examples of so-called 'secondary' narcolepsy*

Encephalitis
   Encephalitis lethargica[269]
   Polioencephalitis[252]
   Encephalitis or para-infectious illness in childhood[233]
Head injury[224, 228, 233, 259]
Cerebral tumour
   3rd ventricle[232]
   Brain stem[217, 265]
   Cerebellum[271]
   Frontal lobe (tuberculoma)[246]
Extracerebral tumour
   Salivary tumour[260]
Cerebrovascular disease
   Vertebrobasilar ischaemia[250]
   Brain stem infarction[272]
   Polycythaemia[247]
Multiple sclerosis[220, 229]
Metabolic and endocrine diseases (obesity, diabetes, hypoglycaemia, acromegaly, diabetes
   insipidus)[224, 256]

Many early reports of apparent 'symptomatic' narcolepsy include descriptions of hypersomnia, stupor, coma or rapid recovery and the presence of cataplexy is often doubtful. We can neglect most, if not all of these accounts.[215, 230–232, 235, 236] At present, about 20% of all patients initially investigated for narcolepsy turn out to have a different condition, usually sleep apnoea or very rarely a structural lesion.[225, 239, 259, 264, 273] Heyck and Hess[239] classified seven of 30 narcoleptics under a symptomatic heading, and Roth[259] listed 51 cases of symptomatic narcolepsy due to encephalitis or head injury, but in many of these instances the difference in presentation from true narcolepsy is considerable.

NARCOLEPSY AND CEREBRAL TUMOURS

Pineal tumours,[216] hypothalamic tumours,[232] third ventricular tumours and cysts[231] and upper brain stem gliomas[217, 265] have all been associated with narcolepsy. The pathology is very diverse, with emphasis on infiltrating rather than focal lesions. Lymphomas, microgliomas, glioblastomas are reported much more frequently than discrete focal tumours as causes of symptomatic narcolepsy. A few of these examples have a superficial resemblance to idiopathic narcolepsy; the patient described by Anderson and Salmon[217] had sleep paralysis and cataplexy due to a microglioma which infiltrated the walls and floor of the third ventricle and the upper brain stem with marked involvement of the locus coeruleus. Stahl *et al.*[265] described a patient with narcolepsy, cataplexy and sleep paralysis accompanying a glioblastoma of the rostral brain stem and hyothalamus. The patient had near-continuous cataplexy with fluctuation in tone and posture accompanied by marked variability in H reflex. This changed in amplitude and was sometimes completely abolished accompanying attacks of cataplexy, which occurred every few seconds. Narcolepsy and cataplexy responded to methylphenidate and clomipramine in this patient.

The association of narcolepsy with tumours outside the upper brain stem and posterior hypothalamus is very doubtful. In a famous French narcoleptic, an agricultural labourer called in his village 'Pierre le dormeur', removal of a cerebellar haemangioblastoma 28 years after the onset of narcolepsy did not affect his sleepiness.[271] Perhaps polycythaemia secondary to the cerebellar tumour (the RBC was 5.9 million) may have increased the severity of idiopathic narcolepsy. There seem to be very few exceptions to the general rule that hemisphere lesions do not cause narcolepsy. Bonduelle and Degos[224] point out that virtually the only example of this is the case of Leychelle et al.,[246] a 63-year-old man who complained of sudden attacks of irresistible sleep which became more and more frequent and were associated with a tuberculoma of the right frontal lobe. However, the subject did not have cataplexy. An example of a tumour outside the brain associated with possible narcolepsy (a mixed salivary tumour situated near the carotid sheath in the right tonsillar fossa) was described by Schlager and Meier.[260]

NARCOLEPSY, ENDOCRINE AND METABOLIC DISEASE

Secondary narcolepsy has been attributed to most endocrine disorders as well as many metabolic diseases. Lack of precision in terminology and confusion of narcolepsy with sleep apnoea accounts for most, if not all, of these reports. Cases with identical symptomatology to idiopathic narcolepsy, associated with intoxication (e.g. two cases of narcolepsy with mercury poisoning and isoniazid respectively[258]) present greater difficulty.

Diabetes insipidus is sometimes described as an accompaniment of narcolepsy. Most, if not all, of these subjects do not have typical narcolepsy, but drowsiness in association with a hypothalamic tumour, syphilis or a vascular lesion, extreme obesity, and sleep apnoea.[224, 255] Narcolepsy has often been described in association with acromegaly, but here drowsiness is probably due to sleep apnoea. There are several accounts of hypersomnia or lethargy (but not real narcolepsy) with either diabetes or hypoglycaemia. Although these may result in drowsiness or stupor, few would go as far as Roberts[256] in attributing a near-epidemic of 'narcolepsy' in Florida negroes to 'functional hyperinsulinism'. Indeed there is some evidence that hypoglycaemia will cause improvement in narcolepsy. Smith and Schneider[263] showed in five patients with narcolepsy–cataplexy that insulin-induced hypoglycaemia resulted in a decrease in drowsiness.

Eating causes sleeping in normal subjects as well as in narcoleptics. Many different foods, not only sugar, will promote sleep.[266] This normal tendency is increased in narcolepsy; excessive postprandial drowsiness, sleep attacks during meals, even sleep regularly provoked by eating a small amount of a specific food, are characteristic of narcolepsy.[243, 274] Suwa and Toru[268] reported a patient with periodic somnolence whose sleep was induced by glucose. Bell[218] was so impressed by these data that she determined the eating habits of narcoleptics to see if their diet was in any way unusual and could account for their excess sleepiness. She found that some narcoleptics claimed that sleepiness was notably reduced whenever they reduced their sugar to lose weight; and a few reported compulsive eating and a craving for sweet foods.[218] However, the appetite of narcoleptics not on tricyclic drugs for cataplexy is usually normal.

MYXOEDEMA AND SLEEP

Myxoedema does not cause narcolepsy but may produce hypersomnolence, torpor, apathy, stupor or coma. The lowered alertness is accompanied by a slowing of EEG rhythms with prominent 5–7 Hz activity and a diminished response to photic stimulation. These changes are all reversed by thyroid treatment.[257] Hypersomnolence in myxoedema is sometimes, but not always, associated with sleep apnoea. Opposite sleep changes occur in hyperthyroidism, where Passouant et al.[251] found an increase in sleep latency, reduction in total sleep time to 5 or 6 h and less stage 3–4 NREM sleep than normal.

ENCEPHALITIS LETHARGICA AND NARCOLEPSY

Wilder, writing in 1928, considered that encephalitis lethargica accounted for 20% of all cases of narcolepsy. Today most physicians have never seen this association and Bonduelle and Degos[224] criticize much of the evidence presented in favour of the diagnosis of post-encephalitic narcolepsy in the literature from 1917 onwards.[215] In at least some instances, the simultaneous pandemic of influenza rather than the epidemic of encephalitis may have been responsible for so-called narcolepsy.

The evidence for encephalitis is often ill-founded and the diagnosis of narcolepsy uncertain. However, encephalitis lethargica was extremely pleomorphic with different clinical features from year to year and between different countries. There is no doubt of the authenticity of post-encephalitic narcolepsy in a few cases of encephalitis lethargica, with a typical history of acute illness, ocular signs, mood and mental changes, parkinsonism within a year of illness, oculogyric crises, and then late appearance of narcolepsy–cataplexy. Unlike post-encephalitic parkinsonism, however, post-encephalitic narcolepsy usually slowly improved (see pp. 81–83).

The frequency of true post-encephalitic narcolepsy has been exaggerated. The condition was uncommon. Many cases of encephalitis lethargica coming to post mortem had severe neuronal loss in the central tegmental field and virtual total destruction of the locus coeruleus without any report of narcolepsy or other sleep disturbance during life.

NARCOLEPSY AND SYPHILIS

Bonduelle and Degos[224] could find only two accounts of the possible association between narcolepsy and syphilis: that of Foix et al.[230] of a patient with syphilis, diabetes insipidus and a bitemporal hemianopia, in which narcolepsy improved, although polyuria did not, with treatment for syphilis; and that of Guillain and Alajouanine[236] in which syphilis caused a state reminiscent of encephalitis lethargica, improving with treatment.

VASCULAR NARCOLEPSY

Brain stem cerebrovascular disease may cause persistent hypersomnia or insomnia, but not true narcolepsy–cataplexy. There are remarkably few reports of 'narcolepsy' following brain stem infarction[272] or occurring as a symptom of cerebrobasilar ischaemia.[250] Roth[258] attributed narcolepsy in only three instances to cerebrovascular disease. Age, evidence of vascular pathology and response to treatment differentiate these cases from true narcolepsy. Niedermeyer et al. described a 56-year-old physician with attacks of sudden daytime sleeping who 10 months later experienced intermittent double vision, slurred speech and vertigo. Cranial arteriography showed marked tortuosity of the basilar artery with ectasia of major arteries. An electroencephalogram was abnormal with recurrent generalized bursts of high-voltage activity. This patient's symptoms were ascribed to vertebrobasilar insufficiency, and on treatment with aspirin attacks stopped.

Sudden sleep attacks are not a characteristic feature of multi-infarct dementia, although in the daytime recordings of patients with advanced cerebrovascular disease abrupt changes from the waking state to stage 2 sleep may be noted, with frequent short NREM sleep stretches.[149]

POST-TRAUMATIC NARCOLEPSY

The reality of narcolepsy following head injury is in doubt. Many cases of post-traumatic narcolepsy described during and after the First World War seem to be mainly, if not entirely, examples of battle neurosis, post-traumatic epilepsy or hypersomnia. Other instances with gradual or late development of hypersomnolence after head injury have little resemblance to narcolepsy or may have been due to unrecognized hydrocephalus. However, Roth[258] described 22 cases of post-traumatic narcolepsy and Bonduelle et al.[222, 223] considered that a man who developed narcolepsy, cataplexy and hypnagogic hallucinations 5 years after a severe head injury was an authentic example of secondary narcolepsy.

NARCOLEPSY AND MULTIPLE SCLEROSIS

There is no doubt of the occurrence of narcolepsy and cataplexy in unequivocal cases of multiple sclerosis.[220, 228, 229, 239, 261, 262, 275] However, it is exceptional for the statistics of multiple sclerosis to include narcolepsy among the many possible manifestations of the disease. In some cases of multiple sclerosis[229] narcolepsy presents at an unusually late age and may regress, in keeping with the hypothesis that multiple sclerosis is the underlying cause, not a chance association. In other instances, narcolepsy–cataplexy may precede the onset of multiple sclerosis by over a decade[248] and it seems probable that here the association is due to chance. Post mortem examination has shown the presence of hypothalamic periventricular plaques in a 39-year-old woman with multiple sclerosis who had isolated sleep episodes but not typical narcolepsy.[226, 235] Polygraphic recording by Schrader et al.[261] in a typical narcoleptic–cataplectic also with multiple sclerosis showed SOREM periods, increase in REM time and disturbed nocturnal sleep.

The explanation for the association between multiple sclerosis and narcolepsy may lie in the overlap of a common genetic determinant for the two conditions, with an increased frequency of HLA B$_7$ and DR$_2$ in both multiple sclerosis[244] and narcolepsy.[221] Thus occasionally the two diseases may concur. The alternative explanation, that brain stem demyelination in multiple sclerosis results in narcolepsy, appears less likely.

EPILEPSY AND NARCOLEPSY (Table 6.13)

Despite Gélineau's statement in his original paper that narcolepsy should be clearly separated from the epilepsies,[234] many authors have associated narcolepsy with epilepsy, impressed by the paroxysmal nature of the attacks, the frequency of auras such as fatigue, vague sensory complaints before sleep episodes and periods of automatic behaviour and cataplexy.[227, 254, 270] Particularly in cataplexy, the stereotyped attacks, loss of muscle tone, facial muscle flickering, tongue protrusion and also daytime hallucinosis may lead to confusion with epilepsy. There are well documented cases of epilepsy and daytime drowsiness occurring in the same individual, and, in rare instances, paroxysmal EEG abnormalities are found in subjects with typical narcolepsy,[254] but in many of these cases epilepsy and sleepiness are linked by a common aetiology, usually trauma,[270] or the drowsiness is due to anti-epileptic drugs. There is no evidence that REM narcolepsy and epilepsy share a common physiological basis, and there is no known genetic link between the two conditions.

SECONDARY CATAPLEXY

Secondary cataplexy, with or without narcolepsy or sleep paralysis, is very rare. Experimental brain lesions at any site do not reliably produce cataplexy in animals, although generalized atonia without PGO spikes or rapid eye movements can be induced by reflex proprioceptive or nocioceptive stimuli in animals with a previous pontine transection at the level of the nucleus

Table 6.13. *Comparison of findings in cataplexy, narcolepsy and epilepsy*

	Cataplexy	Narcolepsy	Epilepsy
Trigger	Laughter	Monotony	Nil
Duration	Seconds	Seconds to hours	Seconds to minutes
Aura	Nil	Nil	Common
Mannerisms, stereotypies	Facial twitches	None	Common
Manipulatory exploratory behaviour	None	None	Common
Repetitive behaviour or vocalization	None	Rare	Common
Hallucinations or illusions	Hypnagogic hallucinations	Hypnagogic hallucinations	Occasional
Depersonalization or familiarity	No	Uncommon	Common
Amnesic episodes	No	Common	Variable
Variability of behaviour from episode to episode	Similar	Some variability	Similar
Episode halted by stimulation	Usual	Common	No
Associated muscle twitching	Yes	Rare	Occasional
Affective changes, resists restraint	No	Rare	Occasional
Post-ictal symptoms, confusion, dysphasia	Sometimes	Rare	Common
EEG findings	Alert – REM	Alert – REM	Specific abnormalities
Drug response	Tricyclic drugs	Amphetamine	Anti-epileptic drugs

reticularis ponto-oralis.[241, 242] Also, electrical stimulation of the descending reticular formation in the medulla will cause atonia.[267] The final common pathway for cataplexy is assumed to involve descending inhibitory and excitatory pathways from the rostral brain stem to the medulla,[240, 253] the inhibitory regions of Magoun and Rhines[249] projecting to the spinal motor neurone.[238] Destruction of the rostral areas of these pathways may have been the anatomical basis for cataplexy in two patients with brain stem lesions (systemic lupus erythematosus: glioma) described by Lascelles *et al.*[245] and Stahl *et al.*[265]

THE KLEINE–LEVIN SYNDROME

In the Indian mythological epic *Rāmāyana*, there is a graphic account of a possible case of the Kleine–Levin syndrome. Kumbhakarna, the younger brother of the demon king Rāvana, used to sleep six months at a stretch, getting up for a short period in which he ate up herds and herds of people and animals and drank an enormous quantity of wine. At this rate, says the epic, he would have consumed all the three worlds within a short period, were he not to be overcome by another long spell of sleep (Plate 2(b)). (Tulsidasa[328] and Prebhakaran *et al.*[318] describe an Indian subject with the Kleine–Levin syndrome.)

Antimoff,[277] Kleine,[301] Lewis[305] and Levin[304] all reported recurring attacks of overeating, drowsiness and anxiety in adolescent boys.

In 1898, J.A. Antimoff reported a youth of 19 who developed a state of drowsiness lasting 7 days, six or eight weeks after being badly frightened by an ill-tempered horse. The patient's own description is available, '. . . deep sleep the entire time. In a dream I see a horse. I am very scared and afraid of everything. My appetite is excellent. I am awake only for meals . . . I sleep deeply during the first two to three days; during the following days I wake frequently and then go to sleep again. Suddenly everything is over.' Similar episodes reappeared every few months and were of variable duration, though the patient ceased to dream about the horse.[287]

In 1925, Kleine, a Frankfurt psychiatrist, described five examples of episodic somnolence, separated by long intervals of normal health. Lewis,[305] in a psychoanalytical study of three problem children, described a boy who, from the age of 10 to 12 had five attacks of sleepiness, weakness, bemusement and gluttony, each lasting 2–12 weeks. In his first attack the boy ate an astonishing amount of raw hamburger steaks. Close observation showed certain peculiarities of behaviour. He would imitate in solitude the antics of Charlie Chaplin. The child's subsequent progress was never traced.[287]

In 1929, Max Levin, a New York psychiatrist, described a 19-year-old patient who showed pathological hunger, together with sleepy attacks. Levin rewrote his original case report in 1936 and drew specific attention to a new syndrome of periodic somnolence and morbid hunger.[304] Critchley and Hoffman[288] introduced the eponymous term Kleine–Levin syndrome to describe this condition.

In 1962, Critchley carried out a detailed analysis of the 15 cases in the literature and added 11 of this own.[287] The main clinical features emphasized by Critchley included the combination of episodic sleep and overeating occurring in adolescent males, with a tendency for recovery to occur eventually. Critchley considered that the overeating was compulsive in nature, and not due to pathological hunger. Fresco et al.[291] reviewed the world literature and found a total of 120 possible examples.

Most of the published case reports do not match the classic description. The initial accounts of the Kleine–Levin syndrome all concerned youths or young men, but since the report of Critchley many cases have been described in women.[289] Billiard et al.[282] found 15 female cases, and Billiard[281] gathered 24 female cases and estimated the male: female ratio at between 4:3 and 4:1. In both sexes atypical examples occur, with late and not adolescent onset, a clear association with menstruation or cyclical depression, the absence of overeating or the presence of very prominent psychiatric features.

Published case reports of Kleine–Levin-like syndromes have included at least four variant syndromes (Table 6.14):

1. a stereotyped functional non-psychiatric disorder with normal physical and mental findings between attacks;

Table 6.14. *The Kleine–Levin syndrome*

Classical form
　Onset in adolescence
　Episodic hypersomnia
　Excessive eating
　Spontaneous recovery (not invariable)
　Male : female ratio 4 : 1 to 4 : 3

Associated features
　Prominent mental and mood changes
　Sometimes hypersexuality in attacks
　Normal mental and physical findings between attacks

Atypical forms
　One or more main symptoms absent

Exclude from diagnosis of Kleine–Levin syndrome
　1. Cases with symptom inversion (e.g. insomnia, not hypersomnia)
　2. Menstrual hypersomnolence
　3. Organic hypothalamic pathology
　4. Psychiatrically determined cases

---

2. a few examples of hypothalamic pathology;
3. menstrual-related hypersomnia, often with cyclical oedema;
4. cyclical depression, with prominent withdrawal, hypersomnia and behavioural alterations.

CLINICAL FEATURES OF THE KLEINE–LEVIN SYNDROME

The Kleine–Levin syndrome is uncommon. The most conspicuous and characteristic symptoms are periodic hypersomnolence and changes in appetite. Behavioural disturbance is inconstant, but usually there is an abnormal mental pattern during attacks with considerable irritability. During each attack, sleep lasts for about 20 h in each 24. The patient is difficult but not impossible to rouse. Spontaneous awakenings do occur as well as arousals to eat, or empty the bladder or rectum. Incontinence is not a feature.

The onset of the Kleine–Levin syndrome in males is usually between the ages of 13 and 18, but onset both earlier (10 years) and later (52 years) has been recorded.

Onset is usually spontaneous, but the condition is sometimes preceded by a feverish illness, stress or overexposure to sunlight. In one patient (case 11 of Critchley), an Arab from Kuwait, attacks came on only in the extremely hot summers of the Persian Gulf.[287] Rosenkotter and Wende[323] observed seven episodes in a single patient, all of which were preceded by a respiratory infection, and Levin[304] reported that, in three of seven patients, symptoms were preceded by fever. Other factors such as drunkenness or seasickness are sometimes implicated.[281]

The start and end of each attack is inconsistent, and may be either rapid or gradual. Each attack lasts from a few days to several weeks (average 5–7 days).

Very prolonged attacks are unusual. One reported episode lasting 52 days seems to have been psychologically determined.[326]

The frequency of attacks is between one every month and one a year. An episode every 6 months is about average, but intervals between attacks are very variable in the same individual.

Between episodes, physical and mental health is entirely normal. There is no relationship between the Kleine–Levin syndrome and epilepsy or other neurological disorder.

The Kleine–Levin syndrome is often thought to be benign and self-limiting with spontaneous recovery in most cases by the age of 30–40 and with no residual sequelae. However, Billiard,[281] in a review of 96 case reports, found that attacks did not cease within the span of follow-up in 43 male subjects (followed up for a mean of 5.6 years) and in 13 female subjects (followed up for up to 9 years). Spontaneous disappearance was verified in 13 male subjects and in six female subjects over follow-up periods from 2 to 4 years. According to Roth, in some cases symptoms never disappear but become permanent.[324]

Familial factors are not important. A mother and son described by Ortiz de Zarate,[313] both with an apparent Kleine–Levin syndrome, were highly atypical, with polyuria and polydypsia.

The mental picture is one of episodic tiredness, lethargy, malaise, irritability and apathy. Immediately before and during each attack a wide range of inappropriate and sometimes bizarre behaviour occurs.[284, 285, 290, 307] There are changes in awareness, speech, mood, cognitive and sexual function. In the great majority of cases, during the attack there is intense irritability and resentment of examination if woken. Grandiose, tearful, disinhibited behaviour is sometimes described, perhaps indicating a frontal component. Speech may be slurred or incoherent, even dysphasic. Disorientation in time and place may be complete, forgetfulness severe and depersonalization is occasionally reported. Dreams, waking fantasies, visual and auditory hallucinations occur, sometimes with a schizophrenic element, as in one of Critchley's patients who felt responsible for all the events of which he was aware, and believed he could stop a clock with his thoughts and control his own hearing and vision.[287] A schizoid behaviour pattern is seen in perhaps a quarter of all attacks.

Mood changes, usually depression or self-disgust, may accompany or follow the attack and last for several days.[322, 329] In two of Gallinek's patients[292–294] severe depression lasted for several weeks after each attack, although the opposite, a period of mood elevation, is also sometimes encountered.[295] Irritability may progress to severe aggression, agitation, frenzy or truculent, noisy, disturbed behaviour, with exhibitionism and inappropriate advances. There is general withdrawal from any social contact and return to bed at the first possible opportunity.

Hypersexuality occurs in a minority of cases, both during and after the attack (23% of male and 20% of females).[281, 316] An army officer cadet, reported by Robinson and McQuillan,[321] masturbated openly, grinning broadly during attacks, but was usually well mannered, quiet and respectful.

Minor features of the attack, occasionally prominent, are headache, sweating and facial congestion. Examination during an attack is usually normal, although pupillary changes, extensor plantar responses, minor reflex abnormalities and nystagmus have all been described.[286] Unexplained fever is reported in between a quarter and a third of all attacks. The temperature increase is usually slight, 0.5–1 °C.

The consumption of unusually large amounts of both raw and cooked foods, sometimes with a voracious appetite, before and during each attack may be very striking. Overeating is often accompanied by considerable and rapid weight increase which may be as great as 5–8 kg. Excessive thirst and polyuria are much less common than compulsive overeating, although a marked diuresis may follow the attack.

On recovery, total or partial amnesia for what has occurred is usual, although disgust at overeating is common and anorexia may persist for some weeks. There may be a short period with depression[293] or sometimes euphoria and sleeplessness.[279, 299, 306, 325]

INVESTIGATIONS IN THE KLEINE–LEVIN SYNDROME

No convincing metabolic or hormonal abnormality has ever been shown and laboratory investigation is usually completely normal, both between and during attacks. Minor changes in urinary ketosteroid excretion may result from alteration in normal circadian patterns of cortisol release, but serum cortisol levels are usually normal with a preserved diurnal rhythm.[298] Glucose tolerance remains normal. Metapyrone–ACTH tests of pituitary function sometimes reveal non-specific abnormalities. The cerebrospinal fluid may show a mild increase in protein content, but is usually normal. The occasional report of a high cerebrospinal fluid 5-HIAA concentration may be due to poor mixing of lumbar and ventricular fluid in drowsy subjects, since the majority of this serotonin metabolite in the lumbar cerebrospinal fluid is derived from spinal, not cerebral, metabolism.

The computerized brain scan findings are usually unremarkable in typical cases.[278]

EEG CHANGES IN THE KLEINE–LEVIN SYNDROME

The EEG between attacks is usually completely normal. A variety of inconstant EEG changes have been reported during sleep attacks.[317] These include:

1. early onset REM periods;[308, 331]
2. decrease in stage 3–4 NREM sleep and also in REM sleep;[327]
3. when REM sleep does occur, frequent interruption by stage 2 NREM sleep and by alpha activity.[302] These EEG abnormalities and in particular early onset REM periods have a superficial resemblance to changes in

endogenous depression.[319] Abnormal respiration has been reported during hypersomnolent attacks, but also during asymptomatic normal periods, and cannot therefore be implicated as the cause of attacks.[303]

4. the multiple sleep latency test during an attack may indicate sleepiness as severe as in narcolepsy or obstructive sleep apnoea.[320]

TREATMENT OF THE KLEINE–LEVIN SYNDROME

Amphetamine has been claimed to reduce the frequency and severity of attacks but does not prevent them altogether.[293] Phenmetrazine and amphetamine both improved the condition of a woman described by Roth[324] but did not shorten the attack duration. Psychotherapy, ECT and neuroleptics are unsuccessful in typical cases. Both MAO inhibitors and tricyclic antidepressant drugs have been tried in cases associated with severe depression.[311] In somewhat atypical cases, seemingly associated with cyclical depression, lithium prophylaxis is sometimes of value. Lithium carbonate 800 mg daily abolished attacks in one patient described by Ogura et al.[309] When lithium was withdrawn, attacks recurred. Abe[276] and Goldberg[296] also reported the successful use of lithium in patients with periodic hypersomnia, but not overeating.

AETIOLOGY OF THE KLEINE–LEVIN SYNDROME

The Kleine–Levin syndrome is generally considered to be a benign functional disorder of limbic or hypothalamic structures, resulting in a combination of appetite and sleep disturbance. The cause is not known. Pai[315] included the Kleine–Levin syndrome amongst the hypersomnias due to neurosis or hysteria, and other attempts have been made to implicate psychosomatic causes.[312] However, although psychiatric features may be prominent during the attack itself, the entirely normal findings between attacks suggest that these are a consequence, rather than a cause, of sleep disturbance. On detailed investigation, small organic lesions in the hypothalamus are sometimes found, or occasionally there is non-specific dilatation of the third ventricle (see, for example Roth,[324] p. 264). The nature of the symptoms, the time of onset at puberty, and the occasional precipitation by fever, heat or light may indicate a disturbance of hypothalamic neurohormonal function, and temperature as well as sleep rhythms are occasionally disturbed.

ATYPICAL CASES OF THE KLEINE–LEVIN SYNDROME

Most case reports of the Kleine–Levin syndrome do not fit the classic description of periodic hypersomnolence and megaphagia occurring in adolescent males and with spontaneous recovery. Fresco et al.[291] in their study of the literature considered that the diagnosis was fully justified in only 58 of 120 published cases. Despite large experience of hypersomnia due to many different causes, some authors report never having seen a typical example of the Kleine–Levin syndrome. Roth found no classic example amongst 569 sleepy patients, but only nine more or less atypical examples with obesity, water retention, depression, amenorrhoea, or evidence of diencephalic damage.[33] Oswald[314] doubted if the syndrome was an independent entity. Some cases have very prominent psychiatric features and are not true examples of the syndrome. Jovanović[300] observed two cases of psychogenic periodic hypersomnia, in one of whom sleep attacks disappeared when the patient received disability payment, only to reappear when he lost them. Occasionally, one component of the syndrome is lacking. Fresco et al.[291] found that 28 of 58 cases of the Kleine–Levin syndrome did not overeat. Rarely, one symptom is replaced by the opposite, e.g. anorexia instead of overeating or insomnia rather than hypersomnia.

The following three case reports illustrate the wide range of problems that may be encountered. (1) Berti Ceroni[280] described a 14-year-old boy who developed hypersomnia and megaphagia lasting 4–5 days after a severe mental shock. The boy recovered but subsequently developed typical narcolepsy–cataplexy with REM sleep onset. (2) Roth[324] described a 32-year-old woman with periodic attacks of hypersomnia, polydipsia and overeating, depression, misery, dependent oedema and mild fever lasting 1–21 days. At first these attacks occurred monthly, but later their frequency increased. At the end of each attack, there was a copious diuresis, weight loss, reduction of appetite and return to normal awareness. (3) Wilder[330] described 30 attacks in a single patient over 30 years. This patient had insomnia, not hypersomnia, with bulimia, polydipsia and disturbed libido. Manic–depressive symptoms were prominent in 20 attacks. Most attacks were short, lasting at most a few weeks, but one lasted for over a year. At the initial presentation a diagnosis of the Kleine–Levin syndrome was considered in all these three cases but modified on subsequent experience to (1) narcolepsy–cataplexy, (2) menstrual narcolepsy, and (3) cyclical bipolar illness.

SLEEP AND THE MENSTRUAL CYCLE

The sleep of normal adult women is different from that of men. Wever[353] showed that under constant conditions and when all external time references were excluded sleep episodes were 1 h 21 min longer in females than in males. In the real world, females between the ages of 20 and 40 go to bed sooner than males, and when elderly go to bed later.[347] Females complain more about their sleep than males.[348] According to Kripke et al.[342] 5.5% of adult men, but 13.6% of adult women report that they suffer from insomnia often or fairly often. The most complaints about their sleep come from middle-aged, non-single females of lower socioeconomic status.[341]

In normal women there is some evidence of minor sleep changes with *the menstrual cycle*, with most stage 3 NREM sleep at the time when oestrogen levels are at a peak, although with no subjective alteration in sleep quality.[333, 339] Hartmann[336, 337] studied the night sleep of women weekly over a 4 month period. REM sleep was lowest during the first two weeks of the menstrual cycle, with an increase towards the middle or end of the cycle. However, Ho[339] and Billiard and Passouant[333] found little alteration in REM sleep at different phases of the menstrual cycle.

The results of sleep studies *in pregnancy* are very variable and often disagree. REM sleep may increase,[350] remain unaltered[340] or decrease (particularly on the first postpartum night). A progressive diminution of stage 4 NREM sleep throughout pregnancy was found by Kurtz *et al.*[343]

Progesterone has been attributed with anaesthetic properties and may induce sleep when given i.v. to both men and women.[349] These authors found that, following a 1 h administration of progesterone 500 mg i.v., sleep occurred in 5–15 min. Heuser[338] gave 200 mg of progesterone 2 h before bedtime and reported that sleep latency was reduced and total sleep time slightly increased. However, physiological changes in progesterone level accompanying the menstrual cycle have not been linked to changes in sleepiness, and in a patient with menstruation-linked hypersomnia described by Sachs *et al.*[352] sleep periods occurred when progesterone levels were low, not high.

Oestrogens have little fundamental effect on sleep, although Billiard and Passouant[333] reported that conjugated oestrogen improved daytime drowsiness in a woman with menstrual-linked hypersomnia. In a similar case reported by Gilligan[335] oestrogen treatment was ineffective and in a further patient with menstrual-related hypersomnia described by Sachs *et al.*[352] oestrogen therapy was only successful when ovulation was inhibited, not otherwise.

Periodic hypersomnia has been linked to *menstruation* since the report of Lhermitte.[344] Lhermitte described a 14-year-old girl who slept deeply for 4 or 5 days beginning the fourth day of her menstrual cycle. When awake the girl overate. The nature of the sleep episode and any possible hormonal disorder were not specified. By 1943 the condition had been described in five or six young girls.[345, 346]

The occurrence of drowsiness at the start of the menstrual cycle has been reported in narcolepsy,[354] essential hypersomnolence[352] and also in the Kleine–Levin syndrome or its variants.[332] Sleep may coincide with ovulatory menstrual cycles that are entirely normal according to hormone analysis and body temperature,[352] or with anovulatory cycles.

About 20 examples of severe menstrual-associated somnolence have now been described, usually in adolescent girls, although the condition may commence later.[351] Overeating or bizarre behaviour are not usually prominent features. In a few examples, the sleep patterns have been relatively or entirely normal, although unusual EEG features have been described in two subjects who had epileptiform discharges during hypersomnolent periods.[334, 352] More usual is the finding of prolonged nocturnal sleep with a diffusely abnormal EEG at the time of waking during attacks, but normal patterns in the interparoxysmal period.[332]

Hypersomnia may cease when ovulation is inhibited by a combination of ethinyloestradiol and lynoestrenol (an oral contraceptive pill).[332, 352] Billiard and his colleagues thought that progesterone triggered the hypersomniac episodes and the beneficial effect of oestrogen in their case was attributed to its inhibitory effect on progesterone secretion.

REFERENCES

DAYTIME DROWSINESS

1. Balter, M.B. & Bauer, M.L. Patterns of prescribing and use of hypnotic drugs in the United States. In: Clift, A.D. (ed.) *Sleep Disturbances and Hypnotic Drug Dependence,* New York: Excerpta Medica (1974) 261–294.
2. Bixler, E.O., Kales, J.D., Scharf, M.B., Kales, A. & Leo, L.A. Incidence of sleep disorders in medical practice: a physician survey. In: Chase, M.H., Mitler, M. & Walter, P.L. (eds.) *Sleep Research, Vol. 5,* Los Angeles: UCLA BIS/BRI (1976) 160.
3. Bixler, E., Kales, A., Soldatos, C., Kales, J. & Healey, S. Prevalence of sleep disorders: A survey of the Los Angeles metropolitan area, *Am. J. Psychiat.* (1979) **136,** 1257–1262.
4. Broughton, R. & Ghanem, Q. The impact of compound narcolepsy on the life of the patient. In: Guilleminault, C., Dement, W.C. & Passouant, P. (eds.) *Narcolepsy,* New York: Spectrum (1976) 201–220.
5. Bruhova, S. & Roth, B. Heredofamilial aspects of narcolepsy and hypersomnia, *Schweiz. Arch. Neurol. Neurochir. Psychiat.* (1972) **110,** 45–54.
6. Coleman, R.M. Diagnosis, treatment and follow-up of about 8000 sleep/wake disorder patients. In: Guilleminault, C. & Lugaresi, E. (eds.) *Sleep/Wake Disorders. Natural History, Epidemiology and Long-Term Evolution,* New York: Raven Press (1983) 87–97.
7. Coleman, R.M., Roffwarg, H.P. & Kennedy, S.J. *et al.* Sleep–wake disorders based on a polysomnographic diagnosis. A national cooperative study, *J. Am. Med. Soc.* (1982) **247,** 997–1003.
8. Coleman, R.M., Zarcone, V.P., Redington, D., Miles, L.E., Dole, K.V., Perkins, W.C., Gananian, M., Moore, B.J., Stringer, J. & Dement, W.C. Sleep–wake disorders in a family practice clinic. In: Chase, M.H., Kripke, D.J. & Walter, P.L. (eds.) *Sleep Research, Vol. 9,* Los Angeles: UCLA BIS/BRI, University of California (1980) 192.
9. Dement, W.C., Carskadon, M.A. & Ley, R. The prevalence of narcolepsy. II. In: Chase, M.H., Stern, W.C. & Walter, P.L. (eds.) *Sleep Research, Vol. 2,* Los Angeles: UCLA BIS/BRI (1973) 147.
10. Dement, W. & Guilleminault, C. Sleep changes in drug dependency; hypersomnia and insomnia – causes, manifestations and treatment. In: Subirana, A., Espadaler, J.M. & Burrows, E.H. (eds.) *10th International Congress of Neurology,* Amsterdam: Excerpta Medica (1973) 42.
11. Detre, T., Himmelhoch, J., Swartzburg, M., Anderson, C.M., Byck, R. & Kupfer, D.J. Hypersomnia in manic–depressive disease, *Am. J. Psychiat.* (1972) **128,** 1303–1305.
12. Guilleminault, C. & Dement, W.C. 235 cases of excessive daytime sleepiness. Diagnosis and tentative classification, *J. Neurol. Sci.* (1977) **31,** 13–27.
13. Guilleminault, C., Phillips, R. & Dement, W. A syndrome of hypersomnia with automatic behaviour, *Electroenceph. Clin. Neurophysiol.* (1975) **38,** 403–413.
14. Hoddes, E., Zarcone, V., Smythe, H. & Dement, W. Quantification of sleepiness: a new approach, *Psychophysiology* (1973) **10,** 431–436.
15. Honda, Y., Asaka, A., Tanimura, M. & Furusho, T. A genetic study of narcolepsy and excessive daytime sleepiness in 308 families with a narcolepsy or hypersomnia proband. In: Guilleminault, C. & Lugaresi, E. (eds.) *Sleep/Wake Disorders: Natural History, Epidemiology and Long-Term Evolution,* New York: Raven Press (1983) 187–199.
16. Honda, Y., Dol, Y., Juji, T. & Satake, M. Narcolepsy and HLA. Positive DR$_2$ as a prerequisite for the development of narcolepsy, *Proc. 6th Annual Meeting of Japanese Society of Biological Psychiatry, Tokyo March 23–24* (1984) 6.

17. Karacan, I., Thornby, J., Anch. M., Holzer, C.E., Warheit, G.L., Schwab, J.J. & Williams, R.L. Prevalence of sleep disturbance in a primarily urban Florida country, *Soc. Sci. Med.* (1976) **10**, 239–244.
18. Kessler, S., Guilleminault, C. & Dement, W.C. A family study of 50 REM narcoleptics, *Acta Neurol. Scand.* (1974) **50**, 503–512.
19. Klimková-Deutschová, E., Macek, Z. & Roth, B. An EEG study of neuroses and pseudoneuroses, *Čas. Lék. Čes.* (1959) **98**, 1213–1218. (in Czech)
20. Kupfer, D.J., Himmelhoch, J.M., Swartzburg, M., Anderson, C., Byck, R. & Detre, T.P. Hypersomnia in manic-depressive disease: a preliminary report *Dis. Nerv. Syst.* (1972) **33**, 720–724.
21. Lavie, P. Sleep habits and sleep disturbances in industrial workers in Israel: main findings and some characteristics of workers complaining of excessive day-time sleepiness, *Sleep* (1981) **4**, 147–158.
22. Michaelis, R. Depressive Verstimmung und Schlafsucht, *Arch. Psychiat. Nervenkr.* (1964) **206**, 345–355.
23. Michaelis, R. Ursachen, klinisches Bild und differential Diagnose der Hypersomnien, *Verhandl inn Med (71 Kongress 1965)*, Munich: J.F. Bergmann (1965) 837–840.
24. Michaelis, R. Zur Typologie der Hypersomnien, *Fortschr. Neurol. Psychiat.* (1965) **33**, 585–599.
25. Mouret, J.R., Renaud, B., Quenin, P., Michel, D. & Schott, B. Monoamines et régulation de la vigilance. 1. Apport et interprétation biochimique des données polygraphiques, *Rev. Neurol.* (1972) **172**, 139–155.
26. Nevšímalová-Bruhová, S. & Roth, B. Heredofamilial aspects of narcolepsy and hypersomnia, *Schweiz. Arch. Neurol. Neurochir. Psychiat.* (1972) **110**, 45–54.
27. Oppel, W.C., Harper, P.A. & Rider, R.V. The age of attaining bladder control, *Pediatrics* (1968) **42**, 614–626.
28. O'Regan, J.B. Hypersomnia and MAOI antidepressants, *Can. Med. Assoc. J.* (1974) **111**, 213.
29. Parkes, J.D. Day time drowsiness, *Lancet* (1981) **2**, 1213–1218.
30. Rechtschaffen, A. & Roth, B. Nocturnal sleep of hypersomniacs, *Activ. Nevr. Sup. (Praha)* (1968) **11**, 229–233.
31. Richardson, G., Carskadon, M., Flagg, W., van der Hoed, J., Dement, W. & Mitler, M. Excessive daytime sleepiness in man: multiple sleep latency measurement in narcoleptic and control subjects, *Electroenceph. Clin. Neurophysiol.* (1978) **45**, 621–627.
32. Roth, B. Functional hypersomnia. In: Guilleminault, C., Dement, W.C. & Passouant, P. (eds.) *Narcolepsy*, New York: Spectrum (1976) 333–351.
33. Roth, B. Narcolepsy and hypersomnia. Review and classification of 642 personally observed cases, *Schweiz. Arch. Neurol. Neurochir. Psychiat.* (1976) **119**, 31–41.
34. Roth, B. Narcolepsy and hypersomnia. In: Williams, R.L. & Karacan, I. (eds.) *Sleep Disorders: Diagnosis and Treatment*, New York: Wiley (1978) 29–59.
35. Roth, B. *Narcolepsy and Hypersomnia*, Basel: Springer Verlag (1980) 1–310.
36. Roth, B., Brůhová, S. & Lehovský, M. REM sleep and NREM sleep in narcolepsy and hypersomnia, *Electroenceph. Clin. Neurophysiol.* (1969) **26**, 172–182.
37. Roth, B. & Nevšímalová, S. Depression in narcolepsy and hypersomnia, *Schweiz. Arch. Neurol. Neurochir. Psychiat.* (1975) **116**, 291–300.
38. Taylor, P.L., Garrick, N.A., Burns, R.S., Tamarkin, L., Murphy, D.L. & Markey, S.P. Diurnal rhythms of serotonin in monkey cerebrospinal fluid, *Life Sci.* (1982) **31**, 1993–1999.
39. Van den Hoed, J., Kraemer, H., Guilleminault, C., Zarcone, V.P., Miles, L.E., Dement, W.C. & Mitler, M.M. Disorders of excessive daytime somnolence: polygraphic and clinical data for 100 patients, *Sleep* (1979) **4**, 23–37.
40. Wyler, A.R., Wilkins, R.J. & Troupin, A.S. Methysergide in the treatment of narcolepsy, *Arch. Neurol.* (1975) **32**, 265–268.

NARCOLEPSY

41. Adie. W.J. Idiopathic narcolepsy: A disease sui generis: with remarks on the mechanism of sleep, *Brain* (1926) **49**, 257–306.
42. Alexiov, A.D. & Roth, B. Some peculiarities of respiration during sleep, *Čs. Neurol. Neurochir.* (1977) **40**, 148–153. (in Czech)

43. Anchors, J.M. & Karnovsky, M.L. Purification of cerebral glucose-6-phosphatase. An enzyme involved in sleep, *J. Biol. Chem.* (1975) **250**, 6408–6416.
44. Anderson, M. & Salmon, M.Y. Symptomatic cataplexy, *J. Neurol. Neurosurg. Psychiat.* (1977) **40**, 186–191.
45. Arvidson, S.B., Eström-Jodal, B., Martinelli, S.A.G. & Niemand, D. Aminophylline antagonises diazepam sedation, *Lancet* (1982) **ii**, 1467.
46. Baraitser, M. & Parkes, J.D. Genetic study of narcoleptic syndrome, *J. Med. Genet.* (1978) **15**, 254–259.
47. Bartels, E.C. & Kuskacioglu, O. Narcolepsy – a possible cause of automobile accidents, *Lahey Clin. Bull.* (1965) **14**, 21–26.
48. Berlucchi, C. Electroencephalographic activity of the isolated hemicerebrum of the cat, *Exp. Neurol.* (1966) **15**, 220–228.
49. Besset, A., Billiard, M., Craste de Paulet, A. & Passouant, P. Correlations between level of alertness and secretion of GH and cortisol during 24 h in 10 narcoleptics, *Electroenceph. Clin. Neurophysiol.* (1977) **42**, 282.
50. Billiard, M., Besset, A. & Cadilhac, J. The clinical and polygraphic development of narcolepsy. In: Guilleminault, C. & Lugaresi, E. (eds.) *Sleep/Wake Disorders: Natural History, Epidemiology and Long-Term Evolution*, New York: Raven Press (1983) 171–185.
51. Billiard, M., Seignalet, J., Besset, A. & Briss, L. Possible association between HLA B7 and narcolepsy, Toronto: *Proceedings Congress on Sleep Research*, May 1984.
52. Birau, N., Meyer, C., Matsubayashi, K. & Meier-Ewert, K.H. Melatonin serum concentration during the nocturnal sleep of narcoleptics, *I.R.C.S. Med. Sci. (Nerv. Syst.)* (1982) **10**, 814.
53. Birchfield, R.L., Sieker, H.O. & Heyman, A. Alterations in blood gases during natural sleep and narcolepsy, *Neurology (Minneap.)* (1958) **8**, 107–112.
54. Bowling, G. & Richards, N.G. Diagnosis and treatment of the narcolepsy syndrome. Analysis of seventy-five case records, *Cleveland Clin. Quart.* (1961) **28**, 38–45.
55. Braffos, O. & Eitinger, L. Psychotic patients with narcolepsy, *Nord. Psykiatr. Tidsskr.* (1963) **17**, 220–226.
56. Broughton, R. Neurology and sleep research, *Can. Psychiat. J.* (1971) **16**, 283–293.
57. Broughton, R. & Ghanem, Q. The impact of compound narcolepsy on the life of the patient. In: Guilleminault, C., Dement, W.C. & Passouant, P. (eds.) *Narcolepsy*, New York: Spectrum (1976) 201–220.
58. Broughton, R. & Mamelak, M. The treatment of narcolepsy–cataplexy with nocturnal gamma hydroxybutyrate, *Can. J. Neurol. Sci.* (1979) **6**, 1–6.
59. Browman, C.P., Gujayarty, K.S., Sampson, M.G. & Mitler, M.M. REM sleep episodes during the maintenance of wakefulness test in patients with sleep apnoea syndrome and patients with narcolepsy, *Sleep* (1983) **6**, 23–28.
60. Browne-Goode, G. Sleep paralysis, *Arch. Neurol. (Chic.)* (1962) **6**, 228–234.
61. Bülov, K. & Ingvar, D.H. Respiration and electroencephalography in narcolepsy, *Neurology* (1963) **13**, 321–325.
62. Caffé, Maladie du sommeil, *J. Connaiss. Méd. Pharmaceut.* (1869) **29**, 323.
63. Carskadon, M.A., Harvey, K., Anders, T. & Dement, W.C. Case report: the development of narcolepsy, *Sleep Res.* (1979) **8**, 174.
64. Cave, H.A. Narcolepsy, *Arch. Neurol. Psychiat. (Chic.)* (1931) **26**, 50–101.
65. Chee, P.H. Ocular manifestations of narcolepsy, *Brit. J. Ophthalmol.* (1968) **52**, 54–56.
66. Comelade, P., Cadilhac, J. & Passouant, P. Temporal epilepsy and narcoleptic seizures, *Rev. Neurol. (Paris)* (1961) **104**, 242–245.
67. Cordeau, J.P. & Mancia, M. Effect of unilateral chronic lesions of the midbrain on the electrocortical activity of the cat, *Arch. Ital. Biol.* (1958) **96**, 374–399.
68. Cordeau, J.P. & Mancia, M. Evidence for the existence of an electroencephalographic synchronization mechanism originating in the lower brain stem, *Electroenceph. Clin. Neurophysiol.* (1959) **11**, 551–564.
69. Dale, R.T. & Langworthy, O.R. The narcoleptic tetrad with spontaneous diplopia and strabismus, *Neurology (Minneap.)* (1964) **14**, 773–775.
70. Daly, D.D. & Yoss, R.E. A family with narcolepsy, *Proc. Mayo Clin.* (1959) **34**, 313–320.
71. Daniels, L.E. Narcolepsy, *Medicine (Baltimore)* (1934) **13**, 1–122.
72. Darke, P.G.G. & Jesson, V. Narcolepsy in a dog, *Vet. Rec.* (1977) **101**, 117–118.
73. Delashaw, J.B., Jr., Foutz, A.S., Guilleminault, C. & Dement, W.C. Effects of pharmacological alterations of acetylcholine on cataplexy in dogs, *Sleep Res.* (1979) **8**, 180.

74. Dell, P. & Puizillout, J.J. Experimental reflex narcolepsy in the cat. In: Guilleminault, C., Dement, W.C. & Passouant, P. (eds.) *Narcolepsy*, New York: Spectrum (1976) 451–472.
75. Dement, W.C. Daytime sleepiness and sleep 'attacks'. In: Guilleminault, C., Dement, W.C. & Passouant, P. (eds.) *Narcolepsy*, New York: Spectrum (1976) 17–42.
76. Dement, W.C., Guilleminault, C. & Mitler, M. Cataplectic attack: polygraphic recording in man and experimental induction in cat, *Neurology* (1973) **23**, 403–404.
77. Dement, W., Zarcone, V., Varner, V., Hoddes, E., Nassau, S., Jacobs, B., Brown, J., McDonald, A., Horan, K., Glass, R., Gonzales, P., Friedman, E. & Phillips, R. The prevalence of narcolepsy, *Sleep Res.* (1972) **1**, 148.
78. Derman, S., Karacan, I., Meyer, J.S. & Sakai, F. Regional cerebral blood flow in narcolepsy, *Sleep Res.* (1979) **8**, 181.
79. Faul, K.F., Barchas, J.D., Foutz, A.S., Dement, W.C. & Holman, R.B. Monoamine metabolite concentrations in the cerebrospinal fluid of normal and narcoleptic dogs, *Brain Res.* (1982) **242**, 137–143.
80. Forbes, C. Narcolepsy, *Lancet* (1894) **1**, 1185.
81. Foutz, A.S., Delashaw, J.B., Jr., Guilleminault, C. & Dement, W.C. Monoaminergic mechanisms and experimental cataplexy, *Ann. Neurol.* (1981) **10**, 369–376.
82. Foutz, A.S., Mitler, M.M., Cavalli-Sforza, L.L. & Dement, W.C. Genetic factors in canine narcolepsy, *Sleep* (1979) **1**, 413–421.
83. Foutz, A.S., Neyman, V. & Dement, W.C. Narcolepsy in equines, *Sleep Res.* (1979) **8**, 186.
84. Gassel, M. & Pompeiano, O. Fusimotor function during sleep in unrestrained cats, *Arch. Ital. Biol.* (1965) **103**, 347–368.
85. Gastaut, M. & Broughton, R. A clinical and polygraphic study of episodic phenomena during sleep, *Rec. Adv. Biol. Psychiat.* (1964) **7**, 197–221.
86. Gelardi, J.A.M. & Brown, J.W. Hereditary cataplexy, *J. Neurol. Neurosurg. Psychiat.* (1967) **30**, 455–457.
87. Gélineau, J.B. De la narcolepsie, *Gaz. Hôp. (Paris)* (1880) **53**, 626–628, 635–637.
88. Gélineau, J.-B.E. *Des peurs maladives ou phobies*, Paris (1894) 74.
89. Gillin, J.C., Horwitz, D. & Wyatt, R.J. Pharmacologic studies of narcolepsy involving serotonin, acetylcholine and monoamine oxidase. In: Guilleminault, C., Dement, W.C. & Passouant, P. (eds.) *Narcolepsy*, New York: Spectrum (1976) 585–603.
90. Gowers, W. *The Borderland of Epilepsy*, London: Churchill (1907) 93.
91. Graves, Observations on the nature and treatment of various diseases, *Dubl. Quart. J. Med. Sci.* (1851) **11**, 1–20.
92. Guilleminault, C. Cataplexy. In: Guilleminault, C., Dement, W.C. & Passouant, P. (eds.) *Narcolepsy*, New York: Spectrum (1976) 125–143.
93. Guilleminault, C. & Anders, T.F. Sleep disorders in children, *Adv. Pediat.* (1976) **23**, 155–174.
94. Guilleminault, C., Billiard, M., Montplaisir, J. & Dement, W.C. Altered states of consciousness in disorders of daytime sleepiness, *J. Neurol. Sci.* (1975) **26**, 377–393.
95. Guilleminault, C. & Dement, W.C. 235 cases of excessive daytime sleepiness, *J. Neurol. Sci.* (1977) **31**, 13–27.
96. Guilleminault, C., Wilson, R.A. & Dement, W.C. A study on cataplexy, *Arch. Neurol.* (1974) **31**, 255–261.
97. Gunne, L.-M. & Lidvall, H.F. The urinary output of catecholamines in narcolepsy under resting conditions and following administration of dopamine, DOPA, and DOPS, *Scand. J. Clin. Lab. Invest.* (1966) **18**, 425–430.
98. Heyck, H. & Hess. R. Zur Narkolepsiefrage: Klinik und Electroenzephalgram, *Fortschr. Neurol. Psychiat.* (1954) **12**, 531–579.
99. Hishikawa, Y. & Kaneko, Z. Electroencephalographic study on narcolepsy, *Electroenceph. Clin. Neurophysiol.* (1965) **18**, 249–259.
100. Hishikawa, Y., Nan'no, H., Tachibana, M., Furuya, E., Koida, M. & Kaneko, Z. The nature of sleep attack and other symptoms of narcolepsy, *Electroenceph. Clin. Neurophysiol.* (1968) **24**, 1–10.
101. Hishikawa, Y., Sumitsuji, N., Matsumoto, K. & Kaneko, Z. H-reflex and EMG of the mental and hyoid muscles during sleep, with special reference to narcolepsy, *Electroenceph. Clin. Neurophysiol.* (1965) **18**, 487–492.
102. Hobson, J.A. Dreaming sleep attacks and desynchronized sleep enhancement. Report of a case of brain stem signs, *Arch. Gen. Psychiat.* (1975) **32**, 1321–1424.
103. Hodes, R. & Dement, W. Depression of electrically induced reflexes (H-reflexes) in man during low voltage EEG 'sleep', *Electroenceph. Clin. Neurophysiol.* (1964) **17**, 617–629.

104. Iijama, S., Wakamatsu, H., Teshima, Y., Sugita, Y. & Hishikawa, Y. Automatic behaviour occurring during the waking state with lowered vigilance in narcoleptics, *Sleep Res.* (1979) **8,** 193.
105. Imlah, N.W. Narcolepsy in identical twins, *J. Neurol. Neurosurg. Psychiat.* (1961) **24,** 158–160.
106. Ingram, W.R., Barris, R.W. & Ranson, S.W. Cataplexy. An experimental study, *Arch. Neurol. Psychiat. (Chic.)* (1936) **35,** 1174–1197.
107. Ishiguro, T., Eto, S. & Suwa, K. Metabolic disorders of monoamine in narcolepsy, *Sleep Res.* (1979) **8,** 194.
108. Janzen, R., Bushart, W. & Wender, G. Hirnbioelektrische Studien und klinische Betrachtungen bei Narkolepsiekranken. In: Jovanovič, U. (ed.) *Der Schlaf,* Munich: J.A. Barth (1969) 207–221.
109. Jovanovič, U.J. Der normale, abnorme und pathologische Schlaf. Polygraphische Untersuchungen, *Verh. Dtsch. Ges. Inn. Med.* Munich: J.F. Bergmann (1965) 807–819.
110. Kannengieser, M.H., Hung, P. & Raynaud, J.P. An *in-vitro* model for the study of psychotropic drugs and as a criterion of antidepressant activity, *Biochem. Pharmacol.* (1973) **22,** 73–84.
111. Keefe, W.P., Yoss, R.E., Martens, T.G. & Daly, D.D. Ocular manifestations of narcolepsy, *Am. J. Ophthalmol.* (1960) **49,** 953–957.
112. Kennedy, A.M. A note on narcolepsy, *Brit. Med. J.* (1929) **1,** 1112–1113.
113. Kessler, S., Guilleminault, C. & Dement, W. A family study of 50 REM narcoleptics, *Acta Neurol. Scand.* (1974) **50,** 503–512.
114. Kleindienst, G. & Usinger, P. Diazepam sedation is not antagonized completely by aminophylline, *Lancet* (1984) **i,** 113.
115. Klemm, W. Neurophysiologic studies on the immobility reflex (animal hypnosis), *Neurosci. Res.* (1971) **4,** 165–212.
116. Knecht, C.D., Oliver, J.E., Redding, R., Selcer, R. & Johnson, G. Narcolepsy in a dog and a cat, *J. Am. Vet. Med. Assoc.* (1973) **162,** 1052–1053.
117. Knott, J.R., Ingram, W.R. & Chiles, W.D. Effects of subcortical lesions on cortical electroencephalogram in cats, *Arch. Neurol. Psychiat. (Chic.)* (1955) **73,** 203–215.
118. Krabbe, F. & Magnussen, G. Familial narcolepsy, *Acta Psychiat. Neurol.* (1942) **17,** 149–173.
119. Kubota, K. & Tanaka, R. The fusimotor activity and natural sleep in the cat, *Brain Res.* (1966) **3,** 198–201.
120. Kuhlo, W. Sleep attacks with apnoea. In: Gastaut, H., Lugaresi, E., Berti Ceroni, G. & Coccagna, G. (eds.) *The Abnormalities of Sleep in Man,* Bologna: Aulo Gaggi (1968) 205–208.
121. Langdon, N., Welsh, K., van Dam, M., Vaughan, R.M. & Parkes, J.D. Genetic markers in narcolepsy, *Lancet* (1984) **ii,** 1178–1180
122. Lascelles, R.G., Mohr, P.D. & Peart, I. Unilateral cataplexy associated with systemic lupus erythematosus, *J. Neurol. Neurosurg. Psychiat.* (1976) **39,** 1023–1026.
123. Levin, M. The pathogenesis of narcolepsy with a consideration of sleep paralysis and localized sleep, *J. Neurol. Psychopath.* (1933) **14,** 1–15.
124. Levin, M. Periodic somnolence and morbid hunger: a new syndrome, *Brain* (1936) **59,** 494–515.
125. Levin, M. Morbid hunger in relation to narcolepsy and epilepsy, *J. Nerv. Ment. Dis.* (1938) **88,** 414–416.
126. Levin, M. Diplopia in narcolepsy, *Arch. Ophthalmol.* (1943) **29,** 942–955.
127. Lhermitte, J. Le sommeil et les narcolepsies, *Prog. Méd.* (1930) **22,** 962–975.
128. Lombard, W.P. (Ref. in de Manacéine[130]) *Am. J. Psychol.* (1888) **1,** 1.
129. Lösner, J. & Zett, W. Angeborene Abduzensparese bei essentieller Narkolepsie, *Psychiat. Neurol. Med. Psychol. (Lpz.)* (1967) **19,** 381–387.
130. de Manacéine, M. In: *Sleep: its Physiology, Pathology, Hygiene and Psychology,* London: Walter Scott (1894) 96.
131. Mankowski, cited in: Devic, M., Aimard, P., Michel, F. & Masquin, N.-O. Étude clinique des narcolepsies – cataplexies essentielles, *Rev. Neurol.* (1967) **116,** 471–490.
132. Maury, Les hallucinations hypnagogiques ou les erreurs des sens dans l'état intermédiaire entre la veille et le sommeil, *Ann. Méd-Psychol.* (1848) **11,** 26–40.
133. Mendelson, W.B., Cain, M., Cook, J.M., Paul, S.M. & Skolnick, P. A benzodiazepine receptor antagonist decreases sleep and reverses the hypnotic action of flurazepam, *Science* (1983) **219,** 414–416.
134. Mendelson, W.B., Owen, C., Skolnick, P., Paul, S.M., Martin, J.V., Ko, G. & Wagner, R. Nifedipine blocks sleep induction by flurazepam in the rat, *Sleep* (1984) **7,** 64–68.

135. Mefford, I.N., Baker, T.L., Boehme, R., Foutz, A.S., Ciaranello, R.D., Barchas, J.D. & Dement, W.C. Narcolepsy: biogenic amine deficits in an animal model, *Science* (1983) **220**, 629–632.
136. Mitchell, S.A. & Cummins, L.E. Idiopathic narcolepsy in one of monozygotic twins. Paper presented at the Association for the Psychophysiological Study of Sleep, Washington DC (1965).
137. Mitchell, S.A. & Dement, W.C. Narcolepsy syndromes: antecedent, contiguous and concomitant nocturnal sleep disordering and deprivation, *Psychophysiology* (1968) **4**, 398.
138. Mitler, M.M. Toward an animal model of narcolepsy–cataplexy. In: Guilleminault, C., Dement, W.C. & Passouant, P. *Narcolepsy*, New York: Spectrum (1976) 387–409.
139. Mitler, M.M. & Dement, W.C. Sleep studies on canine narcolepsy: pattern and cycle comparison between affected and normal dogs, *Electroenceph. Clin. Neurophysiol.* (1977) **43**, 691–699.
140. Mitler, M.M., van den Hoed, J., Carskadon, M.A., Richardson, G., Park, R., Guilleminault, C. & Dement, W.C. REM sleep episodes during the multiple sleep latency test in narcoleptic patients, *Electroenceph. Clin. Neurophysiol.* (1979) **46**, 479–481.
141. Montplaisir, J. Disturbed night sleep. In: Guilleminault, C., Dement, W.C. & Passouant, P. (eds.) *Narcolepsy*, New York: Spectrum (1976) 43–56.
142. Montplaisir, J., de Champlain, J., Young, S.N., Missala, K. Sourkes, T.L., Walsh, J. & Remillard, G. Narcolepsy and idiopathic hypersomnia: biogenic amines and related compounds in CSF, *Neurology (NY)* (1982) **32**, 1299–1302.
143. Mosko, J.B. & Sassin, J.F. The 24-hour rhythm of core temperature in narcolepsy, *Sleep* (1983) **6**, 137–146.
144. Mosko, S.S., Shampain, D.S. & Sassin, J.F. Nocturnal REM latency and sleep disturbance in narcolepsy, *Sleep* (1984) **7**, 115–125.
145. Mouret, J., Debilly, G., Renaud, B. & Blois, R. Narcolepsy and hypersomnia. Diseases or symptoms? Polygraphic and pharmacological studies. In: Guilleminault, C., Dement, W.C. & Passouant, P. (eds.) *Narcolepsy*, New York: Spectrum (1976) 571–584.
146. Nan'no, H., Hishikawa, Y., Koida, H., Takahaski, H. & Koneko, Z. A neurophysiological study of sleep paralysis in narcoleptic patients, *Electroenceph. Clin. Neurophysiol.* (1970) **28**, 382–390.
147. Navelet, Y., Anders, T. & Guilleminault, C. Narcolepsy in children. In: Guilleminault, C., Dement, W.C. & Passouant, P. (eds.) *Narcolepsy*, New York: Spectrum (1976) 171–177.
148. Nevšímalová-Brühová, S. & Roth, B. Heredofamilial aspects of narcolepsy and hypersomnia, *Schweiz. Arch. Neurol. Neurochir. Psychiat.* (1972) **110**, 45–54.
149. Niedermeyer, E. The EEG in diffuse cerebrovascular disorders. In: Remond, A. (ed.) *Handbook of Electroencephalography and Clinical Neurophysiology*, Amsterdam: Elsevier (1972) **14A**, 44–47.
150. Niedermeyer, E., Coyle, P.K. & Preziosi, T.S. Hypersomnia with sudden sleep attacks ('symptomatic narcolepsy') on the basis of vertebrobasilar artery insufficiency. A case report, *Waking Sleeping* (1979) **3**, 361–364.
151. Nygren, A. & Rojdmark, S. Isolated thyrotropin deficiency in a man with narcoleptic attacks, *Acta Med. Scand.* (1982) **212**, 175–177.
152. Ohta, T., Honda, Y., Kameyama, T., Kurita, H. & Takahashi, Y. A long-term prognosis of narcolepsy, *Sleep Res.* (1979) **8**, 206.
153. Oliver, W. *Philosophical Transactions*, London (1704) **24**, No. 304, 2177.
154. Oswald, I. Sleep and its disorders. In: Vinken, P.J. & Bruyn, G.W. (eds.) *Handbook of Clinical Neurology*, *Vol. 3*, Amsterdam: North-Holland (1969) 80–111.
155. Parkes, J.D., Fenton, G., Struthers, G., Curzon, G., Kantameneni, B.D., Buxton, B.H. & Record, C. Narcolepsy and cataplexy. Clinical features, treatment and cerebrospinal fluid findings, *Quart. J. Med.* (1974) **43**, 525–536.
156. Parkes, J.D. & Roy, A. Neurologic, psychiatric and biochemical aspects of Gélineau's syndrome, *Trans. Am. Neurol. Assoc.* (1974) **99**, 103–106.
157. Passouant, P. Problèmes physiopathologiques de la narcolepsie et périodicité du 'sommeil rapide' au cours de nyathémère. In: Gastaut, H., Lugaresi, E., Berti Ceroni, G. & Coccagna, G. (eds.) *The Abnormalities of Sleep in Man*, Bologna: Aulo Gaggi (1968) 177–189.
158. Passouant, P. Historical note. Doctor Gélineau (1828–1906): Narcolepsy Centennial, *Sleep* (1981) **3**, 241–246.
159. Prüll, G. Katamnestiche Erhebungen und therapeutische Erfahrungen bei Narkolepsie kranken, *Nervenarzt.* (1963) **34**, 480–484.

160. Puizzilout, J.J. Reflex triggering of paradoxical sleep by stimulation of the aortic trunk of the vagus: data and hypotheses, *Electroenceph. Clin. Neurophysiol.* (1977) **42**, 282.
161. Rabending, G. & Schmidt, G. Narcolepsy with subclinical spasmodic wave paroxysms in the EEG, *Psychiatr. Neurol. Med. Psychol. (Lpz.)* (1961) **13**, 456–459.
162. Rechtschaffen, A., Wolpert, E.A., Dement, W.C., Mitchell, S.A. & Fisher, C. Nocturnal sleep of narcoleptics, *Electroenceph. Clin. Neurophysiol.* (1963) **15**, 599–609.
163. Redlich, E. Epilegomena zur Narkolepsiefrage, *Z. Ges. Neurol. Psychiat.* (1931) 129–173.
164. Rennert, H. Die Narkolepsie, *Mschr. Psychiat. Neurol.* (1956) **132**, 155–172.
165. Richardson, G.S., Carskadon, M.A., Flagg, W., Van den Hoed, J., Dement, W.C. & Mitler, M.M. Excessive daytime sleepiness in man: multiple sleep latency measurement in narcoleptic and control subjects, *Electroenceph. Clin. Neurophysiol.* (1978) **45**, 621–627.
166. Roberts, H.J. Obesity due to the syndrome of narcolepsy and diabetogenic hyperinsulinism: clinical and therapeutic observations in 252 patients, *J. Am. Geriat. Soc.* (1967) **15**, 721–743.
167. Rosa, R., Kramer, M. & Foright, P. Narcolepsy: symptom frequency and associated disorders, *Sleep Res.* (1979) **8**, 213.
168. Rosenbach, O. (Ref. in de Manacéine[130]) *Z. Klinische Med.* (1881) **2**, 17.
169. Roth, B. *Narcolepsy and Hypersomnia from the Aspect of Physiology of Sleep*, (Státni zdrayotnické nakladatelstvi) Prague (1957) 331.
170. Roth, B. *Narkolepsie und Hypersomnie vom Standpunkt der Physiologie des Schlafes*, Berlin: VEB Volk Gesundheit (1962) 428.
171. Roth, B. *Narcolepsy and Hypersomnia*, Basel: S. Karger (1980) 1–310.
172. Roth, B. & Nevšimalová-Bruhová, S. Eye movements and dreams in REM sleep and NREM sleep in patients with narcolepsy and hypersomnia. In: Zikmund, V. (ed.) *The Oculomotor System and Brain Functions*, London: Butterworth (1973) 425–436.
173. Roth, B. & Nevšimalová, S. Depression in narcolepsy and hypersomnia, *Schweiz. Arch. Neurol. Neurochir. Psychiat.* (1975) **116**, 291–300.
174. Routh, G.S. General anaesthesia and driving, *Lancet* (1979) **1**, 673.
175. Roy, A. Psychiatric aspects of narcolepsy, *Brit. J. Psychiat.* (1976) **128**, 562–565.
176. Rushton, J.G. Sleep paralysis, *Med. Clin. N. Am.* (1944) **28**, 945–949.
177. Rüther, E., Meier-Ewert, K. & Gallitz, A. Zur Symptomatologie des narkoleptischen Syndroms, *Nervenarzt.* (1972) **43**, 640–643.
178. Sakai, K. In: Hobson, J.A. & Brazier, M.A.B. (eds.) *The Reticular Formation Revisited*, New York: *Raven Press* (1980) 427–447.
179. Sakai, F., Meyer, J.S., Karacan, I., Yamaguchi, F. & Yamamoto, M. Narcolepsy: regional cerebral blood flow during sleep and wakefulness, *Neurology* (1979) **29**, 61–67.
180. Scollo-Lavizzari, G. A note on cataplexy with simultaneous EEG recordings, *Eur. Neurol.* (1970) **4**, 57–63.
181. Scollo-Lavizzari, G. Narcolepsy, *Hexagon* (1979) **4**, 10–16.
182. Sitaram, N., Wyatt, R.J., Dawson, S. & Gillin, J.C. REM sleep induction by physostigmine infusion during sleep in normal volunteers, *Science* (1976) **191**, 1281–1283.
183. Slater, I.H., Jones, G.T. & Moore, R.A. Depression of REM sleep in cats by nisoxetine, a potential antidepressant drug, *Psychopharmacol. Comm.* (1976) **2**, 181–188.
184. Sours, J.A. Narcolepsy and other disturbances in the sleep–waking rhythm: a study of 115 cases with review of the literature, *J. Nerv. Ment. Dis.* (1963) **137**, 525–542.
185. Takahashi, Y. & Jimbo, M. Polygraphic study of narcoleptic syndrome with special reference to hypnagogic hallucinations and cataplexy, *Folia Psychiat. Neurol. Jap.* (1963) **7** (Suppl.), 343.
186. Takahashi, K., Takahashi, S., Azumi, K., Honda, Y. & Utena, H. Changes of plasma growth hormone during nocturnal sleep in normals and in hypersomniac patients, *Adv. Neurol. Sci.* (1971) **14**, 743–754.
187. Takahashi, Y., Takahashi, K., Higuchi, T., Niimi, Y., Miyasita, A. & Ishii, Y. Pituitary hormone secretion and narcolepsy. In: Guilleminault, C., Dement, W.C. & Passouant, P. (eds.) *Narcolepsy*, New York: Spectrum (1976) 543–563.
188. Tamura, K., Karacan, I., Thornby, J.I., Ware, J.C., Kaya, N. & Williams, R.L. Relationship of nocturnal penile tumescence (NPT) and REM sleep in narcolepsy, *Sleep Res.* (1979) **8**, 217.
189. Thal, L.J. & Sharpless, N.S. Narcolepsy and hypersomnia (letter), *Neurology* (1983) **33**, 1394.
190. Tharp, B.R. Narcolepsy and epilepsy. In: Guilleminault, C., Dement, W.C. & Passouant, P. (eds.) *Narcolepsy*, New York: Spectrum (1976) 263–281.
191. Thompson, C., Schachter, M. & Parkes, J.D. Drugs for cataplexy, *Ann. Neurol.* (1982) **12**, 63–64.
192. Valley, V. & Broughton, R. Daytime performance deficits and physiological vigilance in

untreated patients with narcolepsy–cataplexy compared to controls, *Rev. Electroenceph. Clin. Neurophysiol.* (1981) **11**, 133–139.

193. van Bogaert, L. Les aspects familiaux des paroxysmes réflexes du tonus, *Ann. Méd-Psychol.* (1936) **94**, 1–14.

194. Vein, A.M. *Syndrome of Hypersomnia (Narcolepsy and Other Forms of Pathologic Sleepiness),* Moscow: Izdatelstvo Meditsina (1966) 236. (in Russian)

195. Vein, A.M. *Disturbances of Sleep and Wakefulness,* Moscow: Izdatelstvo Meditsina (1974) 383. (in Russian)

196. Vizioli, R. Les bases neurophysiologiques de la cataplexie, *Electroenceph. Clin. Neurophysiol.* (1964) **16**, 191–193.

197. Vizioli, R. Discussion on the topic: narcolepsy. In: Gastaut, H., Lugaresi, C., Berti-Ceroni, G. & Coccagna, G. (eds.) *The Abnormalities of Sleep in Man,* Bologna: Aulo Gaggi (1968) 231–234.

198. Vogel, G. Studies in psychophysiology of dreams. III. The dreams of narcolepsy, *Arch. Gen. Psychiat.* (1960) **3**, 421–428.

199. Ware, J.C., Karacan, I., Dervent, A., Meyer, J.S. & Williams, R.L. A case of narcolepsy with attacks precipitated by ingestion of sweet foods, *Sleep Res.* (1979) **8**, 219.

200. Weir Mitchell, S. Remarks on the effects of *Anhehonium Lewinii, Brit. Med. J.* (1896) **2**, 1625–1629.

201. Weitzman, E.D. Twenty-four hour neuroendocrine secretory patterns: observations on patients with narcolepsy. In: Guilleminault, C., Dement, W.C. & Passouant, P. (eds.) *Narcolepsy,* New York: Spectrum (1976) 521–542.

202. Westphal, C. Eigenthümliche mit Einschafen verbundene Anfälle, *Arch. Psychiat. Nervenkr.* (1877) **7**, 681.

203. Wilson, S.A.K. The narcolepsies, *Brain* (1928) **51**, 63–109.

204. Wilson, S.A.K. The narcolepsies. In: Ninian Bruce, A. (ed.) *Neurology,* London: Butterworths (1955) 1680–1694.

205. Wolfenden, W.H. Narcolepsy, *Bull. Post Grad. Comm. Med. Univ. Sidney* (1969) **25**, 64–68.

206. Yoss, R.E. The inheritance of diurnal sleepiness as measured by pupillography, *Proc. Mayo Clin.* (1970) **45**, 426–437.

207. Yoss, R.E. & Daly, D.D. Criteria for the diagnosis of the narcoleptic syndrome, *Proc. Mayo Clin.* (1957) **32**, 320–328.

208. Yoss, R.E. & Daly, D.D. Hereditary aspects of narcolepsy, *Trans. Am. Neurol. Assoc.* (1960) **85**, 239–240.

209. Yoss, R.E. & Daly, D.D. Narcolepsy, *Arch. Int. Med.* (1960) **106**, 168–171.

210. Yoss, R.E. & Daly, D.D. Narcolepsy, *Med. Clin. N. Am.* (1960) **44**, 953–968.

211. Yoss, R.E., Moyer, N.J. & Ogle, K.N. The pupillogram and narcolepsy, *Neurology (Minneap.)* (1969) **19**, 921–928.

212. Zarcone, V. Narcolepsy. A review of the syndrome, *New Engl. J. Med.* (1973) **288**, 1156–1165.

213. Zellweger, H. Narcolepsy and epilepsy: case of narcolepsy with spike and waves in the EEG, *Helv. Paediat. Acta.* (1956) **11**, 269–274.

214. Zorick, F.J., Salis, P.J., Roth, T. & Kramer, M. Narcolepsy and automatic behaviour: a case report, *J. Clin. Psychiat.* (1979) **40**, 194–197.

SECONDARY NARCOLEPSY

215. Alajouanine, T. & Baruk, H. La valeur sémiologique des narcolepsies en dehors de l'encéphalite léthargique, *Prog. Med.* (1926) **17**, 639–645.

216. Alajouanine, T., Lagrange, C. & Baruk, H. Tumeur de la glande pineale diagnosiquée cliniquement chez l'adulte, *Bull. Soc. Med. Hôp. Paris* (1925) **49**, 1309–1314.

217. Anderson, M. & Salmon, M.V. Symptomatic cataplexy, *J. Neurol. Neurosurg. Psychiat.* (1977) **40**, 186–191.

218. Bell, I.R. Diet histories in narcolepsy. In: Guilleminault, C., Dement, W.C. & Passouant, P. (eds.) *Narcolepsy,* New York: Spectrum (1976) 221–227.

219. Benedek, L. & Juba, A. Beitrage zur Pathologie des Diencephalon, *Z. Ges. Neurol. Psychiat.* (1943) **175**, 765–778.

220. Berg, O. & Hanley, J. Narcolepsy in two cases of multiple sclerosis, *Acta. Neurol. Scand.* (1963) **39**, 252–257.

221. Billiard, M., Seignalet, J., Besset, A. & Briss, L. Possible association between HLA B7 and narcolepsy, *Proceedings Congress on Sleep Research,* Toronto, May 1984.

222. Bonduelle, M., Bouygues, P., Delahousse, J. & Faveret, C. Narcolepsie post-traumatique, *Rev. Otoneuro-Ophthalmol.* (1959) **31**, 1–5.

223. Bonduelle, M., Bouygues, P., Delahousse, J. & Faveret, C. Narcolepsie post-traumatique, *Lille Med.* (1959) **4**, 719–721.

224. Bonduelle, M. & Degos, C. Symptomatic narcolepsies: a critical study. In: Guilleminault, C., Dement, W.C. & Passouant, P. (eds.) *Narcolepsy*, New York: Spectrum (1976) 313–332.

225. Brown-Goode, G. Sleep paralysis, *Arch. Neurol.* (1962) **6**, 228–234.

226. Castaigne, P., Escourelle, R., Laplane, D. & Augustine, P. Comas transitoires avec hyperthermie au cours de la sclérose en plaques, *Encephale* (1966) **55** (3), 191–211.

227. Comelade, P., Cadilhac, J. & Passouant, P. Temporal epilepsy and narcoleptic seizures, *Rev. Neurol. (Paris)* (1961) **104**, 252–245.

228. Drake, F.R. Narcolepsy – brief review and report of cases, *Am. J. Med. Sci.* (1949) **218**, 101–114.

229. Ekbom, K. Familial multiple sclerosis associated with narcolepsy, *Arch. Neurol.* (1966) **15**, 337–344.

230. Foix, C., Alajouanine, T. & Dauptain, R. Diabète insipide syphilitique avec hémianopsie bitemporale et crises de narcolepsie. Rétrocession des symptômes associés par le traitement spécifique. Persistance de la polyurie insipide, *Rev. Neurol.* (1922) **29**, 763–766.

231. Francois, H. & Vernier, L. Etude anatomo-clinique d'un cas de tumeur du IIIeme ventricule cérébral, *Rev. Neurol.* (1919) **32**, 921–925.

232. Fulton, J.F. & Bailey, P. Tumours in the region of the third ventricle, *J. Nerv. Ment. Dis.* (1929) **69**, 1–45, 145–164, 261–277.

233. Geisler, E. Narkolepsie und affektiver Tonusverlust bei Kindern, *Med. Wschr. Wochenschr.* (1963) **105**, 2437–2441.

234. Gélineau, J.B. De la Narcolepsie, *Gaz. Hôp.* (1880) **53**, 635–637.

235. Grigoresco, D. Contribution a l'étude des troubles dûs a des lésions des noyaux gris centraux, *Rev. Neurol.* (1932) **2**, 27–45.

236. Guillain, G. & Alajouanine, T. Syphilis du néraxe à forme algique et somnolente simulant l'encéphalite léthargique, *Bull. Soc. Med. Hôp. Paris* (1923) **47**, 380–381.

237. Guilleminault, C. Cataplexy. In: Guilleminault, C., Dement, W.C. & Passoúant, P. (eds.) *Narcolepsy*, New York: Spectrum (1976) 125–143.

238. Guilleminault, C., Wilson, R.A. & Dement, W.C. A study on cataplexy, *Arch. Neurol.* (1974) **31**, 255–261.

239. Heyck, H. & Hess, R. Further results of clinical studies on narcolepsy, *Schweiz. Arch. Neurol. Psychiat.* (1955) **75**, 401–403.

240. Jones, B.E., Harper, S.T. & Halaris, A.E. Effect of locus coeruleus lesions upon cerebral monoamine content, sleep–wakefulness states, and the response to amphetamine in the cat, *Brain Res.* (1977) **124**, 473–496.

241. Jouvet, M. Cataplexie et sommeil paradoxal chez le chat pontique, *C.R. Soc. Biol. (Paris)* (1965) **159**, 383–387.

242. Jouvet, M. Paradoxical sleep. A study of its nature and mechanisms. In: Akert, K., Bally, G. & Schade, J.P. (eds.) *Sleep Mechanisms. Progress in Brain Research, Vol. 19*, Amsterdam: Elsevier (1965) 20–62.

243. Kales, A. & Kales, J.D. Sleep disorders: recent findings in the diagnosis and treatment of disturbed sleep, *New Engl. J. Med.* (1974) **290**, 487–499.

244. Kuwert, E.K. Genetic aspects of multiple sclerosis with special regard to histocompatibility determinants. In: Fog, T. (ed.) *The Histocompatibility in Multiple Sclerosis*, Copenhagen: Munksgaard (1977) 23–37.

245. Lascelles, R.G., Mohr, P.D. & Peart, I. Unilateral cataplexy associated with systemic lupus erythematosus, *J. Neurol. Neurosurg. Psychiat.* (1976) **39**, 1023–1026.

246. Lechelle, P., Alajouanine, T. & Thevenard, A. Deux cas de tumeur du lobe frontal à forme somnolente, *Bull. Soc. Hôp. Med. Paris* (1925) **59**, 1347–1357.

247. Lhermitte, J. & Peyre, E. Narcolepsie–cataplexie: syndrome révélateur et unique de l'érythrémie occulte, *Rev. Neurol.* (1930) **1**, 296–299.

248. Lhermitte, J. & Tornay, A. Le sommeil normal et pathologique, *Rev. Neurol.* (1927) **1**, 751–822, 885–887.

249. Magoun, H.W. & Rhines, R. An inhibitory mechanism in the bulbar reticular formation, *J. Neurophysiol.* (1946) **9**, 165–171.

250. Niedermeyer, E., Coyle, P.K. & Preziosi, T.S. Hypersomnia with sudden sleep attacks ('symptomatic narcolepsy') on the basis of vertebrobasilar artery insufficiency. A case

report, *Waking Sleeping* (1979) **3**, 361–364.

251. Passouant, P., Passouant-Fontaine, T. & Cadilhac, J. L'influence de l'hyperthyroidie sur le sommeil. Étude clinique et expérimentale, *Rev. Neurol.* (1966) **115**, 353–366.

252. Pohl, O. Ein Beitrag zur Pathologie der symptomatischen Narkolepsie, *Deutsch. Z. Nervenheilk.* (1966) **189**, 211–217.

253. Pompeiano, O. Mechanisms responsible for spinal inhibition during desynchronized sleep: Experimental study. In: Guilleminault, C., Dement, W.C. & Passouant, P. (eds.) *Narcolepsy,* New York: Spectrum (1976) 411–449.

254. Rabending, G. & Schmidt, G. Narcolepsy with subclinical spasmodic wave paroxysms in the EEG, *Psychiat. Neurol. Med. Psychol. (Lpz.)* (1961) **13**, 456–459.

255. Riser, M. & Dardenne, J. Narcolepsie et hypoglycémie permanente, *Bull. Soc. Med. Hôp. Paris* (1946) **62**, 413–415.

256. Roberts, H.J. The syndrome of narcolepsy and diabetogenic hyperinsulinism in the American negro: important clinical, social and public health aspects, *J. Am. Geriat. Soc.* (1965) **13**, 852–885.

257. Roberts, D.A. & Schwab, R.S. The cortical alpha rhythm in thyroid disorders, *Endocrinology* (1939) **25**, 75–79.

258. Roth, B. *Narcolepsy and Hypersomnia from the Aspect of Physiology of Sleep,* Prague (1957) 331.

259. Roth, B. *Narcolepsy and Hypersomnia,* Basel: Springer Verlag (1980) 1–310.

260. Schlager, E. & Meier, T. Strange Balinese method of inducing sleep (with some notes about balyans) *Acta. Trop. (Basel)* (1947) **4**, 127–133.

261. Schrader, H., Gotlibsen, O.B. & Skomedal, G.N. Multiple sclerosis and narcolepsy/cataplexy in a monozygotic twin, *Neurology* (1980) **30**, 105–108.

262. Simons, D.J. Narcolepsy. In: Cecil, P.L. & Loob, R.F. (eds.) *A Textbook of Medicine,* Philadelphia: W.B. Saunders (1951) 1382–1384.

263. Smith, S.M. & Schneider, R.A. Narcolepsy and hypoglycaemia, *J. Ment. Sci.* (1959) **105**, 163–170.

264. Sours, J.A. Narcolepsy and other disturbance in the sleep–waking rhythms. A study of 115 cases with review of the literature, *J. Nerv. Ment. Dis.* (1963) **137**, 525–542.

265. Stahl, M., Layzer, R.B., Aminoff, M.J., Townsend, J.J. & Feldon, S. Continuous cataplexy in a patient with a midbrain tumour: the limp man syndrome, *Neurology* (1980) **30**, 115–1118.

266. Stahl, M.L., Orr, W.C. & Bollinger, C. Postprandial sleepiness: objective documentation via polysomnography, *Sleep* (1983) **6**, 29–35.

267. Steriade, M. & Hobson, J.A. Neuronal activity during the sleep–waking cycle, *Prog. Neurobiol.* (1976) **6**, 155–376.

268. Suwa, K. & Toru, M. A case of periodic somnolence whose sleep was induced by glucose, *Folia Psychiat. Neurol. Jap.* (1969) **23**, 253–262.

269. Symmonds, C.P. Narcolepsy as a symptom of encephalitis lethargica, *Lancet* (1926) **ii**, 1214–1215.

270. Tharp, B.R. Narcolepsy and epilepsy. In: Guilleminault, C., Dement, W.C. & Passouant, P. (eds.) *Narcolepsy,* New York: Spectrum (1976) 263–281.

271. Tridon, P., Montaut, J., Picard, L., Weber, M. & Andre, J.M. Syndrome de Gélineau et haemangioblastome kystique de cervelet, *Rev. Neurol.* (1969) **121**, 186–189.

272. van Bogaert, L. Syndrome de la calotte protubérentielle avec myoclonies localisées et troubles du sommeil, *Rev. Neurol.* (1926) **45**, 977–986.

273. Wilder, J. Narkolepsie. In: Bumice, C. & Foerster, H. (eds.) *Handbuch der Neurologie, Vol. 17,* Berlin: Springer Verlag (1935) **193**, 87–141.

274. Zarcone, V. Narcolepsy. A review of the syndrome, *New Engl. J. Med.* (1973) **288**, 1156–1165.

275. Zellweger, H. Narcolepsy and epilepsy: case of narcolepsy with spikes and waves in the EEG, *Helv. Paediat. Acta* (1956) **11**, 269–274.

THE KLEINE–LEVIN SYNDROME

276. Abe, K. Lithium prophylaxis of periodic hypersomnia, *Brit. J. Psychiat.* (1977) **130**, 312–316.

277. Antimoff, J.A., See Critchley, M.[287]

278. Argenta, G. First CT findings in the Kleine–Levin–Critchley syndrome, *Ital. J. Neurol. Sci.* (1981) **2**, 77–79.

279. Barontini, F. & Zappoli, R. A case of Kleine–Levin syndrome. Clinical and polygraphic study, *Proceedings 20th European Meeting on Electroencephalography,* Bologna: Gaggi (1967) 239–245.

332   Sleep and its Disorders

280. Berti Ceroni, G. An episode of hypersomnia and megaphagia and its evaluation in a narcoleptic syndrome. In: Gastaut, H., Lugaresi, E., Berti Ceroni, G. & Coccagna, G. (eds.) *The Abnormalities of Sleep in Man*, Bologna: Aulo Gaggi (1968) 247–249.

281. Billiard, M. The Kleine–Levin syndrome. In: Koella, W.P. (ed.) *Sleep 1980*, Basel: S. Karger (1981) 124–127.

282. Billiard, M., Guilleminault, C. & Dement, W.C. A menstruation-linked periodic hypersomnia: Kleine–Levin syndrome or a new clinical entity? *Neurology (Minneap.)* (1975) **25**, 436–443.

283. Billiard, M. & Passouant, P. Hormones sexuelles et sommeil chez la femme, *Rev. EEG Neurophysiol.* (1974) **4**, 89–106.

284. Billiard, C., Ponsot, G., Lyon, G. & Arfel, G. Syndrome de Kleine–Levin, à propos d'une observation, *Arch. Fr. Pediat.* (1978) **35**, 424–431.

285. Bonkalo, A. Hypersomnia: a discussion of psychiatric implications based on three cases, *Brit. J. Psychiat.* (1968) **114**, 69–75.

286. Bucking, P.H. & Palmer, W.R. New contribution to the clinical aspects and pathophysiology of the Kleine–Levin syndrome, *Much. Med. Wschr.* (1978) **120**, 1571–1572.

287. Critchley, M. Periodic hypersomnia and megaphagia in adolescent males, *Brain* (1962) **85**, 628–656.

288. Critchley, M. & Hoffman, H.L. The syndrome of periodic somnolence and morbid hunger (Kleine–Levin syndrome), *Brit. Med. J.* (1942) **1**, 137–139.

289. Duffy, J.P. & Davison, K. A female case of the Kleine–Levin syndrome, *Brit. J. Psychiat.* (1968) **114**, 77–84.

290. Earle, B.V. Periodic hypersomnia and megaphagia (the Kleine–Levin syndrome), *Psychiat. Quart.* (1965) **39**, 79–83.

291. Fresco, R., Guidicelli, S., Poinso, Y., Tatoosian, A. & Mouren, P. Le syndrome de Kleine–Levin (hypersomnie récurrente des adolescents mâles), *Ann. Med. Psychol.* (1971) **129**, 625–668.

292. Gallinek, A. Syndrome of episodes of hypersomnia, bulimia and abnormal mental states, *J. Am. Med. Assoc.* (1954) **154**, 1081–1083.

293. Gallinek, A. The Kleine–Levin syndrome: hypersomnia, bulimia and abnormal mental states, *World Neurol.* (1962) **3**, 235–241.

294. Gallinek, A. The Kleine–Levin syndrome, *Dis. Nerv. Syst.* (1967) **28**, 448–451.

295. Gilbert, G.J. Periodic hypersomnia and bulimia: the Kleine–Levin syndrome, *Neurology* (1964) **14**, 844–850.

296. Goldberg, M.A. The treatment of Kleine–Levin syndrome with lithium, *Can. J. Psychiat.* (1983) **28**, 491–493.

297. Green, L.N. & Cracco, R.Q. Kleine–Levin syndrome, *Arch. Neurol. (Chic.)* (1970) **22**, 166–175.

298. Hishikawa, Y., Iijima, S., Tashiro, T., Sugita, Y., Teshima, Y., Matsuo, R. & Kanedo, H. Polysomnographic findings and growth hormone secretion in patients with periodic hypersomnia. In: Koella, W.P. (ed.) *Sleep 1980*, Basel: S. Karger (1981) 128–133.

299. Jeffries, J.J. & Lefebvre, A. Depression and mania associated with Kleine–Levin–Critchley syndrome, *Can. Psychiat. Assoc. J.* (1973) **18**, 439–444.

300. Jovanovič, M.J. Die wichtigsten abnormen Schlafsyndrome. In: Jovanovič, U.J. (ed.) *Der Schlaf: Neurophysiologische Aspekte*, Munich: J.A. Barth (1969) 223–231.

301. Kleine, W. Periodische Schlafsucht, *Mschr. Psychiat. Neurol.* (1925) **57**, 285–320.

302. Lavie, P., Gadoth, N., Gordon, C.R., Goldhammer, G. & Bechar, M. Sleep patterns in Kleine–Levin syndrome, *Electroenceph. Clin. Neurophysiol.* (1979) **47**, 369–371.

303. Lavie, P., Klein, E., Gadoth, N., Bental, E., Zomer, J., Bechar, M. & Wajsbort, J. Further observations on sleep abnormalities in Kleine–Levin syndrome: abnormal breathing pattern during sleep, *Electroenceph. Clin. Neurophysiol.* (1981) **52**, 98–101.

304. Levin, M. Periodic somnolence and morbid hunger: a new syndrome, *Brain* (1936) **59**, 494–515.

305. Lewis, N.D.C. The psychoanalytic approach to the problems of children under twelve years of age, *Psychoanal. Rev.* (1926) **13**, 424–443.

306. Lobzin, V.S., Shamrei, R.K. & Churilov, I.K. Pathophysiological mechanisms of periodic hypersomnia and the Kleine–Levin syndrome, *Zh. Nevropatol. Psychiat. Korsakova* (1973) **73**, 1719–1724.

307. Markman, R.A. Kleine–Levin syndrome: report of a case, *Am. J. Psychiat.* (1967) **123**, 1025–1026.

308. Messimy, R., Weil, B. & Safar, J. Sur un cas d'hypersomnie avec troubles des conduites

alimentaires, excitation sexuelle et troubles du comportement, *Sem. Hôp. Paris* (1967) **49**, 3100–3105.

309. Ogura, C., Okuma, T., Nakagawa, K. & Kishimoto, A. Treatment of periodic somnolence with lithium carbonate, *Arch. Neurol. (Chic.)* (1976) **33**, 143–153.
310. Ogura, C., Nakazza, K., Kishimoto, A. & Okuma, T. A case of periodic somnolence improved by lithium carbonate, *Clin. Psychiat.* (1975) **17**, 59–63.
311. O'Regan, J.B. Hypersomnia and MAOI antidepressants, *Can. Med. Assoc. J.* (1974) **213**, 111.
312. Orlosky, M.J. The Kleine–Levin syndrome – a review, *Psychosomatics* (1982) **23**, 609–621.
313. Ortiz de Zarate, J.C. Sindrome de Gélineau (o de Kleine–Levin), *Acta. Neurol. Psiquiat. Argentin.* (1957) **3**, 279–283.
314. Oswald, I. Sleep and its disorders. In: Vinkler, P.J. & Bruyn, G.W. (eds.) *Handbook of Clinical Neurology, Vol. 3*, Amsterdam: North-Holland (1969) 80–111.
315. Pai, M.N. Hypersomnia syndromes, *Brit. Med. J.* (1950) **1**, 522–524.
316. Passouant, P., Cadilhac, J. & Baldy-Moulinier, M. Physio-pathologie des hypersomnies, *Rev. Neurol.* (1967) **116**, 585–629.
317. Popoviciu, L. & Corfariu, O. Etude clinique et polygraphique au cours du nycthémère d'un cas de syndrome de Kleine–Levin–Critchley, *Rev. Roum. Neurol.* (1972) **9**, 221–228.
318. Prebhakaran, N., Murthy, G.K. & Mallya, U.L. A case of Kleine–Levin syndrome in India, *Brit. J. Psychiat.* (1970) **117**, 517–519.
319. Reynolds, C.F., Black, R.S., Coble, P., Holzer, B. & Kupfer, D.J. Similarities in EEG sleep findings for Kleine–Levin syndrome and unipolar depression, *Am.J. Psychiat.* (1980) **137**, 116–118.
320. Reynolds, C.F., Kupfer, D.J., Christiansen, C.L., Auchenbach, R.C., Brenner, R.P., Sewitch, D.E., Taska, L.S. & Coble, P.A. Multiple sleep latency test findings in Kleine–Levin syndrome, *J. Nerv. Ment. Dis.* (1984) **172**, 41–44.
321. Robinson, J.T. & McQuillan, J. Schizophrenic reaction associated with the Kleine–Levin syndrome, *J. Roy. Army Med. Corps.* (1951) **96**, 377–381.
322. Ronald, J. Hypersomnia associated with abnormal hunger. The Kleine–Levin syndrome, *Brit. Med. J.* (1946) **2**, 326–327.
323. Rosenkotter, L. & Wende, S. EEG-Befunde beim Kleine–Levin syndrom, *Mschr. Psychiat. Neurol.* (1955) **130**, 107–121.
324. Roth, B. *Narcolepsy and Hypersomnia*, Basel: S. Karger (1980) 261–262.
325. Sallares, C. & Dillon, C. Sindrom de Kleine–Levin, *Acta Psiquiat. Psicol. Am. Lat.* (1973) **19**, 148–151.
326. Smith, C.M. Comments and observations on psychogenic hypersomnia, *Am. Med. Assoc. Arch. Neurol. Psychiat.* (1958) **80**, 619–624.
327. Takahashi, Y. Clinical studies of periodic somnolence: analysis of 28 personal cases, *Folia Psychiat. Neurol. Jap.* (1967) **67**, 853–889.
328. Tulsidasa *Ramcharitmanasa*, Gorakhpur: Gita Press (1942).
329. Vlach, V. Periodická somnolence, bulimie a psychické poruchy (syndrome Kleineuv–Levinuv), *Čslká. Neurol.* (1962) **25**, 401–405.
330. Wilder, J. A case of atypical Kleine–Levin syndrome, *J. Nerv. Ment. Dis.* (1972) **154**, 69–72.
331. Wilkus, R.J. & Chiles, J.A. Electrophysiological changes during episodes of the Kleine–Levin syndrome, *J. Neurol. Neurosurg. Psychiat.* (1975) **38**, 1225–1231.

SLEEP AND THE MENSTRUAL CYCLE

332. Billiard, M., Guilleminault, C. & Dement, W. A menstruation-linked periodic hypersomnia. Kleine–Levin syndrome or new clinical entity? *Neurology (Minneap.)* (1975) **25**, 436–443.
333. Billiard, M. & Passouant, P. Hormones sexuelles et sommeil chez la femme, *Rev. EEG Neurophysiol.* (1974) **4**, 89–106.
334. Elian, M. & Bornstein, B. The Kleine–Levin syndrome with intermittent abnormality in the EEG, *Electroenceph. Clin. Neurophysiol.* (1969) **27**, 601–604.
335. Gilligan, B.S. Periodic megaphagia and hypersomnia – an example of the Kleine–Levin syndrome in an adolescent girl, *Proc. Aust. Assoc. Neurol.* (1973) **9**, 67–72.
336. Hartmann, E. Dreaming sleep and the menstrual cycle, *J. Nerv. Ment. Dis.* (1966) **143**, 406–416.
337. Hartmann, E. *The Biology of Dreaming*, Springfield, Illinois: Charles C. Thomas (1967).
338. Heuser, G. Hormones and sleep, *Ann. Int. Med.* (1968) **68**, 1086–1088.

339. Ho, A. Sex hormones and the sleep of women. In: Chase, M.H., Stern, W.C. & Walter, P.L. (eds.) *Sleep Research, Vol. 1*, Los Angeles: BIS/BRI UCLA (1972) 184.
340. Karacan, I., Heine, W., Agnew, H.W., Williams, R., Webb, W., Agnew, H. & Ross, J. Characteristics of sleep patterns during late pregnancy and post-partum, *Am. J. Obstet. Gynaecol.* (1968) **101**, 579–586.
341. Karacan, I., Thornby, J.I., Anch, M., Holzer, L., Warleit, G.J. & Williams, R.L. Prevalence of sleep disturbances in a primarily urban Florida country, *Soc. Sci. Med.* (1976) **10**, 239–244.
342. Kripke, D.F., Simons, R.A., Garfinkel, L. & Cuyler, H. Short and long sleep and sleeping pills. Is increased mortality associated? *Arch. Gen. Psychiat.* (1979) **36**, 103–116.
343. Kurtz, D., Lampert, E. & Krieger, J. Hormones, endocrine disease and excessive daytime sleepiness. In: Guilleminault, C., Dement, W.C. & Passouant, P. (eds.) *Narcolepsy*, New York: Spectrum (1976) 367–384.
344. Lhermitte, J. Hypersomnie périodique et menstruation, *Prog. Méd. (Paris)* (1942) **70**, 68–78.
345. Lhermitte, J. & Dubois, E. Crises d'hypersomnie prolongée rhythmées par les règles chez une jeune fille, *Rev. Neurol.* (1941) **73**, 608–614.
346. Lhermitte, J., Hécaen, J. & Bineau, L. Un nouveau cas d'hypersomnie prolongée rhythmée par les règles, *Rev. Neurol.* (1943) **75**, 299–307.
347. Lugaresi, E., Cirignotta, F., Zucconi, M., Mondini, S., Lenzi, P.L. & Coccagna, G. In: Guilleminault, C. & Lugaresi, E. (eds.) *Sleep/Wake Disorders. Natural History, Epidemiology and Long-Term Evolution*, New York: Raven Press (1983) 1–12.
348. McGhie, A. & Russell, S.M. The subjective assessment of normal sleep patterns, *J. Ment. Sci.* (1962) **8**, 642–654.
349. Merryman, W., Boiman, R., Banes, L. & Rotschild, I. Progesterone 'anaesthesia' in human subjects, *J. Clin. Endocrinol. Metab.* (1954) **14**, 1567–1569.
350. Petre-Quadens, O., De Barsy, A., Devos, J. & Sfaello, A. Sleep in pregnancy: evidence of fetal sleep characteristics, *J. Neurol. Sci.* (1967) **4**, 600–605.
351. Roth, B. *Narcolepsy and Hypersomnia from the Aspect of the Physiology of Sleep*, (Státni zdravotnické nakladatelsiví) Prague (1957).
352. Sachs, C., Persson, H.E. & Hagenfeldt, K. Menstruation-linked periodic hypersomnia: a case study with successful treatment, *Neurology (NY)* (1982) **32**, 1376–1379.
353. Wever, R.A. Properties of human sleep–wake cycles: parameters of internally synchronized free-running rhythms, *Sleep* (1984) **7**, 27–51.
354. Wilson, S.A.K. The narcolepsies. In: Ninian Bruce, A. (ed.) *Neurology*, London: Butterworths (1955) 1680–1694.

CHAPTER 7

SLEEP APNOEA AND OTHER RESPIRATORY DISORDERS DURING SLEEP

CONTROL OF BREATHING DURING SLEEP

ANATOMY OF VOLUNTARY PATHWAYS OF RESPIRATION

Respiration whilst waking is under both voluntary and involuntary control. The pathways of the two systems are different. Voluntary pathways originate in the pre-motor cortex. Stimulation here increases respiratory movement, whilst stimulation of the anterior cingulate and posterior orbital areas, as well as the ventromedial aspects of the temporal pole, inhibits breathing. Motor fibres concerned in the voluntary control of respiration decussate in the posterolateral spinal columns to terminate on nuclei of phrenic and intercostal neurones in the anterior horns of the cervical and thoracic cord. Pontine lesions may interrupt these pathways and so abolish the voluntary control of respiration.

ANATOMY OF INVOLUNTARY PATHWAYS OF RESPIRATION

'Respiratory' neurones and neuronal systems involved in sleep mechanisms overlap to some extent in the lower brain stem and pons. The presence of a brain stem respiratory rhythm generator was indicated by early experiments in the goldfish, where medullary cells continue to show rhythmic electrical activity at the same frequency of gill movements, despite removal of higher brain areas. The site of the respiratory oscillator in man is not known with certainty. No cells have been found in the medulla that fit the required criteria for a primary oscillator,[80] and although the nucleus parabrachialis medialis has been considered for this role,[23] Hukuhara[131] in elegant transection experiments showed that this was not so in the cat. Respiratory neurones are mainly concentrated in the medulla, not the pons. Some fire in inspiration, others in expiration.

Pontine neurones may organize upper airway muscle activity in breathing.

The lower medulla contains a high density of respiratory neurones (Fig. 7.2). These are mainly concentrated in:

1. the nucleus ambiguus, with axons to the vagus and glossopharyngeal nerves;

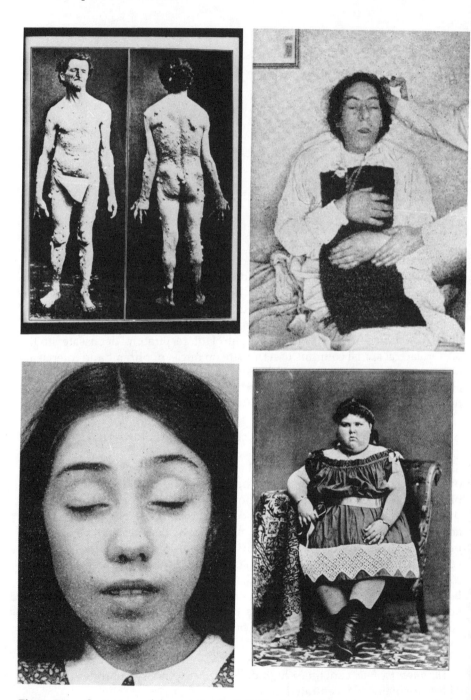

Figure 7.1. *Some causes of sleep apnoea. Top left: Von Recklinghausen's second case; top right: acromegaly (Roxburgh et al.[231]); lower left: bulbar palsy; lower right: hypothalamic lesion and obesity.*

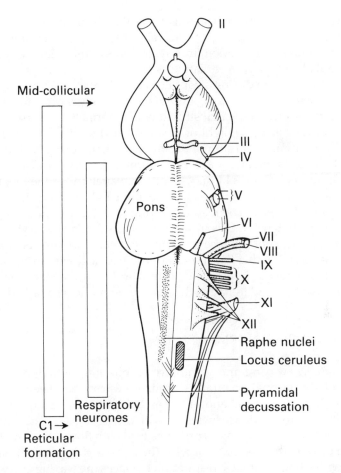

Figure 7.2. *Approximate area of the brain stem from which arousal responses are produced by electrical stimulation and where neurones with firing patterns that correspond to respiration are sited. C1: cervical level 1.*

2. the nucleus ratioambigualis, in the ventrolateral medulla, supplying contralateral intercostal and phrenic motor neurones;
3. the nucleus of the tractus solitarius, supplying contralateral phrenic and intercostal motor neurones.

The relative roles of the efferent tracts (2) and (3) are not known. The nucleus tractus solitarius is the afferent relay station for vagal fibres and indirectly for carotid body afferents. These three areas probably constitute the lower medullary automatic respiratory centre, or at least the respiratory area most resistant to anaesthesia.[131]

Axons from neurones concerned in the involuntary control of respiration descend in the ventrolateral spinal tracts, and are distinct from the more posterior axons of the voluntary respiratory system.

Respiratory muscles receive bilateral innervation from the brain stem nuclei. Bilateral, but not unilateral upper cervical cordotomy, which interrupts the descending automatic ventilation fibre system in the anterolateral spinal cord, causes central alveolar hypoventilation.

Ventilation is reduced during sleep. Loss of voluntary respiratory control is one major cause of respiratory depression during sleep, together with reduction in those environmental stimuli which normally increase respiration whilst awake, such as noise, light or nasal obstruction.[11, 92] The sleeper is less disturbed by environmental stimuli during REM than during NREM stage 1–2 sleep, and needs a greater degree of stimulation for arousal.[212, 213] This difference in arousal threshold may be one explanation for the fact that both physiological and pathological apnoeas during REM sleep are usually longer than during NREM sleep. The result of ventilatory depression during sleep is that arterial oxygen tension falls by approximately 2 kPa in everybody during sleep. This has little consequence in normal subjects and there is little change in oxygen saturation with a flat summit of the haemoglobin–oxygen dissociation curve. However, in hypoxic subjects who lie on the steep slope of the curve whilst awake, a fall in PaO_2 whilst sleeping produces marked desaturation.

BREATHING DURING NORMAL SLEEP

Irregular breathing, waxing and waning of respiration, with apnoeas, due to instability of the normal respiratory control system, has been observed in normal people at sleep onset and in stages 1–2 NREM as well as during REM sleep.[10, 35, 212, 293, 294] Its incidence increases with increasing age.[293, 294] This normal irregular breathing at sleep onset correlates well with fluctuations of PCO_2 and the degree of wakefulness, but not with the degree of hypoxia. It has a close similarity with Cheyne–Stokes' respiration but lacks the waxing and waning as well as the regular quality of this.

Irregular breathing, similar to that of sleep onset, can be produced by mechanical obstruction to the airway as well as by central lesions. By increasing the time over which blood travels from the thorax to the brain, Filehne in 1874 produced periodic respiration in dogs under morphine by gradually constricting and then releasing the arteries conveying blood to the head.[99] Both Cheyne–Stokes breathing during sleep and sleep apnoea occur in normal subjects living at high altitudes; and also both respiratory patterns may result from raised intracranial pressure, distortion and compression of the brain stem, median raphe haemorrhage or tentorial herniation of the medial temporal lobe. Cheyne–Stokes respiration in patients with neurological injuries is most often associated with bilateral lesions of the basal ganglia and deep in the cerebral hemispheres. It also may occur with cardiovascular disease and has been described in apparently healthy persons. Power *et al.*[216] described the presence of Cheyne–Stokes respiration in NREM (but not in REM) sleep in a 63-year-old woman with persistent insomnia, a left hemiplegia and pseudobulbar palsy and CT scan evidence of large right hemisphere cerebral infarct and left-sided cerebellar defect.

Irregular breathing at sleep onset and during NREM sleep is multifactorial in origin, probably due to changes in the hypoxic and hypercapnic ventilatory responses but also to the combination of differences between O_2 and CO_2 control systems (PaO_2 control being linear, $PaCO_2$ hyperbolic with respect to ventilation). Body O_2 stores are much smaller than CO_2 stores, and PaO_2 changes far more rapidly than $PaCO_2$ with ventilation changes.[72]

After sleep onset, in animals, there is a *decrease in ventilation* during NREM sleep, with decreased thoraco-abdominal movement or arterial hypoxaemia and hypercapnia. Both inspiratory and expiratory times are prolonged during sleep in dogs, with a lower tidal volume, and in different species either no change or a slight increase in breathing frequency compared with wakefulness. Quiet sleep in animals delays the transition of the inspiratory–expiratory phase.[224] Data from man have been somewhat conflicting. In an initial study, Newson-Davies *et al.*[189] using magnetometers to avoid the problem of facial instrumentation influencing breathing, found no difference in ventilatory patterns between wakefulness and quiet sleep. Others have shown in normal men, after sleep onset, and with increasing depth of sleep, that there is a slight reduction in minute volume, and occasionally an overall decline in the rate of respiration from the beginning to the end of the night. Respiration is regular and slow, about 12–20 breaths/min, during NREM sleep. As metabolic rate falls slightly during NREM sleep, hypoxaemia and hypercapnia must reflect hypoventilation.

In REM sleep the dominant feature is *extreme variability in ventilation.* Breathing is very irregular with more shallow than deep breaths. Ventilation may be lowest during those periods of REM sleep in which eye movements are most common. Douglas *et al.*[75] found that minute ventilation was lower in REM than NREM sleep, averaging 84% of the level in wakefulness. If a similar degree of hypoventilation occurred when a patient was awake, the resultant hypoxia and hypercapnia would stimulate breathing and return ventilation to normal. However, there is a depression of chemosensitivity during REM sleep which impairs the normal protective mechanisms.

The dysrhythmic nature of breathing in REM sleep may relate to the dysrhythmic nature of REM sleep itself. Medullary respiratory neurone activity in REM sleep shows some correlation with the irregular PGO waves of this sleep stage and perhaps also to irregular rapid eye movements.[199]

CHEMICAL CONTROL OF RESPIRATION DURING SLEEP

The rate and depth of breathing are regulated by a negative feedback control system designed to maintain arterial partial pressures of carbon dioxide (PCO_2: normal values 4.5–6.1 kPa) and oxygen (PO_2: 11–13 kPa) at relatively constant levels. The control system setting is altered during sleep, and all respiratory disorders are made worse during sleep.

Deterioration in breathing during sleep results from a combination of changes in respiratory neurone output to respiratory muscles, the mechanical factors of elevation of the diaphragm in the recumbent position and muscular atonia during sleep, alteration in chemoreceptor sensitivity to PCO_2 and O_2 during sleep, and loss of the normal waking voluntary respiratory drive.[296]

HYPERCAPNIC VENTILATORY RESPONSE

During quiet sleep, hypercapnic ventilatory responses are slightly reduced although Remmers[224] concluded that major changes did not occur. PCO_2 may increase during normal deep sleep to around 7 kPa. Breathing CO_2-enriched gases during normal deep sleep does cause an increase in ventilation but this is less for any given level of end-tidal PCO_2 than during waking. The graph line that relates ventilation to PCO_2 may be shifted to the right and slightly reduced in slope during sleep (Fig. 7.3).[45]

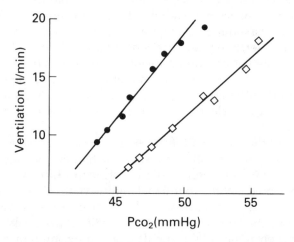

Figure 7.3. *Effect of graded increases in PCO_2 on ventilation during sleep in a healthy young adult. Circles indicate the carbon dioxide response during consciousness, and squares indicate the carbon dioxide response in slow-wave sleep (10 mm Hg = 1.3 kPa). Reprinted with permission from Cherniack.[45]*

The ventilatory responses to breathing oxygen and carbon dioxide are probably broadly similar in REM and NREM sleep in man, and some minute ventilation response to hypoxia is retained during both stages. However, the irregular breathing pattern of REM sleep may apparently mask the respiratory response to changes in PCO_2 during REM sleep. Partial loss of response to the hypercapnic stimulus during REM sleep has been described in dogs, and the response has been shown to be lower in REM than in NREM sleep in adult man.[76] In REM sleep the hypercapnic response is approximately one-third of the level of wakefulness.

HYPOXIC VENTILATORY RESPONSE

Most men live at low altitudes and hypoxaemia is not as important a physiological stimulus to respiration as hypercapnia. However, oxygen tension, both sleeping and waking, is important for respiratory control at high altitudes as well as in chronic lung disease and in patients with neuromuscular disorders affecting the thorax. Initial studies indicated that the respiratory response to hypoxia during sleep is not greatly different from that during wakefulness,[220] although Pappenheimer, in experiments in rats, involving calculations of the alveolar PCO_2 and PO_2, revealed an increased hypoxic responsiveness during NREM sleep.[204] However, more recent investigations in man have shown that the isocapnic ventilatory response to hypoxia decreases during sleep.[71]

In adult men the hypoxic ventilatory response in NREM sleep is approximately two-thirds of that in wakefulness, falling to one-third of the waking level in REM sleep. In adult women, there is no change in the hypoxic ventilatory response between wakefulness and NREM sleep, but the response in REM sleep is about one-half that in the other stages.[72] The reason for this sex difference is not clear. The hypoxic ventilatory response in men reflects metabolic rate although this is not so in women.

MECHANICAL CONTROL OF RESPIRATION DURING SLEEP

Pulmonary stretch reflexes to inflation and deflation of the lungs are mediated by the vagus nerve. In animals, the strength of the Hering–Breuer reflex as shown by the duration of apnoea after lung inflation is increased during slow-wave sleep but decreased during REM sleep. In humans this reflex is strong in babies, but in adults vagal blockade by atropine does not alter the tidal volume or respiratory frequency; and the Hering–Breuer reflex is probably not very important in determining either the frequency of respiration or the tidal volume during either wakefulness or sleep.

The recumbent posture of sleep intensifies any breathing disorder, particularly when the diaphragm is paralysed. In normal awake subjects there is a fall in SaO_2 and rise in PCO_2 in the recumbent as compared with erect posture. This fall is increased during sleep. A number of other mechanical factors during sleep will all aggravate breathing difficulties, including collapse of the tongue backwards, pressure of the abdominal contents on the diaphragm, and flexion or twisting of the neck.

The response to direct mechanical laryngeal, tracheal or bronchial stimulation, inhaled secretions or tracheal aspiration post-surgery, is depressed in both NREM and REM sleep,[212] and the cough reflex is much less strong during sleep than waking. Also, proprioceptive inputs from muscle spindles in the diaphragm and intercostal muscles, and from Golgi tendon organs in the diaphragm, are depressed in sleep. Furthermore, the pattern of ribcage and abdominal movement changes during sleep with, in NREM sleep, relatively more thoracic and less abdominal movement than in waking,[63, 98] although reduction in intercostal muscle tone during sleep may cause a decrease in ribcage movement in some normal adults.[284]

RESPIRATORY MUSCLE TONE DURING SLEEP

Respiratory and skeletal muscle tone is reduced during both slow-wave and REM sleep. The loss of tone in skeletal muscle is most marked in mammals during phasic REM sleep, less severe during tonic REM sleep, and of minor extent during NREM sleep. The respiratory muscles are affected to a lesser extent than the skeletal muscles and although tone is lost in the upper airway muscles and the intercostal muscles,[238] diaphragmatic tone is retained.[224]

The cranial nerves that innervate the tongue, pharyngeal and laryngeal muscles have a sustained activity that coincides with respiration.[225, 267, 296] Phasic tongue movements are sometimes very prominent in human REM sleep[46, 239] and during both very light sleep and REM sleep there is marked periodic waxing and waning of the genioglossus EMG activity which varies with changes in respiration as well as with head position.[194, 236, 237]

AROUSAL RESPONSES TO HYPOXIA AND HYPERCAPNIA

Arousal thresholds to respiratory stimuli in man are difficult to assess, since the instrumentation necessary to deliver the stimulus may both interfere with sleep and contribute to arousal. *Hypoxia* is a poor stimulus to arousal in normal subjects: many normal subjects remain asleep despite an arterial O_2 saturation as low as 70%. *Hypercapnia* is a more potent stimulant, and most subjects arouse before end-tidal PCO_2 has risen by 2 kPa above the level in wakefulness. In normal man there is no difference between sleep stages in the arousal response to either hypoxia or hypercapnia.[76] These arousal responses in normal man contrast with those in many other animal species. Also, arousal responses may be altered by respiratory disease in man. The arousal sensitivity to hypercapnia may be decreased in REM sleep in the sleep apnoea syndrome.[273]

DISORDERS OF RESPIRATION DURING SLEEP

These important conditions are considered here under three headings:

1. Sleep and asthma;
2. Sleep and chronic lung disease;
3. Sleep apnoea syndromes.

References to sections (1) and (2) are listed separately, after the references to the rest of this chapter.

SLEEP AND ASTHMA

In 1698, Dr. John Floyer, describing his own attacks of asthma, wrote 'I have observed the fit always to happen after sleep in the night, when nerves are filled with windy spirits and the heat of the bed has rarefied the spirits and humours'.[314]

Some 4% of the UK population suffers from asthma, and nocturnal asthma may be a more common cause of sleep disturbance than sleep apnoea. In both stable and unstable asthmatics, the condition is made worse by sleep.[320]

Asthma is intimately related to sleep.[311] Patients with asthma are more hypoxic during sleep than are age-matched healthy subjects, and even stable asthmatics sleep poorly, spending more of the night awake or sleeping more lightly than normal subjects. Overnight bronchoconstriction has long been recognized in asthmatics, and about a third of these have their lowest flow rates in the early hours (early morning dips).

Asthma attacks are uncommon in the first hour of sleep,[316] and most occur later at night or in the early morning.[312, 326] Any excess of nocturnal deaths in asthma over that reported in other subjects is controversial, but it has been estimated that there is a 28% higher death rate in asthmatics between midnight and 0800 than at other times, in contrast to only a 5% increase in non-asthmatic deaths.[309]

Asthma and sleep stage
It has proved very difficult to determine the distribution of asthmatic attacks throughout the night. Two studies in asthmatics, one in adults and one in children, have failed to show any correlation between attacks and sleep stage.[317, 318] However, in these studies, patients were taking drugs that might have affected sleep, the respiratory pattern and oxygen saturation were not determined, and respiratory patterns were studied at different phases of the illness. A recent study by Montplaisir et al.[320] has shown clearly that most asthmatic attacks occur during late sleep, with only 15% of attacks in the first third, as compared to 46% of attacks in the last third of the night. Some workers report that attacks of nocturnal wheeze are commoner in REM sleep than in other sleep stages; others disagree.

Respiratory changes during sleep in asthmatics
In asthmatics there is a progressive decrease in FEV throughout the night, amounting to a final 20–50% reduction.[320, 324] However, measurement of FEV demands a cooperative patient who is awake, not asleep. (Although FEV can be determined throughout the *night*, it cannot be determined throughout *sleep*. See the comment on difficulty of respiratory measurements during sleep on p. 379). Despite this decrease in FEV, the degree of oxygen desaturation at night is usually mild, with a mean percentage fall in SaO_2 of only 5–6%.[320] Desaturation may be of greater severity in children than in adults.[325] The degree of hypoxaemia during sleep in asthmatics is linked with the severity of airway

obstruction.[319] Investigators have tried recently to disrupt sleep in patients with nocturnal asthma, but generally have not been able to influence the decrease in FEV or the decrease in SaO_2 that occurs throughout the night.[316]

Arousal responses to irritant stimuli are depressed in REM sleep, and asthmatics, despite attacks, may not awaken during REM sleep.

Causes of nocturnal asthma

Physical factors, allergens and chemical triggers may all contribute to nocturnal asthma. Posture does not seem to play a major role, but the retention of secretions, with decreased mucociliary clearance during sleep, could contribute to air flow limitation during the night and trigger an attack.[311] Aspiration of the gastric contents during sleep may occasionally be a provoking factor.[315] Allergy does not seem to be of primary importance, but the recognition that the house mite faecal pellet, a particle some 20 μm in diameter, is the source of a very high potency antigen in patients with house mite sensitivity, has led to a reappraisal; attacks at night have been demonstrated for as long as a week after a single exposure to allergens.[321]

Histamine inhalation causes bronchoconstriction, with a mean decrease in peak expiratory flow rate of up to 30%, although without any very great drop in SaO_2.[322, 323] This decrease in peak expiratory flow rate due to histamine without great change in SaO_2 resembles the changes occurring naturally in asthma, both waking and sleeping, and histamine release may be one final common mechanism resulting in sleep attacks. It seems unlikely that histamine or other mediators are primarily responsible for asthma at night,[313] although Barnes *et al.*[310] suggested that an increase in histamine level with a decrease in circulating noradrenaline level might account for nocturnal awakenings in asthma. Nocturnal, sleep or posture-related differences in histamine sensitivity have also been implicated.[327] In addition to all these factors, psychogenic factors, with disturbed dreams, may explain why some asthmatics die at night.

The major problem in the prevention of nocturnal asthma is that the most effective drugs, inhaled bronchodilators, do not last long enough to cover the 6–8 h of a normal night's sleep. The use of oral *slow-release theophylline*, or beta-agonists such as *salbutamol*, will cause long-term relief of bronchoconstriction at night, and these drugs can be combined with inhaled bronchodilators both immediately before bedtime and, if necessary, during nocturnal attacks.

SLEEP AND CHRONIC LUNG DISEASE

Arterial oxygen tension falls by about 2 kPa in everybody during sleep due to a reduction in ventilation. In normal subjects this is of no consequence but patients who are hypoxic whilst awake may become much more hypoxic whilst asleep, with arterial PO_2 falling as low as 3.6 kPa. This fall results in marked desaturation in hypoxic patients. Desaturation is particularly marked during REM sleep, and has been reported in many respiratory diseases including chronic bronchitis and emphysema, cystic fibrosis, diaphragmatic palsy, kyphoscoliosis and chronic mountain sickness (see p. 390).

Sleep has an adverse effect on the symptoms of *chronic obstructive pulmonary disease, asthma, chronic bronchitis* and *emphysema,* and also on O_2 saturation in *anaemia.*[338] Arterial oxygen desaturation is increased, sometimes with marked hypoxia during REM sleep, as a result of hypoventilation, a slow rate of respiration, and sometimes central apnoea. In the presence of chronic lung disease, SaO_2 may fall from 85–90% to around 65% during REM sleep. The degree of desaturation is determined by a blunted chemical drive. Patients who start sleep with some degree of hypoxia may show a very marked drop in PO_2 during sleep since they start on the steep part of the curve relating PO_2 to SaO_2.[330, 332, 333, 340] All patients with chronic bronchitis and emphysema who are hypoxic whilst awake thus become much more hypoxic whilst asleep and usually have several intermittent episodes of severe sleep oxygen desaturation every night. The coexistence of sleep apnoea and asthma can result in particularly severe sleep hypoxaemia.[335] Even in chronic stable asthma, irregular breathing during sleep is common.

Sleep hypoxia in chronic lung disease
In obstructive sleep apnoea the fall in arterial SaO_2 during sleep is largely due to apnoea and hypopnoea, but in chronic obstructive pulmonary disease many other factors contribute: suppression of the cough reflex, slowing of mucociliary clearance, sudden falls in cardiac output, cardiac arrhythmias and ventilation–perfusion mismatching, particularly with loss of intercostal muscle activity and alteration in chest wall compliance. This has been shown to be a major cause of sleep desaturation in patients with cystic fibrosis.[337] In most reported instances, sleep hypoxia does not appear to be so severe as to cause brain damage.

Sleep hypercapnia in chronic lung disease
The normal rise in PCO_2 during sleep may be generally aggravated with respiratory disease. Hypercapnia results in cerebral vasodilatation. However, during sleep in chronic bronchitics, the normal vasomotor response to hypercapnia is to some extent suppressed, and any increase in cerebral blood flow, particularly in brain stem areas, may be lower than expected. Some bronchitics have very blunted hypercapnic responses during sleep but most, despite a fall in SaO_2, retain some hypercapnic response.[331]

Sleep and pulmonary hypertension in chronic lung disease
Pulmonary artery pressure increases with sleep and this increase is most pronounced during REM sleep. Unlike the situation in the peripheral circulation, the pulmonary artery pressure increases with hypoxia, and, as in sleep apnoea, sustained nocturnal pulmonary hypertension may develop in patients with chronic obstructive pulmonary disease.[329]

Sleep quality in chronic obstructive pulmonary disease
Sleep quality in chronic obstructive pulmonary disease is often poor, with a reduction in total REM sleep, many arousals and frequent sleep fragmentation. However, patients with chronic hypoxia whilst awake, due to bronchitis or emphysema, may not be woken by further severe sleep oxygen desaturation. As in sleep apnoea, cardiac arrhythmias occur in REM-related hypoxic episodes in chronic bronchitis. A disproportionate number of these patients die at night, but it is not known whether they were indeed asleep, or whether death was due to REM hypoxia-related arrhythmias.

Most patients with severe chronic airflow obstruction do not develop sleep apnoea, and although the cardiovascular consequences of chronic and intermittent airway obstruction are similar, daytime sleepiness is more common with sleep apnoea than with chronic bronchitis. In chronic airway disease apnoeas sometimes do occur during normal sleep[334] but these may be no more common or severe than in normal subjects.[331]

'Blue bloaters' and 'pink puffers'
Tirlapur and Mir[339] reported the occurrence of episodic hypoxaemia during sleep in patients with chronic obstructive airway disease. The frequency and severity of the hypoxaemic episodes were greatest in 'blue bloaters'; i.e. those whose airway obstruction is accompanied by evidence of carbon dioxide retention and cor pulmonale. Tachycardia, ST depression and ventricular ectopics accompanied episodic hypoxaemia. All these features are reduced by low-flow oxygen administration during sleep. This, as well as improving oxygenation, may reduce the number of arousals and improve sleep[336] as well as improve pulmonary blood flow and prolong life. However, oxygen can be dangerous, sometimes causing CO_2 retention and an increase, not a decrease, in the frequency and duration of apnoeic episodes.[328] In contrast to 'blue bloaters', 'pink puffers' have little or no evidence of oxygen desaturation during sleep.

SLEEP APNOEA SYNDROMES

Definitions
The terminology and definition of sleep apnoea are largely founded on experience at Stanford.[113] These important studies have established normal physiological criteria, as well as clearly abnormal breathing patterns during sleep. There is, however, a continuum from normal breathing patterns to grossly disturbed patterns during sleep and these vary with age. Minor degrees of sleep apnoea, as defined below, are nearly always completely asymptomatic; and at certain ages may be entirely normal, not pathological.

It is sometimes difficult to determine the role of sleep apnoea in causing somewhat vague symptomatology, such as minor headache, mild personality disturbances, and failure of libido. However there is no doubt that severe sleep apnoea is an important cause of crippling cardiorespiratory illness as well as daytime drowsiness.

Sleep apnoea may be either normal (less than 30 apnoeas in a night of sleep) or abnormal (over 30 apnoeic episodes, each lasting 10 s or more, during one night of sleep). Most patients with symptomatic sleep apnoea have hundreds of episodes each night. In normal subjects, premenopausal normal weight females usually have less apnoeas during sleep than males of the same age and weight.

Four types of apnoea can be distinguished by respiratory measurements:

1. *Central apnoea.*   Respiratory movements are absent and there is no oronasal airflow.
2. *Obstructive apnoea.*   The diaphragm and chest wall move with changes in intrathoracic pressure, but there is no airflow at the nose or mouth.
3. *Mixed apnoea.*   Respiratory movements and airflow are absent early in the episode, followed by resumption of unsuccessful breathing. The opposite pattern does not occur.
4. *Sub-obstructive apnoea.*   Reduced airflow with increased respiratory effort.

Hypopnoea, like apnoea, may be central, obstructive or mixed. Since mean (or peak) inspiratory or expiratory airflow is seldom measured during sleep, the degree of hypopnea is usually not defined.

The *apnoea index* gives the number of apnoeas occurring during one hour of sleep, and is an estimate of the severity of sleep apnoea. An index of 5 or less is normal in adults.

Diagnosis of pathological sleep apnoea requires the presence of apnoeas in NREM (other than sleep onset) as well as during REM sleep (other than during eye movements – these are not continuous during REM sleep), and apnoeas that occur actually during rapid eye movement are usually not accepted as abnormal.

Hypoventilation is usually defined in terms of oxygen saturation.[87] A decrease in oxygen saturation of more than 4% is regarded as significant by some groups,[26] whereas other workers have used a 10% decrease from a previously stable oxygen saturation.[74]

Distinction of central and obstructive apnoeas

The separation of apnoeas into central, mixed or obstructive types, based on airflow and thoraco-abdominal motion, is somewhat artificial (Fig. 7.4). It implies there may be different mechanisms for the different types of apnoea observed and that sleep apnoea can result from either failure of the brain stem automatic control system of respiration or from mechanical obstruction to the upper airway. However, in one respect, all apnoeas have a central brain stem origin with a prolonged pause in central upper airway motor neurone output at the end of expiration accompanying passive collapse of the oropharyngeal muscles in 'obstructive' as well as in central forms of apnoea.[194] In practice, in most patients with sleep apnoea, both 'central' and 'obstructive' apnoeas occur, although one type usually predominates. The pathogenesis of both types may be similar in the final analysis, although the clinical presentation

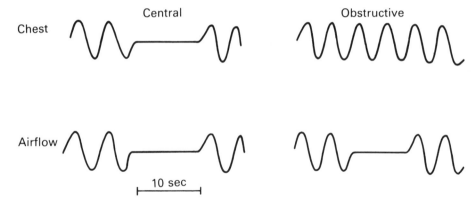

Figure 7.4.   *Schematic diagram indicating the diagnostic features of apnoeas of central and obstructive type, indicating in the upper part of the diagram chest wall movement, measured by a stethogram, and, below, air flow at the nose and mouth, measured by thermocouples. When both airflow and chest movements cease simultaneously apnoeas are classified as 'central' but when chest wall movement continues in the absence of air flow, obstructive apnoeas may be diagnosed. Reprinted with permission from Douglas, M.J.* Respiratory Disease in Practise (1984) 28.

depends on the presence or absence of anatomical narrowing of the upper airway. However, some still consider that the aetiology of central and obstructive apnoeas could be distinct, although this is unlikely. Douglas[72] considered that all types of apnoea had similar mechanisms, a conclusion based on the near universal occurrence of both types of apnoea, both in normal subjects at sleep onset and during REM sleep, as well as in sleep apnoea syndromes, and the observation that there is a parallel reduction in muscle tone in the diaphragm and upper airway opening muscles during obstructive apnoeas.[194]

Over 90% of all cases of sleep apnoea are associated with airway obstruction. Central respiratory failure without airway obstruction accounts for a small minority of cases only. Obstructive sleep apnoea is mainly a male disease occurring in people over 40 and with a steady increase in incidence with age. In contrast, central sleep apnoea occurs in all age groups and has no definite sex distribution.

Physiological sleep apnoea
Brief apnoeas occur in the sleep of normal subjects. These are most common following body movements and during REM sleep.

In *infants* and pre-term babies, recurrent apnoeas occur most frequently in those with the lowest weight[124, 136] and at the lowest gestational age.[12, 12] However, it is usually not clear why apnoeas occur in some babies but not in others.

In normal *children* aged 9–13, between 3 and 40 pauses of 5 s or longer duration occur each night (an average of 17–18 brief apnoeas). Sleep respiration is more regular in girls than in boys.[42]

In *adults*, apnoeas are more frequent with increasing age and are also most common in those who snore or are obese or following alcohol or sedative drug intake.[26, 115, 161, 212, 213] These apnoeas are mainly central, sometimes obstructive. Most are very short, lasting 10 s, and less than 10 episodes occur each night. Normal adult men have more apnoeas than women.[109] In normal subjects, obstructive apnoeas during REM sleep may produce a slight fall in arterial oxygen saturation, but this is rarely more than 2–3%. Central apnoeas during NREM sleep cause insignificant drops in SaO_2.[106]

Although prolonged sleep apnoea is usually considered to be pathological in humans, it may be physiological in some animal species and a means of conserving energy. Elephant seal pups stop breathing every time they fall asleep with bradycardia, and apnoea may last as long as 20 min. On awakening, the pups hyperventilate.

Pathological sleep apnoea

In subjects with sleep apnoea syndromes, episodes of sleep apnoea may last from the minimal conventional duration of 10 s to as long as 100–200 s, with an average of 20–40 s. The total sleep time spent in apnoea is very variable, with a mean of 40–50% in severely affected patients, but sometimes as high as 80%. The frequency and duration of apnoeas and the degree of resulting arterial oxygen desaturation are usually greater during REM than NREM sleep. Because of the skew distribution of REM sleep, apnoeas are more severe in the second than in the first half of the night. Since physiological sleep apnoea is most common in REM sleep, to be certain of the diagnosis of pathological sleep apnoea, repetitive apnoeas should be present during NREM sleep as well as during REM sleep. In fact in patients with severe sleep apnoea there are usually overall more frequent sleep apnoeas during NREM sleep because sleep is so fragmented in these patients by the arousals that very little REM sleep is achieved.

Mechanisms of obstructive sleep apnoea

It has been suggested that obstructive sleep apnoea develops as a result of passive collapse of the hypotonic oropharynx against the negative pressure developed by respiratory muscles.[111, 225, 269] Thus obstructive sleep apnoea may be due to a sleep-induced failure of upper airway opening muscles. During inspiration the pressure within the upper airway is sub-atmospheric to suck air into the lungs. The supraglottic airway is floppy and would collapse during each inspiration without the phasic activity of upper airway opening muscles. These respiratory muscles include the genioglossus, geniohyoid, tensor palatini and the medial pterygoids. Sleep hypotonia in the presence of a narrow airway may be sufficient to permit upper airway collapse.

Fibre-optic endoscopic views have shown that the right and left lateral walls of the oropharynx oppose during episodes of sleep apnoea, commencing with a constriction in the superior oropharynx, midway between the top of the tongue and the naso-oropharyngeal junction.[299] The tongue may close with the soft palate, but not usually with the posterior pharyngeal wall. If the pharyngeal walls collapse for several inspiratory–expiratory cycles, there is loud snoring and deep breathing accompanied by rapid vibration of the soft palate and partial opening of the velopharyngeal sphincters.

In patients with obstructive sleep apnoea, the glottis usually remains open and the vocal cords abduct with each inspiration.[299]

Very rarely, the site of obstruction may be elsewhere. Laryngeal abductor palsy may cause obstruction in the Shy–Drager syndrome,[13] and this may also be the case in the occasional Pickwickian patient.[148, 175]

In normal awake humans, the genioglossal EMG and the diaphragmatic EMG respond similarly to chemical respiratory stimuli, suggesting that upper airway and diaphragm respiratory muscles share similar central control mechanisms.[195, 196] In sleep apnoea this normal balance is disturbed.

Genioglossal EMG activity at the time of resolution of periods of upper airway occlusion is increased out of proportion to the increase in diaphragmatic EMG activity and also out of proportion to the degree of oxygen desaturation. There are differences in the timing and differences in the degree of activation of the other oropharyngeal respiratory muscles, palatal and laryngeal muscles with respiration during sleep[6, 20] and these differences may be important in preventing sleep apnoea.

Compensatory defence mechanisms prevent obstructive sleep apnoea in normal subjects and are of great importance in subjects with critical degrees of airway narrowing. The most important mechanisms involve the laryngeal muscles which respond to hypoxia with dilatation, whilst pharyngeal muscle tone increases in response to a decrease in oxygen saturation, an increase in PCO_2, or arousal. Tonic airway dilatation with arousal depends on the activity of pontomedullary activating regions of the reticular formation.[199]

History of sleep apnoea syndromes

The *Pickwickian syndrome* is a form of obstructive sleep apnoea with obesity, CO_2 retention and diminished ventilatory drive to increase in PCO_2. *Ondine's curse* is a very rare disorder with primary failure of medullary automatic respiratory centres resulting in hypoventilation and central apnoea. The central characters are the fat boy Joe in Dickens's novel (Fig. 7.5) and Hans, the human lover of a Scandinavian water fairy.[57] Here are the case histories and also that of Falstaff.

> Peto: *Falstaff! Fast asleep behind the arras and snorting like a horse.*
> Prince: *Hark, how hard he fetches breath. Search his pockets.*
>   (Shakespeare, Henry IV, Part 1, Act II, Scene iv (see Adler[4]))

> *Mr. Lowton hurried to the door. The object that presented itself to the eyes of the astonished clerk was a boy – a wonderfully fat boy – standing upright on the mat with his eyes closed as if in sleep. He had never seen such a fat boy, in or out of a travelling caravan; and this, coupled with the utter calmness of his appearance, so very different from what was reasonably to have been expected of the inflictor of such knocks, smote him with wonder.*

"What's the matter?" inquired the clerk. The extraordinary boy replied not a word; but he nodded once, and seemed, to the clerk's imagination, to snore feebly. "Where do you come from?" inquired the clerk.

The boy made no sign. He breathed heavily, but in all other respects was motionless.

The clerk repeated the question twice, and receiving no answer, prepared to shut the door, when the boy suddenly opened his eyes, winked several times, sneezed once, and raised his hands as if to repeat the knocking. Finding the door open, he stared about him with astonishment and at length fixed his eyes on Mr. Lowton's face.

"What the devil do you knock in that way for?" inquired the clerk, angrily. "Which way?" said the boy in a slow sleepy voice.

"Why, like forty hackney-coachmen" replied the clerk.

"Because master said I wasn't to leave off knocking till they opened the door, for fear I should go to sleep," said the boy.

(Dickens, C. The Posthumous Papers of the Pickwick Club, *London: Chapman and Hall* (see Burwell et al.[36])

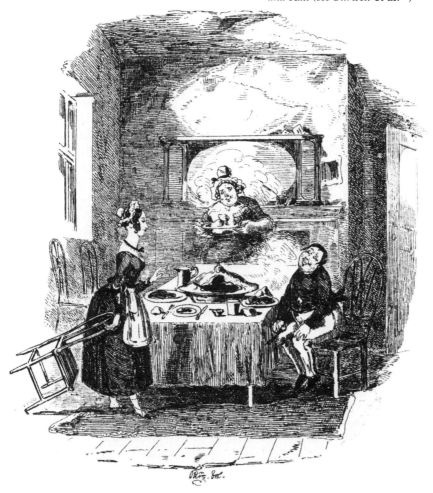

Figure 7.5. *Mary and the fat boy Joe (Charles Dickens:* Pickwick Papers*).*

Ondine: Try to live, Hans. You will forget too.
Hans: Try to live! That's easy to say, isn't it. If only I cared about living! Since
         you went away, I've had to force my body to do things it should do
         automatically. I no longer see unless I order my eyes to see. I don't see the
         grass is green unless I tell them to see it green. And it's not much fun,
         black grass, I can tell you . ˙ . If I relax my vigilance for one moment, I
         may forget to hear or to breathe. He died, they'll say, because he could no
         longer bother to breathe.
         (Giraudoux, J. Ondine, English adaptation by Maurice Valency, New
                                              York: Random House (1954))

GENERAL FEATURES OF SLEEP APNOEA SYNDROMES

SEX INCIDENCE

Central sleep apnoea has an equal sex incidence, but obstructive sleep apnoea is ten times more common in men than women. When obstructive sleep apnoea occurs in women, they are mainly postmenopausal.[161] Male predominance is largely due to the action of androgens and to the different shape of the oropharynx and larynx in men and women. Testosterone causes an increase in appetite, the anabolic state, weight increase and a tendency towards sodium retention, all of which will aggravate sleep apnoea. Additionally, testosterone may result in peripheral oedema, erythrocytosis with a 2–3% increase in the haematocrit due to an increase in erythropoietin activity and direct bone marrow stimulation,[244] and even cor pulmonale in subjects with normal nocturnal respiration.[14, 187, 270]

Sleep apnoea is uncommon in hypogonadal obese males with low testosterone levels.[122] Strumpf et al.[270] reported the development and subsequent resolution of a Pickwickian syndrome with testosterone treatment and withdrawal. Likewise, Sandblom et al.[232] described a 36-year-old male life-long snorer who was moderately obese; he developed sleep apnoea on two separate occasions when given testosterone enanthate 200 mg i.m. weekly for seven months, possibly as a result of further weight gain and oropharyngeal obstruction.[37]

Disordered breathing during sleep is much more common in men than in premenopausal women,[27] and progesterone may 'protect' against the development of obstructive sleep apnoea in women.[126] Progestational agents are said to stimulate breathing,[307] which possibly accounts for the hyperventilation of pregnancy and the luteal stage of menstruation.[70, 97] In addition, progesterone increases the ventilatory responses to hypoxia and hypercapnia in normal subjects, and medroxyprogesterone acetate 60–120 mg/day will sometimes improve central apnoea[169] with a consequent increase in nocturnal oxygen saturation. The effect of progesterone in sleep apnoea is probably due to a number of factors, including central respiratory stimulation, fat redistribution and possibly an improvement in cardiac decompensation due to an increase in glomerular filtration rate and an anti-aldosterone effect.[202, 268] Certainly progesterone has been shown to improve ventilatory drive in central apnoea[276] although the overall effect is slight and progesterone usually does not help patients with obstructive sleep apnoea.[201, 202] According to Strohl et al.[268] progesterone non-responders can be distinguished from responders by the finding of a low resting arterial oxygen tension during wakefulness. At high altitude, progesterone will eliminate the occasional profound drop in SaO_2 during sleep apnoeic episodes, but unlike acetazolamide, progesterone has little or no effect on periodic breathing.[295]

FAMILIAL AND GENETIC FACTORS

The genetics of the various sleep apnoea syndromes are not yet established except in those instances of hereditary disease, such as myotonic dystrophy, which predispose to obstruction, and also possibly to central sleep apnoea. A rare familial disorder in which five members of two generations had the combination of glaucoma and a sleep apnoea syndrome was reported by Walsh and Montplaisir.[291] Respiratory centre sensitivity to hypercapnia may be an inherited trait, and important for the development of sleep apnoea. In a family reported by Strohl et al.[269] the father and two sons had obstructive sleep apnoea, a third son died during sleep at the age of 30, and a fourth asymptomatic son had a child who died suddenly at the age of 4 months, possibly with sleep-related cardiac arrest. However, other familial and genetic factors are usually not very important in obstructive sleep apnoea.

SLEEP APNOEA IN THE ELDERLY

Although sleep apnoea does occur in children[33] it increases in frequency with age in both men and women.[27, 180] The reported incidence of sleep apnoea in the elderly is surprisingly high, although in most cases the condition is completely asymptomatic with a low apnoea index which may be a normal physiological response to ageing.[293] In an elderly population in good health and with no sleep problems, Carskadon and Dement[41] found that seven women and eight men of 40 volunteers (37%) had sleep apnoea, in most cases of central origin. A similar percentage was found by Ancoli-Israel et al.[7] amongst old people, although here sleep-related symptoms were present, and obstructive rather than central apnoea was found in most instances. The size of the problem invites disbelief but all studies have confirmed that sleep apnoea is very common in the elderly: Kries et al.,[147] in a sample of 26 randomly selected men with a mean age of 66 in a hospital medical ward, found that seven (26%) had sleep apnoea; McGinty et al.[164] showed that six of 10 asymptomatic old men had sleep-related breathing disorders; and Pollak et al.[215] reported that, in six elderly subjects with mild chronic obstructive airway disease, five also had sleep apnoea.

Some old people must die in their sleep as a consequence of sleep apnoea, and the 30% increase in mortality rates for all causes during the usual hours of sleep[257] may be partly accounted for by sudden respiratory failure. Kripke and Ancoli-Israel[152] indicated that sleep apnoea may be a common reason why old people die quietly and peacefully and without distress in their sleep.

There is ample documentation that frequent and repetitive airway obstruction with resultant hypoxaemia and hypercapnia, sleep deprivation and fragmentation in young subjects may lead to intellectual and personality changes, irritability, chronic fatigue, inattentiveness and memory impairment. Does the high prevalence of sleep apnoea reported in old people contribute to significant intellectual deterioration and behavioural disturbances in the elderly? At present the data are too limited to allow a firm conclusion. Overall, periods of alveolar hypoventilation and arterial O_2 desaturation during sleep are more severe and prolonged in old than in young subjects and the resting PO_2 decreases with age even during wakefulness.[258] However, severe arterial O_2 desaturation at night is uncommon in the elderly despite occasional sleep apnoea, and this seems unlikely to be of a severity sufficient to impair brain function or result in intellectual deterioration in most instances.[184]

FREQUENCY OF SLEEP APNOEA

Sleep apnoea, as determined by a machine, is very common, but is almost always asymptomatic. The initial studies of Webb[293] and Block et al.[26] indicated that apnoea during sleep was much more common in the general population than originally supposed. Oddly enough, it was studies of snoring that most clearly demonstrated these findings.[152] Lugaresi et al.,[160] believing that the complaint of snoring often indicated the presence of sleep apnoea, found that amongst the inhabitants of the Republic of San Marino 19% of the population aged 30–60 were habitual snorers. However, the incidence of sleep apnoea in the general population has never been formally investigated. Highly indirect evidence for a high prevalence of the syndrome comes from studies in America and Israel which suggest that 4% of the adult population complain of excessive daytime sleepiness, a common cause of which is sleep apnoea.[56, 156] Reynolds et al.[227] reported that of patients seen in a North American sleep disorder clinic because of a sleep disturbance, 18.5% had sleep apnoea, and studies by Lavie,[157] done to estimate the prevalance of sleep disorders in industrial workers in Israel, established that between 1% and 6% of the industrial population had sleep apnoea. However, in no case were apnoeas frequent and most of these subjects were over 40 years of age.

In the United States, Canada, Australia, continental Europe and Japan, the prevalence of symptomatic and asymptomatic sleep apnoea combined is perhaps between 0.01% and 1% of the population. Symptomatic sleep apnoea is still diagnosed only rarely in Britain, sometimes owing to lack of recognition.[8, 167, 246] The high prevalence of symptomatic and asymptomatic sleep apnoea reported from the USA results from the widespread availability of sleep laboratory facilities, but also perhaps from a high prevalence of precipitating factors including obesity, alcoholism and drug abuse – over 8000 tons of hypnotics were consumed in the USA in 1973. Obesity, which is a major risk factor, is present in up to two-thirds of all cases[299] and alcoholism may account for the high prevalence of sleep apnoea reported amongst the Maori of New Zealand. Occasional case reports are not true examples of the syndrome as, for example, an intriguing but phoney Chinese patient with 'sleep apnoea' which was reversed by the transfusion of vital energy![304]

Over 150 patients with sleep apnoea were described in Stanford in 1978, over 450 patients in 1980 and over 800 in 1984.[104, 106, 109] By 1982, sleep apnoea and not narcolepsy was the most common diagnosis in patients investigated for daytime drowsiness in sleep clinics in the United States[56] (sleep apnoea accounted for 43% of such patients, narcolepsy for only 25%).

COURSE AND PROGNOSIS

The natural history of obstructive sleep apnoea is very variable. Worldwide studies, particularly those at Stanford, have established that sleep apnoea, with an apnoea index above 5 but below 40, is mostly an incidental and completely asymptomatic finding. In subjects who are investigated for the complaint of daytime drowsiness and found to have obstructive sleep apnoea, the apnoea index is usually much higher. In the majority of these subjects, symptoms are usually mild and may not progress over 10–20 years of observation unless complicated by severe obesity, alcoholism or the development of serious right heart failure. The situation is different in a small group of severely disabled patients who have frequent and profound drops of arterial SaO_2 at night. A few of these die rapidly and others, mainly the very obese, have severe progressive disability, intractable right heart failure or nocturnal cardiac arrest. Once pulmonary hypertension has developed the outlook is poor, with death in under 4 years in many cases.

It is not clear to what extent severe sleep hypoxia, especially when combined with alcoholism, may damage the brain; in most instances of severe sleep apnoea, treated with tracheostomy, mental changes are reversed by this procedure.

SEDATIVES, HYPNOTICS AND SLEEP APNOEA

Respiratory infection or any ENT abnormality causing airway narrowing will trigger sleep apnoea. Other important precipitants include sedatives, anaesthetics, opiates, benzodiazepines, barbiturates and any other drug that will depress the respiratory centre and cause hypoventilation. All these drugs, and also alcohol, may cause serious respiratory depression in subjects with sleep apnoea and result in an increase in frequency and duration of apnoeic episodes and also an increase in the severity of sleep hypoxia.[140]

In normal subjects benzodiazepines and other hypnotics depress respiration. The degree of depression is dose-dependent. Flurazepam 40 mg, in normal subjects, causes an increase in the number and duration of physiological apnoeic episodes, reduces arousal during hypercapnia, and causes an increase in the degree of oxygen desaturation; although ventilatory responses to hypercapnia and hypoxia are unaltered in this dosage.[69] Nitrazepam has similar effects, but in the doses investigated may depress the ventilatory drive to carbon dioxide, and even precipitate carbon dioxide narcosis in patients with pulmonary disease.[48, 182, 230] Likewise, chlordiazepoxide in therapeutic dosages increases hypercapnia, whilst intravenous diazepam and clonazepam both reduce tidal volume, depress respiratory responses to CO_2 and increase arterial PCO_2.[88, 182, 183]

These changes are of little or no clinical importance in normal subjects, but hypnotics can cause severe respiratory depression in the presence of airway obstruction. The severity of pathologic sleep apnoea is considerably increased by high dosage of benzodiazepines and, in some apparently normal subjects, daytime sleepiness after these drugs may result from unsuspected sleep apnoea as well as from residual drug effects.[177] It is possible, but not proven, that the high mortality, both waking and sleeping, reported in habitual users of sleeping pills, is sometimes associated with sleep apnoea.[153]

Ethanol, like the benzodiazepines, will depress respiration.[278] In patients with sleep apnoea, ethanol 2ml/kg increases both apnoeas and arterial oxygen desaturation. These subjects should avoid alcohol and sleeping pills.

ENT FINDINGS IN SLEEP APNOEA (Fig. 7.6)

Over 90% of all patients with obstructive sleep apnoea have some ENT abnormality. Almost half of a group of patients with obstructive sleep apnoea described by Halperin et al.[117] had a short thick neck, 41% had had some operation on the upper respiratory tract (tonsillectomy, polypectomy, excision of a vocal cord cyst); 25% had chronic vasomotor rhinitis, micrognathia or other mandibular deformity; 18% had a deviated nasal septum, and a similar number a disproportionately large tongue. 14% had chronic sinusitis, 9% a palatal deformity, and 9% hypertrophic tonsils. Many of these factors do not provoke respiratory obstruction by themselves, but may cause a lower pressure in the pharynx than would otherwise occur during inspiration, and thus tip the balance of obstruction.[308] Particularly in infancy and early childhood, nasal obstruction can have a critical effect on ventilation.[146] Heavy snoring due to incomplete airway obstruction may be associated with minor degrees of sleep apnoea, although oxygen desaturation and hypercapnia are usually mild and other features of the sleep apnoea syndrome do not occur.

CLINICAL SYMPTOMATOLOGY OF SLEEP APNOEA SYNDROMES

Patients with sleep apnoea stop breathing intermittently and recurrently during sleep. The condition can be diagnosed with certainty only by watching the patient sleep. However, a very high index of suspicion is raised by a history of loud snoring, gross restlessness and apnoeas during sleep in any patient with daytime drowsiness (Tables 7.1 and 7.2).

Acute or chronic obstruction of the upper airway disturbs normal sleep

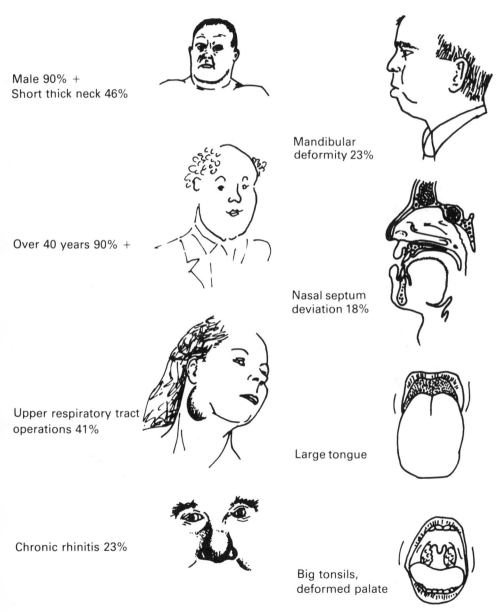

Male 90% +
Short thick neck 46%

Mandibular
deformity 23%

Over 40 years 90% +

Nasal septum
deviation 18%

Upper respiratory tract
operations 41%

Large tongue

Chronic rhinitis 23%

Big tonsils,
deformed palate

Figure 7.6. *ENT findings in sleep apnoea.*

Table 7.1. *Symptomatology in obstructive sleep apnoea*

Snoring	100%
Abnormal sleep behaviour	100%
Altered waking conscious state	78%
Intellectual deterioration	78%
Nocturnal enuresis	
children	majority
adults	30%
Morning headache	36%
Personality deterioration	48%
Sleep disturbance	23%
Sudden death at night	occasional

Data from Guilleminault and Dement[109] and King's College Hospital patients.

Table 7.2. *Features of sleep apnoea*

Cardiovascular and respiratory complications
  Hypoxia
  Hypercapnia
  Pulmonary hypertension
  Right heart failure
  Cardiac arrhythmias
  Systemic hypertension
  Secondary polycythaemia
  Respiratory failure
  Sudden unexplained death

Daytime symptoms
  Drowsiness
  Automatic behaviour
  Morning headache
  Tiredness
  Failure of concentration
  Psychosis
  Depression
  Impotence
  Intellectual deterioration

Night sleep
  Snoring
  Restlessness
  Apnoea
  Multiple arousals
  Nocturnal enuresis
  Somnambulism

physiology. Mechanical obstruction results in snoring, honking or snorting, interrupted by silence (apnoea) which may be of long duration, sometimes over 60 s. Apnoea in turn results in hypercapnia and hypoxia, with secondary cardiac arrhythmias, pulmonary hypertension and cor pulmonale. This can end in death. Much more common clinical sequelae are, however, less serious. Guilleminault and his colleagues have delineated 12 clinical characteristics of sleep apnoea. They found that approximately one half of their cases had seven or more of the following features: snoring, abnormal motor activity during sleep, excessive daytime sleepiness, personality change, deterioration in intellectual capacity, systemic hypertension, sexual problems, abnormal outbursts of irrational behaviour, morning headache, hypnagogic hallucinations, automatic behaviour, and nocturnal enuresis.[110] Many of these problems also occur in children.[112]

NIGHT SLEEP IN CENTRAL SLEEP APNOEA

Clinical symptomatology in *central* and *obstructive* sleep apnoea variants is different. The complaint of insomnia is more common in central sleep apnoea than in obstructive sleep apnoea. In central sleep apnoea, although patients may complain of daytime tiredness and lethargy, they rarely have the same degree of disabling daytime drowsiness as subjects with obstructive sleep apnoea. Also, in central sleep apnoea, the overall degree of sleep distribution at night is less than in obstructive sleep apnoea. Snoring is infrequent and usually not severe, although patients with central sleep apnoea may wake up several times each night, gasping for breath, choking, and sometimes with severe anxiety.

NIGHT SLEEP IN OBSTRUCTIVE SLEEP APNOEA

Sleep is very disturbed with noisy pharyngeal snoring, snorts and honks interrupted by profound periodic silence with apnoea. A pneumatic drill smashing up concrete delivers something like 70–100 dB. Snoring can generate sound ranging in intensity from 69 dB (*Proceedings of the Royal Society of Medicine* (1968) **61,** 575) to 80 dB (*Southern Medical Journal* (1980) **73,** 1035). It is not surprising, therefore, that these patients make intolerable bed partners. The inspiratory snores gradually increase with the increase in airway obstruction followed by a choking inspiratory gasp as the occlusion is overcome. During each apnoea, skeletal muscle tone is reduced and the depth of sleep may briefly increase before arousal terminates some, but not all, episodes.

Gross restlessness, frequent changes in posture, flailing arm movements, twitches of the face and respiratory muscles, jerks of the legs, arms and trunk and tongue movements are often marked; and falls from bed, somnambulism and nocturia may occur. The patient with obstructive sleep apnoea is usually not aware of these frequent and sometimes violent movements, or of any respiratory difficulty during sleep. The usual complaint is one of a poor night's sleep rather than of insomnia, and amnesia for the frequent arousals is the rule.

Most of the night is spent in stage 1–2 NREM sleep, and many patients with severe obstructive sleep apnoea have little or no stage 3–4 sleep.

DAYTIME SYMPTOMS IN SLEEP APNOEA

The overwhelming complaint in sleep apnoea is usually one of daytime drowsiness. Other serious waking symptoms include learning difficulty, failure of concentration, intellectual deterioration and personality change, often accompanied by morning headache, nausea, early morning confusion and constant tiredness.

Daytime sleepiness occurs in up to 80% of patients with sleep apnoea and increases in both severity and frequency with the apnoea index. As in narcolepsy, daytime drowsiness with sleep apnoea may be accompanied by hypnagogic hallucinations, and automatic behaviour occurs in up to 50% of all subjects.[113] Morning arousal can be particularly difficult and sleep drunkenness, grogginess, disorientation, dulling of the senses and motor incoordination occur in between 40% and 60% of subjects. The overall degree of incapacity may be severe and cause major work problems, social difficulties and marital breakdown. Occupational and driving accidents are frequent.

Sudden outbursts of violent behaviour, personality change, anxiety and depressive neurosis have all been attributed to sleep apnoea,[22, 66] but a causative role is sometimes doubtful. Whether sleep apnoea is ever responsible for psychosis in previously non-psychotic individuals is also uncertain, although sleep hypoxia will aggravate previous psychotic tendencies[22] and improvement in sleep with an oropharyngeal airway or tracheostomy will sometimes improve sleep apnoea-associated psychotic features.[170]

Children with sleep apnoea often show a deterioration in school performance and fail to learn.[110] Failure to thrive, nocturnal enuresis, poor weight gain and short stature have been attributed to sleep apnoea in children.[17, 33] There is no evidence that growth failure is due primarily to the sleep disturbance or failure of sleep-onset growth hormone secretion, but failure to learn may result from daytime drowsiness as a consequence of sleep fragmentation at night.

Daytime drowsiness, poor memory and concentration, irritability and personality changes in obstructive sleep apnoea are not due simply to insomnia. These symptoms do not occur or are much less severe in patients with primary insomnia or central sleep apnoea. Also hypoxia alone cannot be the explanation; subjects with chronic obstructive airway disease have persistent hypoxia and carbon dioxide retention, but are rarely as sleepy as patients with obstructive sleep apnoea. According to Weitzman[297] the explanation for daytime drowsiness lies in the frequent shifts of sleep phase occurring throughout the night with loss of stage 3–4 NREM sleep as well as the continuous and marked fluctuation in arterial oxygen saturation and frequent brief arousals. Severe sleep fragmentation seems to be the most important of these factors. Improvement in daytime drowsiness with treatment (e.g. tracheostomy) is accompanied by a rapid reversal of sleep fragmentation with a four-fold decrease in the number of sleep stage changes per hour.[297, 298] Also after tracheostomy, although there may be no overall change in total sleep time, stages 1–2 NREM sleep decrease and stages 3–4 NREM sleep increase (from a mean of 3% to 19% of total sleep time), and this recovery of delta sleep may be important for recovery of normal daytime alertness.

Loss of libido, and difficulty in having an erection with impotence in 48% of male subjects with sleep apnoea, not clearly age-related, nor associated with depression or tricyclic drug treatment, were reported by Guilleminault et al.[115]

CARDIOVASCULAR CHANGES

Cor pulmonale
Apnoea is associated with transient pulmonary hypertension, since hypoxia causes pulmonary arteriolar constriction (not dilatation as elsewhere in the vascular tree). After several years of periodic pulmonary arterial vasoconstriction, sustained rather than intermittent pulmonary hypertension develops. Sleep apnoea thus causes cor pulmonale, sometimes with an increase in pulmonary wedge pressure by 10–20 mmHg.

Systemic hypertension
The relationship of sleep apnoea with systemic hypertension is less well established than with pulmonary hypertension. Obstructive sleep apnoea may be one important factor, together with obesity, alcoholism and increasing age, accounting for the high prevalence of essential hypertension reported in many series of sleep apnoea patients.[214] More than two-thirds of 379 sleep apnoea patients reviewed by Cummiskey had borderline elevation or definitely abnormal systemic blood pressure whilst awake.[106] However, the evidence that sleep apnoea causes systemic hypertension is circumstantial rather than direct. Certainly, following tracheostomy for obstructive sleep apnoea in children, systemic blood pressure may fall, but this is not always the case in adults where in subjects with well documented hypertension improvement is inconstant or insubstantial. Hypertension and sleep apnoea may coexist and both show a predilection for the middle aged and obese subject. Kales et al.[141] found that 30% of a group of hypertensive subjects had mild sleep apnoea.

Cyclical variation in heart rate
Periodic respiratory arrest during sleep leads to a mild to marked cyclical cardiac arrhythmia, with a one-to-one correlation between the number of apnoeas and hypopnoeas, and the number of swings in the heart rate; bradycardia with the apnoea and tachycardia with arousal. A regular pattern of bradycardia, sometimes less than 50 beats/min, alternates with a tachycardia, sometimes more than 120 beats/min. In addition, severe hypoxic episodes may be accompanied by atrial flutter,[16] very severe bradycardia[118] or ventricular premature beats and prolonged asystole.[104] Irregularity of heart beat contributes to a fall in cardiac output during obstructive sleep apnoea.[282]

Cyclical variation in heart rate during sleep apnoea is dependent upon anoxia and mediated via the autonomic nervous system. Thus bradycardia during apnoea may be prevented by giving supplemental oxygen,[171] whilst cardiac arrhythmias are blocked by atropine.[174]

Oxygen desaturation

Each apnoea causes a fall in the oxygen saturation of the blood (Fig. 7.7). Short apnoeas, those lasting 10–20 s only, can cause a fall of SaO_2 from 95% to 80% whilst long apnoeas, those over 1 min in duration, can cause a fall of up to 50%. In contrast to apnoeas, hypopnoeas do not usually cause great arterial O_2 desaturation. The degree of oxygen desaturation may not cause cyanosis and the patient remains pink, but there is often considerable CO_2 retention. Whereas, during normal sleep, arterial PCO_2 rises by O.5 kPa (3–4 mmHg) to around 6.7 kPa (50 mmhg), during sleep apnoea blood PCO_2 measurements may be as high as 9.3 kPa (70 mmHg). Under these circumstances breathing oxygen will abolish hypoxaemia but not hypercapnia.

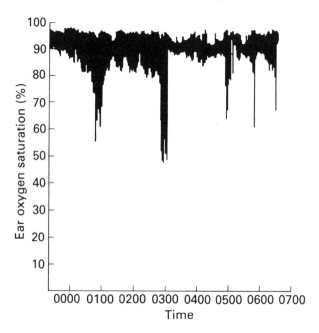

Figure 7.7 *Record of ear oxygen saturation throughout the night in a patient with the sleep apnoea syndrome. The continuously varying oxygen saturation, including some severe episodes of hypoxia, result from the multiple apnoeas. Reprinted with permission from Douglas, N.J.* Respiratory Disease in Practise *(1984) 29.*

Polycythaemia and sleep apnoea

Secondary polycythaemia is a well recognized complication of sleep apnoea.[162] Red cell mass reflects oxygen saturation and nocturnal desaturation probably contributes to the development of polycythaemia. Most patients who develop polycythaemia have some degree of daytime desaturation as well as severe nocturnal hypoxia.[265]

Primary polycythaemia may cause sleep apnoea, but this is very rare. A patient described by Neil *et al.*[188] is of considerable interest in this respect, although atypical and with unusually severe disability. This 39-year-old man had unequivocal polycythaemia rubra vera, leucocytosis, raised leucocyte alkaline phosphatase activity and normal waking arterial oxygen saturation, with splenomegaly. He developed very severe central sleep apnoea, psychotic features, episodes of confusion on waking, progressive difficulty in concentration and daytime drowsiness and, later, severe disorientation, forgetfulness, perseveration and delusions of guilt and annihilation. These features accompanied an increase in haematocrit from 54% to 65%, bilateral papilloedema and high CSF pressure. Waking respiratory function was normal. Phlebotomy, with a reduction in packed cell volume from 65% to 49% over 10 days, caused a dramatic improvement in both confusion and papilloedema, as well as the total disappearance of sleep apnoea.

'Narcolepsy', described by Blood[28] and Johnson and Chalgren[139] in patients with primary or secondary polycythaemia, may have resulted from sleep apnoea. However, sleep disorders are very uncommon in primary polycythaemia, and were not described by Silverstein et al.[251] in any of 511 patients with this disorder. Occasionally polycythaemia may predispose to obstructive sleep apnoea in subjects with a narrow upper airway.

Polycythaemia, both primary and secondary, may reduce brain stem blood flow during sleep and aggravate central sleep apnoea. Cerebral blood flow is reduced in polycythaemia, even with a comparatively low haematocrit; as well as in some patients with sleep apnoea.[178, 281] In the above-reported patient described by Neil and his colleagues, apnoeic episodes occurred only during NREM and not during REM sleep. This highly atypical pattern of apnoeas may have been associated with a further reduction of the normal fall of brain stem blood flow during NREM sleep,[223] whereas brain stem blood flow is normally increased during REM sleep.

SPECIFIC SLEEP APNOEA SYNDROMES

CENTRAL SLEEP APNOEA SYNDROMES (Table 7.3)

Ondine's curse

Ondine's curse, although primarily a hypoventilation, not a sleep apnoea, syndrome, is considered here as the archetypal central respiratory failure syndrome that presents during sleep. Central aeveolar hypoventilation dating from birth can result in total failure of the automatic control of ventilation. It is usually seen in neonates, who initially hypoventilate in quiet sleep, but also later when the child is awake .[65, 133, 176, 243, 245] The infant is cyanosed from birth, but has no cardiac, pulmonary, thoracic or neuromuscular disease to explain the problem. Hypoventilation is usually most marked in REM sleep, and alveolar PCO_2 may be higher than arterial PCO_2. The infant usually responds to external but not to other normal respiratory stimuli. The ventilatory response to endogenous CO_2 is depressed, although peripheral chemoreceptor function may remain intact. The prognosis is very poor and irreversible brain damage can occur. Over 30 such infants have now been described (Fig. 7.8).

In infants with central alveolar hypoventilation, central chemoreceptor function is reduced. The external arcuate nuclei may be absent, and there is

Table 7.3. *Central causes of hypopnoea, periodic and aperiodic breathing and sleep apnoea*

Loss of voluntary motor control	Loss of involuntary motor control	Loss of chemoreceptor control
Respiratory apraxia	Ondine's curse	Chemoreceptor damage
Cheyne–Stokes respiration (with frontal lesions)	Focal low medullary lesions	Afferent nerve damage
Epileptic apnoea	Depressant drugs	Shy–Drager syndrome
Pontine lesions (locked-in syndrome)	Alcohol	Other dysautonomias
Pseudobulbar palsy		Multisystem atrophy and related degenerative brain stem disorders
Selective dorsolateral spinal cord lesions	Selective ventrolateral spinal cord lesions	Surgical removal carotid bodies (e.g. for asthma)

Involvement of CNS ventilatory control mechanisms may cause periodic, aperiodic, or both types of breathing pattern. Most of the above examples do not present as sleep apnoea syndromes, but in many of these disorders the possibility of sleep apnoea should be considered. All respiratory disorders are aggravated during sleep.

sometimes decreased neuronal density in medullary respiratory areas.[89, 158] In the rare syndrome of combined hypoventilation with Hirschsprung's disease (loss of colonic ganglia) there may be a defect of serotonin stem cells in the gut.[260, 261] Several reported infants have shown dysautonomia, decreased heart rate variability, hyperphagia, disturbed diurnal rhythm of urine output, inappropriate ADH secretion, temperature instability. Rarely, Ondine's curse is acquired, as in the initial patient described, and due to focal low medullary lesions involving the automatic respiratory outflow centres.

Hypoxia and hypercapnia can be reversed by positive pressure, assisted ventilation or diaphragmatic pacing. Aminophylline, caffeine and methylphenidate have no effect. Doxapram or progesterone have a minor effect in stimulating breathing and almitrine has a more prolonged effect. Very rarely,

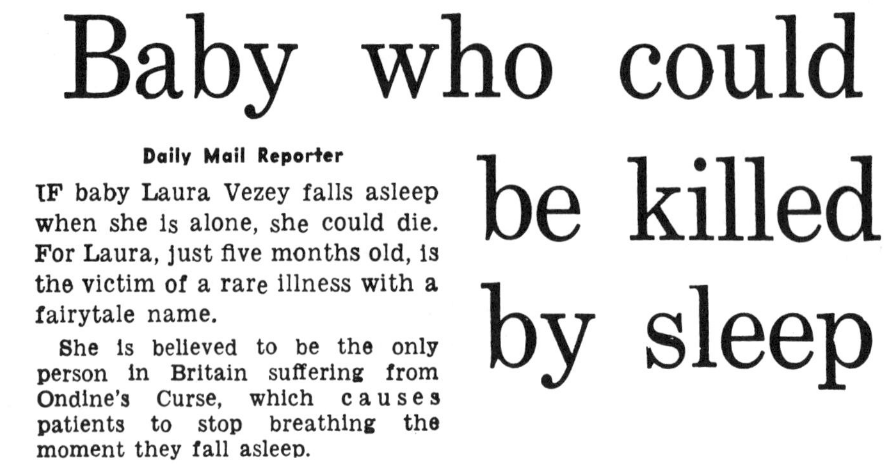

Baby who could be killed by sleep

Daily Mail Reporter

IF baby Laura Vezey falls asleep when she is alone, she could die. For Laura, just five months old, is the victim of a rare illness with a fairytale name.

She is believed to be the only person in Britain suffering from Ondine's Curse, which causes patients to stop breathing the moment they fall asleep.

Figure 7.8. *Central sleep apnoea as a possible cause of cot death. The Daily Mail (1982).*

spontaneous recovery occurs, despite the continued absence of ventilatory response to inhaled CO_2.[190] However, many victims have died in early childhood of pneumonia or cor pulmonale.

Brain stem lesions and sleep apnoea

Low medullary lesions often cause sleep apnoea, although sleep apnoea is sometimes overlooked in the presence of hypopnoea, Cheynes–Stokes breathing and other patterns of periodic respiration, and documented sleep apnoea in association with neurological disease of the posterior fossa is uncommon.

When sleep apnoea results from discrete bilateral lesions of the lower third of the medulla, the clinical picture is characteristic with ninth and tenth cranial nerve palsies, dysphagia, difficulty in coughing, and loss of the cough reflex, snoring, yawning and hiccup, mouth breathing, loss of pharyngeal sensation, and loss of the motor supply to the elevators of the palate, tensors of the vocal cords, intrinsic muscles of the larynx and pharyngeal constrictors. This results in obstructive, as well as central, sleep apnoea.

The different causes of this presentation include brain stem infarction, lateral medullary syndromes,[44] brain stem encephalitis, bulbar poliomyelitis,[128] medullary neoplasms, other acquired lesion, syringomyelia or syringobulbia,[2, 121] olivopontocerebellar atrophy, progressive supranuclear palsy, and palatal myoclonus associated with lesions of the olivodentate system. Sleep apnoea has been documented in Alzheimer's disease;[51, 159, 254] several forms of encephalitis and in particular Western equine encephalitis;[300] post-encephalitic parkinsonism;[62, 266] and Jakob–Creutzfeldt disease.[168, 193, 280] In three of these cases of sleep apnoea with Jakob–Creutzfeldt disease, periods of apnoea during sleep were associated with abrupt cessation of the periodic complexes of this disease and their replacement by 7–9 Hz waves which persisted throughout the apnoea. Likewise, periodic complexes of sub-acute sclerosing leucoencephalitis are altered by ventilatory changes during sleep.[241] Perhaps the sub-cortical pacemakers of these periodic complexes are close to respiratory neurones in the brain stem.

White et al.[300] described a 17-year-old diabetic boy with *Western equine encephalitis*, alveolar hypoventilation, near absence of waking ventilatory responses to hypoxia and hypercapnia, as well as severe sleep apnoea and hypopnoea. As is often the case, the sleep apnoea was noted only by the night nursing staff. After 3 months he eventually recovered.

There have been at least 27 published case reports of chronic alveolar hypoventilation syndromes in *parkinsonism*. These seem to have established that irregular breathing, hypopnoea, rapid breathing, respiratory crises with dyspnoea and possibly sleep apnoea, may all occur as a sequel to postencephalitic,[62, 266] but not idiopathic parkinsonism.

In central sleep apnoea with damage to the automatic respiratory centres, the voluntary control of respiration may assure normal blood gases whilst waking, and periodic daytime apnoea can sometimes be managed by reminding the patient to breathe. However, there is often a progressive impairment first of sleeping and then of waking respiratory control so that assisted ventilation following tracheal intubation or tracheostomy is required. Death may be due to either respiratory failure and infection associated with loss of the cough and swallowing reflex, accumulation and swallowing of secretion with subsequent pneumonia, or to total respiratory arrest during sleep and vagally mediated cardiac arrhythmias with hypoxia.

Narcolepsy and central sleep apnoea
10–15% of patients with *narcolepsy–cataplexy* also have sleep apnoea. This is usually central, rarely obstructive in nature and in most instances there is only a slight increase in the number of nocturnal apnoeas above normal values. The combination of sleep apnoea with narcolepsy–cataplexy may be explained by the close relationship of sleep and respiratory mechanisms; there is no evidence that arousal responses to normal degrees of hypoxia are blunted in narcolepsy.

Cervical cord lesions and sleep apnoea
Bilateral, but not unilateral, interruption of the automatic respiratory outflow pathways to the intercostal muscles and diaphragm by *cervical cordotomy* results in central sleep apnoea. This may follow cervical cord decompression as well as cordotomy,[82, 286] although in the first instance spontaneous normal sleep respiration may be regained 2–4 weeks after operation.

Diaphragmatic paralysis and sleep apnoea
When the diaphragm is paralysed, it may be difficult or impossible to separate central from peripheral apnoeas, with absent respiratory movements under both conditions.

Any neuromuscular disorder that involves the diaphragm may cause sleep apnoea as well as hypopnoea. The diaphragm is the most important muscle of respiration and patients with neuromuscular disorders that affect breathing do not complain of breathlessness until the diaphragm is involved. Ankylosing spondylitis causes rib fixation but does not affect the diaphragm; despite gross reduction in movement of the chest wall, hypoventilation and dyspnoea do not occur. The first and major complaint in diaphragmatic paralysis is dyspnoea on exertion, followed by the development of cor pulmonale, cyanosis, polycythaemia, nightmares, vivid dreams and sleep apnoea. Hypoxia may result in fits in the recumbent position, with a reduction in vital capacity due to the pressure of the abdominal contents on a paralysed diaphragm, but postural or hypoxic fits are rare with other causes of sleep apnoea (however, 'epilepsy' is a rare accompaniment of sleep apnoea and may be related to hypoxia[303]).

When there is pre-existing hypoxia due to neuromuscular, pulmonary or cardiac disease, even a small degree of sleep hypoventilation or apnoea may lead to significant arterial desaturation. This is of particular importance in diaphragmatic paralysis and in myasthenia gravis, poliomyelitis and the

Guillain–Barré syndrome, as well as in other neuromuscular diseases, limb girdle muscular dystrophy, the spinal muscular atrophies, and especially myotonic dystrophy (see p. 373). Hypoventilation and daytime drowsiness occur in all these syndromes. It seems likely that, in addition to hypoventilation, sleep apnoea is a major cause of disability and possibly of death in these conditions.

OBSTRUCTIVE SLEEP APNOEA SYNDROMES (Table 7.4)

'Idiopathic' hypoventilation

The classical description of *'idiopathic' hypoventilation* is one of continuous hypoventilation and sometimes periodic breathing occurring both waking and sleeping, with very depressed ventilatory responses to CO_2, an arterial PCO_2 greater than 6 kPa, normal lungs, an apparently unobstructed airway and no sign of a medullary lesion.[5] Other features resemble very closely those of obstructive sleep apnoea with polycythaemia, lack of energy, headache and breathlessness.

Table 7.4.   *Causes of primary obstructive and combined central–obstructive sleep apnoea syndromes*

Primary obstructive sleep apnoea
   Bone, joint, muscle or soft tissue abnormality resulting in oropharyngeal narrowing

Obstructive cause predominant, although central apnoeas may be frequent
   Myxoedema
   Acromegaly
   Thoracic cage deformity, e.g. kyphoscoliosis
   Neuromuscular disorders
   Myotonia
   Diaphragmatic paralysis

Obstructive and central causes both prominent
   Autonomic neuropathy
   Polycythaemia
   Down's syndrome

The Pickwickian syndrome includes the above features, but also daytime drowsiness, extreme obesity and marked CO_2 retention.

Obstructive sleep apnoea, although described initially in patients with the Pickwickian syndrome, also occurs in subjects who are not obese and do not have waking alveolar hypoventilation, waking CO_2 retention or any abnormality of ventilatory response to changes in the composition of the inspired air. In some of these patients a clear anatomic abnormality of the upper airway can be demonstrated, but this is not always the case. In those patients without clear anatomical obstruction, bronchoscopy and fluoroscopy during sleep have demonstrated that upper airway occlusion is usually due to passive collapse of the pharyngeal walls. An extremely mild form of the disease may be represented by patients who have mainly or entirely REM, not NREM, apnoeas.

Despite differences in presentation, *idiopathic hypoventilation*, the *Pickwickian syndrome* and *obstructive sleep apnoea* are probably all examples of sleep apnoea syndromes rather than different entities. On detailed investigation many patients with so-called idiopathic hypoventilation[84] turn out to have focal medullary lesions, sub-obstructive airway narrowing, low chemoreceptor CO_2 sensitivity or obvious sleep apnoea. Occasionally there is a history of tabes, other forms of neurosyphilis, neuroleptic drug intake, drug-induced parkinsonism or dystonia as well as obesity. The diversity of clinical presentation of sleep apnoea syndromes is probably due to the presence or absence of obesity, differences in the shape of the oropharynx, differences in the chronicity of the cause, and in genetic control of responses to both hypoxia and hypercapnia. Subjects with normal lung function may be divided into groups of high–normal responders and low–normal responders to both hypoxia and hypercapnia.[143] This distribution is under genetic control.[269, 283] However, it is not always clear why some patients with sleep apnoea show diminished ventilatory drive to PCO_2 whilst awake, whereas others show no waking respiratory defect. This may be determined by the duration and severity of the repetitive hypoxic and hypercapnic load whilst sleeping, both of which blunt respiratory drive.

The Pickwickian syndrome

The term *Pickwickian* should be reserved for very obese patients with respiratory failure in the presence of normal lungs and an increased blood PCO_2 level as a cardinal feature of hypoventilation. Most, if not all, of these patients also have sleep apnoea.[129]

Sir William Osler,[203] Sieker *et al.*[250] and Burwell *et al.*[36] all described very sleepy people who were also very fat, and who developed respiratory failure despite apparently near-normal lungs. The idea arose that these patients lacked the strength to move the chest wall or lower the diaphragm. Accompanying heart disease was thought to be due to obesity rather than to be the result of an unusual type of lung disease. Although the patients did not cough, spit or wheeze, and had normal pulmonary gas diffusion, they developed intermittent cyanosis, polycythaemia and right axis deviation, as well as peripheral oedema, venous hypertension and hepatomegaly. Most of these symptoms disappeared as the patients lost weight. The Pickwickian syndrome was thus seen to be associated with curable heart and lung disease, but the association of alveolar hypoventilation with sleepiness seemed inexplicable. Perhaps some central defect might be present, causing voracious appetite and weight increase, as well as drowsiness.

This problem was solved by Gastaut *et al.*[91] who showed that some Pickwickians had sleep apnoea. Many Pickwickians have flow-volume loop evidence of upper airway obstruction, with a narrow oropharynx, due to deposition of fat. However, additional features, not found in other obstructive sleep apnoea syndromes, occur; marked and persistent CO_2 retention, a decrease in total lung volume, a decrease in functional residual capacity, and a decrease in expiratory reserve volume. Careful examination of Pickwickians does not invariably disclose sleep apnoea, and the initial concept of a central appetite and sleep disturbance, rather than upper airway obstruction as the primary cause of symptomatology, may be correct in some instances.

The combination of daytime alveolar hypoventilation with sleep apnoea in obese Pickwickian subjects may be due to the effect of very long-standing recurrent hypoxia on the respiratory centres, eventually diminishing ventilatory drive; although these obese subjects have been considered to lack the strength to breathe. The carbon dioxide tolerance curve of these patients is depressed and shifted to the right, with the result that a higher PCO_2 is required to maintain ventilation in the waking state than in normal subjects.[151] However, diminished ventilatory responses to carbon dioxide inhalation occur in thin as well as obese patients with obstructive sleep apnoea.[52, 285] Sleep apnoea itself may reduce ventilatory drive by causing arousals and thus sleep deprivation and fragmentation, which further decrease ventilatory drive.

Upper airway obstruction
Anatomical narrowing of the upper airways, with passive collapse and occlusion of the respiratory passages due to negative intrathoracic pressure in inspiration, are the major factors causing obstructive sleep apnoea (Fig. 7.9). The alternative hypothesis of active muscle constriction has been considered, but EMG studies usually show atonia, not activation of the occluding muscles. Any factor which narrows the upper airway, including a short mandible or nasal stenosis, will mean that stronger suction (i.e. higher negative pressure) is required for inspiration and thus predispose to obstructive apnoeas.

A highly unusual facial appearance is sometimes found in obstructive sleep apnoea and specific facies may indicate the likely presence of upper airway obstruction. Characteristically the neck is short, thick and protruding, with marked obesity, heavy jowls and micrognathia, the so-called *'bird-like' facies*.[115, 209, 218, 264] Other conditions causing sleep apnoea with characteristic facies include the *Kearns Sayre syndrome* (atypical retinitis pigmentosa, short stature, ovarian agenesis, cardiac conduction defects, with chronic progressive external ophthalmoplegia); the *Pierre Robin syndrome* (cleft palate, unusually large tongue, absent gag reflex); the *Treacher Collins syndrome* (mandibular-facial dysostosis), and *Prader–Willi syndrome* (hypotonia, hypogonadism and mental retardation[116]). A wide variety of other facial and palatal deformities may occur, often accompanied by marked neck deformity.[53] A small or retruded mandible, often associated with palatal, tongue or pharyngeal deformity, is a particular hazard.[137, 138, 249, 290] Pharyngeal hypoplasia, hemifacial microsomia,[249] ankylosis of the temperomandibular joint, osteomyelitis of the mandible or a condylar fracture may also all cause sleep apnoea. However, not all patients with very severe mandibular deformity develop sleep apnoea.

The combination of chest deformity, airway narrowing and medullary compression at the level of the foramen magnum may cause unusually severe

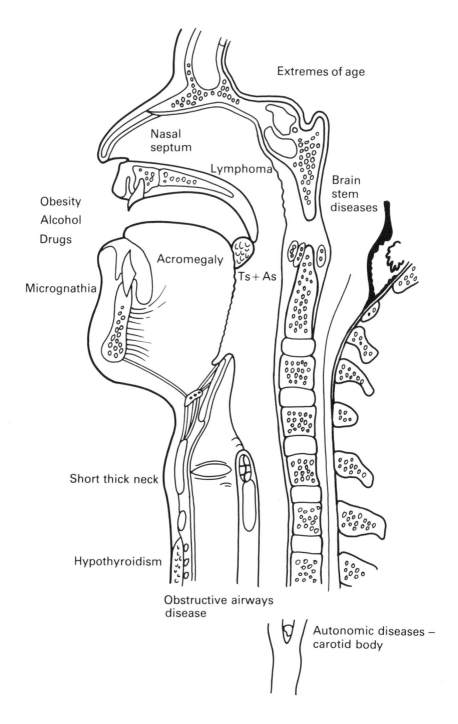

Figure 7.9.   *Common causes of obstructive sleep apnoea. Ts + As: tonsils and adenoids.*

sleep apnoea in *achondroplasia*. Sleep disordered breathing was present in eight of nine achondroplastic children investigated by Stokes *et al.*[262] and five had serious sleep apnoea.

A great number of acquired bone, joint, muscle or soft tissue abnormalities may produce critical upper airway narrowing and sleep apnoea. This may result from simple or gross obesity with fat deposition in the pharynx, or increase in soft tissues in acromegaly, mucopolysaccharidosis or myxoedema. Myxoedema may cause either peripheral obstructive apnoea[279] or predominant central apnoea.[181] Sleep apnoea has been reported following velopalatal surgery for cleft palate, superior vena caval obstruction due to neurofibromatosis, neoplastic lesions of the oropharynx and irradiation-induced fibrosis.[110, 264]

Myotonic dystrophy

About a third of subjects with myotonic dystrophy develop hypoventilation, sleep apnoea and daytime hypersomnia.[19, 40, 54, 93, 108, 211] These breathing problems are due to respiratory muscle stiffness and weakness, airway obstruction and possibly a central respiratory defect. Patients with myotonic dystrophy chronically hypoventilate. The degree of sleep apnoea is usually slight, with an apnoea index of 6–10 central and obstructive episodes each hour.

Hansotia and Frens[119] considered that some patients with myotonic dystrophy may have a central sleep disturbance as well as obstructive sleep apnoea. They described a highly atypical patient who developed 'narcolepsy' – without cataplexy, sleep paralysis or hypnagogic hallucinations – at the age of 20. Two decades later, he developed signs of classic myotonic dystrophy with alveolar hypoventilation and sleep apnoea. Neither of these was severe or apparently sufficient to account for daytime drowsiness in this patient. In more typical cases the severity of daytime drowsiness in myotonic dystrophy may be greater than in other subjects with comparable respiratory muscle stiffness or weakness, or with pure central alveolar hypoventilation syndromes. However, a central sleep disturbance in myotonic dystrophy has not yet been substantiated in the majority of patients.

Treatment of sleep apnoea and daytime drowsiness in the presence of central and obstructive apnoea, muscle dystrophy and myotonia is difficult. Protriptyline and progesterone are usually not very successful in relieving apnoea, and dextroamphetamine and methylphenidate do not greatly increase alertness.[119] Any mechanical obstruction should be removed and continuous nocturnal positive airway pressure is worth a trial. Patients with myotonic dystrophy are very sensitive to anaesthetic and hypnotic drugs, which should be avoided as far as possible.[144]

Acromegaly

The Bible describes the bed, but not the sleep, of giants. Og, the polydactylic King of Basan, was as high as a cedar and had a bedstead of iron (*Deuteronomy* 3:11, *Amos* 2:9, *1 Chronicles* 20:6).

Sleep apnoea can be detected in a tenth to a third of all acromegalics.[113, 179, 210] This is due to airway obstruction with enlargement of the soft tissues of the oropharynx, prognathia and macroglossia.[81] Some, but not all, acromegalics have waking flow-volume loop evidence of upper airway obstruction.[210] Despite sleep apnoea, daytime somnolence is uncommon, occurring in only 2–10% of all patients.[15, 210] As might be expected, growth hormone levels are higher in acromegalics with daytime sleepiness, excessive snoring or both than in those without. In acromegaly, cardiomegaly and congestive heart failure are largely due to ischaemic heart disease and tissue thickening, but severe sleep apnoea may also be partly responsible.

Daytime drowsiness in acromegaly may sometimes be due to central as well as peripheral causes. The following notes on a case of acromegaly are taken from Roxburgh and Collis[231] (see also Fig. 7.1, p. 338).

> Towards the end of July she fell into a very drowsy condition lasting about a fortnight, so that she was unable to do her work. One day she was found asleep on the stairs, and when aroused said she had gone to sleep unintentionally whilst going up. She frequently went to sleep whilst being spoken to. This period of drowsiness was followed by a persistent headache, which remained till her death on September 21st. When this headache first came on, it was very severe and prevented her sleeping ; she took to her bed, and lay groaning day and night unless relieved by morphine injections. Sulphonal, phenacetin, potassium iodide, arsenic, and cannabis indica gave no relief. During the last week in August

In a minority of subjects with severe daytime sleepiness, the apnoea index is low, apparently insufficient to account for serious waking difficulty. Perks *et al.*[210] found no relation between the duration of symptoms of acromegaly and the occurrence of daytime somnolence or excessive nocturnal snoring. Also, although the treatment of acromegaly with bromocriptine or hypophysectomy may result in rapid improvement in daytime drowsiness, this is not always the case, and in a few patients with both acromegaly and daytime drowsiness, growth hormone levels fall with treatment, but daytime somnolence does not improve. These findings led Barnes and his colleagues to suggest that narcolepsy in acromegaly was not always due to acromegalic soft tissue thickening and obstructive apnoea[15] but could result from a central sleep disturbance. However, there is no conclusive evidence that growth hormone has any central actions on sleep or that there is a primary central sleep disturbance in acromegaly. The usual, if not invariable, cause of daytime drowsiness in these subjects is obstructive sleep apnoea.

Down's syndrome
Many patients with Down's syndrome are lethargic and difficult to wake, with rapid intellectual deterioration and acute worsening during infectious illnesses. The early onset of Alzheimer's disease probably explains some of these findings. However, sleep apnoea and progressive pulmonary

hypertension also occur. The oldest patient with Down's syndrome seen at King's College Hospital (aged 52) had a variety of respiratory disturbances in sleep; Cheynes–Stokes respiration, prolonged apnoea and hypopnoea, and also daytime irritability, sleep or stupor for 6 months prior to his death. Likewise, three patients with Down's syndrome described by Clark et al.[50] had prominent sleep respiratory disturbances, with daytime irritability, lethargy, somnolence and cyanosis precipitated by infection, nocturnal seizures aggravated by sleep-induced hypoxia, snoring, enuresis, difficulty in waking, dyspnoea and delirium. In one patient, a boy of 14, the diagnosis of sleep apnoea was suggested by persistent lethargy, hypercapnia and violent flailing efforts during sleep to overcome apparent airway obstruction. Two of these patients had extreme hypertrophy of the tonsils, occluding the hypopharynx, and one a drooping soft palate that touched the base of the tongue, as well as a glottis that prolapsed against the posterior pharyngeal wall. Upper respiratory infection precipitated prolonged and severe obstructive apnoeas during REM sleep. In addition to airway obstruction, there may be a central predisposition to Cheyne–Stokes respiration and apnoeas in Down's syndrome.

The treatment of sleep apnoea in Down's syndrome is difficult. Permanent tracheostomy is probably contraindicated in patients with mental retardation and a poor tolerance of respiratory infection. However, continuous positive airway pressure is seldom achieved for long periods. Prompt antibiotic treatment of respiratory infection may prevent deterioration, and tonsillectomy if appropriate, central stimulants, progesterone or protriptyline may reduce airway obstruction or lessen sleep apnoea.

Autonomic disorders

Patients with familial or acquired dysautonomia have, in addition to autonomic areflexia, abnormal breathing during sleep.[34] A 59-year-old locomotive engineer with the Shy–Drager syndrome, impotence, urinary and faecal incontinence and severe postural hypotension described by Briskin et al.[32] honked like a flock of geese in his sleep and twice required resuscitation. Patients with familial or acquired dysautonomia are often sleepy by day, although seldom to the extent of patients with upper airway obstruction. They may also have periodic respiration whilst awake.[47] The usual sleep complaint in dysautonomia is one of difficulty in getting up in the morning or falling asleep at night and frequent sleep awakenings (sometimes due to nocturia) rather than daytime somnolence, although day sleep attacks, severe confusion and disorientation do occur.[32] If patients with familial dysautonomia are investigated in detail, most turn out to have a respiratory and sleep disorder, both usually mild, with central as well as obstructive sleep apnoea. As in familial dysautonomia, central and peripheral sleep apnoea occurs in some patients with diabetic autonomic neuropathy. This is usually mild and asymptomatic.[221]

The carotid and aortic bodies and medullary intracranial chemoreceptors respond to changes in pH, PCO_2 or PO_2 in the blood and cerebrospinal fluid.

Damage to these systems causes sleep apnoea in dysautonomia. The aortic and more important carotid bodies are specific respiratory chemoreceptors, with an afferent supply by the vagus and glossopharyngeal nerves respectively and efferent supply from the brain stem via the cervical sympathetic nerves. Carotid chemoreceptors respond to arterial hypoxaemia. The response is rapid, within a few breaths. In contrast, central chemoreceptors respond to slow prolonged changes in pH or PCO_2 of the cerebrospinal fluid and brain extracerebral fluid. The medullary intracranial chemoreceptors are outside the blood–brain barrier, separate from the nerve cells of the respiratory centre and localized to the ventrolateral surface of the medulla extending caudally from the pontomedullary junction, bounded medially by the pyramids and laterally by the 8–11th cranial nerve cells.

One major effect of dysautonomia is to abolish the arousal response to hypoxia as a result of carotid body denervation.[31] In theory, this should also produce loss of the Hering–Breuer reflex, loss of the cough reflex and loss of the tracheal mucosa stimulation reflex during both sleep and waking, but this combination does not appear to have been reported in man.

Sleep and breathing in dysautonomia has been reviewed by Guilleminault et al.[103] Many different breathing patterns occur, including irregular respiration, ataxic respiration, obstructive, central or mixed apnoeas. Both the brain stem and the peripheral chemoreceptors are insensitive to normal stimuli. Severe breath-holding spells may occur during childhood and there is an outstanding ability for voluntary breath holding. Many patients suffer from repeated pneumonias and also have an increased liability to hypoxic death. This sometimes occurs suddenly during sleep.[32, 43, 83, 90, 145, 165, 228, 271] Despite the liability to hypoxic death in dysantonomia, the cardiac responses to profound hypoxia are reduced, not increased, and even severe respiratory irregularity may not produce vagally-mediated cardiac arrhythmias as occur in other subjects with sleep apnoea.[90] Therefore the severe alterations in heart rate which are characteristic of other forms of obstructive sleep apnoea do not occur in patients with autonomic areflexia. There is a marked blunting of the normally expected reflex tachycardia in response to hypotension, and only a minimal response to atropine. In contrast, sleep hypoxia does cause a marked rise in pulmonary arterial pressure, suggesting that this is due to local hypoxaemia.[32]

The sleep structure of patients with familial dysautonomia is unusual and differs from the usual pattern in patients with upper airway obstruction.[32, 79, 90] In dysautonomia, there is sometimes a marked decrease in Stage 2 NREM sleep as well as a prolonged REM sleep latency. This may be due to loss of sleep neurones as well as of respiratory neurones in familial dysautonomia. Here, as in multisystem atrophy, spongy changes in the central tegmental tract are found, as well as reductions in sympathetic postganglionic neurones.[207]

Treatment of sleep and respiratory disorders in dysautonomia is difficult. Changes in sleep posture, fludrocortisone, sympathomimetic amines or prevention of venous pooling which may help postural hypotension rarely improve daytime somnolence or prevent sudden death. Tracheostomy results in an increase in the degree of oxygen saturation during sleep, but does not alter total REM time, abolish central apnoeic episodes or prevent respiratory arrest and death during sleep.[32] Weight reduction, acetazolamide, doxapram and protriptyline may provide limited relief.

In patients with dysautonomia, airway obstruction may occur at the larynx and not primarily in the pharynx. There is often a decrease in abduction of the vocal cords due to brain stem or neuronal damage[302] leading to stridor and laryngeal obstruction during sleep.

COT DEATH

In Britain, cot death is the greatest single cause of mortality in the first year of life, excluding the first week after birth. At least 80 causes have been suggested. Sleep apnoea may be responsible for some of these disasters, but its exact role remains very controversial (see e.g. Steinschneider[259]). Cot death occurs mainly in infants under 6 months of age, in winter rather than in summer, and in premature rather than full-term infants. It is more common in boys than girls, in twins than in single infants and in lower than higher socioeconomic class families. Cot death occurs silently during sleep and sometimes apparently after prolonged obstructive apnoea, severe bradycardia or severe arrhythmia.[105, 288] Although sleep apnoea may sometimes be the final event, many other factors lead up to this.

Investigation of the role of sleep apnoea in cot death has centred on the ventilatory responses of near-victims and their relatives. Ventilatory responses to hypoxia and hypercapnia of waking and sleeping infants who are near-miss for cot death (an episode of severe hypoventilation, but not resulting in death) are sometimes depressed.[9, 132] This is also the case in the parents of some, but not all, victims and near-victims of cot death.[1, 306] Also, the respiratory responses to nasal obstruction may be very sluggish in newborn babies.[125]

It is unlikely that cot death is always due to sleep apnoea. Congenital heart disease diagnosed at necropsy is a frequent finding in cot death victims.[3, 21, 38] Infection, influenza, whopping cough, spasmodic croup, patent ductus arteriosus, persistent foetal circulation and recurrent laryngeal nerve entrapment against a dilated and tense pulmonary artery on the aortic arch have all been implicated by Vesselinova-Jenkins.[288]

Prematurity is a major factor in cot death. Henderson-Smart et al.[124] have documented the occurrence of apnoea in premature infants in relation to the development of brain stem myelination and synaptic conduction, and have shown that the brain stem conduction times of auditory evoked responses are slightly longer in babies with apnoea than in those with normal respiration but of a similar age.

From a practical viewpoint, routine sleep and respiratory screening of the parents of infant death victims is unrewarding, but infants who are near-victims of sudden death should have these studies,[102] and periodic assessments of SaO_2 should be made during the first 3 months of life in infants with abnormal respiration at birth.[39] Many apnoea alarms used to detect the cessation of breathing are insensitive, but a successful apnoea monitor has been developed by Stradling.[263]

INVESTIGATIONS AND DIAGNOSIS

It is important to consider sleep apnoea as a common cause of excessive daytime drowsiness,[61] but the presentation is very pleomorphic and the diagnosis is often missed. In most instances, minor degrees of either obstructive or central apnoea are asymptomatic. The possibility of sleep apnoea should be considered in any patient with a low medullary lesion, neuromuscular disorder, autonomic neuropathy or upper airway deformity, as well as in those with unexplained symptoms of daytime drowsiness, personality disturbance or cor pulmonale, and particularly if obese or alcoholic.

If the diagnosis of symptomatic sleep apnoea is suspected on clinical grounds, and confirmed by interview of the patient's sleeping partner, the most important task is to *watch the patient sleep* at night. The diagnosis of symptomatic obstructive sleep apnoea can probably be made in almost all cases from 15 min observation.

The next priority is to sort out which patients to investigate. Screening for sleep apnoea is both costly and time-consuming. In particular, overnight sleep recording facilities are extremely scarce or unobtainable in many parts of the world. If sleep apnoea is suspected on clinical grounds, a few simple screening tests are helpful for initial evaluation (Table 7.5) and may confirm the diagnosis. This preliminary evaluation should include a chest X-ray, an ECG and ENT review to detect cor pulmonale, any cardiac dysrhythmia, and cause for upper airway obstruction.

This can be followed by a daytime polysomnogram. The initial study should include at least four EEG leads, plus two electro-oculogram leads, and a mental electromyogram, nasal and labial themister recording, ECG, record of chest movements, and if available determination of blood gases by arterial sampling, ear oximeter, oxygen skin electrode or mass spectrometer analysis of end-tidal air.

Daytime polysomnograms give much of the information necessary for the diagnosis of sleep apnoea,[95, 96] but there are several drawbacks to such day-sleep recordings, and overall the information they give may be insufficient to substantiate a diagnosis of sleep apnoea, or fully evaluate the severity of this. A minimum of 30 min sleep is needed since the polysomnogram diagnosis of pathologic sleep apnoea requires that apnoea has to occur at other times than during sleep onset (the first 10 min of sleep). Any stimulant medication should be discontinued for at least a week before test. Despite drawbacks, a positive result of daytime polysomnogram studies will confirm the diagnosis of sleep apnoea, but a negative short study does not necessarily exclude this diagnosis.

Table 7.5.   *Evaluation of sleep apnoea – suggested screening procedure for suspected sleep apnoea*

History
Does history indicate this diagnosis is likely?
Are any precipitating factors present (e.g. obesity, chest disease, alcoholism)?
Obtain history from sleeping partner.
Obtain psychiatric assessment if necessary.
How disabled is the patient?

Physical signs
Is there any obvious cause for airway obstruction (e.g. abnormal facies, short neck, acromegaly, skeletal deformity, neuromuscular disorder)?
Is the patient obese?
ENT review.
Chest review – is there evidence of cor pulmonale?
Blood pressure (systemic hypertension?).
Watch (and listen to) the patient during night sleep.

Preliminary tests
Chest X-ray.
ECG.
Daytime EEG.
Simple lung function tests, including flow-volume loop studies and spirometry.

Confirmatory tests
Daytime EEG sleep studies, repeated if necessary.
24 h cardiac tape.

Final evaluation
All-night polysomnography.
Lateral CT scan of oropharynx.

The study of breathing during sleep, by either day or night, is difficult. The use of face masks, nose clips, mouth tubes and some chest movement sensors will affect ventilation. Ear oximeters may have variable accuracy, sensitivity and speed of response, and few laboratories are equipped for mass spectrometer analysis of end-tidal air during normal overnight sleep recordings. Some respiratory function tests, such as the forced expiratory volume, demand an alert, cooperative patient. All these problems limit our understanding of what happens to respiration during sleep, and make the evaluation of sleep apnoea difficult.

The cardiac complications of sleep apnoea can be detected by *24 h ECG recording*, and this usually, but not always, permits the detection of sleep apnoea itself. Thus, a 24 h cardiac tape is most helpful in the preliminary evaluation of sleep apnoea syndromes, and is more readily available than sleep laboratory studies. A pattern of sinus arrhythmia and bradycardia during apnoea, followed by abrupt tachycardia, is characteristic of sleep apnoea, and occurs in asymptomatic as well as symptomatic subjects. However, particularly in the presence of an autonomic neuropathy associated with sleep apnoea, there may be no cyclical variation in heart rate.[104]

More detailed evaluation of sleep apnoea is indicated only under special circumstances, in patients with very severe symptomatology, cor pulmonale, or periodic cardiac arrhythmias, for here the prognosis is poor, and it may be necessary to consider tracheostomy if other treatments are unsuccessful. These patients should have an overnight sleep recording, and, if indicated, lateral CT scans of the oropharynx.

All-night sleep recordings are more valuable than daytime sleep recordings, since they allow prolonged study, and also the distribution of apnoeas throughout the night is skew, owing to the greater prevalence of REM sleep in late than early sleep, with in some patients apnoeas most frequent and severe early in the morning hours. However, the ideal 6–8 h all-night recording can be difficult to achieve because of frequent arousals, and in some patients repeated all-night recordings are necessary for full evaluation, since the severity of apnoeas and the degree of arterial oxygen desaturation may vary between nights. It is sometimes difficult to distinguish inspiratory efforts against an occluded airway from the very different pattern of motion in unobstructed breathing and the absence of movement in central apnoea, when the diaphragm is paralysed (see Fig. 7.4).

The advent of non-invasive respiratory magnetometers, as well as the Respitrace jacket (Respitrace Corporation, 731 Saw Mill River Road, Ardsley, NY 10502, USA), have made respiratory studies easier to do during sleep.[247] The technical procedures for diagnosis and evaluation of sleep apnoea are discussed in detail by Guilleminault[101] and Bornstein.[30]

Lateral CT scans of the neck give impressive evidence of generalized airway narrowing, often extending from the nasophraynx to the epiglottis, in many patients, including Pickwickians, in whom the presence of upper airway obstruction may otherwise seem uncertain. In most instances, narrowing is due to redundant soft tissue. In horizontal sections from the nasopharynx to the hypopharynx, the mean cross-sectional area is around 2.33 cm^2 in patients with no airway problems, but reduced to 0.8 cm^2 in apnoeic patients. At the oropharynx, which is the most common site of narrowing, apnoeic patients have a mean cross-sectional area of approximately 1.9 cm^2 less than that of control subjects.[29] Alternatively to the CT scan, a diagnosis of upper airway obstruction can sometimes be confirmed by fluoroscopy.[255] In a minority of subjects with obstructive sleep apnoea, no definite anatomical obstruction can be found, and the notion of inherently poor pharyngeal dilator activity during sleep has arisen.[106]

Brain stem evoked potentials play no part in sceening or assessment of sleep apnoea, although these may be delayed in some patients with both central and obstructive sleep apnoea, in both the waking and the sleeping state. The latency of brain stem evoked potentials to an auditory stimulus is prolonged in some premature babies with breathing difficulty, as well as in children and adults with sleep apnoea. Very approximately, the latency of conduction delay increases with the severity of sleep apnoea and hypoxia. Normal values are restored when sleep hypoxia is prevented by tracheostomy or by continuous positive airway pressure.[208, 277]

Detailed *pulmonary function studies* in the waking state often show little or no abnormality in patients with sleep apnoea. A characteristic sawtooth appearance of the flow-volume loop curve (Fig 7.10) has been proposed as specific for patients with obstructive sleep apnoea, but not all these patients show this abnormality.[120, 233] The greatest value of flow-volume loop studies is in the investigation of large airway obstruction such as tracheal stenosis, which flattens the loop in inspiration.

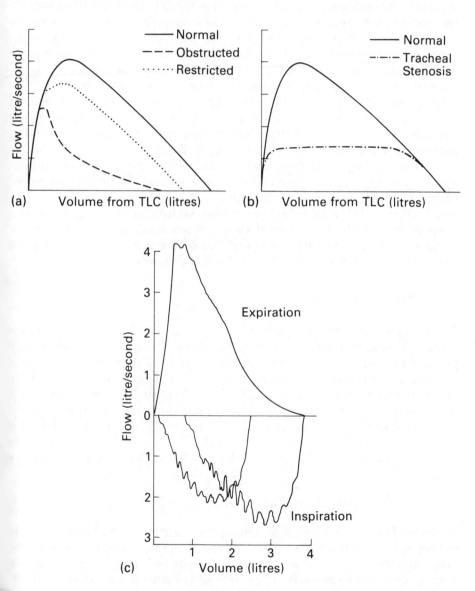

Figure 7.10. *Flow-volume loop patterns: (a) normal, (b) tracheal stenosis, (c) obstructive sleep apnoea. Reprinted with permission from Sanders.*[233]

DIFFERENTIAL DIAGNOSIS

Sleep apnoea is distinguished from *REM narcolepsy* by the behaviour during night sleep, the prominent morning headache, grogginess, persistent daytime tiredness and absence of cataplexy. However, between 10% and 15% of patients with REM narcolepsy have mild sleep apnoea, and the sleep latency is short in both conditions. An early age of onset for narcolepsy, the occurrence of this before sleep apnoea, the presence of cataplexy and a positive family history, as well as the presence of severe narcolepsy but only mild sleep apnoea, may help to characterize those cases of REM narcolepsy in which sleep apnoea also occurs. However, occasionally the diagnosis is difficult, as for example when central sleep apnoea is associated with sleep paralysis.[229]

Obstructive sleep apnoea may be confused with sleep-related *gastro-oesophageal reflux, pharyngeal pouch* or *abnormal swallowing syndromes* (see Parasomnias; Sleep and the Gut), when frequent arousal results from choking, respiratory distress or sometimes chest pain. Patients with these conditions may awake choking, with great anxiety and inability to draw breath, without any history to suggest oesophagitis or any waking swallowing problem. Congestive heart failure, nocturnal angina, Cheyne–Stokes respiration and nocturnal epilepsy are unlikely to be confused with either central or obstructive sleep apnoea syndromes. Central sleep apnoea syndromes are sometimes distinguished from obstructive sleep apnoea syndromes by the more frequent complaint of insomnia, rather than of daytime drowsiness.

TREATMENT (Table 7.6)

The first essential in the treatment of both obstructive and central sleep apnoea is the detection, correction or withdrawal of any obvious cause or associated factor, including obesity, hypnotic drugs, alcohol and chest disease.

Treatment of obstructive apnoea is then aimed at removal, prevention, or bypass of the obstruction, and of central apnoea at stimulation of ventilation unless the cause can be remedied. Treatment of obstructive apnoea is mainly mechanical or surgical, not medical. On the whole, drugs which increase ventilation or reduce apnoea are limited in value, and tracheostomy is sometimes much more effective in reducing obesity than anorectic drugs or dietary control.

MECHANICAL AND SURGICAL METHODS

Mechanical relief of obstructive sleep apnoea causes rapid improvement in wellbeing and daytime drowsiness. The results of respiratory tract surgery in sleep apnoea due to local obstruction, enlarged tonsils, adenoids or micrognathia may be dramatic. Cures may follow relief of nasal obstruction;[19] tonsillectomy, particularly in children;[110] and correction of pharyngeal hypoplasia.[138, 290] Moldofsky *et al.*[185] reported the cure of sleep apnoea in a

Table 7.6.   *Choice of treatment for sleep apnoea*

	Advantages	Disadvantages
Mechanical methods e.g. external ventilation, cuirass respirators Diaphragm pacing	Applicable to treatment of central sleep apnoea	Sometimes may provoke obstruction
CPAP or positive expiratory pressure	Often treatment of choice for obstructive sleep apnoea	Noise sometimes not tolerated, comfortable mask difficult to achieve, sinus infection
Local surgery	Results may be dramatic with local obstruction	
Uvulopalatopharyngoplasty	Radical correction of upper airway obstruction	Severe post-operative discomfort, results uncertain, subsequent nasal regurgitation
Tracheostomy	Immediate and dramatic relief	Local infection, discomfort, very severe psychological problems
Respiratory stimulants e.g. doxapram	Main value short term management of central apnoea	Not pure respiratory stimulant
Central stimulants e.g. amphetamine	Uncertain	Sympathomimetic side effects
Miscellaneous Protriptyline Acetazolamide Progesterone	Possibly modest improvement in SaO_2 and symptoms	Cardiovascular problems and other side effects
Oxygen	May decrease apnoeas	Extreme caution needed, 24–28% O_2 concentration only, monitor PCO_2

patient following surgical correction of a deformed mandible due to osteomyelitis following a dog bite at the age of five; and in other cases of severe jaw deformity, mandibular surgery, osteotomy or advancement will prevent obstructive sleep apnoea.[155]

Surgical removal of redundant oronasopharyngeal tissue in obese subjects, intubation of the oropharynx or nasopharynx to maintain upper airway patency at night if this can be tolerated, and the operation of uvulopalatopharyngoplasty all have a similar aim and all may produce dramatic improvement in obstructive sleep apnoea.[58, 127, 173, 192] *Palatopharyngoplasty* consists of resection of redundant tissue from the lateral pharynx and removal of the uvula. More than 2000 patients are said to have undergone this procedure in Japan for heavy snoring.[252] One problem is the choice of patient for this procedure, and previous careful review of anatomical factors does not always predict results, perhaps because central as well as obstructive factors are present. At present, detailed long-term follow-up studies are lacking. Although the procedure may improve daytime drowsiness, prolonged apnoeas may continue and severe oxygen desaturation persist.

In obese subjects simple loss of weight is sometimes curative,[108] but some patients find this impossible to achieve if the airway obstruction itself is not relieved. Why this should be so is not clear, although it is well established that obese subjects with obstructive sleep apnoea, unable to lose weight before surgery, may achieve this rapidly following tracheostomy.

The management of central apnoea is determined by the availability of mechanical aids to respiration. Diaphragmatic pacing, external ventilation and positive respiration methods have all been developed.[219, 274] Almost 50 years ago, Waud showed that stimulation of the phrenic nerve produced experimental hyperventilation[292] and electrical diaphragmatic pacing by stimulation of the phrenic nerve was established as a practical procedure by Sarnoff et al.[235] This technique has been used successfully over several years to manage central alveolar hypoventilation[55] but requires modification for use in infants and children.[135] The successful use of diaphragmatic pacing demands an intact phrenic nerve and diaphragm. The technique is not always successful in primary alveolar hypoventilation and may induce upper airway occlusion if paradoxical movement of the ribcage occurs with abnormal temporal coordination of inspiratory activation of the upper airway muscles, the ribcage and the diaphragm.[134] Both the treatment of central apnoea with diaphragmatic pacing and the treatment of obstructive apnoea with tracheostomy can increase the alternative type of apnoea but this is usually only temporary.

Diaphragmatic pacing methods, cuirass respirators, rocking beds, etc., are not of value in obstructive sleep apnoea and may aggravate, not relieve, the problem.[85, 242]

CONTINUOUS POSITIVE AIRWAY PRESSURE

Continuous positive airway pressure (CPAP) has now largely replaced tracheostomy in the management of obstructive sleep apnoea, although the exact indications remain a little controversial and CPAP is ineffective in central apnoea. The technique can be used in children and adults, but not always in very young infants.[240] A pressure of 4–10 cm of water (0.45–1.0 kPa) is applied through the nose or mouth continuously throughout sleep to prevent upper airway collapse and resultant airway occlusion. A total seal is not vital, though a silicone rubber sealant has been used in some systems to get an airtight fit around the nose or mouth; this may be poorly tolerated. Alternative ways of giving continuous positive pressure have been developed.[234] To be effective, the system must remain mechanically efficient throughout sleep. Positive pressure with high flow rates is possibly more effective than other systems with end-expiratory pressure alone. CPAP is very effective in the laboratory. Sullivan and his colleagues initially suggested that CPAP was most suitable as an interim therapy whilst other solutions were sought, but successful long-term use of this method at home for up to two years has now been reported on several occasions.[172, 272, 274] Whilst most normal subjects would not tolerate being attached to a noisy machine during sleep, patients with the sleep apnoea syndrome may sleep extremely well, although there are occasional treatment failures[289] and, overall, experience with long-term CPAP at home has not been as successful in the USA as in Australia. Sometimes a marked rebound in REM sleep during the first nights of treatment results in vivid and terrifying dreams.

CPAP through the nose (Figs. 7.11–7.13) will reverse obstructive apnoea and abolish chronic hypercapnia and life-threatening hypoxia in patients with mild to moderate sleep apnoea syndromes. Reversal of daytime hypersomnolence may be dramatic.

CPAP, as well as preventing passive upper airway collapse by abolition of negative transmural pressure, may produce a direct alteration in the underlying loss of muscle tone by upper airway mechanoreceptor stimulation accompanying increase in pressure and flow in the airway.[172]

Search for Goblins

MOTORS from old Goblin vacuum cleaners are set to save respiratory patients from regular journeys to hospital for treatment.

Mrs Lesley Boylan from Witham is helping in the hunt for ten old Goblin motors that can be used in portable ventilator machines.

An anaesthetist at the National Hospital, Queen Square, London, has made two prototype machines using the old motors, she explained.

One patient using one of the two experimental machines is Mrs Boylan's mother, who lives in Norwich.

"I suppose the smaller size is the main advantage of this type of ventilator," said Mrs Boylan, of Blunts Hall Road.

Anyone who can help Mrs Boylan in her search can contact her ·on Witham 512698.

Figure 7.11.   *Vacuum cleaners and sleep apnoea.*

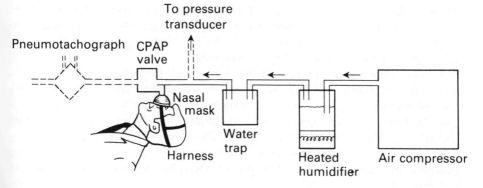

Figure 7.12.   *Positive airway pressure (CPAP) via nasal mask. Reprinted with permission from Rapoport et al.*[219]

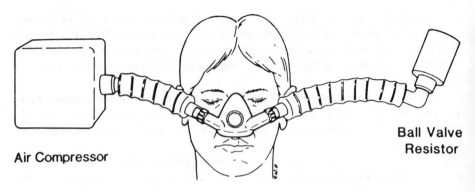

Air Compressor

Ball Valve Resistor

Figure 7.13. *Alternative method for administration of CPAP. Reprinted with permission from Sanders et al.*[234]

Positive expiratory airway pressure (EPAP), like CPAP, can reduce obstructive apnoeas, and stimulation of the face, nostrils and lips, as well as oropharyngeal and laryngeal sensor mechanisms, is probably important for the treatment of obstructive sleep apnoea. It is unlikely that either CPAP or EPAP owe their effects to simple splinting of a hypotonic airway alone.

There are a number of theoretical objections to continuous airway pressure. These are of little practical importance, although both cardiac output and renal function may be reduced with pressures above 10 cm H_2O, and the procedure will aggravate nasal sinus disease and reduce mucosal blood flow.[24, 287] Mechanical failure, causing over-inflation of the lungs, cannot happen with low-pressure systems.

TRACHEOSTOMY

Permanent tracheostomy is a very successful treatment for obstructive sleep apnoea, although it causes frequent and severe problems.[114] Tracheostomy is only indicated for patients with severe arrhythmias, pulmonary hypertension or cor pulmonale, and who cannot tolerate or do not respond to CPAP or EPAP. (At present, any role for palatopharyngoplasty as a definitive alternative to tracheostomy has not been established.) Many patients are reluctant to have a tracheostomy or may refuse.

Perioperative management and technique is all-important.[217] Intubation is more difficult than usual and the tracheostomy must be specifically designed for obstructive sleep apnoea patients.[253] Immediate post-operative complications include breathing difficulties, bleeding, pneumonia and occlusion of the tube with neck fat. Chronic problems include low-grade infection with granulation tissue around the stoma, stomal stenosis, recurrent purulent infection, and, most important, severe psychological and social difficulties.[60]

Relief of airway obstruction by tracheostomy results in a marked and immediate improvement in daytime sleepiness, and the mood improves.

There is occasionally a rapid fall in systemic hypertension, with gradual reversal of polycythaemia and reduction or abolition of cardiac arrhythmias. High values for oxygen saturation during sleep are maintained and although total sleep time may not increase, the fragmentary sleep stage disorganization is reversed.[297]

Following tracheostomy there is an immediate post-operative decrease in the number of obstructive and mixed apnoeas, although central apnoeas and hypopnoeas usually persist for several weeks or months.[106, 107, 297] Additional bonuses include reversal of personality changes, confusion and memory difficulty, although in children with sleep apnoea tracheostomy may not always improve learning difficulty or slight mental disorder.[110]

MEDICAL TREATMENT

Respiratory stimulant drugs such as nikethamide, theophylline, almitrine and doxapram have been used to stimulate breathing in both central and obstructive sleep apnoea, but the usual effect is limited. Most of these central stimulant drugs produce sympathomimetic side effects, increase the liability to cardiac arrhythmias and lead to subsequent respiratory depression on withdrawal. *Aminophylline*, *theophylline* and *ethamivan* (*vanillic acid diethylamide*)[68] reduce the duration, but not the number of obstructive and mixed apnoeas during NREM sleep. *Almitrine*, a stimulant of peripheral chemoreceptors, is of little clinical value.[150] *Doxapram hydrochloride*, which acts directly on the respiratory centre as well as on peripheral chemoreceptors, stimulates respiration and has been used successfully in central sleep apnoea syndromes and following cervical cord decompression.[130] Slow doxapram infusion (1–6 mg i.v./min) causes a sustained and rapid ventilatory increase of 50–100%, with a consequent decrease in PCO_2[163] and is successful for limited periods in central sleep apnoea. However, the patient may have no sleep at all during treatment and some apnoeic attacks still occur.[286]

Passouant[206] suggested using *clomipramine* for central sleep apnoea and bronchodilators for obstructive sleep apnoea, but tricyclic drugs,[149] ephedrine and aminophylline are not of great value.

Strychnine will reduce sleep atonia by blockade of inhibitory post-synaptic potentials and is of theoretical interest in the management of obstructive sleep apnoea. However, strychnine absorption is highly variable. As long as the gastric contents are acid, the strychnine is without effect; when the gastric pH is raised, the drug is highly ionized and absorbed, producing toxic, as well as therapeutic effects.

Amphetamine, *methylphenidate* and *fenfluramine* have been used to prevent daytime drowsiness and control obesity in sleep apnoea syndromes, but both stimulant and anorectic effects are usually limited.[73]

Protriptyline
Protriptyline hydrochloride 20–40 mg p.o. daily reduces the frequency and

duration of apnoeas, leading to improvement in oxygen saturation with reduction in nocturnal awakening and daytime drowsiness in obstructive sleep apnoea syndromes.[49, 256] Further assessment of protriptyline is needed, but it can cause a worthwhile if modest reduction in daytime drowsiness. This action is probably due to a reduction in REM sleep time (which is approximately halved by protriptyline 20 mg) with a consequent reduction in REM apnoea time. The alerting and anorectic effects of protriptyline by day may be of additional value. (Because of this alerting effect, protriptyline is a useful antidepressant for patients with obstructive lung disease.) Perhaps the effect of protriptyline in sleep apnoea is no greater than equivalent REM-suppressant doses of amphetamine, but the two drugs have not been directly compared. Protriptyline treatment of obstructive sleep apnoea has a number of disadvantages. The drug has an atropine-like action and can cause postural hypotension, impotence, possibly epileptiform seizures, tachycardia and palpitations in therapeutic dosages, and dysrhythmias in gross overdosage. It should not be used if any degree of heart block or other cardiac arrhythmias are present.

Oxygen
Low-flow nocturnal oxygen sometimes causes a marked decrease in the number and severity of sleep apnoeas, and an increase in the level of ventilation.[166] Some studies have suggested that apnoeas may be prolonged if oxygen is given during sleep,[106, 107] but most have indicated that the severity of desaturation and the incidence of bradyarrhythmias are decreased.[142, 171, 305] How oxygen causes a decrease in the number of apnoeas is not understood.

In sleep apnoea, and also in chronic obstructive lung disease, arterial O_2 saturation falls during sleep, being lowest during REM sleep. This is associated with poor sleep quality, reduced sleep time, increased sleep stage changes and increased arousal frequency. In 24 patients with chronic obstructive pulmonary disease studied by Fleetham et al.[86] the patients spent a quarter of the night with an SaO_2 more than 5% below waking SaO_2 values. In such subjects, oxygen therapy may have no effect on sleep quality, although arousals are usually associated with sleep arterial oxygen desaturation. Under these circumstances the major stimulus for arousal may be hypercapnia, not hypoxaemia. Despite little or no effect on arousal, oxygen therapy will reduce the severity of nocturnal hypoxaemia in chronic bronchitis and emphysema, as well as in sleep apnoea, although some degree of oxygen desaturation still occurs and it is not established that oxygen will prevent the development of cor pulmonale or secondary polycythaemia.

If oxygen is given to patients with sleep apnoea they must be carefully observed. As in patients with chronic lung disease and hypercapnia, the main stimulus to respiration in long-standing central or obstructive sleep apnoea may be hypoxia rather than hypercapnia. In sleep apnoea the ventilatory response to inhaled CO_2 may be greatly reduced, as compared with the doubling of ventilation, with a rise in PCO_2 of only 2–3 mmHg in normal subjects. The reduced drive results from resetting of the respiratory centre to a higher PCO_2 level and is accompanied by an increase in bicarbonate concentration in the CSF. If these patients are given oxygen, ventilation may cease, with a further rise in PCO_2 to narcotic levels. Because of this, patients with sleep apnoea and hypercapnia should be given oxygen with extreme caution, using 24–28% concentrations only, watching the patient breathe and monitoring blood PCO_2.[25] Oxygen may be of most value in those patients with sleep apnoea who also have chronic bronchitis or emphysema.

Acetazolamide

Acetazolamide, 250 mg eight-hourly, generally but not always prevents severe acute mountain sickness.[100] Symptoms are relieved and hypoxaemia, in particular sleep hypoxaemia, is reduced, although acetazolamide does not always prevent the occasional fatality.[67, 275, 295] The effect of acetazolamide on sleep hypoxia is similar in each sleep stage and the drug produces better sleep at high altitude with elimination of transient oxygen desaturation and reduction in arousals.[275, 295] Acetazolamide counteracts the alkalosis of high altitude, due to inhibition of carbonic anhydrase and promotion of bicarbonate diuresis, with additionally an increase in cerebral blood flow and a reduction in the formation of cerebrospinal fluid.[78, 154, 198] The overall effect of acetazolamide is to reduce periodic breathing at high altitudes with a large improvement in arterial oxygenation, and a reduction in PCO_2 at all levels of hypoxaemia.

Acetazolamide 250 mg p.o. four times a day has been used in a small trial on six patients with symptomatic central apnoea and severe insomnia.[301] In all of the patients there was a decrease in the number of apnoeas and in five of the six there was a decrease in daytime hypersomnolence. Mean arterial pH decreased from 7.42 to 7.34 over 1 week. However, acetazolamide is not always successful, and three patients have been observed with central sleep apnoea that converted to obstructive episodes with acetazolamide,[248] perhaps due to changes in central respiratory drive, with greater inspiratory pressure causing upper airway collapse. Acetazolamide is not tolerated by some patients because of severe paraesthesiae.

SLEEP AT HIGH ALTITUDE

A great many distinguished scientists from Pascal onwards have arranged important experiments at the top of mountains.[226] Sleep has been studied on the windswept high plateau of one of the largest mountain masses in the world, Mount Logan (19 849 feet, 6050 m) in the Canadian Yukon, with fibre-optic ear oximeters, thoracic magnometers and Beckman electroencephalograph machines. During sleep at these altitudes, a cycle of periodic breathing develops, with apnoea, arousal and subsequent return to sleep after several deep breaths.[222] This periodic hypopnoea and apnoea will further increase the degree of hypoxia. At these heights, and particularly during sleep, the steep part of the oxyhaemoglobin dissociation curve is reached[220] and arterial SaO_2 may fall precipitously to a mean level of around 60%. As well as tachycardia, respiratory alkalosis and, after several months, polycythaemia, the carotid body may enlarge, as occurs in Andean animals who live for long periods at high altitudes.[77] Both hypoxia and alkalosis probably contribute to irregular breathing.

Mountain sickness is due to hypoxia, disruption of automatic breathing during sleep, and insomnia. It develops after 6–90 h in lowlanders who rapidly climb high mountains. The symptoms are lethargy, headache, nausea, vomiting and dyspnoea, as well as lightheadedness and discomfort in the chest. There are usually no abnormal physical signs, but a cerebral form may occur (cerebral acute mountain sickness),[67] with ataxia, irritability and abnormal behaviour, drowsiness, hallucination, coma, urinary incontinence, papilloedema, cranial nerve palsies and tremor. Pulmonary features include cough, sputum, basal crepitations, tachypnoea and cyanosis.

The biochemical changes of acute mountain sickness are corrected by bicarbonate excretion by the kidney. Initially, ventilation continues to increase, although all known chemical stimuli to respiration are falling, with a rise in PaO_2, a fall in $PaCO_2$, and an increase in CSF pH. The observed ventilatory drive may be associated with loss of bicarbonate in the brain and CSF with an increased hydrogen ion concentration in the CSF.[18] However, it is still not clear if changes in brain extracellular fluid hydrogen ion concentration are an important drive to breathing in man.[64]

Acclimatization usually takes 5–20 days, and is accompanied by polycythaemia and a change in the oxygen dissociation curve. Polycythaemia, which may take weeks or months to develop fully, results in an increased oxygen transport capacity. The change in the oxygen dissociation curve, which facilitates release of oxygen to the tissues, is due to an increase in the red cell content of 2,3-diphosphoglycerate, a compound which decreases the oxygen affinity of haemoglobin.

A central alveolar hypoventilation syndrome, Monge's disease (soroche or punea) occurs at high altitudes, with some resemblance to Ondine's curse. It is due to failure or loss of acclimatization. There is little or no evidence of lung disease, but cyanosis, finger-clubbing, reduced ventilatory responses to hypoxia, severe polycythaemia with a haematocrit as high as 80% and haemoglobin of 25 g/dl, and heart failure with chronic malaise, headache, dizziness, fatigue and somnolence occur. Descent to low altitude is curative.[186] A somewhat similar condition (Brisket disease) is found in calves which graze at high altitudes in Utah and Colorado: they develop pulmonary hypertension and right heart failure, but not somnolence. Respiratory and sleep disorders at high altitude have not prevented the conquest of Everest: on 8 May 1978, Reinhold Meissner and Peter Habeler, part of an Austrian expedition, became the 62nd and 63rd climbers to reach the summit of Mount Everest, and the first to do so without supplemental oxygen.[226]

REFERENCES

1. Acres, J.C., Sweatman, P., West, P., Brownell, L. & Kryger, M.H. Breathing during sleep in parents of sudden infant death syndrome victims, *Am. Rev. Resp. Dis.* (1982) **125**, 163–166.

2. Adelman, S., Dinner, D.S., Goren, H., Little, J. & Nickerson, P. Obstructive sleep apnea in association with posterior fossa neurologic disease, *Arch. Neurol.* (1984) **41**, 509–510.

3. Adelson, L. & Kinney, R.E. Sudden and unexpected death in infancy and childhood, *Pediatrics* (1956) **17**, 663–697.

4. Adler, J.J. Did Falstaff have the sleep apnoea syndrome? *New Engl. J. Med.* (1983) **308**, 404.

5. Ahmad, M., Cressman, M. & Tomashefski, J.F. Central alveolar hypoventilation syndromes, *Arch. Int. Med.* (1980) **140**, 29–30.

6. Anch, A.M., Remmers, J.E., Sauerland, E.K. & de Groot, W.J. Oropharyngeal patency during waking and sleep in the Pickwickian syndrome: electromyographic activity of the tensor veli palatini, *Electromyog. Clin. Neurophysiol.* (1981) **21**, 317–330.

7. Ancoli Israel, S., Kripke, D.F., Mason, W. & Messin, S. Sleep apnea and nocturnal myoclonus in a senior population, *Sleep* (1981) **4**, 349–358.

8. Apps, M.C. Underdiagnosis of obstructive sleep apnea in Britain, *Lancet* (1983) **1**, 1054.

9. Ariagno, R. Nagel, I. & Guilleminault, C. Waking and ventilatory responses during sleep in infants near-miss for sudden infant death syndrome, *Sleep* (1980) **3**, 351–359.

10. Aserinsky, E. Periodic respiratory pattern occurring in conjunction with eye movements during sleep, *Science* (1966) **150**, 763–766.

11. Asmussen, E. Regulation of respiration: 'the blackbox', *Acta Physiol. Scand.* (1977) **99**, 85–90.

12. Avery, M.E., Fletcher, B.D. & Williams, R.G. (eds.) *The Lung and its Disorders in the Newborn Infant, 4th edn,* Philadelphia: W.B. Saunders (1981).

13. Bannister, R., Gibson, W., Michaels, L. & Oppenheimer, D.R. Laryngeal abductor paralysis in multiple system atrophy. A report on three necropsied cases with observations on the laryngeal muscles and the nuclei ambigui, *Brain* (1981) **104**, 351–368.

14. Bardin, C.W. & Paulsen, C.A. Testes. In: Williams, R.H. (ed.) *Textbook of Endocrinology, 6th edn.* Philadelphia: W.B. Saunders (1981) 335–336.

15. Barnes, A.J., Pallis, C. & Joplin, G.F. Acromegaly and narcolepsy, *Lancet* (1979) **2**, 332–333, 1084.

16. Bartall, H.Z., Tye, K.-H., Roper, P., Desser, K.B. & Benchimol, A. Atrial flutter associated with obstructive sleep apnea syndrome. A case report, *Arch. Int. Med.* (1980) **140**, 121–122.

17. Bate, T.W.P., Price, D.A., Holme, C.A. & McGucken, R.B. Short stature caused by obstructive apnoea during sleep, *Arch. Dis. Child.* (1984) **59**, 78–80.

18. Bauman, J.W., Jr. & Boyle, J. Sleep hypoxemia at high altitudes, *New Engl. J. Med.* (1980) **302**, 813.

19. Benaim, S. & Worster-Drought, C. Myotonia dystrophica, *Med. Illus.* (1954) **8**, 221–226.

20. Berger, R.J. Tonus of extrinsic laryngeal muscles during sleep and dreaming, *Science* (1961) **134**, 840.

21. Bergman, A.B., Ray, C.G., Pomeroy, M.A., Wahl, P.W. & Beckwith, J.B. Studies of the sudden infant death syndrome in King County, Washington. III. Epidemiology, *Pediatrics* (1972) **49**, 860–870.

22. Berrettini, W.H. Paranoid psychosis and sleep apnoea syndrome, *Am. J. Psychiat.* (1980) **137**, 493–494.

23. Bertrand, F. & Hugelin, A. Respiratory synchronizing function of nucleus parabrachialis medialis: Pneumotaxic mechanisms, *J. Neurophysiol.* (1971) **34**, 189–207.

24. Bishop, B., Hirsch, J. & Thursby, M. Volume flow and timing of each breath during positive pressure breathing in man, *J. Appl. Physiol. Resp. Env. Exercise Physiol.* (1978) **45**, 495–501.

25. Block, A.J. Dangerous sleep: oxygen therapy for nocturnal hypoxemia, *New Engl. J. Med.* (1982) **306**, 166–167.

26. Block, A.J., Boysen, P.G., Wynne, J.W. & Hunt, L.A. Sleep apnea, hypopnea and oxygen desaturation in normal subjects – a strong male predominance, *New Engl. J. Med.* (1979) **300**, 513–517.

27. Block, A.J., Wynne, J.W. & Boysen, P.G. Sleep-disordered breathing and nocturnal oxygen desaturation in postmenopausal women, *Am. J. Med.* (1980) **69**, 75–79.

28. Blood, A.M. Polycythaemia vera. Analysis of 41 cases with special emphasis on neurologic and psychiatric manifestations, *Mississippi Doctor* (1950) **28**, 6–12.

29. Bohiman, M.E., Haponik, E.F., Smith, P.L., Allen, R.P., Bleecker, E.R. & Goldman, S.M.

CT demonstration of pharyngeal narrowing in adult obstructive sleep apnea, *A.J.R.* (1983) **140**, 543–548.

30. Bornstein, S.K. Respiratory monitoring during sleeping: polysomnography. In: Guilleminault, C. (ed.) *Sleeping and Waking Disorders: Indications and Techniques* Menlo Park, California: Addison-Wesley (1982) 183–212.

31. Bowes, G., Townsend, E.R., Kozar, L.F., Bromley, S.M. & Phillipson, E.A. Effect of carotid body denervation on arousal response to hypoxia in sleeping dogs, *J. Appl. Physiol.* (1981) **51**, 40–45.

32. Briskin, G.J., Lehrman, K.L. & Guilleminault, C. Shy–Drager syndrome and sleep apnoea. In: Guilleminault, C. & Dement, W.C. (eds.) *Sleep Apnea Syndromes*, New York: Alan R. Liss (1978).

33. Brouillette, R.T., Fernbach, S.K. & Hunt, C.E. Obstructive sleep apnea in infants and children, *J. Pediat.* (1982) **100**, 31–40.

34. Brunt, P.W. & McKusick, V.A. Familial dysautonomia. A report of genetic and clinical studies, with a review of the literature, *Medicine* (1970) **49**, 343–374.

35. Bülow, K. Respiration and wakefulness in man, *Acta Physiol. Scand.* (Suppl. 209) (1963) **59**, 1–110.

36. Burwell, C., Robin, E., Whaley, R. & Bikelman, A. Extreme obesity associated with alveolar hypoventilation: a Pickwickian syndrome, *Am. J. Med.* (1956) **21**, 811–818.

37. Camargo, C.A. Obstructive sleep apnea and testosterone, *New Engl. J. Med.* (1983) **309**, 314.

38. Carpenter, R.G., Gardner, A., McWeeny, P.M. & Emery, J.L. Multistage scoring system for identifying infants at risk of unexpected death, *Arch. Dis. Child.* (1977) **52**, 606–612.

39. Carpenter, R.G., Gardner, A., Jepson, M., Taylor, E.M., Salvin, A., Sunderland, R., Emery, J.L., Pursall, E. & Roe, J. Prevention of unexpected infant death. Evaluation of the first seven years of the Sheffield Intervention Programme, *Lancet* (1983) **1**, 723–727.

40. Carroll, J.E., Zwillich, C.W. & Weil, J.V. Ventilatory response in myotonic dystrophy, *Neurology (Minneap.)* (1977) **27**, 1125–1128.

41. Carskadon, M.A. & Dement, W.C. Respiration during sleep in the aged human, *J. Gerontol.* (1981) **36**, 420–423.

42. Carskadon, M.A., Harvey, K., Dement, W.C., Guilleminault, C., Simmons, F.B. & Anders, T.F. Respiration during sleep in children, *West. J. Med.* (1978) **128**, 477–481.

43. Castaigne, P., Laplane, D., Autret, A., Bousser, M.G., Gray, F. & Baron, J.C. Syndrome de Shy et Drager avec troubles du rhythme respiratoire et de la vigilance, *Rev. Neurol.* (1977) **133**, 455–456.

44. Chaudhary, B.A. Obstructive sleep apnea after lateral medullary syndrome, *S. Med. J.* (1982) **75**, 65–67.

45. Cherniack, N.S. Respiratory dysrhythmias during sleep, *New Engl. J. Med.* (1981) **305**, 325–330.

46. Chokroverty, S. Phasic tongue movements in human rapid eye movement sleep, *Neurology (NY)* (1980) **30**, 665–668.

47. Chokroverty, S., Shard, I.T. & Barron, K.D. Periodic respiration in erect posture in Shy–Drager syndrome, *J. Neurol. Neurosurg. Psychiat.* (1978) **41**, 980–986.

48. Clark, T.J.H., Collins, J.V. & Tong, D. Respiratory depression caused by nitrazepam in patients with respiratory failure, *Lancet* (1971) **2**, 737–738.

49. Clark, R.W., Schmidt, H.S., Schaal, S.F., Boudoulas, H. & Schuller, D.E. Sleep apnoea: treatment with protriptyline, *Neurology* (1979) **29**, 1287–1292.

50. Clark, R.W., Schmidt, H.S. & Schuller, D.E. Sleep-induced ventilatory dysfunction in Down's syndrome, *Arch. Int. Med.* (1980) **140**, 45–50.

51. Coben, L.A., Danziger, W.L. & Berg, L. Frequency analysis of the resting awake EEG in mild senile dementia of Alzheimer type, *Electroenceph. Clin. Neurophysiol.* (1983) **55**, 372–380.

52. Coccagna, G., Cirignotta, F. & Lugaresi, E. The bird-like face syndrome (acquired micrognathia, hypersomnia and sleep apnea). In: Guilleminault, C. & Dement, W.C. (eds.) *Sleep Apnea Syndromes*, New York: Alan R. Liss (1978) 259–271.

53. Coccagna, G., di Donato, G., Verucchi, P., Cirignotta, F., Mantovani, M. & Lugaresi, E. Hypersomnias with periodic apnoeas in acquired micrognathia (a bird-like face syndrome), *Arch. Neurol.* (1976) **33**, 769–776.

54. Coccagna, G., Mantovani, M., Parchi, C., Mironi, F. & Lugaresi, E. Alveolar hypoventilation and hypersomnia in myotonic dystrophy, *J. Neurol. Neurosurg. Psychiat.* (1975) **38**, 977–984.

55. Coleman, M., Boros, S.J., Huseby, T.L. & Brennom, W.S. Congenital central

hypoventilation syndrome. A report of successful experience with bilateral diaphragmatic pacing, *Arch. Dis. Child.* (1980) **55**, 901–903.

56. Coleman, R.M., Roffwarg, H.P., Kennedy, S.J. *et al.* Sleep–wake disorders based on a polysomnographic diagnosis. A national cooperative study, *J. Am. Med. Assoc.* (1982) **247**, 997–1003.

57. Comroe, J.H. Frankenstein, Pickwick and Ondine *Am. Rev. Resp. Dis.* (1975) **111**, 689–692.

58. Conway, W., Fujita, S., Zorick, F., Roth, T., Hartse, K. & Piccione, P. Uvulo-palato-pharyngoplasty in treatment of upper airway apnea, *Am. Rev. Resp. Dis.* (1980) **121**, 121 (abstract).

59. Conway, W., Victor, L., Magilligan, D., Fujita, S., Zorick, F. & Roth, T. Long term experience with tracheostomy for sleep apnoea, *Sleep Res.* (1979) **8**, 176.

60. Conway, W.A., Victor, L.D., Magilligan, D.J., Fujita, S., Zorick, F.J. & Roth, T. Adverse effects of tracheostomy for sleep apnea, *J. Am. Med. Assoc.* (1981) **246**, 347–350.

61. Coverdale, S.G.M., Read, D.J.C., Woolcock, A.J. & Schoeffel, R.E. The importance of suspecting sleep apnoea as a common cause of excessive daytime sleepiness: further experience from the diagnosis and management of 19 patients, *Aust. N.Z. J. Med.* (1980) **10**, 284–288.

62. da Costa, J.L. Chronic hypoventilation due to diminished sensitivity of the respiratory centre associated with parkinsonism, *Med. J. Aust.* (1972) **1**, 373–376.

63. de Manacéïne, M. *Sleep: its Physiology, Pathology, Hygiene and Psychology*, London: Walter Scott (1897).

64. Dempsey, J.A., Skatrud, J.B., Forster, H.V., Hanson, P.E. & Chosy, L.W. Is brain ECF [H⁺] an important drive to breathe in man, *Chest* (1978) **73**, 251–253.

65. Deonna, T., Arczynska, W. & Torrado, A. Congenital failure of automatic ventilation (Ondine's curse), *J. Pediat.* (1974) **84**, 710–714.

66. Derman, S. & Karacan, I. Sleep-induced respiratory disorders, *Psychiat. Ann.* (1979) **9**, 411–425.

67. Dickinson, J.G. Terminology and classification of acute mountain sickness, *Brit. Med. J.* (1982) **285**, 720–721.

68. Dietrich, J., Krauss, A.N., Reidenberg, M., Drayer, D.E. & Auld, P.A. Alterations in state of apneic pre-term infants receiving theophylline, *Clin. Pharmacol. Ther.* (1978) **24**, 474–478.

69. Dolly, F.R. & Block, A.J. Effect of flurazepam on sleep-disordered breathing and nocturnal oxygen desaturation in asymptomatic subjects, *Am. J. Med.* (1982) **73**, 239–243.

70. Doring, G.H. & Loeschcke, H.H. Atmung und Saure-Basengleichgewicht in der Schwangerschaft, *Pflüg. Arch. Ges. Physiol. Mensch. Tier.* (1947) **249**, 437–451.

71. Douglas, N.J. Hypoxic ventilatory response decreases during sleep in normal man, *Am. Rev. Resp. Dis.* (1982) **125**, 286–289.

72. Douglas, N.J. Control of breathing during sleep, *Clin. Sci.* (1984) **67**, 465–471.

73. Douglas, J.G., Gough, J., Preston, P.G., Frazer, I., Haslett, C., Chalmers, S.R. & Munro, J.F. Long-term efficacy of fenfluramine in treatment of obesity, *Lancet* (1983) **1**, 384–386.

74. Douglas, N.J., Leggett, R.J.E., Calverley, P.M.A., Brash, H.M., Flenley, D.C. & Brezinova, V. Transient hypoxaemia during sleep in chronic bronchitis and emphysema, *Lancet* (1979) **i**, 1–4.

75. Douglas, N.J., White, D.P., Pickett, C.K., Weil, J.V. & Zwillich, C.W. Respiration during sleep in normal man, *Thorax* (1982) **37**, 840–844.

76. Douglas, N.J., White, D.P., Weil, J.V., Pickett, C.K. & Zwillich, C.W. Hypercapnic ventilatory response in sleeping adults, *Am. Rev. Resp. Dis.* (1982) **126**, 758–762.

77. Edwards, C.W. The carotid body in animals at high altitude. In: Porter, R. & Knight, J. (eds.) *High Altitude Physiology*, Ciba Foundation Symposium, Edinburgh: Churchill Livingstone (1971).

78. Ehrenreich, D.L., Burns, R.A., Alman, R.W. & Fazekas, J.F. Influence of acetazolamide on cerebral blood flow, *Arch. Neurol.* (1961) **5**, 227–232.

79. Eliashar, I., Lavie, P., Halperin, E., Gordon, C. & Alroy, G. Sleep apneic episodes as indications for adenotonsillectomy, *Arch. Otolaryngol.* (1980) **106**, 492.

80. Euler, C. von, On the central pattern generator for the basic breathing rhythmicity, *J. Appl. Physiol.* (1983) **55**, 1647–1659.

81. Evans, C.C., Hipkin, L.J. & Murray, G.M. Pulmonary function in acromegaly, *Thorax* (1977) **32**, 322–327.

82. Fielding, J.W. 'Ondine's curse'. A complication of upper cervical-spine surgery, *J. Bone Joint Surg.* (1975) **57**, 1000–1001.

83. Filler, J., Smith, A.A., Stone, S. & Dancis, J. Respiratory control in familial dysautonomia, *J. Pediat.* (1965) **66**, 509–516.
84. Fishman, A.P., Goldring, R.M. & Turino, G.M. General alveolar hypoventilation: a syndrome of respiratory and cardiac failure in patients with normal lungs, *Quart. J. Med.* (1966) **35**, 261–275.
85. Fishman, L.S., Samson, J.H. & Sperling, D.R. Primary alveolar hypoventilation syndrome (Ondine's curse). Association with manifestations of hypothalamic disease, *Am. J. Dis. Child.* (1965) **110**, 155–161.
86. Fleetham, J., West, P., Mezon, B., Conway, W., Roth, T. & Kryger, M. Sleep arousals and oxygen desaturation in chronic obstructive pulmonary disease. *Am. Rev. Resp. Dis.* (1982) **126**, 429–433.
87. Flenley, D.C. (Editorial) Hypoxaemia during sleep, *Thorax* (1980) **35**, 81–84.
88. Florez, J. The action of diazepam, nitrazepam and clonazepam on the respiratory centre of decerebrate cats, *Eur. J. Pharmacol.* (1971) **14**, 250–256.
89. Folgering, H., Kuyper, F. & Kine, J.F. Primary alveolar hypoventilation (Ondine's curse syndrome) in an infant without external arcuate nucleus. Case report, *Bull. Eur. Physiopathol. Resp.* (1979) **15**, 659–665.
90. Gadoth, N., Sokol, J. & Lavie, P. Sleep structure and nocturnal disordered breathing in familial dysautonomia, *J. Neurol. Sci.* (1983) **60**, 117–125.
91. Gastaut, H., Tassinari, C.A. & Duron, B. Polygraphic study of the episodic diurnal and nocturnal (hypnic and respiratory) manifestation of the Pickwick syndrome, *Brain Res.* (1966) **1**, 167–186.
92. Gilbert, R., Auchincloss, J.H., Jr., Brodsky, J. & Boden, W. Changes in tidal volume, frequency and ventilation induced by their measurements, *J. Appl. Physiol.* (1972) **33**, 252–254.
93. Gillam, P.M.S., Heaf, P.J.D., Kaufman, L. & Lucas, B.G.B. Respiration in dystrophia myotonica, *Thorax* (1964) **19**, 112–120.
94. Giraudoux, J. *Ondine*, English adaptation by Maurice Valency, New York: Random House (1954).
95. Goode, G.B. & Slyter, H.M. Daytime polysomnogram diagnosis of sleep apnea, *Trans. Am. Neurol. Assoc.* (1980) **105**, 367–370.
96. Goode, G.B. & Slyter, H.M. Daytime polysomnogram diagnosis of sleep disorders, *J. Neurol. Neurosurg. Psychiat.* (1983) **46**, 159–161.
97. Goodlands, R.L., Reynolds, J.G. & Pommerenke, W.T. Alveolar carbon dioxide tension levels during pregnancy and early puerperium, *J. Clin. Endocrinol. Metab.* (1954) **14**, 522–530.
98. Gothe, B., Altose, M.D., Goldman, M.D. & Cherniack, N.S. Effect of quiet sleep in humans on resting and CO_2 stimulated breathing, *J. Appl. Physiol.* (1981) **50**, 724–730.
99. Gowers, W.R. *A Manual of Diseases of the Nervous System*, 2nd edn., Vol. 2, London: Churchill (1893) 129.
100. Greene, M.K., Kerr, A.M., McIntosh, I.B. & Prescott, R.J. Acetazolamide in prevention of acute mountain sickness: a double blind cross over study, *Brit. Med. J.* (1981) **282**, 811–813.
101. Guilleminault, C. Sleep and breathing. In: Guilleminault, C. (ed.) *Sleeping and Waking Disorders: Indications and Techniques*, Menlo Park, California: Addison-Wesley (1982) 155–182.
102. Guilleminault, C., Ariagno, R.L., Forno, L.S., Nagel, L., Baldwin, R. & Owen, M. Obstructive sleep apnoea and near miss for SIDS: 1. Report of an infant with sudden death, *Pediatrics* (1979) **63**, 837–843.
103. Guilleminault, C., Briskin, J.G., Greenfield, M.S. & Silvestri, R. The impact of autonomic nervous system dysfunction on breathing during sleep, *Sleep* (1981) **4**, 263–278.
104. Guilleminault, C., Connolly, S., Winkle, R., Melvin, K. & Tilkian, A. Cyclical variation of the heart rate in sleep apnoea syndrome, *Lancet* (1984) **1**, 126–131.
105. Guilleminault, C. & Coons, S. Near miss sudden infant death infants: a summary of findings, *Electroenceph. Clin. Neurophysiol.* (Suppl.) (1982) **36**, 641–651.
106. Guilleminault, C., Cummiskey, J. & Dement, W.C. Sleep apnea syndrome: recent advances, *Adv. Int. Med.* (1980) **26**, 347–372.
107. Guilleminault, C., Cummiskey, J. & Motta, J. Chronic obstructive airflow disease and sleep studies, *Am. Rev. Resp. Dis.* (1980) **122**, 397–406.
108. Guilleminault, C., Cummiskey, J., Motta, J. & Lynne-Davies, P. Respiratory and haemodynamic study during wakefulness and sleep in myotonic dystrophy, *Sleep* (1978) **1**, 19–31.
109. Guilleminault, C. & Dement, W.C. *Sleep Apnea Syndromes*, New York: Alan R. Liss (1978).

110. Guilleminault, C., Eldridge, F.L., Simmons, F.B. & Dement, W.C. Sleep apnoea in eight children, *Pediatrics* (1976) **58,** 23–30.
111. Guilleminault, C., Hill, M.W., Simmons, F.B. & Dement, W.C. Obstructive sleep apnea: electromyographic and fibreoptic studies, *Exp. Neurol.* (1978) **62,** 48–67.
112. Guilleminault, C., Korobin, R. & Winkle R. A review of 50 children with obstructive sleep apnoea syndrome, *Lung* (1981) **159,** 275–287.
113. Guilleminault, C., van den Hoed, J. & Mitler, M. Clinical overview of the sleep apnoea syndrome. In: Guilleminault, C. & Dement, W.C. (eds.) *Sleep Apnea Syndromes,* New York: Alan R. Liss (1978) 1–12.
114. Guilleminault, C., Simmons, F.B., Motta, J., Cummiskey, J., Rosekind, M., Schroeder, J.S. & Dement, W.C. Obstructive sleep apnoea and tracheostomy: long term follow-up experience, *Arch. Int. Med.* (1981) **141,** 985–988.
115. Guilleminault, C., Tilkian, A.T. & Dement, W.C. The sleep apnoea syndromes, *Ann. Rev. Med.* (1976) **27,** 465–484.
116. Hall, B.D. & Smith, D.W. Prader–Willi syndrome, *J. Pediat.* (1972) **28,** 686–693.
117. Halperin, E., Lavie, P., Alroy, G., Eliashar, I. & Gordon, C. The hypersomnia–sleep–apnoea–syndrome (HSAS): ENT findings, *Sleep Res.* (1979) **8,** 188.
118. Halperin, E., Lavie, P., Klein, E, Zomer, J. & Alroy, G. Sinus arrhythmia and severe bradycardia in sleep apnoea syndrome, *Harefuah J. Isr. Med. Assoc.* (1981) **101,** 207–298.
119. Hansotia, P., & Frens, D. Hypersomnia associated with alveolar hypoventilation in myotonic dystrophy, *Neurology (NY)* (1981) **31,** 1336–1337.
120. Haponik, H.F., Bleecker, E.R., Allen, R.P., Smith, P.L. & Kaplan, J. Abnormal inspiratory flow-volume curves in patients with sleep-disordered breathing, *Am. Rev. Resp. Dis.* (1981) **124,** 571–574.
121. Haponik, E.F., Givens, D. & Angelo, J. Syringobulbia-myelia with obstructive sleep apnea, *Neurology (NY)* (1983) **33,** 1046–1049.
122. Harman, E., Wynne, J.W., Block, A.J. & Malloy-Fisher, L. Sleep-disordered breathing and oxygen desaturation in obese patients, *Chest* (1981) **79,** 256–260.
123. Henderson-Smart, D.J. The effect of gestational age on the incidence and duration of recurrent apnoea in newborn babies, *Aust. Paediat. J.* (1981) **17,** 273–276.
124. Henderson-Smart, D.J., Pettigrew, A.G. & Campbell, D.J. Clinical apnea and brain-stem neural function in preterm infants, *New Engl. J. Med.* (1983) **308,** 353–357.
125. Henderson-Smart, D.J. & Read, D.J.C. Depression of respiratory muscles and defective response to nasal obstruction during active sleep in the newborn, *Aust. Paediat. J.* (1976) **12,** 261–266.
126. Hensley, M.J. Saunders, N.A. & Strohl, K.P. Medroxyprogesterone treatment of obstructive sleep apnoea, *Sleep* (1980) **3,** 441–446.
127. Hernandez, S.F. Palatopharyngoplasty for the obstructive sleep apnea syndrome: technique and preliminary report of results of ten patients, *Am. J. Otolaryngol.* (1982) **3,** 229–234.
128. Hill, R., Robbins, A.W., Messing, R. & Arora, N.S. Sleep apnea syndrome after poliomyelitis, *Am. Rev. Resp. Dis.* (1983) **127,** 129–131.
129. Hishikawa, Y., Furuya, E. & Wakamatsu, H. Hypersomnia and periodic respiration. Presentation of two cases and comment on the physiopathogenesis of the Pickwickian syndrome, *Folia Psychiat. Neurol. Jap.* (1970) **24,** 163–173.
130. Houser, W.C. & Schlueter, D.P. Prolonged doxapram infusion in obesity–hypoventilation syndrome, *J. Am. Med. Assoc.* (1978) **239,** 340–341.
131. Hukuhara, T. Neuronal organization of the central respiratory mechanisms in the brain stem of the cat, *Acta Neurobiol. Exp.* (1973) **33,** 219–244.
132. Hunt, C.E. Abnormal hypercarbic and hypoxic sleep arousal responses in near-miss SIDS infants, *Pediat. Res.* (1981) **15,** 1462–1464.
133. Hunt, C.E., Matalon, S.V., Thompson, T.R., Demuth, S., Loew, J.M., Meiliu, H., Mastri, A. & Burke, B. Central hypoventilation syndrome. Experience with bilateral phrenic nerve pacing in three neonates, *Am. Rev. Resp. Dis.* (1978) **118,** 23–28.
134. Hyland, R.H., Hutcheon, M.A., Perl, A., Bowes, G., Anthonisen, N.R., Zamel, N. & Phillipson, E.A. Upper airway occlusion induced by diaphragm pacing for primary alveolar hypoventilation: implications for the pathogenesis of obstructive sleep apnea, *Am. Rev. Resp. Dis.* (1981) **124,** 180–185.
135. Ilbawi, M.N., Hunt, C.E., De Leon, S.Y. & Idriss, F.S. Diaphragm pacing in infants and children: report of a simplified technique and review of experience, *Am. Thorac. Surg.* (1981) **31,** 61–65.

136. Illingworth, R.S. Cyanotic attacks in newborn infants, *Arch. Dis. Child.* (1957) **32**, 328–332.
137. Imes, N.K., Orr, W.C., Smith, R.O. & Rogers, R.M. Retrognathia and sleep apnea: a life-threatening condition masquerading as narcolepsy, *J. Am. Med. Assoc.* (1977) **237**, 1596–1597.
138. James, D.R. Obstructive sleep apnoea syndrome, *Brit. Med. J.* (1982) **285**, 736.
139. Johnson, D.R. & Chalgren, W.S. Polycythaemia vera and the nervous system, *Neurology (Minneap.)* (1951) **1**, 53–67.
140. Jordan, C. Assessment of the effects of drugs on respiration, *Brit. J. Anaesthesia* (1982) **54**, 763–782.
141. Kales, A., Bixler, E.O., Cadieux, R.J., Schneck, D.W., Shaw, L.C., Locke, T.W., Vela-Buono, A. & Soldatos, C.R. Sleep apnoea in a hypertensive population, *Lancet* (1984) **2**, 1005–1008.
142. Kearley, R., Wynne, J.W., Block, A.J., Boysen, P.G., Lindsey, S. & Martin, C. The effect of low flow oxygen on sleep-disordered breathing and oxygen desaturation. A study of patients with chronic obstructive lung disease, *Chest* (1980) **78**, 682–685.
143. Kellogg, R.H. Central chemical control of respiration. In: Fenn, W.O. & Rahn, H. (eds.) *Handbook of Physiology*, Washington, DC: American Physiological Society (1964) 507–534.
144. Kilburn, K.H., Eagen, J.T. & Heyman, A. Cardiopulmonary insufficiency associated with myotonic dystrophy, *Am. J. Med.* (1959) **26**, 929–935.
145. Koike, Y. Circulatory disturbance of Shy–Drager syndrome – nocturnal polygraphic study, *Rinsho Shinkeigaku* (1981) **21**, 944–951.
146. Konno, A., Togawa, K. & Hoshino, T. The effect of nasal obstruction in infancy and early childhood upon ventilation, *Laryngoscope* (1980) **90**, 699–707.
147. Kreis, P., Kripke, D.F. & Ancoli-Israel, S. Sleep apnea: a prospective study, *West. J. Med.* (1983) **139**, 171–173.
148. Krieger, J., Kurtz, D. & Roeslin, N. Observation fibroscopique directe au cours des apnées hypniques chez un sujet pickwickien, *Nouv. Presse Med.* (1976) **5**, 2890.
149. Krieger, J., Mangin, P. & Kurtz, D. Sleep apnoea syndrome: effects of chlorimipramine in subjects with stable body weight, *Rev. Electroenceph. Neurophysiol. Clin.* (1979) **9**, 250–257.
150. Krieger, J., Mangin, P. & Kurtz, D. Almitrine and sleep apnoea, *Lancet* (1982) **ii**, 210.
151. Krieger, A.J. & Rosomoff, H.L. Sleep-induced apnea, *J. Neurosurg.* (1974) **39**, 168–180.
152. Kripke, D.F. & Ancoli-Israel, S. Epidemiology of sleep apnea among the aged: is sleep apnea a fatal disorder? In: Guilleminault, C. & Lugaresi, E. (eds.) *Sleep/Wake Disorders: Natural History, Epidemiology and Long-Term Evolution*, New York: Raven Press (1983) 137–142.
153. Kripke, D.F., Simons, R.N., Garfinkel, L. & Hammond, E.C. Short and long sleep and sleeping pills, *Arch. Gen. Psychiat.* (1979) **36**, 103–115.
154. Kryger, M., Glas, K. & Jackson, F. Impaired oxygenation during sleep in excessive polycythaemia of high altitude: improvement with respiratory stimulation, *Sleep* (1978) **1**, 3–17.
155. Kuo, P.C., West, R.A., Bloomquist, D.S. & McNeil, R.W. The effect of mandibular osteotomy in three patients with hypersomnic sleep apnea, *Oral Surg.* (1979) **48**, 385–392.
156. Lavie, P. Sleep habits and sleep disturbances in industry workers in Israel: main findings and some characteristics of workers complaining of excessive daytime sleepiness, *Sleep* (1981) **4**, 147–158.
157. Lavie, P. Sleep apnea in Industrial Workers. In: Guilleminault, C. & Lugaresi, E. (eds.) *Sleep/Wake Disorders: Natural History, Epidemiology and Long-Term Evolution*, New York: Raven Press (1983) 127–135.
158. Liu, H.M., Loew, J.M. & Hunt, C.E. Congenital central hypoventilation syndrome: a pathologic study of the neuro-muscular system, *Neurology* (1978) **28**, 1013–1019.
159. Loewenstein, R.J., Weingartner, H., Gillin, J.C., Kaye, W., Ebert, M. & Mendelson, W.B. Disturbances of sleep and cognitive functioning in patients with dementia, *Neurobiol. Aging* (1982) **3**, 371–377.
160. Lugaresi, E., Cirignotta, F., Coccagna, G. & Piana, C. Some epidemiologic data on snoring and cardiocirculatory disturbances, *Sleep* (1980) **3**, 221–224.
161. Lugaresi, E., Coccagna, G. & Cirignotta, F. Snoring and clinical implications. In: Guilleminault, C. & Dement, W.C. (eds.) *Sleep Apnea Syndromes*, New York: Alan R. Liss (1978) 13–21.
162. Lugaresi, E., Coccagna, G. & Mantovani, M. Hypersomnia with periodic apnoeas. In: Weitzman, E.D. (ed.) *Advances in Sleep Research, Vol. 4*, New York: Spectrum (1978) 1–151.
163. Lugliani, R., Whipp, B.J. & Wasserman, K. Doxapram hydrochloride: a respiratory

stimulant for patients with primary alveolar hypoventilation, *Chest* (1979) **76**, 414–419.

164. McGinty, D.J., Arand, D.L. & Littner, M.R. Sleep-related breathing disorders in healthy and hypersomnolent older males, Presented at the 21st Annual Meeting of the Association for the Psychophysiological Study of Sleep, Hyannis, Massachusetts (1981).

165. McKusick, V.A., Norum, R.A., Farkas, H.J., Brunt, P.W. & Mahloudji, M. The Riley–Day syndrome – observations on genetics and survivorship, *Isr. J. Med. Sci.* (1967) **3**, 372.

166. McNicholas, W.T., Carter, J.L., Rutherford, R., Zamel, N. & Phillipson, E.A. Beneficial effect of oxygen in primary alveolar hypoventilation with central sleep apnea, *Am. Rev. Resp. Dis.* (1982) **125**, 773–775.

167. McNicholas, W.T., Tarlo, S.M. & Phillipson, E.A. Is sleep apnoea more common in North America? *Lancet* (1982) **1**, 458.

168. Mandami, M.B., Masdue, J., Ross, E. & Ohara, O. Sleep apnea with unusual EEG changes in Jakob– Creutzfeldt disease, *Electroenceph. Clin. Neurophysiol.* (1983) **55**, 411–416.

169. Martin, R.J. The problem of sleep-related respiratory disorders, *J. Am. Med. Assoc.* (1981) **245**, 1250–1251.

170. Martin, P.R. & Lefebve, A.M. Surgical treatment of sleep apnoea associated psychosis, *Can. Med. Assoc. J.* (1981) **124**, 978–980.

171. Martin, R.J., Sanders, M.H., Gray, B.A. & Pennock, B.E. Acute and long-term ventilatory effects of hyperoxia in the adult sleep apnea syndrome, *Am. Rev. Resp. Dis.* (1982) **125**, 175–180.

172. Mathew, O.P., Abu-Osba, Y.K. & Thach, B.T. Influence of upper airway pressure changes on genioglossus muscle respiratory activity, *J. Appl. Psychiol.* (1982) **52**, 438–444.

173. Mattox, D.E. & Gates, G.A. Alternatives to tracheostomy in sleep apnea, *New Engl. J. Med.* (1983) **308**, 656.

174. Meancock, C.I. Influence of the vagus nerve on changes in heart rate during sleep apnoea in man, *Clin. Sci.* (1982) **62**, 163–167.

175. Megirion, D. & Sherry, J.H. Respiratory functions of the laryngeal muscles during sleep, *Sleep* (1980) **3**, 289–298.

176. Mellins, R.B., Balfour, H.H., Turino, G.M. & Winters, R.W. Failure of automatic control of ventilation (Ondine's curse). Report of an infant born with this syndrome and review of the literature, *Medicine* (1970) **49**, 487–504.

177. Mendelson, W.B., Garnett, D. & Gillin, J.C. Flurazepam-induced sleep apnea syndrome in a patient with insomnia and mild sleep-related respiratory changes, *J. Nerv. Ment. Dis.* (1981) **169**, 261–264.

178. Meyer, J.S., Sakai, F., Karacan, I., Derman, S. & Yamamoto, M. Sleep apnea, narcolepsy and dreaming: regional cerebral hemodynamics, *Ann. Neurol.* (1980) **7**, 479–485.

179. Mezon, B.J., West, B., MacLean, J.P. & Kryger, M.H. Sleep apnea in acromegaly, *Am. J. Med.* (1980) **69**, 615–618.

180. Miles, L.E. & Dement, W.C. Sleep and aging, *Sleep* (1980) **3**, 183.

181. Millman, R.P., Bevilacque, J., Peterson, D.D. & Pack, A.I. Central sleep apnea in hypothyroidism, *Am. Rev. Resp. Dis.* (1983) **127**, 504–507.

182. Model, D.G. Nitrazepam induced respiratory depression in chronic obstructive lung disease, *Brit. J. Dis. Chest.* (1973) **67**, 128–130.

183. Model, D.G. & Berry, D.J. Effects of chlordiazepoxide in respiratory failure due to chronic bronchitis, *Lancet* (1974) **2**, 869–870.

184. Moldofsky, H., Goldstein, R., McNicholas, W.T., Lue, F., Zamel, N. & Phillipson, E.A. Disordered breathing during sleep and overnight intellectual deterioration in patients with pathological aging. In: Guilleminault, C. & Lugaresi, E. (eds.) *Sleep/Wake Disorders: Natural History, Epidemiology and Long-Term Evolution*, New York: Raven Press (1983) 143–150.

185. Moldofsky, H., Kiraly, L., Lue, F., Phillipson, E. & Munro, I.R. Two cases of successful treatment of obstructive sleep apnoea syndrome by correction of oropharyngeal pathology, *Sleep Res.* (1979) **8**, 202.

186. Monge, C.M. & Monge, C.C. *High Altitude Diseases: Mechanisms and Management*, Springfield, Illinois: Charles C. Thomas (1966).

187. Murad, F. & Haynes, R.C. Androgens. In: Gilman, A.G., Goodman, L.S. & Gilman, A. (eds.) *The Pharmacological Basis of Therapeutics*, 6th edn., New York: Macmillan (1980) 1448–1665.

188. Neil, J.F., Reynolds, C.F., Spiker, D.G. & Kupfer, D.I. Polycythaemia vera and central sleep apnoea, *Brit. Med. J.* (1980) **280**, 19.

189. Newsom-Davies, J., Loh, L. & Nodal, J. Effects of CO_2 on the breathing pattern in awake and sleeping man, *Bull. Physiopath.* (1976) **12**, 237.

190. Oliva, P.B., Williams, M.H. & Park, S.S. Alveolar hypoventilation syndrome: case of clinical recovery despite continued absence of ventilatory response to inhaled carbon dioxide, *Am. Rev. Resp. Dis.* (1967) **96**, 805–811.

191. Olsen, K.D., Kern, E.B. & Westbrook, P.R. Sleep and breathing disturbance secondary to nasal obstruction, *Otolaryngol. Head Neck Surg.* (1981) **89**, 804–810.

192. Olsen, K.D., Suh, K.W. & Staats, B.A. Surgically correctable causes of sleep apnea syndrome, *Otolaryngol. Head Neck Surg.* (1981) **89**, 726–731.

193. Onada, M., Koike, K., Hibino, R., Takahashi, A. & Sobue, I. Sleep apnea in Creutzfeldt–Jakob disease and subacute sclerosing panencephalitis – with reference to periodic synchronous discharges, *Rinsho Shinkeigaku* (1978) **18**, 601–607.

194. Önal, E. & Lopata, M. Periodic breathing and the pathogenesis of occlusive sleep apneas, *Am. Rev. Resp. Dis.* (1982) **126**, 676–680.

195. Önal, E., Lopata, M. & O'Connor, T.D. Genioglossal and diaphragmatic EMG responses to CO_2 rebreathing in humans, *J. Appl. Physiol.: Resp. Env. Ex. Physiol.* (1981) **50**, 1052–1055.

196. Önal, E., Lopata, M. & O'Connor, T.D. Diaphragmatic and genioglossal EMG responses to isocapnic hypoxia in humans, *Am. Rev. Resp. Dis.* (1981) **124**, 215–217.

197. Önal, E., Lopata, M. & O'Connor, T. Pathogenesis of apnoea in hypersomnia – sleep apnoea syndrome, *Am. Rev. Resp. Dis.* (1982) **125**, 167–174.

198. Oppelt, W.W., Patlak, C.S. & Rall, D.P. Effect of certain drugs on cerebrospinal fluid production in the dog, *Am. J. Physiol.* (1964) **206**, 247–250.

199. Orem, J. Medullary respiratory neuron activity: relationship to tonic and phasic REM sleep, *J. Appl. Physiol.* (1980) **48**, 54–65.

200. Orem, J. Control of the upper airways during sleep and the hypersomnia–sleep apnoea syndrome. In: Orem, J. & Barnes, C.D. (eds.) *Physiology in Sleep*, New York: Academic Press (1980) 306–307.

201. Orr, W.C., Imes, N.K. & Martin, R.J. Progesterone therapy in obese patients with sleep apnea, *Arch. Int. Med.* (1979) **139**, 109–111.

202. Orr, W.C., Imes, N.K. & Rogers, R.M. Effect of progesterone on the apnea–hypersomnolence syndrome, *Sleep Res.* (1976) **5**, 182.

203. Osler, W. *The Principles and Practice of Medicine, 13th edn.*, New York: Appleton (1938) 544.

204. Pappenheimer, J.R. Sleep and respiration of rats during hypoxia, *J. Physiol.* (1977) **266**, 191–207.

205. Pascal, D. Account of the great experiment concerning the equilibrium of fluids. *The Provincial Letters, Scientific Treatises*, Chicago: Encyclopaedia Britannica (1952) 382–389.

206. Passouant, P. Pathology of sleep, *Experientia* (1980) **36**, 24–26.

207. Pearson, J., Axelrod, F. & Dancis, J. Current concepts of dysautonomia: *Neuropathol. Defects, Ann. N.Y. Acad. Sci.* (1974) **228**, 288.

208. Peled, R., Pratt, H., Schart, B. & Lavie, P. Auditory brainstem evoked potentials during sleep apnea, *Neurology (NY)* (1983) **33**, 419–423.

209. Perks, W.H., Cooper, R.A., Bradbury, S., Horrocks, P., Baldock, N., Allen, A., Vant'Hoff, W., Weidman, G. & Prowse, K. Sleep apnoea in Scheie's syndrome, *Thorax* (1980) **35**, 85–91.

210. Perks, W.H., Horrocks, P.M., Cooper, R.A., Bradbury, S., Allen, A., Baldock, N., Prowse, K. & Vant'Hoff, W. Sleep apnea in acromegaly, *Brit. Med. J.* (1980) **280**, 894–897.

211. Phemister, J.C. & Small, J.M. Hypersomnia in dystrophia myotonica, *J. Neurol. Neurosurg. Psychiat.* (1975) **38**, 979–984.

212. Phillipson, E.A. Respiration during sleep, *Ann. Rev. Physiol.* (1978) **40**, 133–156.

213. Phillipson, E.A. Control of breathing during sleep, *Am. Rev. Respir. Dis.* (1978) **118**, 909–939.

214. Pollak, C.P., Bradlow, H.G., Spielman, A.J. & Weitzman, E.D. A pilot survey of the symptoms of hypersomnia–sleep apnoea syndrome as possible prediction factors for hypertension, *Sleep Res.* (1979) **8**, 210.

215. Pollak, C.P., Pressman, M.R., Appel, D., Spielman, A.J., Chervin, R.D. & Weitzman, E.D. Sleep apnea in elderly insomniacs and effects of flurazepam. In: Chase, M.H., Kripke, D.F. & Walter, P.L. (eds.) *Sleep Research, Vol. 10*, Los Angeles: UCLA BIS/BRI (1981) 222.

216. Power, W.R., Mosko, S.S. & Sassin, J.F. Sleep-stage dependent Cheyne–Stokes respiration after cerebral infarct: a case study, *Neurology (NY)* (1982) **32**, 763–766.

217. Rafferty, T.D., Ruskis, A., Sasaki, C. & Gee, J.B. Perioperative considerations in the management of tracheostomy for the obstructive sleep apnoea patient. Three illustrative case reports, *Brit. J. Anaesth.* (1980) **52**, 619–622.

218. Rajagopal, K.R., Derderian, S.S., Jabbari, B., Burman, K.D. & Hunt K.K. Obstructive sleep apnoea in hypothyroidism, *Am. Rev. Resp. Dis.* (1981) **123**, 188 (abstract).

219. Rapoport, D.M., Sorkin, B., Garay, S.M. & Goldring, R.M. Reversal of the 'Pickwickian syndrome' by long-term use of nocturnal nasal-airway pressure, *New Engl. J. Med.* (1982) **307**, 931–933.
220. Reed, D.J. & Kellogg, R.H. Changes in respiratory response to CO_2 during natural sleep at sea level and at altitude, *J. Appl. Physiol.* (1958) **13**, 325–330.
221. Rees, P.J., Cochrane, G.M., Prior, J.G. & Clark, T.J.H. Sleep apnoea in diabetic patients with autonomic neuropathy, *J. Roy. Soc. Med.* (1981) **74**, 192–195.
222. Reite, M., Jackson, D., Cahoon, R.L. & Weil, J.V. Sleep physiology at high altitude, *Electroenceph. Clin. Neurophysiol.* (1975) **38**, 463–471.
223. Revich, M., Isaacs, G., Evarts, E. & Kety, S. The effect of slow wave sleep and REM sleep on regional cerebral blood flow in cats, *J. Neurochem.* (1968) **15**, 301–306.
224. Remmers, J.E. Effects of sleep on control of breathing. In: Widdicombe, J.G. (ed.) *Respiratory Physiology, III, Vol. 23*, Baltimore: University Park Press (1981) 111–147.
225. Remmers, J.E., de Groot, W.J., Sauerland, E.K. & Anch. A.M. Pathogenesis of upper airway occlusion during sleep, *J. Appl. Physiol.* (1978) **44**, 931–938.
226. Rennie, D. High science, present and future, *New Engl. J. Med.* (1979) **301**, 1343–1344.
227. Reynolds, C.F., III, Coble, P.A., Black, R.S., Holzer, B., Carroll, R. & Kupfer, D.J. Sleep disturbance in a series of elderly patients. Polysomnographic findings, *J. Am. Geriat. Soc.* (1980) **28**, 164–170.
228. Riley, C.M. Familial dysautonomia, *Adv. Pediat.* (1957) **9**, 157.
229. Rosa, R., Kramer, M. & Ebright, P. Central sleep apnoea associated with sleep paralysis: a case report, *Sleep Res.* (1979) **8**, 212.
230. Rudolf, M., Gettes, D.M., Turner, J.A. & Saunders, K.B. Depression of central respiratory drive by nitrazepam, *Thorax* (1978) **33**, 97–100.
231. Roxburgh, R. & Collis, A.J. Notes on a case of acromegaly, *Brit. Med. J.* (1896) **ii**, 63–65.
232. Sandblom, R.E., Matsumoto, A.M., Schoene, R.B. Lee, K.A., Giblin, E.C., Bremner, W.J. & Pierson, D.J. Obstructive sleep apnoea syndrome induced by testosterone administration, *New Engl. J. Med.* (1983) **308**, 508–510.
233. Sanders, M.H., Martin, R.J., Pencock, B.E., Rogers, R.M. The detection of sleep apnoea in the awake patient. The 'saw-tooth' sign, *J. Am. Med. Assoc.* (1981) **245**, 2414–2418.
234. Sanders, M.H., Moore, S.E. & Eveslage, J. CPAP via nasal mask: a treatment for occlusive sleep apnea, *Chest* (1983) **83**, 144–145.
235. Sarnoff, S.J., Gaensler, E.A. & Maloney, J.V. Electrophrenic respiration. IV. The effectiveness of contralateral ventilation during activity of one phrenic nerve, *J. Thorac. Surg.* (1950) **19**, 929–937.
236. Sauerland, E.K. & Harper, R.M. The human tongue during sleep: electromyographic activity of genioglossus muscle, *Exp. Neurol.* (1977) **51**, 160–170.
237. Sauerland, E.K. & Mitchell, S.P. Electromyographic activity of the human genioglossus muscle in response to respiration and to positional changes of the head, *Bull. Los Angeles Neurol. Soc.* (1970) **35**, 69–73.
238. Sauerland, E.K., Orr, W.C. & Hairston, L.E. EMG patterns of oropharyngeal muscles during respiration in wakefulness and sleep, *Electromyog. Clin. Neurophysiol.* (1981) **21**, 307–316.
239. Sauerland, E.K., Sauerland, B.A., Orr, W.C. & Hairston, L.E. Non-invasive electromyography of human genioglossal (tongue) activity, *Electromyog. Clin. Neurophysiol.* (1981) **21**, 279–286.
240. Schmidt-Nowara, W.W. Continuous positive airway pressure for long-term treatment of sleep apnea, *Am. J. Dis. Child.* (1984) **138**, 82–84.
241. Scollo-Lavizzarri, G. Continuous EEG and EMG recordings during night sleep in a case of subacute sclerosing leucoencephalitis, *Electroenceph. Clin. Neurophysiol.* (1968) **25**, 170–174.
242. Seriff, N.S. Alveolar hypoventilation with normal lungs: the syndrome of primary or central alveolar hypoventilation, *Am. N.Y. Acad. Sci.* (1965) **121**, 691–705.
243. Severinghaus, J. & Mitchell, P. Failure of respiratory center automaticity while awake, *Clin. Res.* (1962) **10**, 122–127.
244. Shahidi, N.T. Androgens and erythropoiesis, *New Engl. J. Med.* (1973) **289**, 72–80.
245. Shannon, D.C., Marshland, D.W., Gould, J.B., Callahan, B., Todres, D. & Dennis, J. Central hypoventilation during quiet sleep in two infants, *Pediatrics* (1976) **57**, 342–346.
246. Shapiro, C.M., Caterall, J.R., Oswald, I. & Flenley, D.C Where are the British sleep apnoea patients? *Lancet* (1981) **2**, 523.
247. Sharp, J.T., Druz, W.S., Foster, J.R., Wicks, M.S. & Chokroverty, S. Use of the respiratory

magnetometer in diagnosis and classification of sleep apnea, *Chest* (1980) **77**, 350–353.

248. Shore, E.T. & Millman, R.P. Central sleep apnea and acetazolamide therapy, *Arch. Int. Med.* (1983) **143**, 1278–1280.

249. Shprintzen, R.J., Croft, C.B., Berkman, M.D. & Rakoff, S.J. Velopharyngeal insufficiency in the facio-auriculo vertebral malformation complex, *Cleft Palate J.* (1980) **17**, 132–137.

250. Sieker, H.O., Estes, E.H., Jr., Kelser, G.A. & McIntosh, H.D.A. Cardiopulmonary syndrome with extreme obesity *J. Clin. Invest.* (1955) **34**, 916.

251. Silverstein, A., Gilbert, H. & Wasserman, L.R. Neurologic complications of polycythaemia, *Ann. Int. Med.* (1962) **57**, 909–916.

252. Silvestri, R., Guilleminault, C. & Simmons, F.B. Palatopharyngoplasty in the treatment of obstructive sleep apneic patients. In: Guilleminault, C. & Lugaresi, E. (eds.) *Sleep/Wake Disorders: Natural History, Epidemiology and Long-Term Evolution*, New York: Raven Press (1983) 163–169.

253. Simmons, F.B. 'How I do it' – head and neck. Tracheostomy in obstructive sleep apnea patients, *Laryngoscope* (1979) **89**, 1702–1703.

254. Smallwood, R.G., Vitiello, M.V., Giblin, E.C. & Prinz, P.N. Sleep apnea: relationship to age, sex, and Alzheimer's dementia, *Sleep* (1983) **6**, 16–22.

255. Smith, T.H., Baska, R.F., Francisco, C.B., McGray, G.M. & Kunz, S. Sleep apnea syndrome: diagnosis of upper airway obstruction by fluoroscopy, *J. Pediat.* (1978) **93**, 891–892.

256. Smith, P.L., Haponik, E.F., Allen, R.P. & Bleecker, E.R. The effects of protriptyline in sleep-disordered breathing, *Am. Rev. Resp. Dis.* (1983) **127**, 8–13.

257. Smolensky, M., Halberg, F. & Sargent, F. Chronobiology of the life sequence. In: Ito, S., Ogata, K. & Yoshimura, H. (eds.) *Advances in Climatic Physiology*, Tokyo: Igaku Shoin (1971) 281–318.

258. Sorbini, C.A., Brassi, V., Solinas, E. & Muieson, G. Arterial oxygen tension in relation to age in healthy subjects, *Respiration* (1968) **25**, 3–13.

259. Steinschneider, A. Prolonged apnoea and sudden infant death syndrome: clinical and laboratory observations, *Pediatrics* (1972) **50**, 646.

260. Stern, M., Erttmann, R., Hellwege, H.H. & Kuhn, N. Total aganglionosis of the colon and Ondine's curse, *Lancet* (1980) **i**, 877–878.

261. Stern, M., Hellwege, H.H., Grävinghoff, L. & Lambrecht, W. Total aganglionosis of the colon (Hirschsprung's disease) and congenital failure of autonomic control of ventilation (Ondine's curse), *Acta Paediat. Scand.* (1981) **70**, 121–124.

262. Stokes, D.C., Phillips, J.A., Leonard, C.O., Dorst, J.P., Kopits, S.E., Trojak, J.E. & Brown, D.L. Respiratory complications of achondroplasia, *J. Pediat.* (1983) **102**, 534–541.

263. Stradling, J.R. Apnea alarms, *Lancet* (1980) **1**, 1197.

264. Stradling, J.R., Huddart, S. & Arnold, A.G. Sleep apnoea syndrome caused by neurofibromatosis and superior vena caval obstruction, *Thorax* (1981) **36**, 634–635.

265. Stradling, J.R. & Lane, D.J. Polycythaemia vera and central sleep apnoea, *Brit. Med. J.* (1980) **280**, 404.

266. Strieder, D.J., Baker, W.G., Baringer, J.R. & Kazemi, H. Chronic hypoventilation of central origin: A case with encephalitis lethargica and Parkinson's syndrome, *Am. Rev. Resp. Dis.* (1967) **96**, 501–507.

267. Strohl, K.P., Hensley, M.J., Hallett, M., Saunders, N.A. & Ingram, R.H., Jr. Activation of upper airway muscles before onset of inspiration in normal humans, *J. Appl. Physiol.* (1980) **49**, 638–642.

268. Strohl, K.P., Hensley, M.J., Saunders, N.A., Scharf, S.M., Brown, R. & Ingram, R.H. Progesterone administration and progressive sleep apnoea, *J. Am. Med. Assoc.* (1981) **245**, 1230–1232.

269. Strohl, K.P., Saunders, N.D., Feldman, N.T. & Hallett, M. Obstructive sleep apnea in family members, *New Engl. J. Med.* (1978) **299**, 969–973.

270. Strumpf, I.J., Reynolds, S.F., Vash, P. & Tashkin, D.P. A possible relationship between testosterone, central control of ventilation, and the Pickwickian syndrome, *Am. Rev. Resp. Dis.* (1978) **117**, 183.

271. Sullivan, C.E. Bilateral carotid body resection in asthma: vulnerability to hypoxic death in sleep, *Chest* (1980) **78**, 354.

272. Sullivan, C.E., Berthon-Jones, M. & Issa, F.G. Nocturnal nasal-airway pressure for sleep apnoea, *New Engl. J. Med.* (1983) **309**, 112.

273. Sullivan, C.E. & Issa, F.G. Pathophysiological mechanisms in obstructive sleep apnoea, *Sleep* (1980) **3**, 235–246.

274. Sullivan, C.E., Issa, F.G., Berthon-Jones, M. & Eves, L. Reversal of obstructive sleep apnoea by continuous positive airway pressure applied through the nares, *Lancet* (1981) **1**, 862–865.
275. Sutton, J.R., Houston, C.S., Mansell, A.L., McFadden, M.D., Hackett, P.M., Rigg, J.R. & Powles, A.C. Effect of acetazolamide on hypoxaemia during sleep at high altitude, *New Engl. J. Med.* (1979) **301**, 1329–1331.
276. Sutton, F.D., Zwillich, C.W., Creagh, C.E., Pierson, D.J. & Weil, J.V. Progesterone for outpatient treatment of Pickwickian syndrome, *Ann. Int. Med.* (1975) **83**, 476–479.
277. Synderman, N.L., Johnson, J.T., Moller, M. & Thearle, P.B. Brain-stem evoked potentials in adult sleep apnea, *Ann. Otol. Rhinol. Laryngol.* (1982) **91**, 597–598.
278. Taasan, V.C., Block, A.J., Boysen, P.G. & Wynne, J.W. Alcohol increases sleep apnoea and oxygen desaturation in asymptomatic men, *Am. J. Med.* (1981) **71**, 240–245.
279. Teshima, Y., Sugita, Y., Iijima, S., Wakamatsu, H. & Hishikawa, Y. A study on the nature of hypersomnia in myxoedema, *Sleep Res.* (1979) **8**, 247.
280. Teszner, D. & Foucher, A. Correlations entre les variations de la vigilance, l'activité EEG, la respiration et les clonies dans 1 cas de maladie de Creutzfeldt–Jakob, *Rev. EEG Neurophysiol.* (1978) **8**, 354–360.
281. Thomas, D.J., du Boulay, G.H., Marshall, J., Pearson, T.C., Ross Russell, R.W., Symon, L., Wetherley-Mein, G. & Zilkha, E. Cerebral blood flow in polycythaemia, *Lancet* (1977) **2**, 161–163.
282. Tolle, F.A., Judy, W.V. & Wait, C.B. Reduction in cardiac output during obstructive sleep apnoea, *Chest* (1980) **78**, 543.
283. Turino, G.M. & Goldring, R.M. Sleeping and breathing, *New Engl. J. Med.* (1978) **299**, 1009–1011.
284. Tusiewicz, K., Moldofsky, H., Bryan, A.C. & Bryan, M.H. Mechanics of the rib cage and diaphragm during sleep, *J. Appl. Physiol.* (1977) **43**, 600–611.
285. Valero, A. & Alroy, G. Hypoventilation in acquired micrognathia, *Arch. Int. Med.* (1965) **115**, 307–310.
286. Vella, L.M. Hewitt, P.B., Jones, R.M. & Adams, A.P. Sleep apnoea following cervical cord surgery, *Anaesthesia* (1984) **39**, 108–112.
287. Venus, B., Jacobs, H.K. & Lim, L. Treatment of the adult respiratory distress syndrome with continuous positive airway pressure, *Chest* (1979) **76**, 257–261.
288. Vesselinova-Jenkins, C.K. Model of persistent foetal circulation and sudden infant death syndrome (SIDS), *Lancet* (1980) **2**, 831–834.
289. Wagner, D.R., Pollak, C.P. & Weitzman, E.D. Nocturnal nasal-airway pressure for sleep apnea, *New Engl. J. Med.* (1983) **308**, 461–462.
290. Wallace, J. Obstructive sleep apnoea syndrome, *Brit. Med. J.* (1982) **285**, 736.
291. Walsh, J.T. & Montplaisir, J. Familial glaucoma with sleep apnoea: a new syndrome? *Thorax* (1982) **37**, 845–849.
292. Waud, R.A. Production of artificial respiration by rhythmic stimulation of the phrenic nerves, *Nature* (1937) **140**, 849.
293. Webb, P. Periodic breathing during sleep, *J. Appl. Physiol.* (1974) **37**, 899–903.
294. Webb, P. & Heistand, M. Sleep metabolism and age, *J. Appl. Physiol.* (1975) **38**, 257–262.
295. Weil, J.V., Kryger, M.H. & Scoggin, C.H. Sleep and breathing at high altitude. In: Guilleminault, C. & Dement, W.C. (eds.) *Sleep Apnea Syndromes*, New York: Alan R. Liss (1978) 119–136.
296. Weiner, D., Mitra, J., Salamone, J., Nochomovitz, M. & Cherniack, N.S. Effect of chemical drive on the electrical activity and force of contraction of the tongue and chest wall muscles, *Am. Rev. Resp. Dis.* (1980) **121**, Suppl., 418.
297. Weitzman, E.D. Sleep and its disorders, *Ann. Rev. Neurosci.* (1981) **4**, 381–417.
298. Weitzman, E.D., Kahn, E. & Pollak, C.P. A quantitative analysis of sleep and sleep apnea before and after tracheostomy in patients with the hypersomnic sleep apnea syndrome, *Sleep* (1980) **3**, 407–423.
299. Weitzman, E.D., Pollak, C.P., Borowiecki, B., Burack, B., Shprintzen, R. & Rafoff, S. The hypersomnia–sleep apnoea syndrome: site and mechanism of upper airway obstruction. In: Guilleminault, C. & Dement, W.C. (eds.) *Sleep Apnea Syndromes*. New York: Alan R. Liss (1978) 235–248.
300. White, D.P., Miller, F. & Erickson, R.W. Sleep apnea and nocturnal hypoventilation after Western equine encephalitis, *Am. Rev. Resp. Dis.* (1983) **127**, 132–133.
301. White, D.P., Zwillich, C.W., Pickett, C.K., Douglas, N.J, Findley, L.J. & Weil, J.V. Central sleep apnea. Improvement with acetazolamide therapy, *Arch. Int. Med.* (1982) **142**, 1816–1819.

302. Williams, A., Hanson, D. & Calne, D.B. Vocal cord paralysis in the Shy–Drager syndrome, *J. Neurol. Neurosurg. Psychiat.* (1979) **42**, 151–153.
303. Wyler, A.R. & Weymuller, E.A., Jr. Epilepsy complicated by sleep apnoea, *Ann. Neurol.* (1981) **9**, 403–404.
304. Zhu Songshan. Successful treatment of sleep apnoea syndrome by transfusion of 'vital energy', *Chin. Med. J.* (1980) **93**, 279–280.
305. Zwillich, C.W., Devlin, T., White, D., Douglas, N., Weil, J. & Martin, R. Bradycardia during sleep apnea: characteristics and mechanism, *J. Clin. Invest.* (1982) **69**, 1286–1292.
306. Zwillich, C., McCullough, R., Guilleminault, C., Cummiskey, J. & Weil, J. Respiratory control in the parents of sudden infant death syndrome victims, *Ped. Res. J.* (1980) **14**, 762–764.
307. Zwillich, C.W., Natalino, M.R. & Weil, J.V. The influence of a progestational agent on the control of breathing in man, *Clin. Res.* (1975) **23**, 353A.
308. Zwillich, C., Pickett, C., Hanson, F. & Weil, J. Disturbed sleep and prolonged apnoea in normal man during nasal obstruction, *Am. Rev. Resp. Dis.* (1981) **123**, Suppl., 493.

SLEEP AND ASTHMA

309. Anonymous editorial, Asthma at night, *Lancet* (1983) **1**, 220–222.
310. Barnes, P., Fitzgerald, G., Brown, M. & Dollery, C. Nocturnal asthma and changes in circulating epinephrine, histamine, and cortisol, *New Engl. J. Med.* (1980) **303**, 263–267.
311. Clark, T.J.H. & Hetzel, M.R. Diurnal variation of asthma, *Brit. J. Dis. Chest.* (1977) **71**, 87–92.
312. Cochrane, G.M. & Clark, T.J.H. A survey of asthma mortality in patients between ages 35 and 64 in the Greater London hospitals in 1971, *Thorax* (1975) **30**, 300–305.
313. Drazen, J. Histamine and nocturnal wheezing, *New Engl. J. Med.* (1980) **313**, 278–279.
314. Floyer, J. *A Treatise of the Asthma*, London: Wilkin (1698).
315. Goodall, R.J.R., Earis, J.E., Cooper, D.N., Bernstein, A. & Temple, J.G. Relationship between asthma and gastro-oesophageal reflux, *Thorax* (1981) **36**, 116–121.
316. Hetzel, M.R. & Clark, T.J.H. Does sleep cause nocturnal asthma? *Thorax* (1979) **34**, 749–754.
317. Kales, A., Beall, G.N., Bajor, G.F., Jacobson, A. & Kales, J.D. Sleep studies in asthmatic adults: relationship of attacks to sleep stage and time of night, *J. Allergy Clin. Immunol.* (1968) **41**, 164–173.
318. Kales, A., Kales, J.D., Sly, R.M. Scharf, M.B., Tjiauw-Ling Tan & Preston, T.A. Sleep patterns of asthmatic children: all-night electroencephalographic studies, *J. Allergy Clin. Immunol.* (1970) **46**, 300–308.
319. McFadden, E.R. & Lyons, H.A. Arterial blood gas tension in asthma, *New Engl. J. Med.* (1968) **278**, 1027–1032.
320. Montplaisir, J., Walsh, J. & Malo, J.L. Nocturnal asthma: features of attacks, sleep and breathing patterns, *Am. Rev. Resp. Dis.* (1982) **125**, 18–22.
321. Newman-Taylor, A.J., Davies, R.J., Hendrick, D.J. & Pepys, J. Recurrent nocturnal asthmatic reactions to bronchial provocation tests, *Clin. Allergy* (1979) **9**, 213–219.
322. Poppius, H. & Stenius, B. Changes in arterial oxygen saturation in patients with hyperreactive airways during a histamine inhalation test, *Scand. J. Resp. Dis.* (1977) **58**, 1–4.
323. Randsell, J.W. & Georghiou, P.F. Prolonged methacholine-induced broncho-constriction in dogs, *J. Appl. Physiol.* (1979) **47**, 418–424.
324. Reinberg, A. & Gervais, P. Circadian rhythms in respiratory functions, with special reference to human chronophysiology and chronopharmacology, *Bull. Physiopathol. Resp. (Nancy)* (1972) **8**, 663–675.
325. Smith, T.F. & Hudgel, D. Arterial oxygen saturation during sleep in children with bronchial asthma (abstract), *J. Allergy Clin. Immunol.* (1979) **63**, 155.
326. Turner-Warwick, M. On observing patterns of airflow obstruction in chronic asthma, *Brit. J. Dis. Chest.* (1977) **71**, 73–86.
327. Williams, R.L. Sleep disturbances in various medical and surgical conditions. In: Williams, R.L. & Karacan, I. (eds.) *Sleep Disorders: Diagnosis and Treatment.* New York: Wiley (1978) 285–301.

SLEEP AND CHRONIC LUNG DISEASE

328. Bone, R.C., Pierce, A.K. & Johnson, R.L. Controlled oxygen administration in acute respiratory failure in chronic obstructive pulmonary disease, *Am. J. Med.* (1978) **65**, 896–902.
329. Boyson, P.G., Block, A.J., Wynne, J.W., Hunt, L.A. & Flick, M.R. Nocturnal pulmonary hypertension in patients with chronic obstructive pulmonary disease, *Chest* (1979) **76**, 536–542.
330. Coccagna, G. & Lugaresi, E. Arterial blood gases and pulmonary and systemic arterial blood pressure during sleep in chronic obstructive pulmonary disease, *Sleep* (1979) **1**, 117–124.
331. Fleetham, J.A. & Kryger, M.H. Sleep disorders in chronic airflow obstruction, *Med. Clin. North. Am.* (1981) **65**, 549–561.
332. Fleetham, J.A., Mezon, B., West, P., Bradley, C.A., Anthonisen, N.R. & Kryger, M.H. Chemical control of ventilation and sleep arterial oxygen desaturation in patients with COPD, *Am. Rev. Resp. Dis.* (1980) **122**, 583–589.
333. Guilleminault, C., Cummiskey, J. & Dement, W.C. Sleep apnoea syndrome: recent advances, *Adv. Int. Med.* (1980) **26**, 347–372.
334. Guilleminault, C., Cummiskey, J. & Motta, J. Chronic obstructive airflow disease and sleep studies, *Am. Rev. Resp. Dis.* (1980) **122**, 397–406.
335. Hudgel, D.W. & Shucard, D.W. Co-existence of sleep apnoea and asthma resulting in severe sleep hypoxemia, *J. Am. Med. Assoc.* (1979) **242**, 2789–2790.
336. Kearley, R., Wynne, J.W., Block, A.J., Boysen, P.G., Lindsey, S. & Martin, C. The effect of low flow oxygen on sleep-disordered breathing and oxygen desaturation, *Chest* (1980) **78**, 682–685.
337. Muller, N.L., Francis, P.W., Gurwitz, D., Levison, H. & Bryan, A.C. Mechanism of haemoglobin desaturation during rapid-eye-movement sleep in normal subjects and in patients with cystic fibrosis, *Am. Rev. Resp. Dis.* (1980) **121**, 463–469.
338. Scharf, M.B., Lobel, J.S., Caldwell, E., Cameron, B.F., Kramer, M., de Marchis, J. & Paine, C. Nocturnal oxygen desaturation in patients with sickle cell anaemia, *J. Am. Med. Assoc.* (1983) **249**, 1753–1755.
339. Tirlapur, V.G. & Mir, M.A. Nocturnal hypoxemia and associated electrocardiographic changes in patients with chronic obstructive airways disease, *New Engl. J. Med.* (1982) **306**, 125–130.
340. Wynne, J.W., Block, A.J., Hemenway, J., Hunt, L.A. & Flick, M.R. Disordered breathing and oxygen desaturation during sleep in patients with chronic obstructive lung disease (COPD), *Am. J. Med.* (1979) **66**, 573–579.

PART III

PHARMACOLOGY AND SLEEP

CHAPTER 8

SLEEP NEURO-CHEMISTRY

ACTIVITY OF BRAIN NEUROTRANSMITTER SYSTEMS IN THE CONTROL OF SLEEP AND WAKEFULNESS

Is there a sleep neurotransmitter? The very idea may be false. Before the discovery of REM sleep, the 'wet' physiologists looked for a 'hypnotoxin' or 'sleep juice', associated with the sleep–wake cycle, whilst the 'dry' school explained sleep as a passive state due to inactivity of the reticular formation.[21] These ideas were shown to be superficial by the discovery of REM sleep, the demonstration of the heterogeneity of sleep mechanisms, and the impossibility of explaining sleep–wake behaviour in terms of changes in only two or three brain amines. Very strong cases have been made out for the involvement of *serotonin (5-HT), noradrenaline (norepinephrine), dopamine* and *acetylcholine* in the control of sleeping and waking (reviewed in detail by Jouvet[21] and Gillin *et al.*[13]), but there are many inconsistencies in the results. Many of the data concern cats, not men. Drucker-Colin, writing in 1976, observed that there was no solid demonstration of the important regulation of the sleep–wake cycle by any known neurotransmitter.[6] This is still true today.

5-HT has possessed a great attraction to sleep researchers, but the 5-HT precursor 5-hydroxytryptophan (5-HTP) is not a useful hypnotic in man, despite a role in the regulation of PGO waves in the cat. The *catecholamines* noradrenaline and dopamine have been widely considered to play an essential role in the regulation of sleeping and waking, but neither the noradrenaline precursor dihydroxyphenylserine (DOPS) nor the dopamine precursor dihydroxyphenylalanine (DOPA) greatly alters wakefulness, sleep or REM sleep in man. The importance of *GABA* mechanisms, and the localization of GABA systems concerned in the physiological control of the sleep–wake cycle remains obscure, despite the attribution of the hypnotic effects of benzodiazepines to GABA–chloride channel–benzodiazepine receptor activation. *Anticholinergic* drugs appear to have greater effects on sleep atonia than on sleep–wakefulness itself. Because of all these problems, the 'wet' physiologists have turned to a search for intrinsic or even extrinsic *sleep peptides*, some derived from gut bacteria. However, despite the demonstration of the presence of vasoactive intestinal peptide (VIP) in the suprachiasmatic nucleus, and the assumption that this peptide may be involved in the control of circadian rhythmicity,[7] no known peptide has any proven role in the control of sleeping and waking.

From the monumental survey of Jouvet,[21] the literature on the neurochemistry of sleep is vast. Here we will review briefly the main evidence for the activity of brain monoamine and peptide systems in the regulation of sleep and wakefulness in man. Unfortunately many of the data are conflicting, unsubstantial, uncontrolled or unrepeated, and the number of reliable clues to the neurochemical basis of sleep in man are indeed few. Discussion therefore will be limited to the most important findings and recent developments in the neurochemistry of sleep.

CATECHOLAMINES

NORADRENALINE, SLEEP AND WAKEFULNESS

Cell bodies containing noradrenaline are mostly situated in the brain stem reticular areas,[30] distributed in several nuclei from the medulla to the upper pons. The largest of these nuclei is the locus coeruleus in the pons, which gives rise to an extremely diffuse major ascending projection to the neocortex, thalamus, dorsal hypothalamus and limbic system. The locus coeruleus also innervates the cerebellum, and three separate descending spinal noradrenergic pathways have been identified, in the lateral sympathetic columns and in the dorsal and ventral horns. The remaining noradrenaline neurones in the brain stem are dispersed in several small nuclei in the medulla and pons, with axons which terminate mainly in the hypothalamus and hippocampus. Axons from locus coeruleus neurones possess frequent bifurcations with recurrent collaterals which make contact with the dendrites of brain stem multipolar cells, thus forming an anatomical substrate for collateral inhibition. Thus, when one noradrenaline cell is activated, these collaterals inhibit several neighbouring noradrenaline cells. There is good evidence that these brain stem noradrenaline systems are involved in the control of respiration, blood pressure, other autonomic functions and the maintenance of alertness.

Dopamine neurones are less involved than noradrenaline neurones in sleep–wake mechanisms, and lesions of the major dopamine systems cause only minor alterations in sleep. Dopamine-containing neurones are mainly situated in a few nuclei of the mesodiencephalon, and innervate the neostriatum, n. accumbens and mesolimbic forebrain areas, the frontal cortex and the infundibulum.

The noradrenaline systems of the brain stem show a marked heterogeneity. There is some evidence that these systems are actively involved in the maintenance of wakefulness. (1) Some noradrenaline neurones of the locus coeruleus are active in wakefulness but stop firing in sleep. (2) Kafi et al.[23] have shown that drugs which mimic the action of noradrenaline increase wakefulness in a dose-dependent manner. However, in addition to noradrenaline agonist effects, many of these drugs are also dopamine agonists, or possess mixed agonist–antagonist actions. (3) In contrast to the action of noradrenaline agonists, drugs which decrease the synthesis of noradrenaline, such as the tyrosine hydroxylase inhibitor α-methylparatyrosine (αMPT) and the neuroleptics, reduce wakefulness and in big doses may cause sleep.

Other evidence implicates noradrenaline systems in the control of REM sleep as well as in the maintenance of wakefulness, although here the data are somewhat conflicting. One view suggests that noradrenaline systems are unnecessary for REM sleep, or may even inhibit this, whilst other evidence suggests that the activity of noradrenaline cells is necessary for REM sleep to appear.[10, 34] Two of the best-known theories of how monoamines modify REM sleep are those of Jouvet[21] and Hobson et al.[20]

Jouvet considered that cortical stimulation, mediated by ascending noradrenergic fibre systems, was important for arousal, whilst adrenergic activity in locus coeruleus neurones was related to both the tonic (desynchronization of the EEG, postural atonia, brain temperature elevation) and phasic (PGO waves, REMs, limb twitching, cardiorespiratory abnormalities) aspects of REM sleep. Hobson et al.[20] attempted to explain the cycle of wakefulness, NREM sleep and REM sleep in terms of fluctuations in activity of interconnected brain stem noradrenaline and acetylcholine systems. According to these views, during wakefulness, aminergic inhibition of cholinoceptive neurones of the reticular formation resulted in a low level of resting activity in cholinoceptive neurones in the gigantocellular tegmental field. Then, with the onset of NREM sleep, aminergic inhibition was replaced by excitation, REM periods occurring at the lowest point of inhibition and being accompanied by selective and specific firing of brain stem cholinoceptive neurones.

All the electrophysiological data do not support these ideas, although cholinergic agonists or aminergic antagonists injected into the pontine brain stem can transfer animals from wakefulness into REM sleep. In many areas of the nervous system, the usual pattern of activity in single neurones is similar during wakefulness and during REM sleep, with higher or lower firing rates during NREM sleep. Within brain stem nuclei, there are marked differences in the integrated activity and firing rates of different populations of neurones.[4, 28, 41] Practically any firing pattern can be found. In some dorsal raphe and locus coeruleus neurones, there is a progressive decrease in firing rate from wakefulness to slow-wave to REM sleep. Changes in the activity of single neurones, with the transition from wakefulness to sleep, are sometimes clearly related to reduction in motor activity, not sleep onset itself.[38]

If the animal electrophysiological and pharmacological data are pertinent to man, noradrenergic agonists should increase wakefulness and phenothiazines should promote sleep. This is largely true (Table 8.1). Overall, an increase in sympathetic tone, whatever the cause, is accompanied by a more aroused state. However, the reverse is not always true, and the hypnotic effects of catecholamine antagonists are minor as compared with the benzodiazepines and opiates.

Table 8.1. *Effects on sleep of catecholamines and drugs modifying noradrenaline and dopamine neurotransmission*

Mechanism	Drug	Effect on REM sleep
Synthesis	DOPA	Increase, decrease, no change
	Alpha-methylparatyrosine (αMPT)	Low dose – increase
		High dose – decrease
	DOPS	50–150 mg i.v. no change
Storage	Reserpine	Low dose – increase
Release	Amphetamine	Decrease
Receptor	Dopamine agonists (e.g. ergot alkaloids)	Decrease (also decrease NREM, but bromocriptine causes increase)
	Dopamine antagonists (e.g. phenothiazines)	Low dose – increase
		High dose – decrease
	Noradrenaline antagonists	
	α-blockers (e.g. thymoxamine)	Increase
	ß-blockers (e.g. propranolol)	No change
Inactivation of uptake	Tricyclic drugs	Decrease
Metabolic effect	MAO A and B inhibitors (e.g. phenelzine, deprenyl)	Decrease
	COMT inhibitors (e.g. progesterone)	? Decrease
Postreceptor	Phosphodiesterase inhibitors	Decrease
	Caffeine	
	Theophylline	
	Aminophylline	

DOPA = dihydroxyphenyl alanine, DOPS = dihydroxyphenyl serine,
MAO = mono amine oxidase, COMT = catechol-*O*-methyl transferase.

Many sympathomimetic drugs, e.g. amphetamine, ephedrine and clonidine (which acts as a selective noradrenaline agonist at both pre- and post-synaptic $α_2$ adrenoceptors) increase wakefulness and prevent sleep. In addition, these drugs suppress REM sleep.[1, 13, 16, 18, 29, 35] Tolerance to both the sleep-preventing and REM-suppressant effect develops gradually. In hyperkinetic children on long-term amphetamine treatment, sleep patterns are usually normal after 4–12 weeks.[42] In addition to initial REM suppression, amphetamine and clonidine both abolish REM rebound after REM sleep deprivation.

Clonidine is known to inhibit the firing of noradrenaline neurones in the brain, probably by stimulating $α_2$ adrenoceptors on the cell body. Clonidine decreases presynaptic noradrenaline turnover and release; it also causes a dose-dependent reduction in REM sleep. Svensson *et al.*[39] related REM sleep suppression with clonidine to a reduction in the firing rate of locus coeruleus neurones, and to a decrease in brain noradrenaline release, but it is difficult to determine to what extent REM sleep suppression with clonidine is due to either pre- or post-synaptic mechanisms.[11]

In contrast to clonidine, *piperoxan* is an antagonist of $α_2$ adrenoreceptors. Low doses of this drug depress REM sleep, whilst in high doses (1–20 mg/kg) a dose-dependent facilitation of REM sleep is observed.[12] This dual effect is presumably due to separate pre- and post-synaptic effects on endogenous noradrenaline mechanisms. Inhibition of catecholamine synthesis with αMPT prevents the effects of both low and high doses of piperoxan.

Tricyclic drugs, including imipramine and desipramine, all suppress REM sleep. These drugs increase the availability of noradrenaline at the synaptic level by inhibition of noradrenaline re-uptake, and changes in post-synaptic noradrenaline receptor activation may be involved in REM sleep maintenance. However, Justafre and Gaillard[22] emphasized the complexities of the situation. The activity of many locus coeruleus cells is controlled by α-adreno-ceptor-mediated feedback inhibition,[40] and activation of individual adrenergic systems sometimes results in a decrease, not an increase, in locus coeruleus neuronal firing rates.[33]

Catecholamine antagonists such as haloperidol and pimozide have mainly opposite effects on sleep to those of sympathomimetic drugs. These neuroleptics, and also reserpine and αMPT, cause drowsiness and an increase in REM sleep, although the results are a little variable. *Reserpine* in low doses blocks the synthesis of all brain amines, and causes drowsiness and an increase in REM sleep with both acute and chronic administration.[5, 19] *Chlorpromazine* and *pimozide* have surprisingly little effect on wakefulness in doses which have major neuroleptic effects, although low doses of chlorpromazine (under 1 mg/kg) enhance REM sleep, and high doses suppress REM sleep. Like chlorpromazine, αMPT in low doses causes REM enhancement, and in high doses suppression of REM sleep.[23] (High dosages of αMPT are needed in animals to clearly depress endogenous brain catecholamine formation.) All these drugs interfere with dopamine as well as noradrenaline in the brain; however, Oswald *et al.*[34] reported that the α-adrenoceptor antagonist thymoxamine, which has little or no effect on dopamine systems, induces REM sleep, whilst ß-receptor blockage (e.g. propranolol 120 mg/day) has little or no effect. These findings suggest that the primary effect of neuroleptic drugs on REM sleep is due to noradrenaline, not dopamine, receptor blockade.

There have been only a few studies of sleep–wake changes in the composition of the cerebrospinal fluid in man, and it is difficult to relate the relevance of any reported changes in the concentration of catecholamine metabolites in lumbar or ventricular fluid to changes in activity within small areas of brain stem nuclei (see also p. 149). Wyatt *et al.*[43] reported that the noradrenaline metabolite 3-methoxy-4-hydroxyphenylglycol, and the dopamine metabolite homovanillic acid, were present in higher concentrations in the ventricular fluid of demented patients during REM sleep than during NREM sleep. What this represents in synaptic terms is, however, not clear.

Diseases of the noradrenaline and dopamine systems of the brain stem in man cause surprisingly little disruption of the sleep–wake cycle, and neither the putative noradrenaline precursor l-DOPS nor the dopamine precursor DOPA have major effects on sleep or wakefulness in man. The best studied of these conditions has been Parkinson's disease.

In *idiopathic Parkinson's disease*, dopamine levels in the caudate, putamen and substantia nigra are at most a tenth of normal, and noradrenaline levels in brain stem nuclei, diencephalon and limbic structures are also conspicuously reduced. Poor sleep is a feature of Parkinson's disease, although at least in the early illness there is little or no disturbance of arousal mechanisms. It seems likely that loss of noradrenaline rather than dopamine in brain stem nuclei is responsible for some of the sleep difficulties described, but this question will not be solved until sleep in parkinsonism due to 1-methyl-4-phenyl-1, 2, 3, 6-tetrahydropyridine (MPTP) toxicity (which damages the substantia nigra, but spares the locus coeruleus[3]) has been studied in detail.

Sleep disruption in parkinsonism takes six main forms: frequent arousal, altered dreams, nocturnal vocalization, involuntary myoclonic movements, somnambulism despite akinesia, and excessive daytime sleepiness.[32] These problems are due, at least in part, to stiffness and immobility, as well as to anticholinergic or dopaminergic drugs, and are seen in patients with unilateral as well as with bilateral parkinsonism.[31] The most frequent complaint is one of insomnia. Polygraphic studies confirm there is a decrease in total sleep time, a delay in sleep induction, with many awakenings, and a decrease in both stage 4 NREM and REM sleep. Sleep spindles are unusually rare. Some patients have disruption of the whole circadian sleep–wake cycle, with sleep distributed throughout the entire 24 h rather than consolidated at night, although this is uncommon. Parkinsonian patients with myoclonic jerking during the day due to levodopa invariably have similar jerking at night.[25]

Levodopa, and to a lesser extent amantadine, reverse some of the sleep disturbances of Parkinson's disease, with an increase in total sleep duration and occasionally an increase in stage 4 of NREM sleep. However, the effect of levodopa on REM sleep in Parkinson's disease is variable. A further suppression rather than increase may occur, and this can progress to total sleep suppression as dosage is increased.[2, 8, 14, 17, 24, 44] In some instances, insomnia with levodopa results from sickness due to the drug,[26] whilst improved sleep may depend on increased mobility and wellbeing. However, there is little doubt that levodopa has a fundamental if slight effect on sleep as well as on motor function in Parkinson's disease, with the return of sleep spindles that are obvious to the naked eye accompanying treatment.[36] Levodopa causes a 1–2% increase in brain noradrenaline levels as well as increase in dopamine levels, and sleep changes caused by the drug may result from the increase in noradrenaline, not dopamine.

The putative noradrenaline precursor DOPS 50–100 mg i.v., given with a decarboxylase inhibitor, has no effect on the sleep of normal humans, but high doses of DOPS will reduce sleep in animals.[15, 27] There is controversy as to what extent DOPS is converted to noradrenaline in the human brain.

ACETYLCHOLINE

ACETYLCHOLINE AND SLEEP

Acetylcholine is synthesized from dietary choline and acetyl coenzyme A. The neurotransmitter content of the brain can be altered by changing the plasma composition,[66] and brain acetylcholine levels are increased by eating a choline- or lecithin-rich diet, at least in rats.[45] However, diets rich in choline or lecithin, cholinergic, anticholinergic or anticholinesterase drugs do not greatly affect sleep, the sleep–wake cycle or wakefulness in man.

The main cell bodies of acetylcholine neurones in the brain originate in the brain stem from the nucleus basalis of Meynart and the diagonal band of Broca. Shute and Lewis[61] identified two general pathways of cholinergic tracts, a dorsal tegmental pathway innervating in particular the non-specific nuclei and nucleus reticularis of the thalamus, and a ventral tegmental pathway ascending to the lateral nuclei of the hypothalamus, the striatum, septal nuclei and hippocampus.

ACETYLCHOLINE AND WAKEFULNESS

Centrally acting cholinergic and anticholinergic drugs have minor effects on wakefulness. Hyoscine (scopolamine), benztropine, biperiden and procyclidine sometimes cause drowsiness, whilst orphenadrine may produce increased wakefulness and euphoria, not sedation. These sedative or alerting effects with different anticholinergic drugs are partially dose-dependent. Anticholinergic drug toxicity results in a phase of excitement before eventual coma. Cholinergic and anticholinergic drugs that do not enter the brain (e.g. neostigmine and methscopolamine) have no effect on any aspect of sleep.[60]

Choline, lecithin, anticholinergic and cholinergic drugs have limited effects on memory as well as on wakefulness. These two effects may be linked. In some strains of mice with high learning ability, Mandel et al.[54] demonstrated genetically controlled high levels of acetylcholinesterase and choline acetylase. Detailed studies of sleep and wakefulness in these animals were not reported. In man, hyoscine may reduce awareness and impair the transition from short-term to long-term memory stores, and benzhexol (trihexyphenidyl) in a dose as low as 2 mg p.o. will impair the learning of a short story by old people.[46, 57] Hyoscine causes an immediate, not a delayed, impairment of memory before any subsequent alteration in REM sleep (see below) has occurred. In contrast, muscarinic and nicotinic cholinergic agonists, and anticholinesterases such as physostigmine, facilitate learning in animals, although the effects depend on the test used, the species involved and the type of agonist given.[49] It seems likely that memory impairment following hyoscine or any improvement with physostigmine is related to reduction or increase in wakefulness respectively, although amylobarbitone and amphetamine do not have quite the same effect on memory as anticholinergic and cholinergic drugs respectively.[47]

ACETYLCHOLINE AND REM SLEEP

Muscarinic and nicotinic cholinergic agonists and anticholinesterases increase REM sleep and alter REM sleep latency, but the results are slight and inconstant. Centrally acting anticholinesterases such as physostigmine usually increase REM sleep,[50, 63] and Stoyva and Metcalf[64] suggested that industrial workers who were exposed to organophosphorus compounds with anticholinesterase properties had unusually prolonged REM sleep periods. These findings may be relevant to the sleep disturbance, memory loss and reduction in brain acetylcholine and acetyltransferase levels in Alzheimer's disease,[58] but at present there is no evidence that either REM sleep lack or deficiency of acetylcholine is directly associated with mental impairment in Alzheimer's disease or any other form of dementia.

Although cholinergic and anticholinergic drugs have only slight effects on wakefulness, REM sleep and the sleep–wake cycle, sleep atonia and the atonia of cataplexy are altered by these drugs, and cholinergic systems play an essential role in the maintenance of both tonic and phasic components of REM sleep.

ACETYLCHOLINE AND SLEEP ATONIA

Pompeiano[56] produced a state of tonic depression of extensor and flexor spinal reflexes in the cat, similar to that seen during REM sleep, by intravenous infusion of physostigmine in precollicular decerebrate animals. When small amounts of carbachol are directly injected into the pons of intact animals, a profound atonia, similar to that of REM sleep, develops.[62] Cataplexy, like sleep atonia, is increased by physostigmine and also by arecoline (an acetylcholine-related compound from betel nuts), at least in dogs and ponies, and improved by cholinergic blockade using atropine or hyoscine (scopolamine).[48, 51] Despite this evidence for the involvement of acetylcholine systems in sleep atonia, the role of noradrenaline neurones in the locus coeruleus may be as or more important.

ACETYLCHOLINE AND PGO WAVES

As well as causing atonia, minute injections of carbachol into the dorsal pontine tegmentum will trigger PGO spikes in animals.[55] Physostigmine will facilitate, and atropine will suppress, PGO spikes produced by a number of other manoeuvres. These include reserpinization,[65] REM sleep deprivation[52, 59] and collicular and pontine transection.[53]

SEROTONIN

SEROTONIN AND SLEEP

Serotonin (5-hydroxytryptamine, 5-HT) is derived from the dietary amino acid L-tryptophan, which is hydroxylated to 5-hydroxytryptophan (5-HTP) by the enzyme tryptophan hydroxylase. 5-HTP is decarboxylated by L-aromatic acid decarboxylase to 5-HT. Breakdown of 5-HT results in the formation of the acidic metabolite, 5-hydroxyindoleacetic acid (5-HIAA), present in the CSF and the urine. CSF 5-HIAA determination from samples obtained at lumbar puncture gives little or no index of turnover of 5-HT in the brain; values mainly reflect spinal serotonin metabolism.

L-Tryptophan is present in normal diets in amounts of about 0.5–2 g/day. Eating high-tryptophan diets has little effect in raising brain 5-HT levels, since tryptophan hydroxylase is easily saturated, although 5-HTP, particularly if combined with a peripheral decarboxylase inhibitor (benserazide or carbidopa), will increase 5-HT levels in the brain. L-Tryptophan is actively taken up into 5-HT neurones by means of a neutral amino acid carrier mechanism. Changes in brain 5-HT level can occur rapidly, within hours of a meal. Infants fed tryptophan enter both active and quiet sleep sooner than infants on a normal diet.[98]

Dahlstrom and Fuxe[72] and more recently Poitras and Parent[87] have delineated a widespread distribution of serotonin throughout the brain stem. Nerve cell bodies in the median raphe nuclei of the rostral pons give rise to ascending fibres which innervate the basal ganglia, hypothalamus, thalamus, hippocampus, limbic forebrain and areas of the cortex, whilst 5-HT cell bodies in the medulla oblongata give rise to descending bulbospinal serotoninergic axons which terminate in the lower medulla and the spinal cord. Midline brain stem raphe nuclei contain a very high concentration of serotonin, but other neurotransmitters are present here as well.

There are striking circadian changes in brain 5-HT concentration. Levels are 1–2 times higher sleeping than waking in brain stem nuclei, and 20 times higher in the CSF in primates[90] (see p. 149). The concentration of the 5-HT metabolite 5-HIAA in ventricular fluid is higher during slow-wave sleep in man than during wakefulness.[97]

L-TRYPTOPHAN AND SLEEP

The makers of L-tryptophan-containing medicines warn that these may cause drowsiness. The evidence for this is inconclusive. In children with phenylketonuria, the concentration of 5-HT in blood and the central nervous system is low, but sleep is normal.[89] High plasma tryptophan concentrations occur in patients with carcinoid tumours, but these patients are not usually hypersomniac. There is some evidence that 5-HT is depleted in the central nervous system of depressed patients, and abnormal tryptophan metabolism may occur in patients who are pyridoxine deficient and in women taking oral contraceptives, although it is difficult to relate brain 5-HT concentration to any disturbance of sleeping or waking under these circumstances. However, both brain 5-HT levels and sleep may be reduced in thiamine deficiency.[71]

In man, L-tryptophan has only a limited and uncertain action on sleep and is not a useful hypnotic. Nicholson and Stone[85] compared the effects of L-tryptophan 2, 4 and 6 g with placebo on night-time sleep in normal volunteers. In these dosages, L-tryptophan had little or no effect on sleep, although higher doses, comparable to those used in animal experiments, have not been investigated in man. In studies by Williams et al.[94] and Griffiths et al.[75] L-tryptophan was found to increase slightly both slow-wave sleep and REM sleep. Likewise, Wyatt et al.[95] found an increase in slow-wave sleep with tryptophan, but a decrease in REM sleep.

5-HYDROXYTRYPTOPHAN AND SLEEP

Reports of the action of 5-HTP on sleep are as conflicting as those of L-tryptophan (Table 8.2). Usually some effect is reported, but this may be either an increase in REM sleep[82, 86] or an increase in slow-wave sleep.[67, 100] In REM narcolepsy, 5-HTP does not alter total sleep time.[99]

Table 8.2.   *Effect of drugs which modify serotonin transmission on sleep in man*

Mechanism	Drug	Effect
Synthesis	L-Tryptophan	Dramatic abolition post-hypoxic myoclonus (in wakefulness)
		Variable effects on sleep
	5-Hydroxytryptophan	Restores sleep in PCPA-treated subjects and in some hyposomniacs with brain stem disease
	Parachlorphenyl-alanine (PCPA)	Inhibits sleep
Storage	Reserpine	Increase in total sleep time, REM sleep
Release	Amphetamine	Decrease in REM sleep
	Fenfluramine	
Receptor	LSD	Reduce REM latency, increase REM length
	Methysergide	Decrease REM sleep
		No change delta sleep
Inactivation of uptake	Tricyclic antidepressants	Decrease REM sleep

Drugs that alter the synthesis, storage and release of 5-HT in the brain have only slight effects on sleep in man. However, 5-HT synthesis inhibition using p-chlorphenylalanine (PCPA) usually reduces REM sleep in patients with carcinoid syndrome. Similar results have been obtained in patients with Huntington's chorea, cluster headache and generalized dystonia, and also in normal subjects.[96] 5-HTP (but not L-tryptophan) will restore REM sleep. As with 5-HT synthesis inhibition, 5-HT receptor blockade with methysergide decreases REM sleep in man but does not change delta sleep.[83]

Fischer-Perroudan et al.[74] reported that 5-HTP 2–12 g/24 h given to a totally insomniac patient with the clinical diagnosis of Morvan's fibrillary chorea (see p. 243) increased total sleep, restored slow-wave sleep and caused the appearance of some REM sleep. However, this response was rapidly lost. In another patient with only 4 h sleep per night following a traumatic brain stem lesion, Guilleminault et al.[76] found that 5-HTP caused an increase in total sleep time and in NREM sleep. (No control was used in either of these examples.)

Animal studies reviewed by Jouvet[78] and Morgane and Stern,[84] often involving very high doses of 5-HTP, give clearer evidence of the importance of 5-HT in sleep mechanisms than is seen in man. Destruction of the raphe system containing 80% of serotonergic neurone perikarya, the application of 5-HT to brain stem neurones and studies of 5-HT neuronal activity all suggest that brain stem 5-HT systems are involved in both slow-wave and REM sleep. Lesions of the dorsal and medial raphe nuclei which decrease 5-HT levels in the brain stem of cats cause an initial decrease in total sleep and particularly REM sleep. However, these sleep changes are rapidly reversed, and although 5-HT levels drop to 5–10% of normal after 3 weeks, sleep may have returned to normal at this time.

Direct application of 5-HT to the area postrema, which is outside the blood–brain barrier, increases synchronization of the EEG in paralysed cats,[68] whilst reserpine, which depletes 5-HT but also catecholamines, suppresses both REM and NREM sleep in cats.[78] Brooks and Gershon[69] showed that NREM sleep could be restored by 5-HTP. All these observations provide the basis for the serotonergic theory of sleep and imply that 5-HT acts as a hypnogenic transmitter. However, better knowledge of serotonergic neurones has revealed that some of these are actually most active, and 5-HT release is most abundant, not during sleep, but during wakefulness. Unit neuronal recording has discovered that the spontaneous firing rate of some dorsal raphe neurones decreases as the animal passes from wakefulness to slow-wave to REM sleep.[91] However, in most instances the firing rate of single raphe neurones is not strongly linked to the initiation or maintenance of NREM sleep.

The present evidence does not suggest a major role of serotonin in the initiation or maintenance of either NREM or REM sleep. The major importance of serotonin for sleep may be in the motor sphere, the regulation of PGO waves during REM sleep, and the maintenance of sleep atonia. Several years ago, Jouvet reported that cats with bilateral lesions of the pontine tegmentum had REM sleep without atonia.[79] In these cats the pattern of raphe nuclei discharge during paradoxical sleep may be reversed from normal, with very high firing rates during this sleep phase.[92] In normal animals, the usual decrease in dorsal raphe nuclei output during REM sleep may be related to the decreased motor output that characterizes this stage of sleep and to central motor inhibition.[77]

Evidence for a possible motor function of raphe 5-HT neurones was obtained by Dement et al.[73] in cats treated with PCPA. They found that the cat was not only insomniac, but that phasic PGO activity, formerly confined to the REM period, migrated first into NREM sleep and then into the waking state. Recently, Sallanon et al.[88] have shown that paradoxical sleep can be restored to PCPA-pretreated insomniac cats by cerebrospinal fluid transfer from normal cats.

Although 5-HTP is not a useful hypnotic, it does have a major effect on one possible sleep-associated disorder. At least 100 patients with post-hypoxic myoclonus and two patients with palatal myoclonus have been reported to respond to 5-HTP, which sometimes results in total abolition of muscle jerking during wakefulness.[70, 80, 81, 93] Some of these subjects have reduced or absent REM sleep. However, despite a search for selective damage to serotonin neurones in the dorsal raphe of the brain stem in post-hypoxic myoclonus, this has not been shown convincingly, and the effect of 5-HTP on sleep in these patients is unknown.

ENDOGENOUS SLEEP FACTORS

Legendre and Piéron[126] deprived dogs of sleep for many days. They found that cerebrospinal fluid from these sleep-deprived dogs, injected into the cisterna magna of normal dogs, made the recipients sleepy for 2–4 h following transfusion. Other investigators have found similar results. These experiments led to the idea of a *hypnotoxin*, an endogenous substance produced by the body during wakefulness, and promoting sleep when conditions allowed. In addition to sleep-promoting factors produced during wakefulness or by sleep deprivation, other investigators have searched for sleep-inducing factors produced during sleep itself. A number of these sleep-promoting substances, some of which are neuropeptides, have been identified in the cerebrospinal' fluid, blood or urine of animals and men. However, in no instance is there any clear evidence of a definite physiological role in sleep promotion, and it is puzzling that either wakefulness or sleep can result in the production of such a compound. As well as neuropeptides, a wide range of other substances have been considered for a hypnotoxic role, including many hormones and even prostaglandins: thus Ueno *et al.*[179] demonstrated that prostaglandin D_2 induced sleep when microinjected into the preoptic area of conscious cats.

The very idea of a physiological hypnotoxin in man has been questioned by the findings of Lenard and Schulte[127] and Webb[182] of independent sleep in Siamese twins with a common circulation (Fig. 8.1). Also dogs with two heads, one implanted artificially into the circulation, sleep at different times.[108] Experimental design in the search for a hypnotoxin is not beyond criticism. Naturally sleepy animals have been used, many curious species have been investigated, and sleep deprivation of both rabbits and slaughterhouse cattle has been produced by a 12 h truck drive to the biochemical laboratory. In the experiments of Legendre and Piéron, control CSF occasionally produced sleep, and sleep was very atypical, accompanied by raised intracranial pressure and hyperthermia. There is thus considerable scepticism about many of the endogenous 'sleep factors' which have been described.

Sleep factors in the blood, cerebrospinal fluid and brain have been proposed by the groups of Monnier, Pappenheimer and Uchizono. These findings have been extensively reviewed by Drucker-Colin[111] and Mendelson *et al.*[136], who describe the biochemical procedures and methodological details used. However, the search for a sleep peptide in the blood or cerebrospinal fluid has been disappointing as yet, perhaps because no such compound exists.

NEUROPEPTIDES

The effect of many different neuropeptides on sleep has been systematically investigated. The results are conflicting, although may be important in the circadian control of the sleep–wake cycle.[160] Riou *et al.*[156] reported that angiotensin II, arginine vasopressin, substance P, neurotensin, ß-endorphin, enkephalins and cholecystokinin octapeptide (CCK-8) had no effect on the sleep of rats. In contrast to these results, VIP (100 ng given by intracerebroventricular route) promoted the onset of sleep. REM sleep occurred when VIP was injected during the light period, and both NREM and REM sleep occurred when VIP was injected during the dark period. In addition to promoting natural sleep, VIP reversed the insomnia produced by 5-HT synthesis inhibition. Sleep induction by VIP and other neuropeptides depends on the species investigated, the dose given, the route of administration and the experimental method. Drowsiness or sleep has been reported following arginine vasotocin,[130, 142] CCK-8,[129, 159] ß-endorphin[121] and αMSH.[128] Sleep induction with αMSH was attributed to the effect of this peptide on hypothalamic and mesencephalic dopamine neurones. The tendency of sleep to shift to more delta sleep following intracerebroventricular injection in rats[123] must be considered in the evaluation of these results.

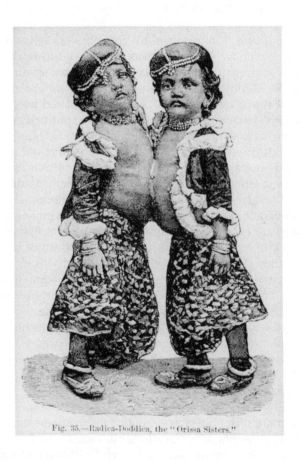

Fig. 35.—Radica-Doddica, the "Orissa Sisters."

Figure 8.1.   *Siamese twins may have a common circulation, but sleep at different times.*

REM SLEEP FACTORS

The search for endogenous REM sleep-promoting factors in Jouvet's laboratory has given most interesting results. CSF transfer experiments have shown that CSF from REM sleep-deprived cats restores REM sleep to donor cats made insomniac by PCPA. PCPA blocks 5-HT synthesis, and in cats reduces slow-wave and REM sleep. When spinal fluid from REM sleep-deprived cats was infused into PCPA-treated cats, REM sleep increased in all of 10 animals, although spinal fluid from normal, not REM sleep-deprived, cats occasionally had similar results. The effects of CSF transfer from totally sleep-deprived cats and the results of transfusion of CSF to normal, not PCPA-treated, cats were not described.[161]

DELTA SLEEP-INDUCING PEPTIDE

Between 1963 and 1965, Monnier and his collaborators isolated a nonapeptide from the brain of rabbits. This factor was produced during sleep, initiated by slow electrical stimulation of intralaminary thalamic nuclei. When the circulation of the stimulated rabbit was connected to a recipient rabbit, the second rabbit went to sleep.[137, 138] A factor was isolated by dialysis from the stimulated rabbit's blood which has since been purified, determined and synthesized, and is now commercially available.

Delta sleep-inducing peptide (DSIP) sometimes induces slow-wave sleep in rabbits, rats and mice and REM sleep in cats.[119, 153, 168] However, DSIP does not reliably induce sleep in all species or all studies,[120, 174] and the effect is independent of the dose, or the dose–response curve is bell-shaped. The effect of DSIP has proved difficult to evaluate in man. Sleep is inconstant and, when it does occur, the latency is surprisingly long, over 2 h.[111] Schlerschlicht et al.[164, 165] reported that DSIP had similar effects in man to those of benzodiazepines, inducing sedation and reversing drug-induced insomnia; Schneider-Helmert[167] reported that DSIP given i.v. to healthy human volunteers and insomniacs promoted sleep and had an anxiolytic effect in neurotic patients. However, any effect is very sensitive to the infusion rate.

The problem with DSIP as a sleep factor is the inconstancy of sleep production, and the terminology may be misleading as a specific effect on sleep has not been shown, although electrophysiological experiments have shown that DSIP inhibits thalamic neurones.[142] Schoenenberger and Monnier[168] showed that the amino acid sequence of DSIP was Trp–Ala–Gly–Gly–Asp–Ala–Ser–Gly–Glu; and radioimmunoassay methods for the determination of DSIP were developed by Kastin et al.[120] The highest content of DSIP in rat brain occurs in the thalamus. The peptide has not yet been isolated from the human brain although DSIP-like material is present in human blood and milk, and an artificial structural gene for DSIP has been synthesized and the respective bacteria have been cloned.

SLEEP-PROMOTING SUBSTANCE FROM THE BRAIN

Uchizono and his colleagues extracted by water dialysis a sleep promoting substance (SPS) from the brain stem of rats that had been sleep-deprived for 24 h by repeated electroshock. The initial factor sample was obtained from the brain stems of 1000 sleep-deprived rats, but this produced enough material for studies on only four animals.[139, 140, 177, 178] SPS is reported to produce delayed REM sleep, but it has not yet been chemically identified, and Mendelson et al.[136] were unable to detect any sleep-promoting factor produced in the brain stem of sleep-deprived animals.

PAPPENHEIMER'S FACTOR 'S'

Pappenheimer discovered a sleep-promoting factor in the cerebrospinal fluid during an attempt to repeat the experiments of Legendre and Piéron.[146] Goats were sleep-deprived by electric shock and noise. Goat cerebrospinal fluid was then withdrawn over the subsequent 5 h and given by intracerebroventricular injection in rats. In the first experiment, only reduced locomotor activity occurred in the rats, although this was subsequently related to EEG synchronization, sleep and alteration in body temperature.[115, 145] As the experiments progressed, Krueger et al.[125] extracted a small peptide (MW 300–500) from the cerebrospinal fluid, and a similar factor was identified in the brain stem of slaughterhouse cattle, as well as in the whole brains of sleep-deprived rabbits. An identical factor occurs in human urine.[124] In addition, a cerebrospinal fluid excitatory factor ('waking' factor) was identified. Intraventricular infusion of Pappenheimer's sleep factor into rats, cats, rabbits and squirrel monkeys sometimes induces slow-wave sleep,[124] but attempts to reproduce these experiments have not always been successful. Ringle and Herndon,[155] using cerebrospinal fluid from electroshock sleep-deprived rabbits, found no change in locomotor activity in recipient animals.

Factor S is a small glucopeptide that has been provisionally identified from urine extractions as a muramyl peptide (muramic acid, Ala, Gln, Glu and diaminopimelic acid in molar ratios 1:2:1:1:1). Muramyl peptides are sub-units of polymeric peptidoglycans present in the cell walls of bacteria and plants, but not present in mammalian cells, although diaminopimelic acid is a normal component of human urine, derived from the gut bacteria and vegetable food.

The relationship between the cell walls of bacteria and the regulation of sleep and also body temperature is very unexpected. Pappenheimer[144] considered that high-affinity receptors for muramyl peptides must be present in the brain, presumably in the anterior hypothalamus for temperature regulation and in more caudal somnogenic regions; and that muramyl peptides, isolated from the urine, were natural endogenous sleep-inducing modulators. By way of hypothesis, Pappenheimer said: 'I suggest that the muramic acid and diaminopimelic acid found in mammalian sleep factor derive from bacteria taken in with food and may be regarded as akin to any of the essential amino acids or vitamins which cannot be synthesized by mammalian cells'.

HORMONAL AND OTHER FACTORS THAT MODIFY SLEEP

Growth hormone and sleep

Growth hormone enters many areas of the brain after intraperitoneal injection[171] and it has been considered that the release of growth hormone during slow-wave sleep triggers subsequent REM sleep. An increase in deep sleep occurs in some growth hormone deficient dwarves[181] and a decrease in some acromegalics,[107] but no constant change in REM sleep has been identified in dwarves or giants. A few aged normal subjects, as well as some but not all acromegalics, preserve fairly normal sleep patterns despite absence of sleep-onset growth hormone release.[103, 162] There is no compelling evidence for a physiological role of growth hormone in the control of sleep onset or REM sleep. In initial studies in man, Mendelson et al.[135] found that high doses of human growth hormone (5 units) but not low doses (2 units) increased REM sleep time and decreased delta sleep, but subsequently these results have not been confirmed. Sleep-related growth hormone release can be abolished by methscopolamine with no alteration in slow-wave sleep; or increased by piperidine, again without any change in sleep.[132, 133]

Although growth hormone appears to have little or no effect on sleep, growth hormone active metabolites may influence sleep. Injections of growth hormone into cats, rabbits and humans are sometimes followed by a variable and apparently dose-dependent increase in REM sleep 3 h after injection, corresponding to the time of growth hormone metabolite synthesis.[113, 135, 170]

Antidiuretic hormone and sleep

It has been suggested frequently in the last decade that ADH has important actions on memory and sleep, in addition to the tubular and vasopressor effects. In laboratory animals, arginine vasotocin and lysine vasotocin improve learned behaviour and possibly also increase REM sleep. The evidence that ADH has any physiological role in learning or sleep mechanisms in man is much less conclusive, although at least one study suggests that ADH slightly improves sleep, attention and memory in normal man.[183]

Arginine vasotocin will induce slow-wave sleep but abolish REM sleep in animals. Pavel et al.[151] found that arginine vasotocin, in homeopathic doses of 10^{-6} pg (about 600 molecules) injected into the third ventricle of cats, promoted sleep, but these results have not always been confirmed.[174] Pavel[148] reported that the effects of vasotocin on sleep in cats were mediated by serotonin mechanisms, since combination of vasotocin with a serotonin re-uptake blocking drug (fluoxetine) increased slow-wave sleep, whilst combination with the 5-HT receptor antagonist metergoline abolished slow-wave sleep.

ADH has little or no effect on sleep in man. Arginine vasotocin 2–12 mg s.c. does not induce sleep in normal subjects,[106] although it may reduce REM sleep in narcoleptics and in symptomatic hypersomniacs according to Popoviciu.[154] Pavel *et al.*[150] reported that vasotocin, possibly synthesized in the pineal gland. [147, 149] but not demonstrated by Dogterom *et al.*[110] or by Negro-Vilar *et al.*, [141] was released into the cerebrospinal fluid of man during REM sleep; and considered that arginine vasotocin would induce REM periods in narcoleptics. The effects of ADH on learning in animals may be due to an increase in alertness, and be mediated via CSF pathways, and by modulation of neurotransmission in catecholamine systems distributed throughout the dorsal noradrenergic bundle.[173]

The effect of ADH on memory in animals is long-term[122] and is independent of both vasopressor and antidiuretic activity, since desglycinamide lysine vasopressin (DGLVP), which has no classic endocrine effect, has actions on memory which are similar to those of the whole molecule.[101] However, the experimental design here is critical. Male rats, trained to chase female rats in a T maze, choose the correct turning more often after DGLVP, but DGLVP may not alter memory under other experimental conditions.

In rats with hereditary diabetes insipidus and with low vasopressin content in the posterior pituitary, sleep is shorter and learning poorer than in heterozygous litter mates.[109] However, the sleep disturbance, if not the poor memory, may be due simply to the search for water. Men with hypothalamic diabetes insipidus do not have any gross sleep or memory disturbance, apart from frequent arousals with drinking and micturition.

ACTH and sleep
ACTH sometimes causes humans to feel more awake. This may be secondary to elevation of mood.

ACTH infusion sometimes delays the onset of subsequent REM sleep periods in normal volunteers, although ACTH has no effect on the sleep of patients with Addison's disease.[116] If ACTH does have any effect on sleep in man, it is probably mediated by cortisol release from an intact adrenal cortex. In animals, Sawyer[163] found that the circadian periodicity of REM sleep was abolished by adrenalectomy but restored by cortisol. Jouvet[118] showed there was a progressive decline in REM sleep following removal of the pituitary and hypothalamus in cats. This was restored by ACTH and posterior pituitary extract. In animals, ACTH may facilitate a selective arousal state, particularly of limbic–midbrain structures, resulting in increased attention and perception, but ACTH has only slight effects on arousal in man.

Luteinizing hormone (LH) and sleep
A number of studies have investigated the effects of oestrogen, progesterone and LH-releasing hormone (LH-RH) on sleep. Minor changes in sleep pattern occur with puberty and with menstruation,[105] but overall LH has little direct effect on sleep. Mendelson *et al.*[131] showed that LH-RH administration as an intravenous dose of 100 µg over an 8 h period does not affect sleep, although LH is secreted during sleep in pubertal boys and girls.[102]

Proteins and sleep

Inhibition of protein synthesis may reduce or alter REM sleep in animals, and also cause memory blockade, although there is little data available in man. Anisomycin, which interrupts protein synthesis, produces a specific decrease in phasic events (PGO waves) rather than tonic events (sleep atonia) during REM sleep, or shortens REM sleep.[114, 158] However, PGO spikes during sleep are not altered by chloramphenicol treatment, despite reduction in protein synthesis.[112] The protein-synthesis inhibitor cycloheximide has been reported both to increase and to decrease REM sleep.[152, 172] REM sleep suppression and memory blockade due to protein synthesis inhibition may depend on inhibition of enzymes involved in catecholamine synthesis. Horne[117] considered that protein synthesis during sleep was important for brain macromolecule synthesis, although sleep, because of the fasting state, may be a time of tissue breakdown rather than of tissue repair. The rate of protein synthesis throughout the body is related to food intake, not to sleep.

Calcium and sleep

The effects of calcium and calcitonin on sleep have been reviewed by Mendelson et al.[136] In animals, the intracerebral administration of *calcium* may induce sleep-like states with alteration in behaviour and changes in the EEG.[175, 176, 180] Carman and Wyatt[104] gave synthetic salmon *calcitonin* to a group of psychiatric patients, and reported that this had a tranquillizing and depressant effect, although with a reduction in nocturnal sleep. However, Mendelson et al[136] reported that calcitonin (140 MRC units) caused only minor changes in the sleep of normal young volunteers. The calcium antagonist *nifedipine* has been shown to reverse benzodiazepine-induced sedation in animals.[134]

Interferon

Highly purified human leucocyte interferon A, produced by recombinant DNA technology, causes dose-dependent reversible CNS toxicity, profound somnolence, lethargy, confusion and visual hallucinosis. Somnolence is accompanied by increased slow-wave activity in electroencephalograms, but unlike normal sleep this has a frontal predominance and subjects become non-responsive to waking stimuli.[169] Somnolence is a major dose-limiting factor with all interferons investigated, and is probably due to a non-specific encephalopathy rather than to true sleep. A similar condition occurs in many patients with toxic confusional states, with cytotoxic drugs, and in hepatic encephalopathy.[143]

REFERENCES

ACTIVITY OF BRAIN NEUROTRANSMITTER SYSTEMS

CATECHOLAMINES

1. Autret, A., Minz, M., Beilleyaire, T., Cathala, H.P. & Castaigne, P. Suppression of paradoxical sleep by clonidine in man, *C.R. Acad. Sci.* (1976) **283**, 955–957.
2. Azumi, K., Jinnai, S. & Takahashi, S. The effects of l-dopa on sleep pattern and SPR in normal adults, *Sleep Res.* (1972) **1**, 40.
3. Burns, R.S., Markey, S.P., Philips, J.M. & Chiueh, C.C. The neurotoxicity of 1-methyl-4-phenyl-1,2,3,6-tetrahydropyridine (MPTP) in the monkey and man, *Can. J. Neurol. Sci.* (1984) **11**, 166–168.
4. Chu, N.S. & Bloom, F.E. Activity patterns of catecholamine-containing pontine neurones in the dorso-lateral tegmentum of unrestrained cats, *J. Neurobiol.* (1975) **5**, 527–544.
5. Coulter, J.D., Lester, B.K. & Williams, H.L. Reserpine and sleep, *Psychopharmacologia* (1971) **19**, 134–147.
6. Drucker-Colin, R.R. Is there a sleep transmitter? *Prog. Neurobiol.* (1976) **6**, 1–22.
7. Fahrenkrug, J. & Emson, P.C. Vasoactive intestinal polypeptide: functional aspects. *Brit. Med. Bull.* (1982) **38**, 265–270.
8. Fram, D.H., Murphy, D.L., Goodwin, F.K., Brodie, H.K.H., Bunney, W.E.J. & Snyder, F. L-dopa and sleep in depressed patients. *Psychophysiology* (1970) **7**, 316–317.
9. Gaillard, J.-M. Pharmacologie du sommeil chez l'homme. *Confront. Psychiat.* (1977) **15**, 103–150.
10. Gaillard, J.-M. Paradoxical sleep as a functional response to the activity of brain catecholaminergic neurones. In: Chase, M.H. & Weitzman, E.D. (eds.) *Sleep Disorders: Basic and Clinical Research*, Lancaster: MTP (1983) 307–317.
11. Gaillard, J.-M. & Kafi, S. Involvement of pre- and post-synaptic receptors in catecholaminergic control of paradoxical sleep in man, *Eur. J. Pharmacol.* (1979) **15**, 83–89.
12. Gaillard, J.-M. & Kafi, S. Effect of alpha-adrenoceptor antagonist piperoxane on rat waking and paradoxical sleep. In: Koella, W.P. (ed.) *Sleep 1982*, Basel: S. Karger (1982) 267–269.
13. Gillin, J.C., Mendelson, W.B., Sitaram, N. & Wyatt, R.J. The neuropharmacology of sleep and wakefulness. *Ann. Rev. Pharmacol. Toxicol.* (1978) **18**, 563–579.
14. Gillin, J.C., Post, R.M., Wyatt, R.J., Goodwin, F.K., Snyder, F. & Bunney, W.E. REM inhibitory effect of l-dopa infusion during human sleep, *Electroenceph. Clin. Neurophysiol.* (1973) **35**, 181–186.
15. Gillin, J., Post, R., Wyatt, R.J., Snyder, F., Goodwin, F. & Bunney, W.E. Infusion of threodihydroxyphenylserine (DOPS) and 5-hydroxytryptophan (5HT) during human sleep, *Sleep Res.* (1972) **1**, 45.
16. Gillin, J.C., van Kammen, D.P., Graves, J. & Murphy, D.L. Differential effects of d- and l-amphetamine on the sleep of depressed patients, *Life Sci.* (1975) **17**, 1233–1240.
17. Greenberg, R. & Perlman, C.A. L-dopa, parkinsonism and sleep, *Psychophysiology* (1970) **7**, 314.
18. Haig, J.R., Schroeder, C.S. & Schroeder, S.R. Effects of methylphenidate on hyperactive children's sleep. *Psychopharmacologia* (1975) **37**, 185–188.
19. Hartmann, E. & Cravens, J. The effects of long term administration of psychotrophic drugs on human sleep. II. The effects of reserpine, *Psychopharmacologia* (1973) **33**, 169–184.
20. Hobson, J.A., McCarley, R.W. & McKenna, T.M. Cellular evidence bearing on the pontine brain-stem hypothesis of desynchronized sleep control, *Prog. Neurobiol.* (1976) **6**, 280–376.
21. Jouvet, M. The role of monoamines and acetyl-choline containing neurones in the regulation of the sleep–waking cycle. *Ergebn. Physiol.* (1972) **64**, 166–307.
22. Justafre, J.-C. & Gaillard, J.-M. Diminution du sommeil paradoxal chez le rat sous antidépresseur tricyclique: rôle de l'inhibition collatérale, *Rev. EEG Neurophysiol.* (1981) **11**, 228–235.
23. Kafi, S., Bouras, C., Constantinidis, J. & Gaillard, J.-M. Paradoxical sleep and brain catecholamines in the rat after single oral repeated administration of alpha-methyl-paratyrosine, *Brain Res.* (1977) **135**, 123–134.
24. Kales, A., Ansel, R.D., Markham, C.H., Scharf, M.D. & Tan, T.L. Sleep in patients with

Parkinson's disease and normal subjects prior to and following levodopa administration, *Clin. Pharmacol. Ther.* (1971) **12**, 397.

25. Klawans, H.L., Goetz, C. & Bergen, D. Levodopa-induced myoclonus, *Arch. Neurol.* (1975) **32**, 331–334.

26. Klingler, M. A glimpse into Roche research: antiparkinson treatment, *Int. J. Clin. Pharmacol. Ther. Toxicol.* (1982) **20**, 190–193.

27. Kubikowski, P. & Kadzielawa, K. The electroencephalographic analysis of the central action of dihydroxyphenylserine, *Acta Physiol. Pol.* (1973) **24**, 41–49.

28. McGinty, D.J., Harper, R.M. & Fairbanks, M.K. Neuronal unit activity and the control of sleep state. In: Weitzman, E.D. (ed.) *Advances in Sleep Research*, New York: Spectrum (1974) 173–216.

29. Mendelson, W.B., Gillin, J.C. & Wyatt, R.J. *Human Sleep and its Disorders,* New York/London: Plenum Press (1977) 36–42.

30. Moore, R.Y. The reticular formation: monoamine neurone systems. In: Hobson, J.A. & Brazier, M.A.B. (eds.) *The Reticular Formation Revisited,* New York: Raven Press (1980) 67–81.

31. Myslobodsky, M., Mintz, M., Ben-Mayor, V. & Radwan, H. Unilateral dopamine deficit and lateral EEG asymmetry: sleep abnormalities in hemi-Parkinson's patients, *Electroenceph. Clin. Neurophysiol.* (1982) **54**, 227–231.

32. Nausieda, P.A., Glantz, R., Weber, S., Baum, R. & Klawans, H.L. Psychiatric complications of levodopa therapy of Parkinson's disease. In: Hassler, R.G. & Christ, J.F. (eds.) *Advances in Neurology, Vol. 40,* New York: Raven Press (1984) 271–277.

33. Nybäch, H.V., Walters, J.R., Aghajanian, G. & Roth, R.H. Tricyclic antidepressants: effects on the firing rates of brain noradrenergic neurones, *Eur. J. Pharmacol.* (1975) **2**, 107–110.

34. Oswald, I., Thacore, V.R., Adam, K., Brezinova, V. & Burack, R. Alpha-adrenergic receptor blockage increases human REM sleep, *Brit. J. Clin. Pharmacol.* (1975) **2**, 107–110.

35. Post, R.M., Gillin, J.C., Wyatt, R.J. & Goodwin, F.K. The effect of orally administered cocaine on sleep of depressed patients, *Psychopharmacologia* (1974) **37**, 59–66.

36. Puca, F.M., Briccolo, A. & Turella, G. Effect of L-dopa or amantadine on sleep spindles in parkinsonism, *Electroenceph. Clin. Neurophysiol.* (1973) **35**, 327–330.

37. Sagales, T. & Erill, S. Effects of central dopaminergic blockage with pimozide upon the EEG stages of sleep in man, *Psychopharmacologia* (1975) **41**, 53–56.

38. Siegel, J.M. & McGinty, D.J. Pontine reticular formation neurones: relationship of discharge to motor activity, *Science* (1977) **196**, 678–680.

39. Svensson, T.H., Bunney, B.S. & Aghajanian, G.K. Inhibition of both noradrenergic and serotonergic neurones in the brain by the alpha-adrenergic agonist clonidine, *Brain Res.* (1975) **92**, 291–306.

40. Svensson, T.H. & Usdin, T. Feedback inhibition of brain noradrenaline neurones by tricyclic antidepressants: alpha receptor mediation, *Science* (1978) **202**, 1089–1091.

41. Trulson, M.E. & Jacobs, B.L. Raphe unit activity in freely moving cats: correlation with level of behavioural arousal, *Brain Res.* (1979) **163**, 135–150.

42. Watson, R., Hartmann, E. & Schildkraut, J.J. Amphetamine withdrawal: affective state, sleep patterns and MHPG excretion, *Am. J. Psychiat.* (1972) **129**, 263–269.

43. Wyatt, R.J., Cantor, F., Gillin, J.C., Gordon, E., Karoum, F., McCullough, D., Neff, N., Ommaya, A., Rauscher, F.P., Seaborg, J.B. & Slaby, A. Ventricular fluid metabolites of phenolic amines and catecholamine. In: Usdin, E. & Sandler, M., (eds.) *Trace Amines in the Brain,* New York: Dekker (1976) 209–231.

44. Wyatt, R.J., Chase, T.N., Scott, J., Snyder, F. & Engelman, K. Effect of l-dopa on the sleep of man, *Nature* (1970) **228**, 999–1001.

ACETYLCHOLINE

45. Cohen, E.L. & Wurtman, R.J. Brain acetylcholine control by dietary choline, *Science* (1976) **191**, 561–562.

46. Crow, T.J. & Grove-White, I.G. An analysis of the learning deficit following hyoscine administration to man, *Brit. J. Pharmacol.* (1973) **49**, 322–327.

47. Crow, T.J., Grove-White, I.G. & Ross, D.G. The specificity of the action of hyoscine on human learning, *Brit. J. Clin. Pharmacol.* (1976) **2**, 367–368.

48. Delashaw, J.B., Foutz, A.S., Guilleminault, T.C. & Dement, W.C. Cholinergic mechanisms and cataplexy in dogs, *Exp. Neurol.* (1979) **66**, 745–757.

49. Drachman, D.A. & Sahakian, B.J. Memory and cognitive function in the elderly. A preliminary trial of physostigmine, *Arch. Neurol.* (1980) **37**, 674–675.
50. Grob, P. & Harvey, J.C. Effect in man of the anticholinesterase compound sarin (isopropyl methyl phosphoro-fluoridate), *J. Clin. Invest.* (1958) **37**, 350–368.
51. Guilleminault, C. & Foutz, A.S. Muscle inhibition and cataplexy. In: Chase, M.H. & Weitzman, E.D. (eds.) *Sleep Disorders: Basic and Clinical Research,* Lancaster: MTP (1983) 137–143.
52. Jacobs, B.L., Henricksen, S.J. & Dement, W.C. Neurological bases of the PGO waves, *Brain Res.* (1972) **48**, 406–411.
53. Magherini, P.C., Pompeiano, O. & Thoden, U. The neurochemical basis of REM sleep. A cholinergic mechanism responsible for rhythmic activities of the vestibulo-oculomotor system, *Brain Res.* (1971) **35**, 565–569.
54. Mandel, P., Ayad, G., Hermetet, J.C. & Ebel, A. Correlation between choline acetyl-transferase and learning ability in different mice strains and their offspring, *Brain Res.* (1974) **72**, 65–70.
55. Mitler, M.M. & Dement, W.C. Cataplectic-like behaviour in cats after micro injection of carbachol in pontine reticular formation, *Brain Res.* (1974) **68**, 335–343.
56. Pompeiano, O. Reticular control of the vestibular nuclei: physiology and pharmacology, *Prog. Brain Res.* (1972) **37**, 614–618.
57. Potamianos, G. & Kellett, J.M. Anticholinergic drugs and memory: the effect of benzhexol on memory in a group of geriatric patients, *Brit. J. Psychiat.* (1982) **140**, 470–472.
58. Reisine, T.D., Bird, E.D. & Spokes, E. Pre and postsynaptic neurochemical alterations in Alzheimer's disease, *Trans. Am. Soc. Neurochem. (1978)* **9**, 203.
59. Ruch-Monachan, M.A., Jalfie, M. & Haefely, W. Drugs and PGO waves in the lateral geniculate body of the curarized cat, *Arch. Int. Pharmacodyn. Ther.* (1976) **219**, 251–346.
60. Sagales, T., Erill, S. & Domino, E.F. Differential effects of scopolamine and chlorpromazine on REM and NREM sleep in normal male subjects, *Clin. Pharmacol. Ther.* (1969) **10**, 522–529.
61. Shute, C.C.D. & Lewis, P.R. The ascending cholinergic reticular system: neocortical, olfactory and subcortical projections, *Brain* (1967) **90**, 497–520.
62. Silberman, E.K., Vivaldi, E., Garfield, J., McCarley, R.W. & Hobson, J.A. Carbachol triggering of desynchronized sleep phenomena: enhancement via small volume infusions, *Brain Res.* (1980) **191**, 215–224.
63. Sitaram, N., Wyatt, R.J., Dawson, S. & Gillin, J.C. REM sleep induction during sleep in normal volunteers, *Science* (1976) **191**, 1281–1283.
64. Stoyva, J. & Metcalf, D. Sleep patterns following chronic exposure to cholinesterase-inhibiting organophosphate compounds, *Psychopharmacology* (1968) **5**, 206.
65. Vimont-Vicary, P. *La suppression des différents états de sommeil. Etude compartementale, EEG, et neuropharmacologique chez le chat,* thesis, University of Lyon (1965) 95.
66. Wurtman, R.J. Choline and lethicin in brain disorders. In: Barbeau, A., Growden, J.H. & Wurtman, R.J. (eds.) *Nutrition and the Brain, Vol. 5,* New York: Raven Press (1979) 1–12.

SEROTONIN

67. Autret, A., Minz, M., Bussel, B., Cathala, H.P. & Castaigne, P. Human sleep and 5-HTP. Effects of repeated high doses and of association with benserazide (RO 04 4602), *Electroenceph. Clin. Neurophysiol.* (1976) **41**, 408–413.
68. Bronzino, J.D., Morgane, P.J. & Stern, W.C. EEG synchronization following application of serotonin to area postrema, *Am. J. Physiol.* (1972) **223**, 376–383.
69. Brooks, D.C. & Gershon, M.D. Amine repletion in the reserpinized cat: Effect upon PGO waves and REM sleep *Electroenceph. Clin. Neurophysiol.* (1977) **42**, 35–47.
70. Chadwick, D., Hallett, M., Jenner, P. & Marsden, C.D. Serotonin and action myoclonus – a review. In: Legg, N.J. (ed.) *Neurotransmitter Systems and their Clinical Disorders,* London: Academic Press (1978) 151–165.
71. Crespi, F. & Jouvet, M. Sleep and indolamine alterations induced by thiamine deficiency, *Brain Res.* (1982) **248**, 275–283.
72. Dahlstrom, A. & Fuxe, K. Evidence for the existence of monoamine-containing neurones in the central nervous system: I. Demonstration of monoamines in the cell bodies of brain stem neurones, *Acta Physiol. Scand.* (1964) **62** Suppl. 232, 1–55.
73. Dement, W., Zarcone, V., Ferguson, J., Cohen, H., Pivik, T. & Barchas, J. Some parallel

findings in schizophrenic patients and serotonin-depleted cats. In: Siva, D.V. (ed.) *Schizophrenia – Current Concepts and Research*, New York: P.J.D. Publications (1969) 775–811.

74. Fischer-Perroudan, C., Mouret, J. & Jouvet, M. Sur un cas d'agrypnie (4 mois sans sommeil) au cours d'une maladie de Morvan. Effet favorable due 5-hydroxytryptophane, *Electroenceph. Clin. Neurophysiol.* (1974) **36**, 1–18.
75. Griffiths, W.J., Lester, B.K., Coulter, J.D. & Williams, H.L. Tryptophan and sleep in young adults. *Psychophysiology* (1972) **9**, 345–356.
76. Guilleminault, C., Cathala, J.P. & Castaigne, P. Effects of 5-hydroxytryptophan on sleep of a patient with brain stem lesion, *Electroenceph. Clin. Neurophysiol.* (1973) **34**, 177–184.
77. Jacobs, B.L., Heym, J., Steinfels, G.F. & Trulson, M.E. Activity of brain serotonergic neurones. In: Chase, M. & Weitzman, E.D. (eds.) *Sleep Disorders: Basic and Clinical Research,* Lancaster: MTP (1983) 573–589.
78. Jouvet, M. The role of monoamines and acetylcholine-containing neurones in the regulation of the sleep–waking cycle, *Ergebn. Physiol.* (1972) **64**, 166–307.
79. Jouvet, M. & Delorme, G. Locus coeruleus et sommeil paradoxal, *C.R. Soc. Biol.* (1965) **159**, 895–899.
80. Lhermitte, F., Peterfalvi, M., Marteau, R., Gazengel, J. & Serdara, M. Analyse pharmacologique d'un cas de myoclonus d'intention et d'action postanoxique, *Rev. Neurol.* (1971) **124**, 21–31.
81. Magnussen, E., Dupont, A. & De Fine Olivarius, B. Palatal myoclonus treated with 5-hydroxytryptophan and a decarboxylase inhibitor, *Acta Neurol. Scand.* (1977) 251–253.
82. Mandell, M.P., Mandell, A.J. & Jacobsen, A. Biochemical and neurophysiological studies of paradoxical sleep, *Recent Adv. Biol. Psychiat.* (1965) **7**, 115–122.
83. Mendelson, W.B., Reichman, J. & Uthmer, E. Serotonin inhibition and sleep, *Biol. Psychiat.* (1975) **10**, 459–464.
84. Morgane, P.J. & Stern, W.C. Chemical anatomy of brain circuits in relation to sleep and wakefulness, *Adv. Sleep Res.* (1974) **1**, 1–131.
85. Nicholson, A.N. & Stone, B.M. L-tryptophan and sleep in healthy man, *Electroenceph. Clin. Neurophysiol.* (1979) **47**, 539–545.
86. Oswald, I., Ashcroft, G.W., Berger, R.J., Eccleston, D., Evans, J.I. & Thacore, V.R. Some experiments in the chemistry of normal sleep, *Brit. J. Psychiat.* (1966) **112**, 391–399.
87. Poitras, D. & Parent, A. Atlas of the distribution of monoamine-containing nerve cell bodies in the brain stem of the cat, *J. Comp. Neurol.* (1978) **179**, 699–718.
88. Sallanon, M., Buda, C., Janin, M. & Jouvet, M. Restoration of paradoxical sleep by cerebrospinal fluid transfer to PCPA pretreated insomniac cats, *Brain Res.* (1982) **251**, 137–147.
89. Schulte, F.J., Karsen, J.H., Engelbart, S., Bell, E.F., Castell, R. & Lenard, H.G. Sleep patterns in hyperphenylalanemia: A lesson serotonin learned from phenylketonuria, *Pediat. Res.* (1973) **7**, 588–599.
90. Taylor, P.L., Garrick, N.A., Burns, R.S., Tamarkin, L., Murphy, D.L. & Markey, S.P. Diurnal rhythms of serotonin in monkey cerebrospinal fluid, *Life Sci.* (1982) **31**, 1993–1999.
91. Trulson, M.E. & Jacobs, B.L. Raphe unit activity in freely moving cats: correlation with levels of behavioural arousal, *Brain Res.* (1979) **163**, 135–150.
92. Trulson, M.E., Jacobs, B.L. & Morrison, A.R. Raphe unit activity in normal cats and pontine lesioned cats displaying REM sleep without atonia, *Brain Res.* (1981) **226**, 75–91.
93. Williams, A., Goodenberger, D. & Calne, D.B. Palatal myoclonus following herpes zoster ameliorated by 5-hydroxytryptophan and carbidopa, *Neurology* (1978) **28**, 358–359.
94. Williams, H.L., Lester, B.K. & Coulter, J.B. Monamines and the EEG stages of sleep, *Activ. Nerv. Sup. (Praha)* (1969) **11**, 188–192.
95. Wyatt, R.J., Engelman, K., Kupfer, D.J., Fram, D.H., Sjoersdma, A. & Snyder, F. Effects of l-tryptophan (a natural sedative) on human sleep, *Lancet* (1970) **2**, 842–846.
96. Wyatt, R.J., Engelman, K., Kupfer, D.J., Scott, J., Sjoersdma, A. & Snyder, F. Effects of parachlorphenylalanine on sleep in man, *Electroenceph. Clin. Neurophysiol.* (1969) **27**, 529–532.
97. Wyatt, R.J., Neff, N.H., Vaughan, J., Franz, J. & Ommaya, A. Ventricular fluid 5-hydroxyindoleacetic acid concentrations during human sleep, *Adv. Biochem. Psychopharmacol.* (1974) **11**, 193–197.
98. Yogman, M.W. & Zeisel, S.H. Diet and sleep patterns in newborn infants, *New Engl. J. Med.* (1983) **39**, 1147–1149.
99. Zarcone, V.P., Hoddes, E. & Smythe, H. Oral 5-hydroxytryptophan effects on sleep. In:

Barchas, J. & Usdin, E. (eds.) *Serotonin and Behaviour*, New York: Academic Press (1973) 499–509.
100. Zarcone, V., Kales, A., Scharf, J., Tjiauw-Ling-Tan, Simmons, J.Q. & Dement, W.C. Repeated oral injection of 5-HTP, *Arch. Gen. Psychiat.* (1973) **28**, 843–846.

ENDOGENOUS SLEEP FACTORS

101. Bohus, B. Effect of desglycinamide-lyside vasopressin (DG-LVP) on sexually motivated T-maze behaviour in the male rat, *Horm. Behav.* (1977) **8**, 52–61.
102. Boyar, R., Finkelstein, J., Roffwarg, H., Kapen, S., Weitman, E. & Hellman, J. Synchronization of augmented luteinizing hormone secretion with sleep during puberty, *New Engl. J. Med.* (1972) **287**, 582–586.
103. Carlson, H.E., Gillin, J.C., Corden, P. & Snyder, F. Absence of sleep-related growth hormone peaks in aged normal subjects and in acromegaly, *J. Clin. Endocrinol. Metab.* (1972) **34**, 1102–1105.
104. Carman, J.G. & Wyatt, R.J. Use of calcitonin in psychotic agitation or mania, *Arch. Gen. Psychiat.* (1979) **36**, 72–75.
105. Carskadon, M.A., Harvey, K., Duke, P., Anders, T.F., Litt, I.F. & Dement, W.C. Pubertal changes in daytime sleepiness, *Sleep* (1980) **2**, 453–460.
106. Coculescu, M., Serbanescu, A. & Temeli, E. Influence of arginine vasotocin administration on nocturnal sleep of human subjects, *Waking Sleeping* (1979) **3**, 1–5.
107. Cryer, P.E. and Daughaday, W.A. Regulation of growth hormone secretion in acromegaly, *J. Clin. Endocrinol. Metab.* (1969) **29**, 386–393.
108. De Andres, I., Gutierrez-Rivas, E. & Nava, E. Independence of sleep–wakefulness cycle in an implanted head 'encephaloisole'. *Neurosci. Lett.* (1976) **2**, 13–18.
109. De Wied, D. & Bohus, B. Modulation of memory processes by neuropeptides of hypothalamic–neurohypophyseal origin. In: Brazier, M.A.B. (ed.) *Brain Mechanisms in Memory and Learning: from the Single Neuron to Man*, New York: Raven Press (1979) 139–150.
110. Dogterom, J., Pevet, P., Buijs, R.M., Snijdewint, S.M. & Swaab, D.J. Vasopressin oxytocin and vasotocin in pineal gland, subcommisural organ and foetal pituitary: failure to demonstrate vasotocin in mammals, *Acta Endocrinol. (Copenh.)* Suppl. **225**, 413.
111. Drucker-Colin, R. Endogenous sleep peptides. In: Wheatley, D. (ed.) *Psychopharmacology of Sleep*, New York: Raven Press (1981) 53–72.
112. Drucker-Colin, R.R., Dreyfus-Cortes, G. & Bernal-Pedraza, J.G. Differences in multiple unit activity discharge frequency during short and long REM sleep periods: effects of protein synthesis inhibition, *Behav. Neurol. Biol.* (1979) **26**, 123–127.
113. Drucker-Colin, R.R., Spanis, C.W., Hunyani, J., Sassin, J.F. & McGaugh, J.C. Growth hormone effects on sleep and wakefulness in the rat, *Neuroendocrinology* (1975) **18**, 1–8.
114. Drucker-Colin, R.R., Zamora, J., Bernal-Pedraza, J. & Sosa, B. Modification of REM sleep and associated phasic activities by protein synthesis inhibitors, *Exp. Neurol.* (1979) **63**, 458–467.
115. Fencl, V., Koski, G. & Pappenheimer, J.R. Factors in cerebrospinal fluid from goats that affect sleep and activity in rats, *J. Physiol.* (1971) **216**, 565–589.
116. Gillin, J.C., Jacobs, L.S., Snyder, F. & Henkin, R.I. Effects of ACTH on sleep of normal subjects and patients with Addison's disease. *Neuroendocrinology* (1974) **15**, 21–31.
117. Horne, J.A. Human sleep and tissue restitution: some qualifications and doubts, *Clin. Sci.* (1983) **65**, 569–578.
118. Jouvet, M. Paradoxical sleep – a study of its nature and mechanism, *Prog. Brain Res.* (1965) **18**, 20–62.
119. Kafi, S. & Gaillard, J.M. The delta-sleep-inducing peptide (DSIP) increases duration of sleep in rats, *Neurosci. Lett.* (1979) **13**, 169–172.
120. Kastin, A.J., Nissen, C., Schally, A.V. & Coy, D.M. Radioimmunoassay of DSIP-like material in rat brain, *Brain Res. Bull.* (1978) **3**, 691–695.
121. King, C. Effects of beta-endorphin and morphine on the sleep–wakefulness behaviour of cats, *Sleep* (1981) **4**, 259–262.
122. Krieger, D.T. & Martin, J.B. Brain peptides (second of two parts), *New Engl. J. Med.* (1981) **304**, 944–951.
123. Krueger, J.M. Sleep-promoting factor S: characterization and analogs. In: Koella, W.P. (ed.) *Sleep 1982*, Basel: S. Karger (1983) 107–109.

124. Krueger, J.M., Bacsik, J. & Garcia-Arraras, J. Sleep-promoting material from human urine and its relation to factor S from brain, *Am. J. Physiol.* (1980) **238**, E116–126.
125. Krueger, J.M. Pappenheimer, J.R. & Karnovsky, M.L. Sleep-promoting factor S: purification and properties, *Proc. Nat. Acad. Sci. USA* (1978) **75**, 5235–5238.
126. Legendre, R. & Piéron, H. Recherches sur le besoin de sommeil consécutif à une vielle prolongée, *Z. Allgem. Physiol.* (1913) **14**, 235–262.
127. Lenard, H.G. & Schulte, F.J. Polygraphic sleep study in craniopagus twin, *J. Neurol. Neurosurg. Psychiat.* (1972) **35**, 756–760.
128. Lichtensteiger, W., Monnet, F. & Felix, D. Peptide effects on mammalian and invertebrate dopamine neurones. In: Kopin, I.J. & Barchas, J.D. (eds.) *Catecholamines, Vol. 2,* New York: Pergamon (1979) 1086–1088.
129. Mansbach, R.S. & Lorenz, D.N. Cholecystokinin (CCK-8) elicits prandial sleep in rats, *Physiol. Behav.* (1983) **30**, 179–183.
130. Mendelson, W.B., Gillin, J.C., Pisner, G. & Wyatt, R.J. Arginine vasotocin and sleep in the rat, *Brain Res.* (1980) **182**, 246–249.
131. Mendelson, W.B., Gold, P.W., Slater, S., Gillin, J.C. & Goodwin, F.K. LH-RH administration and human sleep, *Sleep Res.* (1978) **7**, 122.
132. Mendelson, W.B., Jacobs, L.C., Sitaram, N., Wyatt, R.J. & Gillin, J.C. Methscopolamine inhibition of sleep-related growth hormone secretion, *J. Clin. Invest.* (1978) **61**, 1683–1690.
133. Mendelson, W.B., Lantigua, R.A., Wyatt, R.J., Gillin, J.C. & Jacobs, L.S. Piperidine enhances sleep-related and insulin-induced growth hormone secretion: further evidence for a cholinergic secretory mechanism, *J. Clin. Endocrinol. Metab.* (1981) **52**, 409–415.
134. Mendelson, W.B., Owen, C., Skolnick, P., Paul, S.M., Martin, J.V., Ko, G. & Wagner, R. Nifedipine blocks sleep induction by flurazepam in the rat, *Sleep* (1984) **7**, 64–68.
135. Mendelson, W.B., Seater, S., Gold, P. & Gillin, J.C. The effect of growth hormone administration on human sleep: a dose response study, *Biol. Psychiat.* (1980) **15**, 613–618.
136. Mendelson, W.B., Wyatt, R.J. & Gillin, J.C. Whither the sleep factors? In: Chase, M.H. & Weitzman, E.D. (eds.) *Sleep Disorders: Basic and Clinical Research,* Lancaster: MTP (1983) 281–305.
137. Monnier, M., Dudler, L., Gaechter, R., Maier, P.F., Tobler, H.J. & Schoenenberger, G.A. The delta sleep-inducing peptide (DSIP): comparative properties of the original and synthetic nonapeptide, *Experienta* (1977) **33**, 548–552.
138. Monnier, M., Dudler, L., Gaechter, R. & Schoenenberger, G.A. Delta sleep-inducing peptide (DSIP): EEG and motor activity in rabbits following intravenous administration, *Neurosci. Lett.* (1977) **6**, 9–13.
139. Nagasaki, H., Iriki, M., Inone, S. & Uchizono, K. The presence of sleep-promoting material in the brain of sleep-deprived rats, *Proc. Jap. Acad.* (1974) **50**, 241–246.
140. Nagasaki, H., Kitahama, K., Valatx, J.L. & Jouvet, M. Sleep-promoting substance (SPS) and delta sleep-inducing peptide (DSIP) in the mouse, *Brain Res.* (1980) **192**, 276–280.
141. Negro-Vilar, A., Sanchez-Franco, F., Kwintkowski, M. & Samson, K.W. Failure to detect radioimmunoassayable arginine vasotocin in mammalian pineals, *Brain Res. Bull.* (1979) **4**, 789–792.
142. Normanton, J.R. & Gent, J.P. Comparison of the effects of two 'sleep' peptides, delta-sleep-inducing peptide and arginine-vasotocin, on single neurones in the rat and rabbit brain stem, *Neuroscience* (1983) **8**, 107–114.
143. Obrecht, R., Okhomina, F.O.A. & Scott, D.F. Value of EEG in acute confusional state, *J. Neurol. Neurosurg. Psychiat.* (1979) **42**, 75–77.
144. Pappenheimer, J.R. Induction of sleep by muramyl peptides, *J. Physiol. (Lond.)* (1983) **336**, 1–11.
145. Pappenheimer, J.R., Koski, G., Fencl, V., Karnovsky, M.L. & Krueger, J. Extraction of sleep promoting factor S from cerebrospinal fluid and from brains of sleep deprived animals, *J. Neurophysiol.* (1975) **38**, 1299–1311.
146. Pappenheimer, J.R., Miller, T.B. & Goodrich, C.A. Sleep-promoting effects of cerebrospinal fluid from sleep-deprived goats, *Proc. Nat. Acad. Sci.* (1967) **58**, 513–517.
147. Pavel, S. Evidence for the presence of lysine vasotocin in the pig pineal gland, *Endocrinology* (1965) **77**, 812–817.
148. Pavel, S. Pineal vasotocin and sleep: involvement of serotonin-containing neurones, *Brain Res. Bull.* (1979) **4**, 731–734.
149. Pavel, S., Goldstein, R., Ghinea, E. & Calb, M. Chromatographic evidence of vasotocin biosynthesis by cultured pineal cells from rat foetuses, *Endocrinology* (1977) **100**, 205–208.

150. Pavel, S., Goldstein, R., Popoviciu, L., Corfariu, O., Földes, A. & Farkas, E. Pineal vasotocin: REM sleep dependent release into cerebrospinal fluid of man, *Waking Sleeping* (1980) **3**, 347–352.

151. Pavel, S., Psatta, A. & Goldstein, R. Slow-wave sleep induced in cats by extremely small amounts of synthetic and pineal vasotocin injected into the third ventricle of the brain, *Brain Res. Bull.* (1977) **2**, 251–254.

152. Pegram, V., Hammond, D. & Bridgers, W. The effect of protein synthesis inhibition on sleep in mice, *Behav. Biol.* (1973) **9**, 377–382.

153. Polc, P., Schneeberger, J. & Haefely, W. Effect of the delta sleep-inducing peptide (DSIP) on the sleep–wakefulness cycle of cats, *Neurosci. Lett.* (1978) **9**, 33–36.

154. Popoviciu, L. Effects of arginine vasotocin on REM sleep in narcoleptics and in symptomatic hypersomniacs, *Electroenceph. Clin. Neurophysiol.* (1982) **53**, 325–328.

155. Ringle, D. & Herndon, B. Effects on rats of csf from sleep deprived rabbits, *Pflug. Arch.* (1969) **306**, 320–328.

156. Riou, F., Cespuglio, R. & Jouvet, M. Endogenous sleep promoting substances. Paper given at 6th European General Congress of Sleep Research, 23–26 March 1982, Zurich. See Borbély, A. *Trends Pharmacol. Sci.* (1982) **3**, 350.

157. Rohatiner, A.Z.S., Prior, P.F., Burton, A.C., Smith, A.T., Balkwill, F.R. & Lister, T.A. Central nervous system toxicity of interferon, *Brit. J. Cancer* (1983) **3**, 419–422.

158. Rojas-Ramirez, J.A., Aguilar-Jiminez, E., Poseda-Andrews, A., Bernal-Pedraza, J. & Drucker-Colin, R.R. The effects of various protein synthesis inhibitors on the sleep–wake cycle of rats, *Psychopharmacology* (1977) **53**, 147–150.

159. Rojas-Ramirez, J.A., Crawley, J.N. & Mendelson, W.B. Electroencephalographic analysis of the sleep-inducing action of cholecystokinin, *Neuropeptides* (1982) **3**, 129–138.

160. Sachs, J., Ungar, J., Waser, P.G. & Borbély, A. Factors in cerebrospinal fluid affecting motor activity in the rat, *Neurosci. Lett.* (1976) **2**, 83–86.

161. Sallanon, M., Buda, C., Janin, M. & Jouvet, M. L'insomnie provoquée par la *p*-chlorphénylalanine chez le chat. Sa réversibilité par l'injection intraventriculaire de liquide céphalorachidien prélevé chez des chats privés de sommeil paradoxical, *C.R. Acad. Sci. (Paris)* (1981) **292**, 113–117.

162. Sassin, J.F., Hellman, L. & Weitzman, E.D. A circadian pattern of growth hormone secretion in acromegalics, *Sleep Res.* (1972) **1**, 189.

163. Sawyer, C.H. Some effects of hormones on sleep, *Exp. Med. Surg.* (1969) **27**, 177–186.

164. Schlerschlicht, R., Bonetti, E.P. & Toh, C.C. Effects of intracerebroventricularly injected 'nerveside' on free behaviour and EEG-activity of rats: a pilot study, *Arch. Int. Pharmacol. Ther.* (1979) **239**, 221–229.

165. Schlerschlicht, R., Schneeberger, J. & Haefely, W. Delta sleep-inducing peptide (DSIP) antagonizes morphine insomnia in cats, *Sleep Res.* (1979) **8**, 84.

166. Schnedorf, J.G. & Ivy, A.C. An examination of the hypnotoxin theory of sleep, *Am. J. Physiol.* (1939) **125**, 491–505.

167. Schneider-Helmert, D. 6th European Congress of Sleep Research 23–26 March 1982, Zurich. Endogenous sleep promoting inhibition. See Borbély, A. *Trends Pharmacol. Sci.* (1982) **3**, 320.

168. Schoenenberger, G.A. & Monnier, M. Characterization of a delta-electro-encephalogram-(sleep)-inducing peptide, *Proc. Nat. Acad. Sci. USA* (1977) **74**, 1282–1286.

169. Smedley, H., Katrak, M., Sikora, K. & Wheeler, T. Neurological effects of recombinant human interferon, *Brit. Med. J.* (1983) **286**, 262–264.

170. Stern, W.C., Jalowiec, E., Shabshalowitz, H. & Morgane, P.J. Effect of growth hormone on sleep–waking pattern in cats, *Horm. Behav.* (1975) **6**, 189–196.

171. Stern, W.C., Miller, M., Resnick, O. & Morgane, P.J. Distribution of 125-labelled rat growth hormone in regional brain areas and peripheral tissue of the rat, *Am. J. Anat.* (1975) **144**, 503.

172. Stern, W.C., Morgane, P.J., Panksepp, J., Solovick, A.J. & Jalowiec, J.E. Elevation of REM sleep following inhibition of protein synthesis, *Brain Res.* (1972) **47**, 254–258.

173. Telegdy, G. & Kovács, G.L. Role of monoamines in mediating the action of hormones on learning and memory. In: Brazier, M.A.B. (ed.) *Brain Mechanisms in Memory and Learning: from the Single Neuron to Man*, New York: Raven Press (1979) 249–268.

174. Tobler, I. & Borbély, A. Effect of delta sleep inducing peptide (DSIP) and arginine vasotocin (AVT) on sleep and motor activity in the rat, *Waking Sleeping* (1980) **4**, 139–153.

175. Tobler-Kost, I. Sleep regulation in the rat: neurochemical mechanisms and the effect of night–dark schedules. Inaugural dissertation, Philosophischen-Doktorwurde, Philosophischen Fakultät II der Universität Zurich (1980).

176. Toszeghi, P., Tobler, I. & Borbély, A. Cerebral ventricular infusion of excess calcium in the rat: effects on sleep states, behaviour, and cortical EEG, *Eur. J. Pharmacol.* (1978) **51,** 407–416.

177. Uchizono, K., Higashi, A., Triki, M., Nagasaki, H., Ishikawa, M., Komoda, Y., Inoni, S. & Honda, K. Sleep-promoting fractions obtained from brain-stem in sleep-deprived rats. In: Ito, M. (ed.) *Integrative Control Functions of the Brain, Vol. 1,* Tokyo: Kodansha LTA/ Amsterdam: Elsevier (1978) 392–396.

178. Uchizono, K., Inoni, S., Iriki, M., Ishikawa, M., Komoda, Y. & Nagasaki, H. Purification of the sleep-promoting substance from sleep-deprived rat brain. In: Walter, R. & Menhofer, J. (eds.) *Peptide Chemistry, Structure and Biology,* Michigan: Ann Arbor Publ. (1975) 667–671.

179. Ueno, R., Ishikawa, Y., Nakayama, T. & Hayaisho, O. Prostaglandin D2 induces sleep when microinjected into the preoptic area of conscious rats, *Biochem. Biophys. Res. Commun.* (1982) **109,** 576–582.

180. Veale, W.L. & Myers, R.D. Emotional behaviour, arousal and sleep produced by sodium and calcium perfusion within the hypothalamus of the cat, *Physiol. Behav.* (1971) **7,** 601–607.

181. Vogel, G.W., Rudman, D., Thumond, A., Barrowclough, B., Giesler, D. & Hickman, J. Human growth hormone and slow-wave sleep. *Psychophysiology* (1972) **9,** 102.

182. Webb, W.B. The sleep of conjoined twins, *Sleep* (1978) **1,** 205–211.

183. Weingartner, H., Gold, P., Ballenger, J.C., Smallberg, S.A., Summers, R., Rubinow, D.R., Post, R.M. & Goodwin, F.K. Effects of vasopressin on human memory functions, *Science* (1981) **211,** 601–603.

CHAPTER 9

DRUGS AND THE TREATMENT OF INSOMNIA

HYPNOTICS
MANAGEMENT OF INSOMNIA
BENZODIAZEPINES

HYPNOTICS

More prescriptions are written for hypnotic–anxiolytic drugs than for any other class of compound. In the United States, over 8000 tons of benzodiazepines were prescribed in 1977; and 27 million of 128 million drug prescriptions in 1976 – about one thousand million doses – were for their hypnotic effect. However, the number of hypnotic prescriptions was much lower in 1976 than in 1971. In the last decade, benzodiazepines have almost completely replaced barbiturates. In 1971, flurazepam accounted for only 7% of all hypnotics prescribed in the USA but in 1977 for 53%.[28, 42, 64]

All known hypnotics promote sleep and inhibit wakefulness. The effects on sleep and wakefulness cannot be separated. All hypnotic drugs shorten sleep latency, reduce nocturnal wakefulness, increase total sleep time and decrease body movements during sleep, and all cause difficulty in arousal. All hypnotics are general CNS depressants and not specific sleep-promoting compounds, and in large enough doses or with long-acting compounds, all depress waking function. There are short- and long-term costs as well as benefits. The aim of a good night's sleep should be to improve vigour the next day – this has rarely been demonstrated as a consequence of hypnotic drug use.

MANAGEMENT OF INSOMNIA (Tables 9.1 and 9.2)

Drug treatment for insomnia is all too often casual and incorrect. In many forms of insomnia, *non-hypnotic* drugs are better than hypnotics. In post-encephalitic parkinsonism, for example, *amphetamines* may actually improve sleep. In

Table 9.1. *Duration of clinical effect and specific uses of selected benzodiazepine hypnotics*

Drug	Duration of sedative effect (h)	Particular use
Triazolam (0.125–0.25 mg)	3–4	Onset insomnia
Temazepam (10–30 mg) ⎫ Lormetazepam (0.5–1 mg) ⎬	6–8	Nocturnal awakenings
Nitrazepam (2.5–10 mg)	8–12	Early morning waking
Flurazepam (15–30 mg)	12 or more	Persistent sedation

Table 9.2.   *Management of insomnia*

Physiological variants of normal	
1. Advanced age (sleep apnoea, myoclonus, anxiety, depression, general medical illness and musculoskeletal pain all common)	(a) Sleep hygiene (b) Long-acting hypnotic with anxiolytic effect may be preferred by patient (c) Audiotapes: e.g. *Sleep without Drugs* (Gerald Bennett, clinical psychologist, 120 Rochdale Road, Todmorden, OL14 7NA, UK)
2. Transient and situational pain or anxiety	(a) Analgesics (b) Diazepam 5–10 mg
3. Sleep–wake cycle disturbances, e.g. jet flight or shiftwork	e.g. travel London–New York: take medium-acting hypnotic, go to bed 2100, get up 0600
4. Short sleepers (no complaint of insomnia)	No treatment
'Pseudo' insomnia	
1. Misinterpretation	Polysomnogram for diagnosis
2. Delusion of sleeplessness	Explain to patient
3. Hypochondriasis	
4. Need for a lot of sleep	
Psychiatric disorders and insomnia	
1. Endogenous depression	Sedative tricyclic (rarely stimulant antidepressant, e.g. protriptyline in presence of hypersomnia)
2. Severe anxiety:	
Onset insomnia	triazolam; chloral hydrate
Maintenance insomnia	temazepam (or nitrazepam)
Early morning waking	nitrazepam
Mixed onset and maintenance insomnia	nitrazepam, flunitrazepam
3. Psychosis	Antipsychotic
Parasomnia with insomnia	
1. Obstructive sleep apnoea	Relieve obstruction
2. Sleep myoclonus	Benzodiazepine
3. Bed wetting	Buzzer and pad
Medical disorders and insomnia, e.g.	
1. Ulcer pain	Cimetidine
2. Nocturnal angina	Nifedipine
3. Nocturnal asthma	Salbutamol
4. Parkinsonism	Levodopa
Drug-induced insomnia	Withdraw alcohol, coffee, tea, cola or chronic hypnotic overdose
Periodic insomnia	Check for endocrine disorder
Insomnia in special circumstances	
Childhood	Behavioural therapy
Pregnancy	No drug if possible
'Psychophysiological' in adults	Relieve stress, regular relaxation, sleep hygiene

The most important management of insomnia is removal or treatment of the cause, and alteration of inappropriate sleep habits. Hypnotics are often not the answer. If hypnotics are given, use short courses and low doses. Try alternate night therapy. Keep the treatment under review. Benzodiazepines and other hypnotics may increase nocturnal confusion, agitation and restlessness in elderly patients, and in children may displace night terrors to the daytime. Behavioural therapy and non-hypnotic drugs where appropriate are often more successful than hypnotics. Stop hypnotics on hospital discharge.

endogenous depression after a 2–3 week latency *antidepressant drugs* are the correct treatment. *Phenothiazines* or *haloperidol* will improve sleep in psychotics and *phenytoin* is of value when paroxysmal nightmares are a manifestation of psychomotor attacks. *Beta-adrenergic antagonists* will improve disturbed sleep in hyperthyroidism, *cimetidine* in peptic ulcer. Patients with pseudo-insomnia who complain of poor sleep but who have normal polysomnogram studies usually require no treatment, but it is possible that such patients need more sleep than normal and so a hypnotic may be appropriate.

When hypnotics are necessary, benzodiazepines are the drugs of choice, mainly on account of their effectiveness and high therapeutic index.[28] The choice of drug for sleep-onset insomnia (e.g. triazolam) and sleep-maintenance insomnia (e.g. temazepam) will be different, whilst if early morning waking is a problem, flurazepam will induce sleep of long duration. Many insomniacs are anxious during the day, and the anxiolytic effects of long-acting benzodiazepines such as flurazepam are of value to them. Hypnotics should not be prescribed indiscriminately. Ideally they should be reserved for short courses of treatment in the acutely distressed. The prescribing of hypnotics to children, except for occasional use, such as for night terrors and somnambulism, is not justified.

Data on the efficacy and toxicity of benzodiazepine hypnotics after single doses and during repeated use come from both controlled clinical trials and from sleep laboratory studies. Insomniacs are a heterogeneous group, and the two types of studies sometimes conflict, but two broad generalizations are possible. Benzodiazepine hypnotics are effective in the treatment of most types of insomnia; and most patients do not need long-term treatment.[23] Benzodiazepines are best given in short courses. After a good night's sleep, the drugs can be omitted for 2–3 nights. The hazards of well monitored treatment with hypnotic drugs are very small,[8] although true physiological addiction to benzodiazepines may nonetheless occur.[21]

Four groups of subjects should not take benzodiazepines or other hypnotics except in very low doses. These subjects include the pregnant, alcoholics, those who have to get up and function in the middle of the night, and those with symptomatic sleep apnoea.[57] Most benzodiazepines will increase the severity of sleep apnoea, although triazolam and flurazepam are said to be suitable in low doses,[28] i.e. 125 µg and 15 mg respectively.

The near total replacement of the 50 or more previously available *barbiturates* by the *benzodiazepines* has resulted from their lower toxicity rather than from any superior hypnotic effect. In particular, benzodiazepines cause less respiratory and cardiac depression than barbiturates, although overdosage will cause respiratory failure.

Barbiturates produce tolerance to their central and metabolic effects with an increase in metabolism and elimination following the induction of hepatic microsomal enzymes, so that the effectiveness of a constant dose of, for example, phenobarbitone rapidly wanes. Tolerance to benzodiazepines does occur, but is less marked and never complete. Barbiturates were (and are) very effective hypnotics. Many derivatives of barbituric acid were once available, mainly distinguished by their duration of action. However, barbiturates have many drawbacks with frequent cumulation, physical dependence, withdrawal symptoms and, in mild overdosage, causing profound sleep and respiratory depression followed by cardiovascular collapse and death. However, there is little evidence for the once widespread idea that barbiturates specifically weakened the memory so that the first dose was forgotten, repeated doses being taken from the bedside bottle. This problem is not confined to hypnotic drugs alone.

Chloral was the first hypnotic (1868) and is still useful today. It was introduced by Liebrich who knew that alkaline solutions liberated chloroform, and hoped, wrongly, that chloral would have the same effect. Although a gastric irritant, chloral hydrate 0.5–1 g is widely used and has a rapid onset of action. *Dichloralphenazone* (adult dose 650 mg tablets or elixir containing 225 mg/5 ml) and *triclofos sodium* 1–2 g (adult dose) cause fewer gastro-intestinal upsets than chloral hydrate. In both children and the elderly, elixirs of these drugs are useful hypnotics and allow for exact dose titration (chloral hydrate dose in children 30–50 mg/kg up to a maximum single dose of 1 g). Chloral should be taken well diluted to minimize gastro-intestinal disturbances, and may cause skin rashes as well as contact sensitivity.

Chlormethiazole (tablets of chlormethiazole base 192 mg: 2 tablets at bedtime) has the advantage of rapid elimination, and is a useful hypnotic in the elderly because of its freedom from hangover. As with all hypnotics, dependence may occur after a week or so of treatment.

BENZODIAZEPINES

Benzodiazepines (Table 9.3) were first synthesized by Leo Sternbach in 1933, and in 1956 his pharmacologist colleague, Lowell Randell, found that chlordiazepoxide had tranquillizing effects in animals.[25] The first benzodiazepine to be introduced for clinical use was chlordiazepoxide in 1960–1961, and this spawned a series of vastly successful drugs used in the treatment of insomnia, but also in the management of anxiety, tension, epilepsy, muscle spasm and a variety of psychosomatic disorders.

The mode of action of benzodiazepines remained unknown for almost two decades. With the discovery of gamma-aminobutyric acid (GABA) as the predominant inhibitory neurotransmitter in the CNS, and the demonstration that benzodiazepines facilitate inhibitory synaptic transmission at GABA-ergic synapses, it appeared that the hypnotic action of benzodiazepines was largely dependent on GABA mechanisms with selective reduction of excitatory inputs to cerebral neurones,[26] although non-GABA mechanisms may also be important. Previously Taylor and Laverty[66] and Wise et al.[75] had related the anxiolytic effects of benzodiazepines to changes in catecholamine metabolism and reduction in serotonin turnover in the brain.

Table 9.3. *Selected benzodiazepine hypnotics*

Approved name	Therapeutic adult dose (mg)		Major active metabolite	Elimination half-life* (h)
	Main effect hypnotic–sedative (single dose)	Main effect anxiolytic (per 24 h)		
Midazolam (induction anaesthetic)				1.5–2.5
Flurazepam	15–30		Hydroxymethylflurazepam	24–100†
Triazolam	0.125–0.25		None	2–4.5
Chlordiazepoxide		30–100	Desmethylchlordiazepoxide	5–30
Temazepam	10–30		None	4–8
Lorazepam		1–10	None	10–22
Nitrazepam	2.5–10		None	18–28
Clonazepam	1–4	2–6	None	22–38
Clobazam		20–30	N-desmethylclobazam	18–22
Diazepam	10	10–60	Desmethyldiazepam	20–100

*Duration of clinical action may be much shorter than elimination half-life.
†Metabolite half-life.

30–40% of all synapses in the mammalian CNS are GABA-ergic. Most GABA-ergic neurones are interneurones. The GABA content is highest in the substantia nigra, globus pallidus and hypothalamus. GABA levels are very low or undetectable outside the brain.

Several types of GABA receptor exist.[7] These are blocked by two classes of convulsant agent, GABA receptor antagonists (e.g. bicuculline) or drugs that block chloride channels (e.g. picrotoxin).

GABA and benzodiazepine binding sites can be anatomically separated, but there is considerable evidence that they are functionally linked. Dr. Michael Kuhar of Johns Hopkins University has developed methods of visualizing benzodiazepine binding sites by microscopy and autoradiography.[38, 77] Visualization has revealed that most if not all benzodiazepine binding sites are coupled to binding glycoprotein localized at GABA-ergic receptors.[69] Animal studies have revealed pre-synaptic benzodiazepine binding sites on 5-HT neurones, but very large doses of benzodiazepines are required to affect these systems and their function is unknown.

Intracellular recording studies have shown that, in the presence of GABA, a change in the permeability to chloride ion occurs at benzodiazepine receptor sites except when the benzodiazepine site is occupied.[16] Benzodiazepines modulate the action of the brain GABA-ergic inhibitory system by three mechanisms: (1) increasing the affinity of the GABA receptor; (2) improving the interaction of GABA with its receptor; or (3) improving the coupling between GABA receptor activation and chloride channel opening.[25]

Three kinds of benzodiazepine receptor, both neuronal and extraneuronal, have been recognized by autoradiography, termed BZD1, 2 and 3. No functional differences have yet been attributed to the different BZD receptor types, and it is not certain if any selectivity of effects of different benzodiazepines on sleep, muscle relaxation, sedation and ataxia can be attributed to any selectivity of receptor binding. These BZD receptors have a widespread but selective distribution in the brain stem, lamina 4 of the cortex, choroid plexus and around the ventricles, cerebellum, substantia nigra, and outside the brain in the stomach wall.[63, 64] Little is known of the function of extraneuronal benzodiazepine receptors. Perhaps cortical lamina 4 is a site where sensation can be eliminated on going to sleep. Many other drugs that cause sedation, opiates, barbiturates and serotonin, as well as benzo-diazepines, have binding sites here.

Most benzodiazepines show little or no receptor selectivity, although quazepam (but not its metabolites) preferentially attaches to BZD1 receptors.

No definite endogenous ligand for benzodiazepine receptors has yet been found in man. None of the various brain constituents so far isolated fills this role. Melatonin or its metabolites do bind to the benzodiazepine receptor, but the melatonin content in the brain is very low and it is unlikely that melatonin is a natural sleep-promoting compound. However, the search continues for a natural arousal-reducing, anticonvulsant and anxiolytic substance (or a substance with opposite effects; increasing attention, causing paroxysmal activity and anxiety).

NON-BENZODIAZEPINE HYPNOTICS

New classes of non-benzodiazepine hypnotic and anxiolytic drugs have recently been identified with a cyclopyrrolone structure. These novel compounds interact with benzodiazepine receptors and have similar hypnotic effects to ordinary benzodiazepines, although their chemical structure is quite different. Also they have somewhat different binding sites from benzodiazepines.[48, 76, 78]

BENZODIAZEPINE ANTAGONISTS

The introduction of highly specific benzodiazepine receptor antagonists such as the imidazobenzodiazepine derivative Ro 15-1788 has been a milestone in pharmacological research.[5] A number of drugs will antagonize benzo-diazepine-induced sedation or act as non-specific or specific benzodiazepine receptor antagonists.[67] These include amphetamine, naloxone,[55] protein modulators,[24] the calcium antagonist nifedipine[45] and a number of ß-carboline derivatives.[60]

Ro 15-1788 will immediately wake up patients severely intoxicated with benzodiazepines.[60] Normal awareness occurs within a few seconds of injection of the antagonist after flunitrazepam, followed 3–4 h later by a return of sleep. In addition to the reversal of benzodiazepine-induced sedation, some ß-carbolines have intrinsic alerting effects, and may also produce severe anxiety. The benzodiazepine receptor antagonist 3-hydroxymethyl-ß-carboline, which blocks sleep induction by flurazepam, by itself causes a dose-dependent increase in sleep latency in the rat.[43] Other benzodiazepine antagonists produce convulsions or a seizure-like EEG pattern in animals, or severe anxiety likened to a horror trip in man.

N-methyl-ß-carboline-3-carboxamide, a non-benzodiazepine that acts on brain benzodiazepine receptors, causes severe anxiety and panic, reversed by benzodiazepines. Dorow et al.[13] reported the effect of a 400 mg oral dose of this compound. 'The first drug effects lasted for 2 min and were accompanied by facial flushes, tremor and cold sweat. After 25 min a stronger attack started, with feelings of severe anxiety, inability to concentrate, and increasing inner tension and excitation. The volunteer tried to counteract these frightening symptoms with heavy breathing and stereotyped rocking movements. At all times, expressing himself in terse phrases, he was fully conscious and coherent in thought and speech. He later described his sensations as an impending fear of death or annihilation.' Within 90 s of an injection of lormetazepam 1 mg these symptoms faded.

ANXIOLYTIC AND HYPNOTIC EFFECTS OF BENZODIAZEPINES

Most hypnotic drugs also relieve anxiety (and most central stimulant drugs also produce anxiety). Drug effects on anxiety and alertness are difficult to separate, and most if not all benzodiazepines have anxiolytic as well as hypnotic effects. With most benzodiazepines, any selectivity of the behavioural effect depends entirely on pharmacokinetic factors. These include the dose (anxiolytic at low dose, hypnotic at high dose), the pattern of metabolism (many benzodiazepines are converted to the same metabolite, desmethyldiazepam, which has a very long half-life and is an effective anxiolytic), and the duration of brain receptor binding. The anxiolytic or hypnotic use of benzodiazepines is also determined by the pattern of research development and of clinical testing. Both anxiolytic and hypnotic actions are sustained for at least 6 months during long-term benzodiazepine use.[15]

However, not all the apparent differences between the anxiolytic and hypnotic effects of benzodiazepines may depend on pharmacokinetic factors. Oxazepam is not a very effective sleep-inducer, and anxiety may be reduced in doses that do not cause somnolence. With two short-acting drugs, triazolam 0.5–1 mg and temazepam 30 mg, temazepam may cause the least residual impairment for equal hypnotic effect.[4] A few clinical studies suggest that the incidence of drowsiness is lower with prazepam and other intermediate half-life benzodiazepines such as lorazepam and aprazolam than with other benzodiazepines in equivalent anxiolytic doses[3, 9] although these results are not entirely consistent, and results with prazepam probably depend on the slow appearance of desmethyl metabolites in the blood.[22]

Mechanism of anxiolytic effect

Two main theories of anxiolytic drug action have been suggested. (1) Redmond and Huang[56] suggested that the noradrenergic activity of locus coeruleus neurones was high in anxiety, and reduction in this played an important role in the anxiety-lowering role of benzodiazepines. A role for the locus coeruleus in anxiety is based on the results of lesion experiments in animals and of pharmacological experiments which alter the firing rate of locus coeruleus neurones. Locus coeruleus neuronal impulse flow is decreased by diazepam and other benzodiazepine anxiolytics and hypnotics. (2) Another theory considers that the anxiolytic effect of benzodiazepines is due to actions on GABA neurones throughout the CNS.[27] Neither theory may be correct. The non-benzodiazepine drug buspirone is an effective anxiolytic but causes an increase, not a decrease, in locus coeruleus impulse flow; it also does not potentiate GABA inhibition.[59]

BENZODIAZEPINE PHARMACOKINETICS

Pharmacodynamically, benzodiazepines are nearly identical. The differences between them arise from their different pharmacokinetics. The most important factors governing the choice of benzodiazepines in the treatment of insomnia therefore are the *dose,* the individual drug *rate of absorption,* the *bioavailability,* the *distribution half-life* (most relevant for single-dose effects), and the *elimination half-life* (most important with chronic treatment) (Table 9.4). There is

Table 9.4.   *Comparative effects of benzodiazepines with short and long half-lives*

	Elimination half-life	
	Short	Long
Tolerance	Rapid	Effective for several weeks
Early morning insomnia	Common	No
Daytime insomnia	Yes	No
Daytime anxiety	May occur	None
Daytime sedation	Slight	Moderate
Withdrawal anxiety and insomnia	Massive increase in sleep latency	Minor increase in sleep latency or no change
		Little or no rebound insomnia

no clear direct relationship between plasma benzodiazepine concentration and the clinical sedative or anxiolytic effect, but overall the behavioural effects closely mirror the pharmacokinetic properties.

Standard analytical methods for benzodiazepines allow measurements of only one compound at a time. This is essential for kinetic investigation of the parent drug, but is not satisfactory when the correlation to clinical effects is being assessed. Benzodiazepine binding equivalents in plasma do not always reflect brain levels at the receptor site, but plasma levels of benzodiazepine radio-receptor assay active material (i.e. parent compound and/or active metabolite[12]) may correlate better with clinical effects than measurement of parent drug.[30] In some instances, EEG studies are a more useful guide to clinical effects than plasma half-life studies, since they reflect persistence of the compound or active metabolites within the brain. Johnson and his colleagues have shown that the central action of benzodiazepines as indicated by increase in sleep spindles does not always match with the plasma benzodiazepine level, although it probably reflects the degree of benzodiazepine receptor activation in the brain.[32]

ABSORPTION AND SLEEP ONSET

Sleep induction by benzodiazepines depends entirely on the rate of absorption from the gut. This depends on the lipophilicity of the drug and also on drug formulation and capsulation. Most benzodiazepines are rapidly absorbed from the gastro-intestinal tract, but absorption is slowed by food as well as by antacids, so hypnotics should be given on an empty stomach. Blood–brain passage is less important, since this is rapid with all investigated benzodiazepines.

The absorption rate following i.m. injection of many benzodiazepines is slower than following oral administration.

In the treatment of sleep-onset insomnia the relative absorption rates parallel the clinical efficacy of *flurazepam* (rapidly absorbed), *triazolam* (intermediate absorption rate) and *temazepam* (slow absorption in hard gelatine formulation).[11, 17, 18] The time the medication is taken relative to going to bed is therefore of great importance.

The times to peak plasma concentration (t_{max}) with different benzodiazepines differ slightly. In healthy young adults, average values are *triazolam* 60 min, *lormetazepam* 90 min and *oxazepam* 120 min, although there are very wide individual differences with each drug.

BIOAVAILABILITY AND SLEEP MAINTENANCE

The duration of the clinical action of benzodiazepines in single-dose studies depends on the extent of benzodiazepine distribution, but drug accumulation becomes important with multiple doses. Accumulation is determined by metabolic clearance and elimination half-life. A long half-life by itself does not necessarily imply a long duration of sedation, nor does a short half-life imply a' short duration of action. The dose may be as or more important than the half-life since this will largely determine the degree of receptor binding in the brain.

Some short-acting benzodiazepine derivatives (e.g. *oxazepam, lorazepam, lormetazepam*) are almost completely inactivated by conjugation by one step in the liver, and have few residual morning-after effects. Indeed, rapidly eliminated benzodiazepines may result in early morning insomnia.[37, 39] Other drugs (e.g. flurazepam, nitrazepam) produce persistent long-acting metabolites and cause definite impairment in alertness, motor performance and cognitive function the morning after.

Benzodiazepine metabolism varies with the patient's ability to handle the drug and is largely age-dependent. The elimination half-life of diazepam in healthy male subjects may increase three- to four-fold from the age of 20 to 80, and the bioavailability of the drug is therefore greatly increased.

It is possible to obtain benzodiazepines with practically any half-life from the ultra-short *midazolam* (1–2 h) and *triazolam* (3 h) to *desmethyldiazepam* (80–100 h).

METABOLISM

Most benzodiazepines are metabolized in the liver and some produce numerous active metabolites. The pattern of metabolism of the different drugs is very similar and desmethyldiazepam has a central position. This substance is pharmacologically active and has a very long half-life, up to 100 h, which may explain the frequent persistence of hangover following for example diazepam, whilst in contrast temazepam which does not form this metabolite causes much less prolonged sedation. Benzodiazepines are mainly transformed in the liver by conjugation with attachment of the molecule to glucuronic acid and excretion in the urine of pharmacologically inactive metabolites. Acetamides, not glucuronides, are the major metabolites of the 7-nitro compounds. All 3-hydroxylated benzodiazepines (*temazepam, lormetazepam* and *oxazepam*) which are readily glucuronidized in the 3-position have similar elimination half-lives of 8–10 h in healthy young subjects. Although most of the biotransformation of the benzodiazepines takes part in the liver, Mahon *et al.*[41] showed rapid biotransformation of flurazepam in the small intestine in man.

The accumulation of active metabolites complicates the pharmacology of certain benzodiazepines. Failure of hepatic detoxication in cirrhosis or viral hepatitis will prolong the activity of some benzodiazepines, which then increase the degree of encephalopathy.

INDIVIDUAL BENZODIAZEPINES

Temazepam
With temazepam, the major metabolite is the inert glucuronide conjugate. Smaller amounts of temazepam are metabolized by N-demethylation to yield oxazepam, which then appears in the urine as oxazepam glucuronide. Divoll et al.[11] suggested that because temazepam is metabolized by conjugation rather than oxidation its metabolic pathway is less likely to be influenced by factors such as old age. In practice, any clinical advantage of temazepam over flurazepam or triazolam in old people has not been established. The Scherer soft gelatine capsule of temazepam in a solution of propylene glycol has a considerably shorter time to concentration peak (t_{max} = 50 min) than temazepam in hard gelatine capsules (t_{max} = 86 min).

Temazepam has been said not to accumulate, with a short half-life and with effects restricted to the night of ingestion. This is not strictly correct. The mean half-life of temazepam[11] is somewhere between 13 and 14 h, and in some individuals is longer than 30 h. As with all intermediate-acting benzodiazepines, big doses of temazepam (30–60 mg) are more likely to cause hangover effects than low doses (10–20 mg).

Triazolam
Triazolam is metabolized principally by hepatic microsomal oxidation. The rate of hepatic clearance is high, depending on liver blood flow as well as the activity of hepatic microsomal enzymes. Brotizolam[47] and midazolam[20] have similar pharmacokinetic profiles. All these drugs are rapidly or very rapidly eliminated following single oral doses, and would not be expected to accumulate. With triazolam, the half-life is between 1.5 and 5 h and any given dose is almost totally eliminated after 12–15 h. Non-accumulating hypnotics of this type have a number of advantages and disadvantages. The rapid elimination results in no hangover effect, but with very short-acting compounds early morning rebound insomnia and anxiety occur, and the disappearance of all the drug plus metabolites from the blood within a day of stopping long-term treatment may cause severe rebound of symptoms on drug withdrawal.[35, 36] Abrupt withdrawal may cause confusion, toxic psychosis, convulsions or a condition resembling delirium tremens, as well as sweating and diarrhoea. Long-term treatment should therefore be stopped slowly.

Flurazepam
Flurazepam produces a complex mixture of short-acting and long-acting metabolites. Hydroxyethylflurazepam and flurazepam aldehyde are both very

rapidly eliminated but desalkylflurazepam is eliminated very slowly with a half-life of from 40 to 150 h but as long as 500 h in the elderly.[19] With repeated dosing, steady-state levels of this metabolite are reached after 2–3 weeks, and accumulation causes impairment of waking performance although plasma desalkylflurazepam concentration does not parallel daytime drowsiness.[18] Single doses of flurazepam 15 mg will cause a full night's sleep with little residual impairment, but with 30 mg an anxiolytic effect is obvious the day after.

DRUG INTERACTIONS WITH BENZODIAZEPINES

Several drugs (e.g. *spironolactone, phenobarbitone*) stimulate the metabolism of benzodiazepines, but benzodiazepines by themselves are only weak hepatic microsomal enzyme inducers and, unlike barbiturates, benzodiazepines can be given quite safely with oral anticoagulants. The extent of plasma albumin binding varies from only a few percent with flurazepam to nearly 99% with diazepam, but competition for this with other drugs is clinically unimportant. The sedative effects of benzodiazepines are increased by combination with centrally acting *neuroleptics, tranquillizers, sedative antidepressants, hypnotics, analgesics, anaesthetics* and *alcohol*. In healthy young subjects given small doses of temazepam or loprazolam, moderate doses of alcohol produce no more than an additive effect and do not necessarily prolong the effects of benzodiazepines as they may do in the elderly and alcoholic. The elimination half-life of desmethyldiazepam is increased by *cimetidine*, and interactions between this drug and benzodiazepines are clinically important.

PREGNANCY, BREAST FEEDING

There is no evidence about the safety of benzodiazepines in pregnancy, nor is there any evidence from animal work that the drugs are free of hazard. Prolonged administration of low doses or high doses of benzodiazepines in the last trimester has been reported to produce irregularities in the fetal heart beat, and hypotonia, poor sucking and hypothermia in neonates.

Benzodiazepines cross the placenta and enter milk. Diazepam and nitrazepam are found in human milk at between 10% and 50% of the plasma concentration. Use during lactation should be avoided.

SIDE EFFECTS OF BENZODIAZEPINES

The non-sedative effects of benzodiazepines are usually not clinically important. Effects on *blood pressure* and *heart rate* are minor. Triazolam causes an increase in sleeping heart rate of around 2 beats/min. In normal dosages in normal subjects, there is little evidence of *respiratory depression*, although nitrazepam will cause an increase in PCO_2 in chronic bronchitics[58] and clinical doses of flurazepam may induce the sleep apnoea syndrome in patients previously with minor apnoea only.[44] Oswald and Adam[49] made the interesting observation that benzodiazepines cause a small *loss of body weight*.

Diazepam but not other benzodiazepines causes dose-dependent transient *analgesia* after intravenous administration. Hormonal effects are negligible. The decrease in the amount of slow-wave sleep seen after benzodiazepines is not associated with any decrease in sleep-related growth hormone output.[2] *Unpredictable effects* of benzodiazepines are rare. Stimulation rather than sedation may occur in elderly or psychotic individuals with paradoxical aggressive outbursts, excitement, confusion and the uncovering of depression with suicidal tendencies. Hypnagogic hallucinations at sleep onset are not unusual, and nitrazepam sometimes causes nightmares.

BENZODIAZEPINE EFFECTS ON THE EEG

Different benzodiazepines have similar effects on sleeping and waking. Waking, alpha activity is decreased, and there is often an increase in high-voltage fast activity over all parts of the brain, particularly over the anterior areas.

The amplitude and latency of cortical components of somatosensory evoked potentials may be changed by benzodiazepines although short latency components of visual and auditory potentials are not greatly altered.

All benzodiazepines cause striking EEG changes during sleep. With long-acting benzodiazepines these may persist at least 5 days, sometimes longer, and are probably directly related to the presence of active drug or metabolites in the brain. There is an overall decrease in the number of sleep-stage shifts throughout the night. In addition to these changes in normal sleep pattern, benzodiazepines induce hippocampus waves that never occur in spontaneous sleep.

There is no convincing evidence that any benzodiazepine has a specific effect on any stage of sleep. All shorten sleep latency, reduce night awakenings and increase total sleep time. The increase in total sleep time with benzodiazepines is greatest in subjects with previous short sleep times, least in those with prolonged sleep.

Benzodiazepines decrease NREM stages 1, 3 and 4, increase stage 2 sleep, increase the latency to REM sleep, and diminish REM sleep. These effects are similar to those of barbiturates but less marked. The reduction of REM sleep with benzodiazepines is accompanied by a decrease in the frequency of eyeball movements. Usually there is a reduction but sometimes an increase in the number of REM cycles, with a reduction in the number of epochs containing either single REM episodes or REM bursts. REM latency has considerable inherent variability and the response to benzodiazepines may be erratic with either a decrease or an increase in latency during chronic use.

REM sleep reduction by benzodiazepines is often most conspicuous during the first third of the night, and during chronic administration a late-night REM sleep rebound sometimes develops with short acting compounds[2] similar to that which develops after protracted use of barbiturates.[34] REM rebound on drug withdrawal is dose-related, obvious after large (20–60 mg nightly) but not after small (5 mg) doses of nitrazepam, other benzodiazepines and non-benzodiazepine hypnotics.[33, 51]

EEG measurements and in particular enhancement of fast frequencies (12.5–30 Hz), sleep latency and sleep quality are of value as an index of the CNS activity of different benzodiazepines. With lormetazepam, flunitrazepam and flurazepam there is a sound correlation between benzodiazepine activity in the plasma and an increase in ß frequencies in the EEG.[52]

THE DAY AFTER BENZODIAZEPINES

Using an exact dose schedule of nitrazepam 2.5–10 mg in two groups of subjects, light and deep sleepers, Peck *et al.*[53] showed that light sleepers felt more refreshed after nitrazepam 5 mg, and day performance improved rather than deteriorated, whilst all subjects were impaired after 10 mg. In practice, this fine tuning is very unlikely to be achieved in normal clinical practice. More recently Dement *et al.*[10] have shown that short-acting benzodiazepines (triazolam 0.5 mg) at bedtime are sometimes followed by increased alertness the next day whilst long-acting benzodiazepines (flurazepam 30 mg) are followed by increased daytime sleepiness. However, better sleep due to benzodiazepines is rarely followed by better waking performance the next day, unless this is impaired due to anxiety. In most subjects given both short- and long-term benzodiazepines, minor impairments in waking motor skills and vigilance tasks can be detected if the test used is sensitive enough. Residual effects may be more severe in subjects who usually sleep lightly than in those who are deep sleepers.[53] Impairment in skill is often but not always recognized by the subject.[6]

Benzodiazepines affect many different performance tasks the next day. Those investigated have included proof reading ability, the absolute auditory threshold, short- and long-term memory, the discrimination conditioning of the eyelid response, the speed of recognition of hidden words, the duration of visual after-images, saccadic eye movements, a rudder control task, memory of a telephone number, digit span, and the speed of putting caps on to ballpoint pens.[31] Performance in all these tasks is affected by many variables, including personality, memory and motivation, as well as by alertness. Overall, restful undisturbed sleep will produce an improvement of psychological performance whilst disturbed poor sleep causes a deterioration the next day. The effect of benzodiazepines can go either way; improved performance with better sleep, impaired performance with residual drug after-effects. In one study the ability to drive a car the next morning was found to be impaired after *flurazepam* 30 mg, but actually increased after *lormetazepam* 1.5 mg. Short-acting compounds without active metabolites in low doses have a profound advantage over long-acting accumulating compounds when morning vigilance is necessary.[74]

Physiological studies are less sensitive than behavioural studies to detect hangover effects of benzodiazepines. In drug-free conditions, the amplitude of some components (N200, P300) of evoked somatosensory potentials may be related to the state of alertness, excitation or perhaps even anxiety; their amplitude is proportional to the size of a bet (US $) in a computerized gambling task.[62] The long-acting metabolite of flurazepam, N-desalkylflurazepam, will reduce the amplitude of visual evoked potential components, but the effect is slight and non-specific.

Are serious accidents ever directly attributable to the residual effects of benzodiazepine hypnotics? Certainly gross amnesic states with lapses of memory and concentration, similar to senile dementia, can follow big doses of benzodiazepines in the elderly; and perhaps younger people should not drive to work or use risky industrial machinery the morning after big doses of benzodiazepines.

All hypnotics at some doses produce decrements in performance next day. Higher doses consistently produce more decrement than lower doses. The severity of post-hypnotic hangover and sedation depends on the drug, the dose and the patient's ability to eliminate benzodiazepines; basically on how much active compound remains in the brain after overnight drug distribution and clearance. The least likelihood of prolonged sequelae occurs with those drugs that are rapidly eliminated by biotransformation such as *triazolam*, or with those drugs with rapid and extensive transference to the peripheral tissues, such as *diazepam*. It is generally believed that long-acting drugs produce a greater impairment of waking performance the next day than short-acting drugs. The most important factor here, however, may be the size of dose rather than the elimination half-life.

BENZODIAZEPINE WITHDRAWAL

Withdrawal of hypnotics after long-term use almost always leads to a recrudescence of the original symptoms, difficulty in sleeping and anxiety. Although rebound insomnia was initially described with barbiturates, there is no doubt of its occurrence with benzodiazepines, but the frequency and severity vary.[46] Insomnia and anxiety usually lasts 2–3 weeks.[54] Rebound symptoms may be at least twice as severe as those initially present. Oswald *et al.*[50] found that for 2–3 weeks after lormetazepam withdrawal in poor sleepers, sleep latency and quality were worse than base line values.

Withdrawal symptoms can be minimized by tapering rather than stopping treatment (particularly important with drugs with short half-lives) and by ß-adrenergic blocking drugs.[1, 68]

Benzodiazepine withdrawal phenomena can occur whilst a drug is being administered (early morning insomnia and daytime anxiety) as well as on withdrawal (rebound insomnia and rebound anxiety).[35, 37] These effects, which are probably related to rapid drug elimination and drug-induced changes in benzodiazepine receptor sensitivity, may be entirely unexpected by the patient. The greatest degrees of disturbance are caused by the abrupt withdrawal of short half-life drugs (e.g. triazolam, midazolam and lormetazepam). Following withdrawal of long-acting benzodiazepines, anxiety, excess sensitivity to light and sound, systolic hypertension, tremulousness, autonomic overactivity, sweating and sometimes psychosis and epilepsy occur. Other undesirable side-effects of benzodiazepines, impairment of memory and sometimes psychiatric symptomatology with feelings of anxiety, confusion, depersonalization and hallucinations[70] may be related more to the direct effect of the drug than to drug withdrawal.

DEPENDENCE UPON AND TOLERANCE TO HYPNOTICS

Benzodiazepine hypnotics remain effective as sleeping pills for at least 6 months of continued use,[50] although they do produce adaptation and tolerance.[21] There is some evidence that benzodiazepines lose anxiolytic as well as hypnotic efficacy owing to receptor site changes as well as to enzyme induction and alteration in drug metabolism. Although most benzodiazepines do not induce their own metabolism, chlordiazepoxide, diazepam and flurazepam appear to do so, so that during repeated administrations the steady-state concentration in plasma may fall to negligible levels in the case of flurazepam, and the elimination half-life of the desamino metabolite also decreases.[29, 40]

Dependence on benzodiazepine hypnotics is not a major clinical problem, although Clift[8] indicated the importance of frequent review by the prescribing doctor. In the barbiturate era, Willcox[73] suggested that hypnotics should never be used each night and no more than six doses of barbiturates should ever be prescribed. Dependence and addiction to hypnotics are most likely in patients with a history of alcoholism or drug abuse, and in patients with severe personality disorders.

BENZODIAZEPINES IN THE ELDERLY

The metabolism and elimination of CNS depressant drugs is decreased in many elderly people who have a low renal glomerular filtration rate, possibly reduced hepatic blood flow and decreased activity of hepatic drug-metabolizing enzymes. Overall, benzodiazepine dosage should be at least halved in the elderly, and even then daytime alertness may be seriously impaired. The elimination half-life for diazepam is increased 60% in the elderly, and the apparent volume of distribution of the drug is also increased. In contrast, the elimination of oxazepam (which does not depend on desmethylation) is not altered by ageing.

Old people take sleeping pills much more often than young adults.[14] The theoretical choice of hypnotic in the elderly is undoubtedly a short-acting benzodiazepine given in low dosage. However, Wheatley[72] argues that many old people respond poorly to the short-acting drugs and prefer the longer-acting nitrazepam and flurazepam, not only on grounds of hypnotic efficacy but also for general daytime reduction of anxiety. One study has shown that lormetazepam 0.5 mg (with an intermediate elimination half-life of 5–15 h) is a suitable hypnotic in insomniacs over 55, increasing total sleep time by about 25 min without early morning rebound insomnia or clinically significant adverse effects.[71] However, rebound insomnia may follow long-term lormetazepam withdrawal.

The overall choice of benzodiazepine, both for the young and the old, lies between non-accumulating hypnotics with short half-lives, few adverse daytime sequelae, but an increased likelihood of rebound insomnia on drug withdrawal; and longer-acting compounds which cause more troublesome daytime drowsiness but fewer problems on withdrawal.

As an endpiece the following remedy for agoraphobia from E.-B. Gélineau is given:

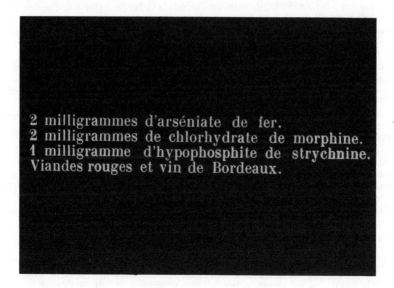

2 milligrammes d'arséniate de fer.
2 milligrammes de chlorhydrate de morphine.
1 milligramme d'hypophosphite de strychnine.
Viandes rouges et vin de Bordeaux.

REFERENCES

1. Abernethy, D.R., Greenblatt, D.J. & Shader, R.I. Treatment of diazepam withdrawal syndrome with propranolol, *Ann. Int. Med.* (1981) **94**, 354–355.
2. Adam, K., Adamson, L., Brezinova, V., Hunter, W.M. & Oswald, I. Nitrazepam: lastingly effective but trouble on withdrawal, *Brit. Med. J.* (1976) **1**, 1558–1560.
3. Ameer, B. & Greenblatt, D.J. Lorazepam: a review of its clinical pharmacological properties and therapeutic uses, *Drugs* (1981) **21**, 161–200.

4. Bond, A. & Lader, M. After-effects of sleeping drugs. In: Wheatley, D. (ed.) *Psychopharmacology of Sleep*, New York: Raven Press (1981) 177–197.
5. Bonetti, E.P., Pieri, L., Cumin, R., Schaffner, R., Pieri, M., Gamzu, E.R., Muller, R.K.M. & Haefely, W. Benzodiazepine antagonist Ro 15-1788: neurological and behavioural effects, *Psychopharmacology* (1982) **78**, 8–18.
6. Borland, R.G. & Nicholson, A.N. Comparison of the residual effects of two benzodiazepines (nitrazepam and flurazepam hydrochloride) and pentobarbitone sodium on human performance, *Brit. J. Clin. Pharmacol.* (1975) **2**, 9–17.
7. Browner, M., Ferkany, J.W. & Enna, S.J. Biochemical identification of pharmacologically and functionally distinct GABA receptors in brain, *J. Neurosci.* (1981) **1**, 514–518.
8. Clift, A.D. Factors leading to dependence on hypnotic drugs, *Brit. Med. J.* (1972) **3**, 4–7.
9. Cohn, J.B. Multicentre double-blind efficacy and safety study comparing aprazolam, diazepam and placebo in clinically anxious patients, *J. Clin. Psychiat.* (1981) **42**, 347–351.
10. Dement, W., Seidel, W. & Carskadon, M. Daytime alertness, insomnia and benzodiazepines, *Sleep* (1982) **5**, S28–45.
11. Divoll, M., Greenblatt, D.J., Harmatz, J.S. & Shader, R.I. Effect of age and gender on' disposition of temazepam, *J. Pharmacol. Sci.* (1981) **70**, 1104–1107.
12. Dorow, R. Pharmacokinetic and clinical studies with a benzodiazepine radio receptor assay. In: Hindmarch, I., Ott, H. & Roth, T. (eds.) *Sleep, Benzodiazepines and Performance*, Berlin: Springer Verlag (1984) 105–118.
13. Dorow, R., Horowski, R., Paschelke, G., Amin, M. & Braestrup, C. Severe anxiety induced by FG 7142, a ß-carboline ligand for benzodiazepine receptors, *Lancet* (1983) **2**, 98–99.
14. Dunnell, K. & Cartwright, A. *Medicine Takers, Prescribers and Hoarders*, London: Routledge and Kegan Paul (1972).
15. Fabre, L.F., McLendon, D.M. & Stephens, A.G. Comparison of the therapeutic effect, tolerance and safety of ketazolam and diazepam administered for six months to out patients with chronic anxiety neuroses, *J. Int. Med. Res.* (1981) **9**, 191–198.
16. Gallager, D.W. Benzodiazepines and gamma-aminobutyric acid, *Sleep* (1982) **5**, S3–11.
17. Greenblatt, D.J., Divoll, M., Abernethy, D.R., Moschitto, L.J., Smith, R.B. & Shader, R.I. Reduced clearance of triazolam in old age: relation to antipyrine oxidizing capacity, *Brit. J. Clin. Pharmacol.* (1983) **15**, 303–309.
18. Greenblatt, D.J., Divoll, M., Abernethy, D.R. & Shader, R.I. Benzodiazepine hypnotics: kinetics and therapeutic options, *Sleep* (1982) **5** Suppl. S18–S27.
19. Greenblatt, D.J., Divoll, M., Harmatz, J.S., MacLaughlin, D.S. & Shader, R.I. Kinetics and clinical effects of flurazepam in young elderly non-insomniacs, *Clin. Pharmacol. Ther.* (1981) **30**, 475–486.
20. Greenblatt, D.J., Lockniskar, A., Ochs, H.R. & Lauven, P.M. Automated gas chromatography for studies of midazolam pharmacokinetics, *Anesthesiology* (1981) **55**, 176–179.
21. Greenblatt, D.J. & Shader, R.I. Dependence, tolerance and addiction to benzodiazepines: clinical and pharmacokinetic considerations, *Drug Metab. Rev.* (1978) **8**, 13–28.
22. Greenblatt, D.J. & Shader, R.I. Prazepam and lorazepam, two new benzodiazepines, *New Engl. J. Med.* (1978) **299**, 1342–1344.
23. Greenblatt, D.J., Shader, R.I. & Abernethy, D.R. Current status of benzodiazepines (second of two parts), *New Engl. J. Med.* (1983) **309**, 410–416.
24. Guidotti, A., Toffano, G. & Costa, E. An endogenous protein modulates the affinity of GABA and benzodiazepine receptors in rat brain, *Nature* (1978) **275**, 553–555.
25. Haefely, W. Alleviation anxiety – the benzodiazepine saga. In: Parnham, M.J. & Bruinvals, J. (eds.) *Discoveries in Pharmacology, Vol. 1, Psycho- and Neuro-pharmacology*, Amsterdam: Elsevier (1983) 269–306.
26. Haefely, W., Kulcsar, A., Möhler, H., Pieri, L., Polc, P. & Schaffner, R. Possible involvement of GABA in the central actions of benzodiazepines, *Adv. Biochem. Psychopharmacol.* (1975) **14**, 131–151.
27. Haefely, W., Polc, P., Pieri, L. & Schaffner, R. Effects of benzodiazepines on the electrical activity of the central nervous system: Correlation with synaptic pharmacology. In: Saletu, B., Berner, B. & Hollister, L. (eds.) *Neuropsychopharmacology*, Oxford: Pergamon Press (1979) 449–458.
28. Harvey, S.C. Hypnotics and sedatives. In: Gilman, A.G., Goodman, L.S. & Gilman, A. (eds.) *The Pharmacological Basis of Therapeutics*, New York: Macmillan (1980) 339–375.
29. Hasegawa, M. & Matsubara, I. Metabolic fates of flurazepam. 1. Gas chromatographic

determination of flurazepam and its metabolites in human urine and blood using electron capture detector, *Chem. Pharmacol. Bull. (Tokyo)* (1975) **23**, 1826–1833.

30. Horowski, R. & Dorow, R. Die Bedeutung pharmakokinetischer Befunde für die klinische Wirkung von Benzodiazepinen, *Internist* (1982) **23**, 632.

31. Hindmarch, I. Psychological performance models as indicators of the effects of hypnotic drugs on sleep. In: Hindmarch, I., Ott, H. & Roth, T. (eds.) *Sleep Benzodiazepines and Performance*, Berlin: Springer Verlag (1984) 58–68.

32. Johnson, L.C., Spinweber, C.L., Seidel, W.F. & Dement, W.C. Sleep spindle and delta changes during chronic use of a short-acting and a long-acting benzodiazepine hypnotic, *Electroenceph. Clin. Neurophysiol.* (1983) **55**, 662–667.

33. Kales, A., Kales, J., Scharf, M.B. & Tjiauw-Ling, T. All-night EEG studies of chloral hydrate, flurazepam and methaqualone, *Arch. Gen. Psychiat.* (1970) **23**, 219–225.

34. Kales, A., Preston, T.A., Tjiauw-Ling, T. & Allen, C. Hypnotics and altered sleep–dream patterns, *Arch. Gen. Psychiat.* (1970) **23**, 211–218.

35. Kales, A., Scharf, M.B. & Kales, J.D. Rebound insomnia: a new clinical syndrome, *Science* (1978) **201**, 1039–1041.

36. Kales, A., Scharf, M.B., Kales, J.D. & Soldatos, C.R. Rebound insomnia: a potential hazard following withdrawal of certain benzodiazepines, *J. Am. Med. Assoc.* (1979) **241**, 1692–1695.

37. Kales, A., Soldatos, C.R., Bixler, E.O. & Kales, J.D. Early morning insomnia with rapidly eliminated benzodiazepines, *Science* (1983) **220**, 95–97.

38. Kuhar, M. Autoradiographic localization of drugs and neurotransmitter receptors in the brain, *Trends Neurosci.* (1981) **4**, 60–64.

39. Lader, M.H. Insomnia and short-acting benzodiazepine hypnotics, *J. Clin. Psychiat.* (1983) **44**, 47–53.

40. Linnoila, M., Korttila, M. & Mattila, M.J. Effect of food and repeated injections on serum diazepam levels, *Acta Pharmacol. Toxicol. (Copenh.)* (1975) **36**, 181–186.

41. Mahon, W.A., Inaba, T. & Stone, R.M. Metabolism of flurazepam by the small intestine, *Clin. Pharmacol. Ther.* (1977) **22**, 228–233.

42. Mendelson, W.B. *The Use and Misuse of Sleeping Pills*, New York: Plenum Press (1980).

43. Mendelson, W.B., Cain, M., Cook, J.M., Paul, S.M. & Skolnick, P. A benzodiazepine antagonist decreases sleep and reverses the hypnotic action of flurazepam, *Science* (1983) **219**, 414–416.

44. Mendelson, W.B., Garnett, D. & Gillin, J.C. Flurazepam-induced sleep apnoea syndrome in a patient with insomnia and mild sleep-related respiratory changes, *J. Nerv. Ment. Dis.* (1981) **169**, 261–264.

45. Mendelson, W.B., Owen, C., Skolnick, P., Paul, S.M., Martin, J.V., Ko, G. & Wagner, R. Nifedipine blocks sleep induction by flurazepam in the rat, *Sleep* (1984) **7**, 64–68.

46. Nicholson, A.N. Hypnotics: rebound insomnia and residual sequelae, *Brit. J. Clin. Pharmacol.* (1980) **9**, 223–225.

47. Nicholson, A.M., Stone, B.M. & Pascoe, P.A. Studies on sleep and performance with a triazolo-1, 4-thienodiazepine (brotizolam), *Brit. J. Clin. Pharmacol.* (1980) **10**, 75–81.

48. Nielsen, M. & Braestrup, C. Ethyl ß-carboline-3-carboxylate slows differential benzodiazepine receptor interaction, *Nature* (1980) **286**, 606–607.

49. Oswald, I. & Adam, K. Benzodiazepines cause small loss of body weight, *Brit. Med. J.* (1980) **281**, 1039–1040.

50. Oswald, I., French, C., Adam, K. & Gilham, J. Benzodiazepine hypnotics remain effective for 24 weeks, *Brit. Med. J.* (1982) **284**, 860–863.

51. Oswald, I. & Priest, R.G. Five weeks to escape the sleeping-pill habit, *Brit. Med. J.* (1965) **2**, 1093–1095.

52. Ott, H. Are electroencephalographic and psychomotor measures sensitive in detecting residual sequelae of benzodiazepine hypnotics? In: Hindmarch, I., Ott, H. & Roth, T. (eds.) *Sleep Benzodiazepines and Performance*, Berlin: Springer Verlag (1984) 133–151.

53. Peck, A.W., Bye, C.E. & Claridge, R. Difference between light and sound sleepers in the residual effect of nitrazepam, *Brit. J. Clin. Pharmacol.* (1977) **4**, 101–108.

54. Petursson, H. & Lader, M.H. Withdrawal from long-term benzodiazepine treatment, *Brit. Med. J.* (1981) **283**, 643–645.

55. Pitt-Miller, P. Reversal of flunitrazepam-induced drowsiness with naloxone, *Anaesthesia* (1982) **37**, 1216.

56. Redmond, D.E. & Huang, Y.H. New evidence for a locus coeruleus norepinephrine connection with anxiety, *Life Sci.* (1979) **25**, 2149–2162.

57. Roth, T., Zorick, F., Wittig, R. & Roehrs, T. Pharmacological and medical considerations in hypnotic use, *Sleep* (1982) **5**, S46–52.
58. Rudolf, M., Geddis, D.M., Turner, J.A.McM. & Saunders, K.B. Depression of central respiratory drive by nitrazepam, *Thorax* (1978) **33**, 97–100.
59. Sanghera, M.K. & German, D.C. The effects of benzodiazepine and non-benzodiazepine anxiolytics on locus coeruleus unit activity, *J. Neural Transmiss.* (1983) **57**, 267–279.
60. Scollo-Lavizzari, G. First clinical investigation of the benzodiazepine antagonist Ro 15-1788 in comatose patients, *Eur. Neurol.* (1983) **22**, 7–11.
61. Stone, B.M. Diazepam and its hydroxylated metabolites: studies on sleep in healthy men, *Brit. J. Clin. Pharmacol.* (1979) **8**, 57S.
62. Sutton, S. P300 – Thirteen years later. In: Begleiter, H. (ed.) *Evoked Brain Potentials and Behaviour*, New York: Plenum Press (1979).
63. Tallman, J.F. Benzodiazepines: from receptor to function in sleep, *Sleep* (1982) **5**, S12–17.
64. Tallman, J., Paul, S., Skolnick, P. & Gallager, D. Receptors for the age of anxiety: molecular pharmacology of the benzodiazepines, *Science* (1980) **207**, 274–281.
65. Tallman, J.F., Thomas, J.W. & Gallager, D.W. GABA-ergic modulation of benzodiazepine binding site sensitivity, *Nature* (1978) **274**, 383–385.
66. Taylor, K.M. & Laverty, R. The effect of chlordiazepoxide, diazepam and nitrazepam on catecholamine metabolism in regions of the rat brain, *Eur. J. Pharmacol.* (1969) **8**, 296–301.
67. Tenen, S.S. & Hirsch, J.D. Beta-carboline-3-carboxylic acid ethyl ester antagonizes diazepam activity, *Nature* (1980) **288**, 609–610.
68. Tyrer, P., Rutherford, D. & Huggett, T. Benzodiazepine withdrawal symptoms and propranolol, *Lancet* (1981) **1**, 520–522.
69. Understall, J., Kuhar, M., Niehoff, D. & Palacios, J. Benzodiazepine receptors are coupled to a subpopulation of gamma-aminobutyric acid (GABA) receptors: evidence from a quantitive autoradiographic study, *J. Pharmacol. Exp. Ther.* (1981) **218**, 797–804.
70. van der Kroef, C. Reactions to triazolam, *Lancet* (1979) **2**, 526.
71. Vogel, G.W. Sleep laboratory studies of lormetazepam in older insomniacs. In: Hindmarch, I., Ott, H. & Roth, T. (eds.) *Sleep Benzodiazepines and Performance*, Berlin: Springer Verlag (1984) 69–78.
72. Wheatley, D. (ed.) *Psychopharmacology of Sleep*, New York: Raven Press (1981) 246.
73. Willcox, W.H. The clinical and pathological effects of hypnotic drugs of the barbiturate acid and sulphonyl groups, *Proc. Roy. Soc. Med.* (1927) **20**, 1479–1486.
74. Willumeit, H.P., Ott, H. & Neubert, W. Simulated car driving as a useful technique for the determination of residual effects and alcohol interaction after short- and long-acting benzodiazepines. In: Hindmarch, I., Ott, H. & Roth, T. *Sleep Benzodiazepines and Performance*, Berlin: Springer Verlag (1984) 183–192.
75. Wise, C.D., Berger, B.D. & Stein, L. Benzodiazepines: anxiety-reducing activity by reduction of serotonin turnover in the brain, *Science* (1972) **177**, 180–183.
76. Young, W.S. & Kuhar, M.J. Autoradiographic localization of benzodiazepine receptors in the brains of human and animals, *Nature* (1979) **280**, 393–394.
77. Young, W.S. & Kuhar, M.J. Autoradiographic localisation of benzodiazepine receptors in the rat brain, *J. Pharmacol. Exp. Ther.* (1980) **212**, 337–346.
78. Young, W.S., Niehoff, D., Kuhar, M.J., Beer, B. & Lippa, P. Multiple benzodiazepine receptor localization by light miscroscopic radiohistochemistry, *J. Pharmacol. Exp. Ther.* (1981) **216**, 425–430.

CHAPTER 10

AMPHETA-MINES AND OTHER DRUGS IN THE TREATMENT OF DAYTIME DROWSINESS AND CATAPLEXY

AMPHETAMINE

Amphetamine was first synthesized in 1887, but its psychostimulant action was not recognized until 1927 when Alles showed that the drug was a safer and also a cheaper alternative to ephedrine, which was in short supply.[2] Amphetamine is a powerful central nervous system stimulant drug. It will increase effort, elevate mood, prevent fatigue, increase vigilance and prevent sleep, stimulate respiration and cause immediate electrical and behavioural arousal from natural or drug-induced sleep. When exceptional endeavour is required, as for example in astronauts, with preservation of concentration and alertness, amphetamine will prolong effort and increase performance. By British law, dexamphetamine (dextroamphetamine, $(+)$-α-methylphenethyl-amine) must be included in the emergency supplies of lifeboats, and in the Second World War amphetamines were dispensed to both military and industrial personnel in belligerent countries. However, fatigue cannot be delayed indefinitely and its onset may be catastrophic.

The anorectic effect of amphetamine was discovered by chance. Prinzmetal and Bloomberg[135] noted that one of their patients being treated for narcolepsy by amphetamine, who was also overweight, lost a significant amount of weight on the drug. Lesses and Myerson[97] gave the racemic mixture d,l-amphetamine to 17 obese patients with very gratifying results. Not only did most patients lose weight but the drug also increased the patients' sense of wellbeing.

Alles' discovery followed the encephalitis lethargica epidemic and it was quickly found that amphetamine had an antiparkinsonian as well as a stimulant effect.[38, 106, 129, 161] However, from the onset the problem was obvious; because of the euphoria amphetamine produced, widespread abuse rapidly occurred in many countries. In the war, amphetamine had been supplied to paratroopers and commandos. British troops alone were issued with 72 million tablets. In Japan, methylamphetamine initially issued to munition factory workers flooded the civilian market at the end of the war.

The development of highly competitive sport with increased drug taking coincided with the period of amphetamine abuse, but also the development of sensitive gas chromatographic measurements of amphetamine and related drugs in the blood.[27] Amphetamines will improve the performance of athletes even at the peak of fitness, as well as of racehorses and greyhounds, but the price is disqualification if detected. A peak of amphetamine abuse occurred in the 1960s. Since then many countries have restricted or banned distribution. However, difficulties in supply have caused problems for narcoleptics who need rather than abuse these drugs.

CENTRAL STIMULANT EFFECTS OF AMPHETAMINE

The central stimulant effects of amphetamine are thought to be due to cortical stimulation and stimulation of the reticular activating system. Amphetamine causes a dose-related increase in subjective arousal with in high doses, irritation, aggression, agitation and sometimes violence. These results are different from person to person depending on the setting, mental state and personality of the individual. Indeed, a few subjects experience drowsiness, not increased alertness.[166] In a study of Danish office workers, Bahnsen et al.[9] reported that a third of those given amphetamines described an increase in alertness with difficulty in getting off to sleep, as compared to 6% of those given placebo. Lasagna et al.[95] found that amphetamine 20 mg s.c. given to 20 normal male subjects caused 12 of them to feel definitely more alert, although Hurst et al.[82] found that less than a third of subjects given d-amphetamine 15 mg thought the drug was stimulant.

MOTOR PERFORMANCE

The usual effect of dexamphetamine 10–30 mg is to produce wakefulness, alertness, self-confidence, ability to concentrate, sometimes elation and euphoria, talkativeness and increase in motor activity. More work can be done, but the number of errors is not necessarily decreased. Physical performance is also improved. In military field studies as well as in athletes the benefit is greatest when performance has been reduced by fatigue or lack of sleep. Smith and Beecher[157] found that athletes could swim and run faster and put the shot further 2 h after amphetamine 14 mg/70kg. In addition to an increase in twitch tension, amphetamine causes a fine *tremor*; familial tremor becomes much more obvious. Other motor effects of amphetamine are only seen in high dosage. *Orofacial dyskinesia* has been described as a sign of amphetamine addiction.[104] Unlike neuroleptic-induced tardive dyskinesia, orofacial dyskinesia with amphetamines is quickly reversed on drug withdrawal. *Choreo-athetosis* has been reported with methylphenidate,[51] and a curious motor disorder called *'punding'* by Rylander[144] is occasionally seen in addicts on big doses of amphetamines who develop choreiform or complex stereotyped behaviour (assembling or dismantling machinery, clocks or motors, or polishing their nails for hours on end). Although amphetamine usually produces *motor hyperactivity*, hyperactivity in children with brain damage may improve with amphetamine.[145] Amphetamine together with atropine produces a much greater increase in locomotor activity than amphetamine alone.

PSYCHOMOTOR EFFECTS OF AMPHETAMINE

Psychomotor performance is usually improved by amphetamine,[155] but this result is only seen for simple, not complex, tasks. Holliday[79] found that 66 young, tired students solved a greater number of simple arithmetic problems with less errors when given dexamphetamine 10 mg than 66 similar students who were given a placebo. Whatever the actual results of amphetamine on psychomotor performance tests may be, subjects often think they have done better than they have, and judgement is impaired.[158]

AMPHETAMINES AND MOOD

In controlled studies designed to evaluate the euphoriant effects of amphetamines, Lasagna *et al.*[95] compared amphetamine to pentobarbitone, morphine, heroin and placebo in 20 normal subjects. 13 of the 20 subjects considered that amphetamine was the most pleasant of these. However, prolonged use or large doses are nearly always followed by mental depression and fatigue.

AMPHETAMINE PSYCHOSIS

High doses of amphetamine cause psychosis although this is rarely seen with therapeutic dosages in narcoleptics. In addicts on large amphetamine doses (e.g. dexamphetamine 100–300 mg daily), a condition resembling paranoid schizophrenia with disturbances in perception, visual hallucinations, overt psychotic behaviour and paranoid delusions develops. Amphetamine psychosis usually rapidly resolves on stopping the drug.[33] Strangely, amphetamines are said not to increase alertness in schizophrenics,[66] but this may be the result of personality factors, not due to a basic defect of arousal or amphetamine handling in schizophrenics. In a few subjects, possibly those with incipient schizophrenia, amphetamine psychosis is chronic despite amphetamine withdrawal.[4] During psychotic episodes, the urinary excretion of catecholamines may be considerably raised.[87] The occurrence of psychosis is independent of plasma amphetamine concentration although this is usually very high. It may depend more on the accumulation of metabolites than of amphetamine.[99] Overall, amphetamine psychosis is much more frequent in psychotic patients or in drug addicts than in narcoleptics or those given amphetamine to control obesity.

AMPHETAMINE AND APPETITE

Amphetamine reduces appetite: a dog, but not a man, will stop eating entirely if given amphetamine an hour before the daily meal. Amphetamine reduces hunger in most but not all subjects.[14] Weight loss in obese humans is almost entirely due to reduced food intake with drug-induced loss of acuity of smell and taste, and only slightly to increased metabolism and increased physical activity.[73] Hollister[80] reported that the consumption of a standard chocolate milk shake was reduced in seven out of 12 normal male subjects given dexamphetamine 2.5 h previously. The greatest suppression of appetite occurs when plasma drug levels are highest.

How does amphetamine reduce hunger? The site of action is probably in the lateral hypothalamic feeding centre. Injection of amphetamine into this area, but not into ventromedial satiety areas, reduces food intake.[19] Peripheral actions of amphetamine on glucose metabolism are of secondary importance.[14] Tolerance to the anorectic effect of amphetamine develops rapidly, perhaps the reason why anorexia and weight loss do not occur during the long-term treatment of narcolepsy. When overeating is due to psychological factors, it is usually not limited by amphetamine.

AMPHETAMINES AND SLEEP

The need for sleep is reduced by amphetamines but it cannot be avoided indefinitely. Amphetamine reduces the frequency of attention lapses and microsleeps that impair performance after prolonged sleep deprivation, and improves the execution of tasks needing sustained attention. The effects of amphetamine are greatest when the person is sleepy. Moruzzi and Magoun[112] suggested that the alerting effect of amphetamine was due to the action on the reticular formation. There is a lot of evidence that amphetamines cause EEG arousal by actions at this site.[55] Dexamphetamine causes a fall in the threshold for EEG arousal elicited by electrical stimulation of the reticular formation.

Amphetamine increases the latency of onset of REM sleep, and suppresses this sleep phase from over 20% to less than 10% of total sleep time.[140] Amphetamine has less marked effects on other sleep stages.[90] Very low amphetamine plasma concentrations lead to obvious EEG effects.[111] Amphetamine derivatives (with the exception of fenfluramine) cause similar EEG changes, a reduction of REM sleep and an increase in wakefulness.[116-118] Waking, amphetamine causes a shift towards higher EEG frequencies; and sleeping, a reduction in delta sleep.

During prolonged amphetamine treatment, tolerance to the suppression of REM sleep occurs although some reduction of this sleep phase remains obvious. On stopping amphetamine, there is a considerable REM sleep rebound with short REM latency and increase in total sleep time, and up to 2 months may be needed for normal sleep patterns to return.[121, 123]

DEXAMPHETAMINE AND LEVAMPHETAMINE

Smith and Davis[159] found that dexamphetamine was at least twice as potent as the laevorotatory isomer levamphetamine in elevating mood in normal subjects. In elicitation of other CNS excitatory effects, the dextrorotatory isomer is 2–4 times more potent than the laevorotatory isomer. Hartman and Cravens[74] demonstrated that dexamphetamine had a greater effect on sleep than levamphetamine, and the effects of sleep deprivation are reversed more by dexamphetamine than by levamphetamine.[75] Passouant et al.[130] reported that dexamphetamine was two to three times more potent a stimulant than levamphetamine in narcoleptics, although levamphetamine was effective and sometimes satisfactory in patients who had not responded to dexamphetamine, or in whom this isomer caused dose-limiting side effects. Schwab and Passouant[149] described nine narcoleptics, in six of whom levamphetamine gave complete control of narcolepsy and in three partial control, with apparently less side-effects than from previous treatment with dexamphetamine. Similarly, Parkes and Fenton[126] showed that both isomers were effective in narcolepsy with no very great difference in therapeutic index. However, animal studies suggest that levamphetamine is slightly more potent than dexamphetamine in its cardiovascular action. With other phenylethylamines, the dextrorotatory isomer usually has a greater central stimulant effect than the laevorotatory isomer. In the extreme case of isopropylamphetamine, the dextrorotatory but not the laevorotatory isomer is a central stimulant drug. With naturally occurring catecholamines, laevorotatory adrenaline and noradrenaline are 7–20 times more potent than the unnaturally occurring dextrorotatory isomers.[17, 148]

Dexamphetamine and levamphetamine have several pharmacological differences. Dexamphetamine is more effective in increasing the concentration of homovanillic acid in the rat striatum than levamphetamine,[88] and the two isomers have different effects on catecholamine release,[109] dopamine and noradrenaline re-uptake[35, 168] and serotonin receptors.[31] The two isomers also have different effects on neuronal activity in the reticular formation.[139] The effects of amphetamine isomers have been investigated in parkinsonism and behaviour disorders[164] as well as in narcolepsy. Amphetamine psychosis is produced by approximately the same cumulative dosage of each isomer,[5, 165] whereas dexamphetamine is more potent than levamphetamine in the treatment of narcolepsy, parkinsonism, aggression and restlessness in hyperkinetic children and Gilles de la Tourette's syndrome.[7, 105]

SYMPATHOMIMETIC EFFECTS OF AMPHETAMINES

In man, amphetamine causes indirect alpha and beta adrenoceptor stimulation in the sympathetic nervous system resulting in systolic and diastolic hypertension, variable increase or decrease in heart rate (most often slowing), hyperthermia, mydriasis and contraction of the bladder sphincter, and, in high doses, cardiac arrhythmias. Tolerance to the cardiovascular effects develops rapidly, and with normal therapeutic doses in narcolepsy (e.g. dexamphetamine 10–60 mg daily) there is little or no change in cardiac output or cerebral blood flow. However, amphetamine has been associated with hypertensive crises, acute myocardial infarction[119] and intracranial haemorrhage amongst drug abusers.[40, 41, 45, 151] Amphetamine stimulates the respiratory centre in animals with increase in the rate and depth of respiration, but this is not conspicuous in usual doses in man.

AMPHETAMINE PHARMACOKINETICS

Amphetamine is well absorbed from the gastrointestinal tract. 30–80% of an oral dose is excreted unchanged in the urine. The metabolism and urinary excretion of amphetamine is pH dependent. At a low urinary pH little amphetamine is metabolized, but at a high urinary pH the aminoalkyl group undergoes oxidative deamination with the formation of benzoic acid. Thus at urinary pH 5 the elimination half-life of amphetamine is short, about 5 h, but at pH 7.3 this increases to 21 h.[13] Excretion is delayed and clinical effects are prolonged by sodium bicarbonate,[156] shortened by ammonium chloride. The remainder of a dose of amphetamine is hydroxylated in the liver and metabolized to phenylacetone and *p*-hydroxynorephedrine which may function as a false neurotransmitter. The accumulation of this metabolite has been held responsible for psychotic symptoms after prolonged use.[6]

Dring *et al.*[44] studied the fate of ^{14}C-amphetamine in three men each given 5 mg orally (about 0.07 mg/kg). 60% of the ^{14}C was excreted in one day and 90% in 4 days. 30% of radioactivity was accounted for by unchanged drug, 21% as total benzoic acid and 3% as hydroxyamphetamine.

Following oral administration of dextroamphetamine 10–20 mg, peak plasma concentrations of 400–900 nmol/l appear 3–4 h after administration (equivalent to peak plasma levels of 30–60 ng/ml following amphetamine 30 mg p.o.[47] These plasma drug levels are similar with dexamphetamine and levamphetamine and are determined by dosage as well as by urinary amphetamine output.[181] A comparison of benzamphetamine hydrochloride 75 mg as a single dose with the same formulation and total drug dosage, but given in 15 mg portions, shows that the latter drug regime, similar to that produced by sustained-release preparations, causes a more gradual and delayed response over a 12 h period.[147] Plasma amphetamine levels correlate with changes in alertness and also with anorectic effects[18] but not with psychotic symptoms.

AMPHETAMINE INTERACTIONS

Alteration in the activity of hepatic microsomal enzyme systems by the intake of other drugs or by disease can cause alterations in amphetamine metabolism. *Phenothiazines* prevent the central effects of amphetamines but also alter their metabolism. Thus *chlorpromazine, trifluoperazine, perphenazine* and *thioproperazine* increase the half-life of amphetamine in the brain but inhibit central behavioural effects, stereotyped behaviour in animals and euphoria in man. In contrast, *chlordiazepoxide, diazepam* and *diethyldithiocarbamate*, which increase amphetamine tissue levels, may prolong amphetamine-induced stereotyped face and mouth movements in animals[93] and possibly increase effectiveness in man. Several other drugs affect the central and peripheral effects of amphetamines by different mechanisms. *Monoamine oxidase (MAO) A inhibitors, nialamide, pargyline* and *tranylcypromine* inhibit the removal of amphetamine by the liver and potentiate all the effects.[169] Patients treated with these monamine oxidase inhibitors should not therefore take amphetamines. However, amphetamine is not a substrate for MAO B, and the *MAO B inhibitor eldepryl* can be safely combined with amphetamine; indeed, a small percentage of eldepryl is interconverted to amphetamine in the brain.

Tricyclic drugs inhibit the metabolism of amphetamine and enhance the behavioural effects, although the danger of interaction has been overstressed. The combination of amphetamine with tricyclic drugs may theoretically increase blood pressure, but amphetamine 10–60 mg (and also methylphenidate 10–60 mg and mazindol 2–8 mg) has been safely given with *imipramine* and *clomipramine* 10–100 mg daily[167, 184] in the combined treatment of narcolepsy–cataplexy. The dosage of amphetamine required to control narcolepsy is reduced by approximately a third by the simultaneous administration of tricyclic drugs.[30] In contrast to tricyclic drugs and to MAO A inhibitors, *haloperidol, reserpine* and *atropine* have no effect on amphetamine hydroxylation in the animal liver,[98] although they may reduce the central effects.

AMPHETAMINE TOLERANCE

Tolerance to the *central stimulant effect* of amphetamine develops in 30–40% of all subjects after a few days or weeks of repeated intake. Tolerance to the *anorexigenic effect* develops eventually in the majority of subjects. Tolerance may result from increased tissue affinity and changes in receptor sensitivity.[175] Some chronic amphetamine abusers handle amphetamine in an identical manner to drug-naive subjects, but in others who have taken amphetamine for long periods, the elimination half-life is longer and the apparent volume of distribution is higher.

NEUROCHEMICAL BASIS FOR THE CENTRAL ACTION OF AMPHETAMINE IN MAN

Amphetamine freely enters the brain in man, and the concentrations in cerebrospinal fluid and plasma are similar.[8] However, there are regional intracerebral differences in distribution and effects. Selective amphetamine accumulation occurs in a wing-shaped area of the mesencephalic reticular formation, revealed by autoradiography[132] and there are marked differences in the effect of amphetamine on adrenaline accumulation in different brain regions, with little or no effect in the striatum, hippocampus or cortex, but a marked reduction in the hypothalamus, medulla and cerebellum.[58] Amphetamine promotes the release of noradrenaline to a greater extent in the amygdala and hypothalamus than other areas.[48]

There is considerable evidence that the major central effects of amphetamine are mediated via catecholamine mechanisms.[28, 29, 34, 71, 137] Acetylcholine and serotonin mechanisms are less important.[39]

Amphetamine causes release of extragranular amines from central dopamine and noradrenaline neurones, and in high dosages (5–10 mg/kg) also from central serotonin neurones. This results in depletion of brain noradrenaline, but not of brain serotonin.[22, 23] The effect of amphetamine on catecholamine release is considerable. Besson et al.[16] showed that very low concentrations of amphetamine (10^{-6} mol/l) increased release of dopamine, synthesized from tyrosine by as much as 400–450%. Amphetamines also cause a partial inhibition of re-uptake of noradrenaline and dopamine.[56] Axelrod[8] showed that the re-uptake block caused by amphetamines was accompanied by a three-fold increase in noradrenaline and a two-fold increase in adrenaline metabolism.

Dexamphetamine causes a marked reduction in the firing rate of dopamine and noradrenaline neurones in the brain. In the locus coeruleus, the spontaneous activity of noradrenaline neurones is reduced to half to quarter of the previous firing rate by dexamphetamine 0.2 mg/kg.[64] Dopamine neurones of the area compacta and ventral tegmental region of the brain stem show a similar inhibition.[25, 26] Inhibition of neuronal firing is dependent on post-synaptic feedback pathways, since it is prevented by pretreatment with the inhibitor of tyrosine hydroxylase, αMPT. Indirect stimulation of catecholamine receptors caused by amphetamines thus leads to slowing of the firing rate of catecholamine neurones.

MODE OF ACTION OF AMPHETAMINES

Are the behavioural effects of amphetamine due to noradrenaline and dopamine release in the brain? This has been investigated by determining how specific receptor blocking drugs alter the central responses to amphetamine (these responses may differ between species and at different ages).[102] *Dopamine receptor blockade* with pimozide (or with chlorpromazine after several doses) will reduce or prevent the stimulant but not the anorectic effect of dexamphetamine 10–20 mg in normal volunteer subjects, and of extremely large doses (200 mg) in addicted subjects.[86, 153, 154] In contrast, *beta receptor blockade* by propranolol has no effect on amphetamine-mediated behaviour whilst *alpha receptor blockade* by phenoxybenzamine slightly increases the behavioural effects of amphetamines. Hormonal responses to amphetamine (potentiation of levodopa-induced release of growth hormone, and elevation of corticosteroids[15, 124]) are attenuated by adrenergic blockade.[141]

Catecholamine synthesis inhibition, like dopamine receptor blockade, will prevent most of the behavioural effects of amphetamine in man. Treatment with αMPT, an inhibitor of tyrosine hydroxylase and hence of catecholamine synthesis, prevents the effects of amphetamine in animals[163, 177] and amphetamine-induced euphoria in man, although tolerance develops rapidly.[67] However, catecholamine precursors – L-DOPA and DOPS – do not cause increased alertness or euphoria, and the central stimulant effects of amphetamine are probably due, at least in part, to non-catecholamine mechanisms.

Amphetamines alter *cerebral energy metabolism,* with an increase in the incorporation of glucose into brain glycogen and increase in activity of the cerebral enzymes, glycogen phosphorylase and synthetase[114] and depletion of glutamic oxaloacetic transaminase and glutamic pyruvate transaminase, both enzymes which are involved in the regulation of brain energy metabolism. Amphetamines cause variable alterations in ribonucleic acid and protein metabolism in the rat brain[42] with, in the plasma and a number of body tissues, an increase in concentration of free fatty acids.[70, 131] None of these metabolic changes has been definitely associated with behavioural effects; they may all be secondary to changes in blood flow or catecholamine systems caused by amphetamines.[114]

AMPHETAMINES IN HYPERKINETIC CHILDREN

It has been estimated that up to 5% of children may be hyperkinetic[162] and amphetamines have a dramatic effect in quieting a high proportion of these.[1, 21] However, the idea that amphetamine has a specific effect on motor hyperactivity in brain-damaged children has been questioned. In formal studies, stimulant drugs certainly increase learning ability and improve behaviour in over half all such children,[91] but exactly similar responses may appear in normal children.[138, 176] The calming effect of amphetamines in hyperkinetic children appears paradoxical but may be largely secondary to an improvement in awareness with better concentration.[94]

TREATMENT OF NARCOLEPSY

Practically all the known drugs that act on the central nervous system (hypnotics, anti-epileptics and vitamins as well as central stimulants) have been tried at some time or other as possible treatments for narcolepsy. With the exception of amphetamine and related compounds with a phenylethylamine structure most of these drugs are not very effective. The earliest successful treatment in Europe may have been with *caffeine*.[178] The sympathomimetic amines were introduced in the 1930s (*ephedrine,*[85] *benzedrine,*[135, 171] *dexamphetamine*[134]). Prinzmetal and Bloomberg[135] first used *racemic amphetamine* in narcolepsy because of the observation by Alles[2] that the respiratory stimulant and analeptic effect of the drug was much greater than those of noradrenaline given systemically in amounts with a similar pressor effect, whilst overall the blood pressure raising potency of racemic amphetamine in high dosage was only 1/200 to 1/100 of that of noradrenaline. This treatment was far more effective than ephedrine, previously used for over four millenia as a stimulant in China.

Methylamphetamine, one of the most powerful stimulant drugs known, was used to treat narcolepsy by Eaton.[46] *Levamphetamine*, less potent than d-amphetamine (but according to Passouant, Schwab *et al.*[130, 149] with a greater therapeutic index than dexamphetamine) had a brief vogue in the 1960s. Yoss and Daly[183] recommended *methylphenidate* as the phenylethylamine of choice to treat narcolepsy, stressing the low incidence of peripheral sympathomimetic stimulation, although the drug was not compared to any other compound or placebo. A few drugs without the phenylethylamine structure are effective in narcolepsy but are usually less potent than amphetamine (e.g. *gamma-hydroxybutyrate*,[24] *mazindol*[128]). Table 10.1 shows, in alphabetical order, some of the other drugs that have been investigated, usually with limited or no success, or as in the case of *MAO A inhibitors*[179] associated with severe long-term management problems.

Table 10.1.   *Drugs used in the treatment of narcolepsy*

Amantadine[49]
Ascorbic acid[172]
Aspartic acid[127]
Carbamazepine[136]
Clonazepam[125]
Clonidine[125]
Dihydroxyphenylserine (DOPS)[68]
Glutamate[125]
5-Hydroxytryptophan (5-HTP)[184]
Levodopa (L-DOPA)[68]
Methysergide[180]
Opiates[72]
Thiamine[172]
Yohimbine[89]

PRACTICAL TREATMENT OF NARCOLEPSY

Most narcoleptics need to adapt their work and their lives to their sleep attacks. One or two planned day naps lasting 30–60 min usually after lunch and after tea are a good idea, and Roth[143] recommends a good sleep over the weekends. Shiftwork is usually unsuitable although it is sometimes easier to take a nap during night than day work. In addition to planning their lives, occupation and travel, a low to moderate dose of one of the available CNS stimulant drugs is usually necessary. No definite superiority of any single drug has been proven; all compounds of this class cause sympathomimetic side-effects, produce tolerance, and all have a potential misuse. Depending on drug availability in different countries, it is advisable to start with one of the less potent compounds (e.g. *mazindol* 2–8 mg daily in two divided doses at 0800 and 1200, or *fencamfamin* 20–30 mg twice daily) and reserve *methylphenidate* (10–60 mg daily) or *dexamphetamine* (10–60 mg daily) for those who do not respond well to less potent alternatives. Low rather than high doses (which only produce irritability, talkativeness and often sweating, but no further improvement in narcolepsy) should be aimed for. In 31 narcoleptics described by Guilleminault et al.[65] dexamphetamine dose ranged from 10 to 300 mg daily. Although six patients were taking doses higher than 100 mg daily, these were not more effective than lower doses in the control of narcolepsy and had the paradoxical effect of increasing rather than reducing daytime drowsiness. Three of these subjects improved with a lowering of amphetamine dosage. A small number of narcoleptics, however, continue to take high amphetamine dosage (150–300 mg daily), usually as a result of tolerance. Some narcoleptics undoubtedly misuse amphetamine for its euphoriant effect and show marked toxicity.

Approximately one third of all narcoleptics have a good and sustained response to *dexamphetamine* 10–30 mg daily, the response is satisfactory in one third, whilst the remainder report little improvement in their symptoms. These results are dependent more on plasma amphetamine level than on age, duration of narcolepsy or severity of attacks.

If tolerance to amphetamine occurs, this should be withdrawn for a 1–2 week period or another drug tried.

Some central stimulant drugs are slightly more cumulative than others (e.g. magnesium pemoline, fencamfamin) and the full effect may not be seen initially on starting treatment. A useful guide to dosage is a patient sleep diary. Narcolepsy is usually made worse by any daytime *sedative*, and long half-life *hypnotics, phenothiazines*, sedative *antihistamines* or *alcohol* will greatly increase daytime drowsiness although a pre-night sleep medium half-life hypnotic (e.g. temazepam 10–20 mg) may prevent night sleep fragmentation and improve alertness the following day.

SIDE-EFFECTS OF AMPHETAMINE (Table 10.2)

Serious problems with long-term amphetamine use are uncommon in most narcoleptics. The main complaints with dexamphetamine 20–30 mg daily are *minor irritability, sweating, difficulty in getting off to sleep* and sometimes *mood elevation, talkativeness* and *hyperactivity*. The acute administration of d,l-amphetamine 40 mg p.o. or s.c. causes a rise in *systolic blood pressure* of 10–60 mg,[171] but tolerance to the cardiovascular effects develops rapidly and chronic administration does not result in irreversible hypertension. The incidence of hypertension, angina and cerebrovascular disease is very similar in amphetamine-treated narcoleptics and age-, sex and weight-matched controls.[125]

Connell[33] reviewed the possible *teratogenicity* of amphetamine, but

Table 10.2.   *Side-effects of amphetamines in narcoleptics reported by 60 narcoleptic patients on long-term amphetamine treatment.*

Anorexia	2	Dyspepsia	2
Nausea	2	Temper	25
Irritability	26	Jittery	13
Insomnia	6	Palpitations	13
Headache	25	Muscle jerks	12
Oro-facial dyskinesia	3	Chorea	1
Psychosis	1	Tremor	1
Sweat	2	Hallucinations	1
Rash	1	No side effects	14

concluded that this was unlikely despite reports of cardiovascular malformations in the offspring of three women who had taken amphetamines early in pregnancy.

The possibility that amphetamine abuse may cause permanent *structural brain damage* was considered after the Japanese epidemic of abuse following the Second World War,[96] but this claim has never been substantiated. *Necrotizing angiitis,* indistinguishable from that of polyarteritis nodosa, has been associated with the abuse of high doses of methylamphetamine, and, in a single subject, with intravenous abuse of amphetamine. Other vascular complications of amphetamine are discussed on p. 463.

ALTERNATIVES TO AMPHETAMINE

Phenmetrazine
A number of alternative compounds to amphetamine have been produced both for the treatment of narcolepsy and the management of obesity, in the hope that these might prove to be less addictive or have a wider therapeutic ratio than amphetamine. Most of these have a phenylethylamine structure. *Phenmetrazine,* one of the first of these compounds to be introduced in the 1950s, was initially thought to have some anorectic effect but less of a stimulant action, but the drug was soon found to cause elevation of mood and psychosis, and like amphetamine came to be widely misused.[50, 103] Phenmetrazine 25–75 mg daily in 1–3 divided doses, like dexamphetamine, is effective in the treatment of narcolepsy.[20]

Methylamphetamine and methylphenidate
Methylamphetamine and *methylphenidate* may have greater central and less peripheral effects then dexamphetamine although methylamphetamine will cause myocardial depression[142] and methylphenidate causes fairly frequent sympathomimetic effects. Some phenylethylamines have different effects on alertness and on appetite, but the effect obtained largely depends on whether the subject is a normal volunteer, an obese weightwatcher or a sleepy narcoleptic. However, *methylamphetamine* and *methylphenidate* appear to have more stimulant than anorectic effect, *amphetamine* has both actions, and *fenfluramine* mainly causes appetite suppression. As well as differences in

Table 10.3. *Structure and activities of catecholamine and non-catecholamine stimulant drugs*

	β CH	α CH	NH	Benzenering substitutions
Adrenaline	OH	H	CH$_3$	3OH, 4OH
Noradrenaline	OH	H	H	3OH, 4OH
Dopamine	H	H	H	3OH, 4OH
Phenylethylamine	H	H	H	
Dexamphetamine	H	CH$_3$	H	

Drug	Average daily dose (mg) in obesity or narcolepsy	Stimulant potency	Anorexic effect	Sympathetic stimulation
Dexamphetamine (Dexedrine)	10–40	++	++	++
Methylphenidate (Ritalin)	10–40	++	+	+
Phenmetrazine (Preludin)	25–75	++	+++	+
Fencamfamin (Reactivan)	20–60	+	++	+
Phentermine (Duromin)	15–30	+	+	+
Diethylpropion (Apisate, Tenuate)	75–150	+	++	+
Mazindol (Teronac)	2–6	+	++	±
Fenfluramine (Ponderax)	20–40	±	+++	±

This table does not give an exact comparison of the behavioural effects of different drugs. These differ from person to person. Direct comparisons in narcolepsy are lacking. The effects are subjective and depend on drug dosages, urinary pH, presence or absence of psychological factors, obesity or sleep disturbance, and may be different in acute and chronic use. However, most of these drugs with the exception of fenfluramine are effective in narcolepsy.

behavioural effects, the pharmacological actions of different phenyl-ethylamines differ. Frey and Magnusson[54] showed that *p-chloramphetamine* and other chlor-substituted derivatives of amphetamine had similar central effects but unlike methylamphetamine lowered the concentration of serotonin, not of noradrenaline, in the brain. Methylamphetamine is a much more potent stimulant than these halogenated compounds.

Yoss and Daily[183] suggested that of the available drugs *methylphenidate,* a piperidine derivative related to amphetamine, and a mild central stimulant, 10–60 mg daily was the treatment of choice for narcoleptics. It produced good or excellent symptomatic relief in 49 of 60 patients, and had a better therapeutic index than dexamphetamine, i.e. a greater difference between the dose necessary to prevent narcolepsy and that causing severe side effects. Guilleminault et al.[65] also considered that methylphenidate gave at least as good control of narcolepsy as dexamphetamine in patients who had had both treatments, with little reduction of appetite or increase in blood pressure.

Similar claims have been made for methylamphetamine, but the widespread misuse of this highly stimulant drug has led to severe legal restriction on its manufacture, sale and prescription. Despite these claims, the pharmacological properties of methylphenidate and methylamphetamine are essentially similar to those of other amphetamine derivatives and, allowing for equivalence of dosage, the potential for abuse and also the therapeutic index are probably not greatly different.[46, 182] Millichap[107, 108] claimed that methylphenidate was superior to amphetamine in the treatment of hyperkinetic children considered to have mild brain damage, but this result may have been dose-dependent. High methylphenidate doses inhibit growth in children[145] and increase heart rate.[91] Like amphetamine, methylamphetamine and methylphenidate will cause acute visual hallucinosis.[100]

Magnesium pemoline

Pemoline (40–120 mg daily) has similar behavioural effects to those of methylphenidate (20–60 mg daily) although pemoline has mainly been considered as an appetite suppressant. Its main interest is its long half-life, and it can be given once daily. Like other CNS stimulant drugs, pemoline will reverse benzodiazepine and antihistamine-induced drowsiness[115] and interacts with MAO A inhibitors.

Fenfluramine

Fenfluramine has been considered to be an appetite-suppressant drug lacking any stimulant property. This is not strictly correct, although fenfluramine does not have the same euphoriant effect as amphetamine and because of this can be readily distinguished by addicts.[63] Fenfluramine does sometimes cause increased alertness, not drowsiness,[81] and drug withdrawal is often followed by depression, not elevation of mood.[122] No formal trial of fenfluramine has been reported in narcoleptics, but it is unlikely to be very effective and the EEG effects differ from those of amphetamine, although both drugs reduce REM sleep.[53] Any specific effects of fenfluramine in obesity may be due partly to a peripheral, not a central, action. Turner[170] showed that fenfluramine enhanced the uptake of glucose by skeletal muscle *in vitro*, an effect blocked by the 5-HT antagonist methysergide.

Other CNS stimulant drugs

Diethylpropion (75–150 mg daily) was introduced as an anorectic drug, thought to have less stimulant effect than amphetamine. For a given anorectic effect, diethylpropion has less stimulant action in normal volunteers and causes less locomotor hyperactivity in animals.[78]

Phentermine (Ionamin 15–30 mg daily) is a similar compound which lowers hunger and may be less stimulant than dextroamphetamine.[150]

Fencamfamin (Reactivan, 20–60 mg daily) is a fairly potent stimulant. In direct comparisons, fencamfamin 20 mg is approximately as potent as dex-amphetamine 10 mg in the control of narcolepsy and may have a more sustained action (Shindler, unpublished studies).

The use of the phenylethylamine derivatives has been mainly decided by the course of their clinical development; whether to control obesity, prevent hyperkinesis in children, control depression or fatigue, or to treat narcolepsy. However, all have common properties. They will all cause insomnia, restlessness, agitation, tachycardia, dizziness as well as tolerance, psychotic episodes and amphetamine-type dependence particularly in vulnerable personalities.[37, 83] The usual EEG effects and suppression of REM sleep are in most cases less marked than with amphetamine. Morselli et al.[110] showed that normal volunteers given phentermine 30 mg (with an elimination half-life, at average urinary pH, of 7-8 h) had only slight changes in the subsequent sleeping EEG.

In a narcoleptic on a normal diet and with a urinary pH of 5, the alerting effect of a single oral dose of *dexamphetamine* 10 mg lasts for 3-5 h, and of *mazindol* 2-4 mg slightly longer (5-6 h), whilst *magnesium pemoline* and *fencamfamin* only produce their full effect after 1-2 days of treatment. The elimination half-life of these compounds is shorter at low urinary pH. The average elimination half-life for *diethylpropion*[11] and its active metabolites is about 4-5 h and for *phentermine*[12] is 7-8 h.

Monoamine oxidase inhibitors

Two monoamine oxidase isoenzymes, MAO A and MAO B have been characterized. In the human brain, noradrenaline is a substrate for MAO A and dopamine for MAO B. Many MAO inhibitors show selectivity of enzyme inhibition although this may be dose-dependent, as with pargyline which inhibits MAO B in low doses, both enzymes in high doses. In contrast, eldepryl inhibits only MAO B. Both MAO A and MAO B inhibitors have been investigated in narcolepsy.

Baumgarten[10] treated narcoleptics with the MAO A inhibitor *nialamide* combined with ephedrine, with the assumption that nialamide would block deamination of the catecholamines released by ephedrine and thus prolong the alerting effect. However, the combination is potentially hazardous. Wyatt et al.[179] used the MAO A inhibitor *phenelzine* alone, and this successfully abolished both narcolepsy and cataplexy for up to a year in patients with previously intractable narcolepsy; although this finding remains to be confirmed. Phenelzine has less stimulant action than other MAO inhibitors and the usual effect on normal sleep is slight.[3, 57, 120] However, MAO A inhibitors do cause a minor degree of REM sleep suppression.[32]

The MAO B inhibitor *eldepryl* shows partial interconversion (10-40%) to amphetamine in the brain and might be expected to have some alerting effect in narcoleptics. However, with low dosages that have been investigated (5-10 mg daily, sufficient to cause inhibition of MAO B for 7-14 days) there is no obvious effect.[146]

Mazindol

Mazindol behaves pharmacologically like amphetamine but has a different chemical structure.[61] Mazindol 2-4 mg p.o. has few cardiac and vasopressor effects. In these doses mazindol produces central stimulation, a reduction in appetite and increase in alertness, but little or no change in mood.[60, 62, 69, 174] Mazindol 2-4 mg causes a minor increase in critical flicker fusion measures.[76]

Tolerance to mazindol is uncommon and abuse potential may be low.[36, 59]

The pharmacokinetics of mazindol have proved hard to evaluate since the active drug and its metabolites cannot be easily distinguished, with a combined elimination half-life of approximately 30–50 h. However, the usual clinical effect of a single oral dose is short, with a peak increase in alertness in narcoleptics at 2 h and some residual improvement at 6 h following mazindol 2–4 mg p.o.

The effects of mazindol on sleep are somewhat unusual. REM sleep is reduced but, unlike amphetamine, mazindol in low doses does not reduce total sleep time (Spiegel, see Parkes and Schachter[128]). In the treatment of narcolepsy, mazindol 2 mg is approximately equipotent to d-amphetamine 10–15 mg, causing a slight increase in alertness without subsequent depression, anxiety or irritability. Vespignani et al.[173] gave mazindol 2–5 mg per day to eight narcoleptics for 15–41 months with good results in six but minor side effects (dry mouth, irritability) in three. Mazindol, like all sympathomimetic drugs, will potentiate the pressor effects of catecholamines. It may cause anorexia, gastro-intestinal discomfort, insomnia, nervousness, dizziness, dry mouth, nausea, constipation, urinary retention and occasionally angioneurotic oedema, peripheral oedema and vomiting. Violent tremors have also been reported.[101]

The lack of euphoria and irritability is a notable feature in narcoleptics on mazindol. Götestam and Gunne[63] found in a group of prisoners who had previously abused amphetamine that mazindol did not produce the pleasant high or drugged feeling caused by amphetamine, and de Felice et al.[52] showed that mazindol could be withdrawn without features of physical or psychological dependence. However, the effects of high mazindol dosage on mood have not been investigated.

Ephedrine and caffeine

Ephedrine, obtained from the herb *ma huang*, has been used for at least 4000 years in China as a central stimulant. Ephedrine 30–60 mg 2–4 times daily causes increased alertness and prevents sleep in narcoleptics[43, 84, 85] but the effect is less than that of amphetamine 10–20 mg 2–3 times daily, and toxic side effects, tachycardia, sweating and headache are not uncommon. Very high ephedrine dosages (750–1000 mg daily) were used to treat narcolepsy by Sigwald et al.[152] but these doses may produce severe toxicity. Caffeine citrate[92] is a less potent alternative to ephedrine. The amount of caffeine in six cups of coffee has about the same alerting effect as dexamphetamine 5 mg.

Gamma-hydroxybutyrate

Unlike the drugs previously discussed, gamma-hydroxybutyrate (GHB) is a sedative, not a stimulant.[160] It occurs naturally in the brain and in the 1960s had a brief vogue as an intravenous anaesthetic, although results were inconsistent and anaesthesia was often followed by withdrawal hallucinosis, euphoria and disinhibition, tremor and involuntary movements. The neuropharmacological actions of GHB are complex, with an increase in dopamine and acetylcholine but not GABA levels in the brain, and an inhibition of firing in dopaminergic neurones. Taken orally, GHB has less dramatic behavioural effects than when given intravenously. GHB and its metabolite, gamma-butyrolactone, are unique in promoting day sleep accompanied by an increase, not a decrease, in REM sleep.

Broughton and his colleagues have investigated the use of GHB in narcolepsy to improve disturbed night sleep. Broughton and Mamelak[24] gave GHB 50 mg/kg every 24 h by mouth in divided nightly doses for up to 20 months to 16 patients with narcolepsy–cataplexy, and reported that in all subjects nocturnal GHB resulted in a reduction in day sleep attacks as well as improvement in night sleep. The patients had to be given several doses of GHB each night since this is rapidly eliminated and a single oral dose of GHB promotes sleep for only a short period (2–4 h). Despite GHB, small morning doses of methylphenidate remained necessary.

In contrast to the beneficial results of oral GHB in narcolepsy, Price et al.[133] reported that intravenous use was followed by a very high incidence of side-effects, impaired motor control, visual hallucinosis, slurred speech and nystagmus, euphoria and disinhibition, with precipitation of sleep apnoea in one subject. If nocturnal sleep disturbance is an important cause of daytime drowsiness in narcolepsy, a short-acting oral nocturnal benzodiazepine may be as effective as GHB in improving night sleep and reducing day sleep.

TREATMENT OF CATAPLEXY (Table 10.4)

Tricyclic drugs prevent cataplexy and also sleep paralysis, although they do not usually abolish other forms of sudden atonia or drop attacks. *Imipramine, desipramine (desmethylimipramine)* and in particular *clomipramine* reduce or abolish cataplexy in over two-thirds of all narcoleptics.[77] Cataplexy is abolished with low drug doses (e.g. clomipramine 10 mg daily), smaller than those usually necessary for an antidepressant effect, and the effect on cataplexy is obvious within 24 h of starting treatment. Withdrawal may be followed by a severe rebound of cataplexy lasting 3–4 days, and occasionally status cataplecticus. A small minority of subjects develop tolerance to tricyclics within 2–12 weeks of starting treatment. Even in low doses, these drugs can cause delayed ejaculation in males, with a gradual increase in weight in both sexes during long-term treatment. All these tricyclic drugs have an anticholinergic effect, and all inhibit REM sleep to a minor degree, although sleep returns to normal during chronic treatment with clomipramine. Clomipramine, a halogenated derivative of imipramine is five times more potent than the parent compound in the ability to block serotonin re-uptake, but less potent than other tricyclic drugs in the ability to block noradrenaline re-uptake. Whether these differences account for the high activity of clomipramine in cataplexy is unknown.

A few other drugs are sometimes successful in cataplexy. Cataplexy is most

Table 10.4. *Practical treatment of narcolepsy–cataplexy*

Narcolepsy	Average 24 h dose (mg)	Cataplexy	
Mazindol	2–6	Clomipramine	10–100
Dexamphetamine	10–60	Desipramine	25–100
Methylphenidate*	10–60	Imipramine	25–100
Other phenylethylamines e.g. fencamfamin	20–60	Clonazepam	1–4
Protriptyline	20–60	Anticholinergicst e.g. benzhexol (trihexyphenidyl)	5–15
Propranololt	40–120	Fluoxetine*	20–60
Gammahydroxybutyrate (GHB)*			
MAO inhibitorst			

* Not generally available in the UK.
t Ineffective in the author's experience.

Different drugs are needed to treat narcolepsy and cataplexy, although cataplexy usually improves somewhat with CNS stimulant drugs. Combined stimulant–tricyclic treatment is often necessary. Stimulants are not listed in order of potency, but in order of suggested therapeutic trial. Short to medium acting benzodiazepines (e.g temazepam) or nocturnal GHB may improve night sleep and allow for a reduction in day-stimulant dosage.

frequent when subjects are tired, so amphetamine is partially effective. *5-HTP*, alone or combined with a decarboxylase inhibitor, the MAO A inhibitor *phenelzine,*[179] *clonazepam*, and *fluoxetine* (Langdon and Shindler, unpublished data) all sometimes reduce cataplexy. Anticholinergic drugs usually do not abolish human cataplexy, despite their high efficacy in dogs.

As an endpiece, the following treatment for ecstasy from Gould and Pyle (1897) is given:

> **Treatment.**—The means of treatment, though not differing essentially from those proper for catalepsy, require, nevertheless, special mention of some particulars. The influence of moral force in preventing and curing ecstasy is well marked, and many instances are on record in which epidemics of it have been arrested by arguments addressed to the fears of the subjects. I have several times aborted and prevented ecstatic manifestations by making preparations to cauterize the region of the spine with a red-hot iron.

Over the last century medical treatment has been transformed, but will the genetic engineer of tomorrow look upon the benzodiazepines as we today regard the red-hot poker?

REFERENCES

1. Alexandris, A. & Lundell, R.W. Effect of thioridazine, amphetamine and placebo on the hyperkinetic syndrome and cognitive area in mentally deficient children, *Can. Med. Assoc. J.* (1968) **98**, 92–96.
2. Alles, G.A. The comparative physiological actions of dl-ß-phenylisopropylamines: Pressor effects and toxicity, *J. Pharmacol. Exp. Ther.* (1933) **47**, 339–354.
3. Akindele, M.O., Evans, J.L. & Oswald, I. Monoamine oxidase inhibitors, sleep and mood, *Electroenceph. Clin. Neurophysiol.* (1970) **29**, 47–56.

4. Angrist, B. & Gershon, S. Behavioural profile of a potent new psychotoxic compound, *Psychopharmacologia* (1973) **30**, 109–116.
5. Angrist, B.M., Shopsin, B. & Gershon, S. Comparative psychotomimetric effects of stereoisomers of amphetamine, *Nature (Lond.)* (1971) **234**, 152–153.
6. Angrist, B., Shopsin, B. & Gershon, S. Metabolites of monoamines in urine and cerebrospinal fluid after large doses of amphetamine administration, *Psychopharmacologia* (1972) **26**, 1–9.
7. Arnold, L., Kirilcuk, V., Corson, S.A. & Corson, E. Levoamphetamine and dextroamphetamine: differential effects on aggression and hypertension in children and dogs, *Am. J. Psychiat.* (1973) **130**, 165–170.
8. Axelrod, J. Amphetamine: metabolism, physiological disposition and its effects on catecholamine storage. In: Costa, E. & Garattini, S. (eds.) *Amphetamines and Related Compounds,* New York: Raven Press (1970) 207–216.
9. Bahnsen, P., Jacobsen, E. & Thesleff, H. The subjective effect of ß-phenyl isopropylaminsulfate on normal adults, *Acta. Med. Scand.* (1938) **97**, 89–131.
10. Baumgarten, H.G. Die behandlung der Narkolepsie mit Nialamid und Ephedrin, *Klin. Kschr.* (1968) **46**, 334–335.
11. Beckett, A.H. A comparative study of the phamacokinetics of fenfluramine, ethylamphetamine, diethylproprion and their metabolites, *Curr. Med. Res. Opin.* (1979) **6**, Suppl. 1, 107–117.
12. Beckett, A.H. & Brooks, L.G. The metabolism and urinary excretion in man of phentermine, and the influence of N-methyl and p-chloro substitution, *J. Pharm. Pharmacol.* (1971) **23**, 288–294.
13. Beckett, A.H., Rowland, M. & Turner, P. Influence of urinary pH on excretion of amphetamine, *Lancet* (1965) **i**, 303.
14. Bernstein, L.M. & Grossman, M.I. An experimental test of the glucostatic theory of regulation of food intake, *J. Clin. Invest.* (1956) **35**, 627–633.
15. Besser, G.M., Butler, P.W.P., Landon, J. & Rees, L. Influence of amphetamines on plasma corticosteroid and growth hormone levels in man, *Brit. Med. J.* (1969) **4**, 528–530.
16. Besson, M.J., Cheramy, A., Gauchy, C. & Glowinski, J. In vivo spontaneous and evoked release of newly synthesised dopamine in the cat caudate nucleus, *Adv. Neurol.* (1974) **5**, 69–78.
17. Biel, J.H. Structure-activity relationship of amphetamines and derivatives. In: Costa, E. & Garattini, S. (eds.) *Amphetamines and Related Compounds,* New York: Raven Press (1970) 3–19.
18. Blundell, J.E., Campbell, D.B., Lesham, M. & Toyer, R. Comparison of the time course of the anorectic effect of fenfluramine and amphetamine with drug levels in blood, *J. Pharm. Pharmacol.* (1975) **27**, 187–192.
19. Blundell, J.E. & Lesham, M.D. Hypothalamic lesions and drug-induced anorexia, *Postgrad. Med. J.* (1973) **51**, Suppl. 1, 45–54.
20. Bochnik, H.J. & Spiegelberg, U. Klinische und experimentelle EEG-Untersuchungen bei Gesunden, Epileptikern und anderen Hirnkranken mit Preludin (2-phenyl-3-methyltetrahydro-1,4-oxazinhydrochloride), *Psychopharmacologia (Berlin)* (1960) **1**, 493–505.
21. Bradley, C. The behaviour of children receiving benzedrine, *Am. J. Psychiat.* (1937) **94**, 577–585.
22. Breese, G.R., Cooper, B.R. & Mueller, R.A. Evidence for involvement of 5-hydroxytryptamine in the actions of amphetamine, *Brit. J. Pharmacol.* (1974) **52**, 307–314.
23. Breese, G.R., Kopin, I.J. & Weise, V.K. Effects of amphetamine derivatives on brain dopamine and noradrenaline, *Brit. J. Pharmacol.* (1970) **38**, 537–545.
24. Broughton, R. & Mamelak, M. The treatment of narcolepsy and cataplexy with nocturnal gamma hydroxybutyrate, *Can. J. Neurol. Sci.* (1979) **6**, 1–6.
25. Bunney, B.S., Aghajanian, G.K. & Roth, R.H. L-DOPA, amphetamine and apomorphine: comparison of effects on the firing rate of rat dopaminergic neurones, *Nature (New Biol.)* (1973) **245**, 123–124.
26. Bunney, B.S., Walters, J.R., Roth, R.H. & Aghajanian, G.K. Dopaminergic neurones: effect of antipsychotic drugs and amphetamine on single cell activity, *J. Pharmacol. Exp. Ther.* (1973) **185**, 560–571.
27. Campbell, D.B. Gas chromatographic measurement of levels of fenfluramine and norfenfluramine in human plasma, red cells and urine following therapeutic dose, *J. Chromatog.* (1970) **49**, 442–447.
28. Carlsson, A. Amphetamine and brain catecholamines. In: Costa, E. & Garattini, S. (eds.)

Amphetamines and Related Compounds, New York: Raven Press (1970) 289–300.

29. Carlsson, A., Lindqvist, M., Fuxe, K. & Hamberger, B. The effect of (+)-amphetamine on various central and peripheral catecholamine-containing neurones, *J. Pharm. Pharmacol.* (1966) **18,** 128–130.
30. Carlton, P.L. Potentiation of the behavioural effects of amphetamines by imipramine, *Psychopharmacologia* (1961) **2,** 364–376.
31. Cheng, H.C. & Long, J.P. Effects of d- and l-amphetamine on 5-hydroxytryptamine receptors, *Arch. Int. Pharmacodyn. Ther.* (1973) **204,** 124–131.
32. Cohen, R.M., Pickar, D., Garnett, D., Lipper, S., Gillin, J.C. & Murphy, D.L. REM sleep suppression induced by selective monamine oxidase inhibitors, *Psychopharmacology (Berlin)* (1982) **78,** 137–140.
33. Connell, P.H. *Amphetamine Psychosis,* Maudsley Monograph, London: Oxford University Press (1958).
34. Costa, E., Groppetti, A. & Naimzada, M.K. Effects of amphetamine on the turnover rate of brain catecholamines and motor activity, *Brit. J. Pharmacol.* (1972) **44,** 742–751.
35. Coyle, J.T. & Snyder, S.H. Catecholamine uptake by synaptosomes in homogenates of rat brain: stereospecificity in different areas, *J. Pharmac. Exp. Ther.* (1969) **170,** 221–231.
36. Craddock, D. Anorectic drugs, *Drugs* (1976) **11,** 378–393.
37. Csillag, E.R. Stimulant drugs – their use and misuse, *Med. J. Aust.* (1971) **1,** 968.
38. Davis, P.L. & Stewart, W.B. The use of benzedrine sulfate in postencephalitic parkinsonism, *J. Am. Med. Assoc.* (1938) **110,** 1890–1892.
39. Deffenu, G., Bartolini, A. & Pepeu, G. Effect of amphetamine on cholinergic systems of the cerebral cortex of the cat. In: Costa, E. & Garattini, S. (eds.) *Amphetamines and Related Compounds,* New York: Raven Press (1970) 357–368.
40. Delaney, P. & Estes, M. Intracranial haemorrhage from amphetamine abuse, *Neurology (Minneap.)* (1980) **30,** 1125–1128.
41. Delaney, P. & Estes, M. Intracranial haemorrhage with amphetamine abuse, *Neurology (NY)* (1981) **31,** 1059–1060.
42. Dewar, A.J. & Winterburn, A. Amphetamine and RNA and protein metabolism in rat brain, *Brain Res.* (1973) **59,** 459–470.
43. Doyle, J.B. & Daniels, L.E. Symptomatic treatment for narcolepsy, *J. Am. Med. Assoc.* (1931) **9,** 1370–1372.
44. Dring, L.G., Smith, R.L. & Williams, R.T. The metabolic fate of amphetamines in man and other species, *Biochem. J.* (1970) **116,** 425–435.
45. D'Souza, T. & Shraberg, D. Intracranial hemorrhage associated with amphetamine use, *Neurology (NY)* (1981) **31,** 922–923.
46. Eaton, L.M. Treatment of narcolepsy with desoxyephedrine hydrochloride, *Proc. Mayo Clin.* (1943) **18,** 262–264.
47. Ebert, M.H., Von Kammen, D.P. & Murphy, D.L. Plasma levels of amphetamine and behavioural response. In: Gottschalk, L.A. & Merlis, S. (eds.) *Pharmacokinetics of Psychoactive Drugs,* New York: Spectrum (1976) 157–169.
48. Ebstein, R.P., Ebstein, B.S. & Samuel, D. Differential sensitivity of amygdala and hypothalamus to amphetamine-induced release of norepinephrine, *J. Neurochem.* (1972) **19,** 2703–2705.
49. Ersmark, B. & Lidvall, H.F. Trial with amantadine in narcolepsy, *Psychopharmacologia* (1973) **28,** 308.
50. Evans, J. Psychosis and addiction to phenmetrazine, *Lancet* (1959) **2,** 152–155.
51. Extern, I. Methylphenidate-induced choreo-athetosis, *Am. J. Psychiat.* (1978) **135,** 252–253.
52. de Felice, E.A., Chaykin, L.B. & Cohen, A. Double-blind clinical evaluation of mazindol, dextroamphetamine and placebo in treatment of exogenous obesity, *Curr. Ther. Res.* (1973) **15,** 358–366.
53. Fink, M., Shapiro, D.M. & Itil, T.M. EEG profiles of fenfluramine, amobarbital and dextroamphetamine in normal volunteers, *Psychopharmacologia* (1971) **22,** 369–373.
54. Frey, H.H. & Magnussen, M.P. Different central mediation of the stimulant effects of amphetamine and its *p*-chloro analogue, *Biochem. Pharmacol.* (1968) **17,** 1299–1307.
55. Fujimori, M. & Himwich, H.E. Electroencephalographic analyses of amphetamine and its metoxyderivatives with reference to their sites of EEG alerting in the rabbit brain, *Int. J. Neuropharmacol.* (1969) **8,** 601–613.
56. Fuxe, K. & Ungerstedt, U. Histochemical, biochemical and functional studies on central monoamine neurones after acute and chronic amphetamine administration. In: Costa, E. &

Garattini, S. (eds.) *Amphetamines and Related Compounds,* New York: Raven Press (1970) 257–288.

57. Gillin, J.C., Horwitz, D. & Wyatt, R.J. Pharmacologic studies of narcolepsy involving serotonin, acetylcholine and monoamine oxidase. In: Guilleminault, C., Dement, W.C. & Passouant, P. (eds.) *Narcolepsy,* New York: Spectrum (1976) 585–603.

58. Glowinski, J., Axelrod, J. & Iversen, L.L. Regional studies of catecholamines in the rat brain. IV. Effects of drugs on the disposition and metabolism of H^3-norepinephrine and H^3-dopamine, *J. Pharmacol. Exp. Ther.* (1966) **153**, 30–41.

59. Gogerty, J.H. 57th Annual Meeting of American Societies for Experimental Biology, 15–20 April 1973.

60. Gogerty, J.H., Honlitan, W., Galen, M., Eden, P. & Penberthy, C. Neuropharmacological studies on an imidaze-isoindole derivative, *Fed. Proc.* (1968) **27**, 501.

61. Gogerty, J.H., Penberthy, C., Iorio, L.C. & Trapold, J.H. Pharmacological analysis of a new anorectic substance; 5-hydroxy-5-(4′chlorophenyl)-2,3-dihydro-5H-imidazo-(2,1-a) isoindole (mazindol), *Arch. Int. Pharmacodyn.* (1975) **214**, 285–307.

62. Gogerty, J.H. & Trapold, J.H. Chemistry and pharmacology of mazindol, *Triangle* (1976) **15**, 25–36.

63. Götestam, K.G. & Gunne, L.M. Subjective effects of two anorexigenic agents; fenfluramine and AN448 in amphetamine-dependent subjects, *Brit. J. Addict.* (1972) **67**, 39–44.

64. Graham, A.W. & Aghajanian, G.K. Effects of amphetamine on single cell activity in a catecholamine nucleus, the locus coeruleus, *Nature (Lond.)* (1971) **234**, 100–102.

65. Guilleminault C., Carskadon, M. & Dement, W.C. On the treatment of rapid eye movement narcolepsy, *Arch. Neurol.* (1974) **30**, 90–93.

66. Gunne, L.M. & Änggård, E. Pharmacokinetic studies with amphetamines – relationship to neuropsychiatric disorders, *J. Pharmacokinet. Biopharmacol.* (1973) **1**, 481–495.

67. Gunne, L.M., Anggård, E. & Jönsson, L.E. Clinical trials with amphetamine-blocking drugs, *Psychiat. Neurol. Neurochir. (Amst.)* (1972) **75**, 225–226.

68. Gunne, L.M. & Lidvall, H.F. The urinary output of catecholamines in narcolepsy under resting conditions and following administration of dopamine, DOPA and DOPS, *Scand. J. Clin. Lab. Invest.* (1966) **18**, 425–430.

69. Hadler, A.J. Mazindol, a new non-amphetamine anorexigenic agent, *J. Clin. Pharmacol.* (1972) **12**, 453–458.

70. Hajos, G.T. & Garattini, S. A note on the effect of (+) and (−) amphetamine on lipid metabolism, *J. Pharm. Pharmacol.* (1973) **25**, 418–419.

71. Hanson, L.C.F. Evidence that the central action of (+) amphetamine is mediated via catecholamines, *Psychopharmacologia (Berlin)* (1967) **10**, 289–298.

72. Harper, J.M. Gélineau's narcolepsy relieved by opiates, *Lancet* (1981) i, 92.

73. Harris, S.C., Ivy, A.C. & Searle, C.M. The mechanism of amphetamine-induced loss of weight, *J. Am. Med. Assoc.* (1947) **134**, 1468–1475.

74. Hartmann, E. & Cravens, J. Sleep: effects of d- and l-amphetamine in man and in the rat, *Psychopharmacology* (1976) **50**, 171–175.

75. Hartmann, E., Orzack, M.H. & Branconnier, R. Sleep deprivation deficits and their reversal by d- and l-amphetamine, *Psychopharmacology* (1977) **53**, 185–189.

76. Hedges, A. AN 448 on critical flicker frequency and heart rate in man, *S. Afr. Med. J.* (1972) **46**, 139.

77. Hishikawa, Y., Ida, H., Nakai, K. & Kaneko, Z. Treatment of narcolepsy with imipramine (Tofranil) and desmethylimipramine (Pertofran), *J. Neurol. Sci.* (1966) **3**, 453–461.

78. Hoekenga, M.T., O'Dillon, R.H. & Leyland, H.M. A comprehensive review of diethylpropion hydrochloride. In: Garattini, S. & Samanin, R. (eds.) *Central Mechanisms of Anorectic Drugs,* New York: Raven Press (1978) 391–404.

79. Holliday, A.R. The effects of d-amphetamine on errors and correct responses of human beings performing a simple intellectual task, *Clin. Pharmacol. Ther.* (1966) **7**, 312–322.

80. Hollister, L.E. Hunger and appetite, after single doses of marihuana, alcohol and dextroamphetamine, *Clin. Pharmacol. Therap.* (1971) **12**, 44–49.

81. Holmstrand, J. & Johnson, J. Subjective effects of two anorexigenic agents – fenfluramine and AN 448 in normal studies, *Postgrad. Med. J.* (1975) **51**, 183–186.

82. Hurst, P.M., Weidner, M.F., Radlow, R. & Ross, S. Drugs and placebos: drug guessing by naval volunteers, *Psychol. Rep.* (1939) **33**, 683–694.

83. Isbell, H. & Chrusciel, T.L. Dependence liability of 'non-narcotic' drugs, *Bull. WHO* (1970) **43**, Suppl. 1, 66.

84. Janota, O. Discussion of a paper by Pelnář: Narcolepsie avec cataplexie, *Rev. Neurol.* (1930) **47**, 427–428.
85. Janota, O. Symptomatische Behandlung der pathologischen Schlafsucht, besonders der Narkolepsie, *Med. Klin.* (1931) **27**, 278–281.
86. Jönsson, L.E. Pharmacological blockade of amphetamine: effects in amphetamine dependent subjects, *Eur. J. Clin. Pharmacol.* (1972) **4**, 206–211.
87. Jönsson, L.E., Lewander, T. & Gunne, L.M. Amphetamine psychosis: urinary excretion of catecholamines and concentrations of homovanillic acid (HVA) and 5-hydroxyindole acetic acid (5HIAA) in the cerebrospinal fluid, *Res. Comm. Chem. Path. Pharmacol.* (1971) **2**, 355–369.
88. Jori, A., Dolfini, E., Tognini, G. & Garattini, S. Differential effects of amphetamine, fenfluramine and norfenfluramine stereoisomers on the increase of striatum homovanillic acid in rats, *J. Pharm. Pharmacol.* (1973) **25**, 315–318.
89. Jovanovič, U.J. Suggestion for the treatment of sleep disturbances and conclusions. In: Koella, W.P. & Levin, M. (eds.) *Sleep: Physiology, Biochemistry, Psychology, Pharmacology, Clinical Implications*, Basel: S. Karger (1973) 145–163.
90. Kay, D.C., Blackburn, A.B., Buckingham, J.A. & Karacan, I. Human pharmacology of sleep. *In:* Williams, R.L. & Karacan, I. (eds.) *Pharmacology of Sleep*, New York: Wiley (1976) 83–210.
91. Knights, R.M. & Hinton, G.S. The effects of methylphenidate (Ritalin) on the motor skills and behaviour of children with learning problems, *J. Nerv. Ment. Dis.* (1969) **148**, 643–653.
92. Lader, M. Comparison of amphetamine sulphate and caffeine citrate in man, *Psychopharmacologia (Berlin)* (1969) **14**, 83–94.
93. Lal, S., Sourkes, T.L. & Missala, K. The effect of certain tranquillisers, chlorpromazine metabolites and diethyldithiocarbamate on tissue amphetamine levels in the rat, *Arch. Int. Pharmacodyn. Ther.* (1974) **207**, 122–130.
94. Lasagna, L. & Epstein, L.C. The use of amphetamines in the treatment of hyperkinetic children. In: Costa, E. & Garattini, S. (eds.) *Amphetamines and Related Compounds*, New York: Raven Press (1970) 849–863.
95. Lasagna, L., Von Felsinger, J.M. & Beecher, H.K. Drug induced mood changes in man. Observations on healthy subjects, chronically ill patients and past addicts, *J. Am. Med. Assoc.* (1955) **157**, 1006–1020.
96. Lemere, F. The danger of amphetamine dependence, *Am. J. Psychiat.* (1966) **123**, 569–572.
97. Lesses, M.F. & Myerson, A. Benzedrine sulphate as an aid to the treatment of obesity, *New. Engl. J. Med.* (1938) **218**, 119–124.
98. Lewander, T. Influence of various psychoactive drugs on the *in vivo* metabolism of d-amphetamine in the rat, *Eur. J. Pharmacol.* (1969) **6**, 38–44.
99. Lewander, T. On the accumulation of p-hydroxynorephedrine in noradrenaline neurones during chronic administration of amphetamine in the rat in relation to amphetamine tolerance, *Psychiat. Neurol. Neurochir.* (1972) **75**, 215–218.
100. Lucas, A.R. & Weiss, M. Methylphenidate hallucinosis, *J. Am. Med. Assoc.* (1971) **217**, 1079–1081.
101. Maclay, W.P. & Wallace, M.G. A multicentre general practice trial of mazindol in the treatment of obesity, *Practitioner* (1977) **218**, 431.
102. Marley, E. & Stephenson, J.D. Actions of dexamphetamine and amphetamine-like amines in chickens with brain transections, *Brit. J. Pharmacol.* (1971) **42**, 522–542.
103. Martin, W.R., Sloan, J.W., Sapira, J.D. & Jasinski, D.R. Physiologic, subjective and behavioural effects of amphetamine, methamphetamine, ephedrine, phenmetrazine and methylphenidate in man, *Clin. Pharm. Therap.* (1971) **12**, 245–258.
104. Mattson, R.H. & Calverley, J.R. Dextroamphetamine-sulfate-induced dyskinesias, *J. Am. Med. Assoc.* (1968) **204**, 400–402.
105. Meyerhoff, J.L. & Snyder, S.H. Gilles de la Tourette's disease and minimal brain dysfunction: amphetamine isomers reveal catecholamine correlates in an affected patient, *Psychopharmacologia* (1973) **29**, 211–220.
106. Miller, E. & Nieburg, H.A. Amphetamines. Valuable adjuncts in treatment of parkinsonism, *N.Y. State J. Med.* (1973) **73**, 2657–2661.
107. Millichap, J.G. Drugs in management of hyperkinetic and perceptually handicapped children, *J. Am. Med. Assoc.* (1968) **206**, 1527–1530.
108. Millichap, J.G. Drugs in management of minimal brain dysfunction, *Ann. N.Y. Acad. Sci.* (1973) **205**, 321–334.
109. Moore, K.E. Toxicity and catecholamine releasing action of d- and l-amphetamine in isolated and aggregated mice, *J. Pharmac. Exp. Ther.* (1963) **142**, 6.

110. Morselli, P.L., Maggini, C., Placidi, G.F., Gemini, R. & Tegnini, G. An integrated approach to the clinical pharamacology of anorectic drugs. In: Garattini, S. & Samanin, R. (eds.) *Central Mechanisms of Anorectic Drugs*, New York: Raven Press (1978) 243.
111. Morselli, P.L., Placidi, G.F., Maggini, C., Gomeni, R., Guazelli, M., De Listio, G., Standen, S. & Tognori, G. An integrated approach for the evaluation of psychotropic drugs in man, *Psychopharmacologia* (1976) **46**, 211–217.
112. Moruzzi, G. & Magoun, H.W. Brain stem reticular formation and activation of the EEG, *Electroenceph. Clin. Neurophysiol.* (1949) **1**, 455–473.
113. Nahorski, S.R. & Rogers, K.J. The incorporation of glucose into brain glycogen and the activation of cerebral glycogen phosphorylase and synthetase: some effects of amphetamine, *J. Neurochem.* (1974) **23**, 579–587.
114. Nahorski, S.R. & Rogers, K.J. The role of catecholamines in the action of amphetamines and l-dopa on cerebral energy metabolism, *Neuropharmacology* (1975) **14**, 283–290.
115. Newlands, W.J. The effects of pemoline on antihistamine-induced drowsiness, *Practitioner* (1980) **224**, 1199–1201.
116. Nicholson, A.N. & Stone, B.M. Effect of some stimulants on sleep in man, *Brit. J. Pharmacol.* (1979) **66**, 476P.
117. Nicholson, A.N. & Stone, B.M. Heterocyclic amphetamine derivatives and caffeine on sleep in man, *Brit. J. Clin. Pharmacol.* (1980) **9**, 195–203.
118. Nicholson, A.N., Stone, B.M. & Jones, M.C. Wakefulness and reduced rapid eye movement sleep: studies with prolintane and pemoline, *Brit. J. Clin. Pharmacol.* (1980) **10**, 465–472.
119. Orzel, J.A. Acute myocardial infarction complicated by chronic amphetamine use, *Arch. Int. Med.* (1982) **142**, 644.
120. Oswald, I. Sleep and its disorders. In: Vinken, P.J. & Bruyn, G.W. (eds.) *Handbook of Clinical Neurology, Vol. 3*, Amsterdam: North-Holland (1969) 80–111.
121. Oswald, I. Effects on sleep of amphetamine and its derivatives. In: Costa, E. & Garattini, S. (eds.) *Amphetamines and Related Compounds*, New York: Raven Press (1970) 865–871.
122. Oswald, I., Lewis, S.A., Dunleavy, D.L.F., Brezinova, V. & Briggs, M. Drugs of dependence but not of abuse: fenfluramine and imipramine, *Brit. Med. J.* (1971) **3**, 70–73.
123. Oswald, I. & Thacore, V.R. Amphetamine and phenmetrazine addiction. Physiological abnormalities in the abstinence syndrome, *Brit. Med. J.* (1963) **2**, 427–431.
124. Panda, J.N. & Ray, A.K. Effect of chronic use of d-amphetamine on transaminase activity of brain, *Int. J. Exp. Biol.* (1973) **II**, 345–347.
125. Parkes, J.D., Baraitser, M., Marsden, C.D. & Asselman, P. Natural history, symptoms and treatment of the narcoleptic syndrome, *Acta Neurol. Scand.* (1975) **52**, 337–353.
126. Parkes, J.D. & Fenton, G.W. Levo(−) amphetamine and dextro(+) amphetamine in the treatment of narcolepsy, *J. Neurol. Neurosurg. Psychiat.* (1973) **36**, 1076–1081.
127. Parkes, J.D., Fenton, G., Struthers, G., Curzon, G., Kantameneni, B.D., Buxton, B.H. & Record, C. Narcolepsy and cataplexy. Clinical features, treatment and cerebrospinal fluid findings, *Quart. J. Med.* (1974) **43**, 525–536.
128. Parkes, J.D. & Schachter, M. Mazindol in the treatment of narcolepsy, *Acta Neurol. Scand.* (1979) **60**, 250–254.
129. Parkes, J.D., Tarsy, D., Marsden, C.D., Bovill, K.T., Phipps, J.A. Rose, P. & Asselman, P. Amphetamines in the treatment of Parkinson's disease, *J. Neurol. Neurosurg. Psychiat.* (1975) **38**, 232–237.
130. Passouant, P., Schwab, R.S., Cadilhac, J. & Baldy-Moulinier, M. Narcolepsie-cataplexie. Étude du sommeil de nuit et du sommeil de jour. Traitement par une amphétamine lévogyre, *Rev. Neurol.* (1964) **III**, 415–426.
131. Pinter, E.J. & Pattee, C.J. Fat mobilizing action of amphetamine, *J. Clin. Invest.* (1968) **47**, 394.
132. Placidi, G.F., Masuoka, D.T. & Earle, R.W. Distribution of ^{14}C amphetamine in mouse brain: an autoradiographic study, *Brain Res.* (1972) **38**, 399–405.
133. Price, P.A., Schachter, M., Smith, S.J., Baxter, R.C.H. & Parkes, J.D. Gamma-hydroxybutyrate in narcolepsy, *Ann. Neurol.* (1981) **9**, 198.
134. Prinzmetal, M. & Alles, G.A. Central nervous system stimulant effects of dextro-amphetamine sulphate, *Am. J. Med. Sci.* (1940) **200**, 665–673.
135. Prinzmetal, M. & Bloomberg, W. The use of benzedrine for the treatment of narcolepsy, *J. Am. Med. Assoc.* (1935) **105**, 2051–2054.
136. Pruzinski, A. & Szulc-Kuberska, J. Carbamezepine in the treatment of narcolepsy, *Pol. Tyg. Lek.* (1973) **28**, 1244–1245.
137. Randrup, A. & Munkvad, I. Biochemical, anatomical and psychological investigations of

stereotyped behaviour induced by amphetamines in several animal species and man. In: Costa, E. & Garattini, S. (eds.) *Amphetamine and Related Compounds,* New York: Raven Press (1970) 695–713.

138. Rapoport, J.L., Buchsbaum, M.S., Zahn, T.P., Weingartner, H., Ludlow, C. & Mikkelsen, E.J. Dextroamphetamine: cognitive and behavioural effects in normal prepubertal boys, *Science* (1978) **199,** 560–563.

139. Rebec, G.U. & Groves, P.M. Differential effects of the optical isomers of amphetamine on neuronal activity in the reticular formation and caudate nucleus of the rat, *Brain Res.* (1975) **83,** 301–318.

140. Rechtschaffen, A. & Maron, L. The effect of amphetamine on the sleep cycle, *Electroenceph. Clin. Neurophysiol.* (1964) **16,** 438–445.

141. Rees, L., Butler, P.W.P., Gosling, C. & Besser, G.M. Adrenergic blockade and the corticosteroid and growth hormone responses to methylamphetamine, *Nature (Lond.)* (1970) **228,** 565–566.

142. von Rossum, J.M. Mode of action of psychomotor stimulant drugs, *Int. Rev. Neurobiol.* (1970) **12,** 307–383.

143. Roth, B. *Narcolepsy and Hypersomnia,* Basel: S. Karger (1980) 18.

144. Rylander, G. Psychosis and the punding and choreiform syndromes in addiction to central stimulant drugs, *Psychiat. Neurol. Neurochir.* (1972) **75,** 203–212.

145. Safer, D., Allen, R. & Barr, R. Depression of growth in hyperactive children on stimulant drugs, *New Engl. J. Med.* (1972) **287,** 217–220.

146. Schachter, M. & Parkes, J.D. Deprenyl in narcolepsy, *Lancet* (1978) **i,** 831.

147. Schlagel, C.A. & Sanborn, E.C. Comparative pharmacodynamic activity of single and divided doses of benzphetamine hydrochloride, *J. Pharmacol. Sci.* (1969) **58,** 1453–1456.

148. Schoot, van der, J.B., Ariends, E.J, von Rossum, J.M. & Hurkmans, J.T.

148. Schoot, van der, J.B., Ariens, E.J, von Rossum, J.M. & Hurkmans, J.T. Phenylisopropylamine derivatives, structure and action, *Arzneimittel-Forsch.* (1962) **12,** 902–907.

149. Schwab, R.S. & Passouant,, P. Scientific exhibit at the American Neurological Association, Atlantic City, New Jersey, 15–17 June 1964.

150. Seaton, D.A., Rose, K. & Duncan, L.J.P. A comparison of the appetite suppressing properties of d-amphetamine and phentermine, *Scot. Med. J.* (1964) **9,** 482–485.

151. Shukla, D. Intracranial hemorrhage associated with amphetamine use, *Neurology (NY)* (1981) **32,** 917–918.

152. Sigwald, J., Julou, L., Bouttier, D. & Thomas, J. Thérapeutique de l'hypersomnie, *Rev. Neurol.* (1967) **116,** 631–646.

153. Silverstone, J.T., Fincham, J., Wells, B. & Kyriakides, M. The effect of pimozide on amphetamine induced arousal, euphoria and anorexia in man, *Neuropharmacology* (1980) **19,** 1235–1237.

154. Silverstone, J.T. & Kyriakides, M. Clinical pharmacology of appetite. In: Silverstone, T. (ed.) *Drugs and Appetite,* London: Academic Press (1982) 107.

155. Silverstone, J.T. & Wells, B. Clinical psychopharmacology of amphetamine and related compounds. *In:* Caldwell, J. (ed.) *Amphetamine and Related Stimulants,* Boca Raton, Florida: CRC Press (1980).

156. Smart, J.V. & Turner, P. Influence of urinary pH on the degree and duration of action of amphetamine on the critical flicker fusion frequency in man, *Brit. J. Pharmacol. Chemother.* (1966) **26,** 468–472.

157. Smith, G.M. & Beecher, H.K. Amphetamine sulphate and athletic performance. 1. Objective effects, *J. Am. Med. Assoc.* (1959) **170,** 524–557.

158. Smith, G.M. & Beecher, H.K. Drugs and judgement: effects of amphetamine and secobarbital on self-stimulation, *J. Psychol.* (1964) **58,** 397–405.

159. Smith, R.C. & Davis, J.M. Comparative effects of d-amphetamine, l-amphetamine and methylphenidate on mood in man, *Psychopharmacology* (1977) **53,** 1–12.

160. Snead, O.C. Gamma hydroxybutyrate, *Life Sci.* (1977) **20,** 1935–1944.

161. Solomon, P.S., Mitchell, R.S. & Prinzmetal, M. The use of benzedrine sulphate in postencephalitic Parkinson's disease, *J. Am. Med.Assoc.* (1937) **108,** 1765–1770.

162. Sroufe, L.A. & Stewart, M.A. Treating problem children with stimulant drugs, *New Engl. J. Med.* (1973) **289,** 407–413.

163. Svensson, T.H. The effect of inhibition of catecholamine synthesis on dexamphetamine induced central stimulation, *Eur. J. Pharmacol.* (1970) **12,** 161–167.

164. Taylor, K.M. & Snyder, S.H. Amphetamine: differentiation by d and l isomers of behaviour

involving brain norepinephrine or dopamine, *Science* (1970) **168**, 1487–1489.

165.   Taylor, K.M. & Snyder, S.H. Differential effects of d- and l-amphetamine on behaviour and on catecholamine disposition in dopamine and norepinephrine-containing neurones of rat brain, *Brain Res.* (1971) **28**, 295–309.

166.   Tecce, J.J. & Cole, J.O. Amphetamine effects in man: paradoxical drowsiness and lowered electrical brain activity (CNV), *Science* (1974) **185**, 451–453.

167.   Thompson, C., Schachter, M. & Parkes, J.D. Drugs for cataplexy, *Ann. Neurol.* (1982) **12**, 63–64.

168.   Thornburg, J.E. & Moore, K.E. Dopamine and norepinephrine uptake by rat brain synaptosomes: relative inhibitory potencies of l- and d-amphetamine and amantadine, *Res. Comm. Chem. Path. Pharmacol.* (1973) **5**, 81–89.

169.   Trinker, F.R. & Rand, M.J. The effect of nialamide, pargyline and tranylcypramine on the removal of amphetamine by the perfused liver, *J. Pharm. Pharmacol.* (1970) **22**, 496–499.

170.   Turner, P. Peripheral mechanisms of action of fenfluramine, *Curr. Med. Res. Opin.* (1979) **6**, Suppl. 1, 101–106.

171.   Ulrich, H. Narcolepsy and its treatment with benzedrine sulfate, *New Engl. J. Med.* (1937) **217**, 696–701.

172.   Vein, A.M. *Disturbances of Sleep and Wakefulness*, Moscow: Izdatelstvo Meditsina (1974) 383.

173.   Vespignani, H., Barroche, G., Escaillas, J.P. & Weber, M. Importance of mazindol in the treatment of narcolepsy, *Sleep* (1984) **7**, 274–275.

174.   Wallace, A.G. AN 448 sandoz (mazindol) in the treatment of obesity, *Med. J. Aust.* (1976) **1**, 343.

175.   Weiner, W.J., Goetz, C.G., Nausieda, P.A. & Klawans, H.L. Amphetamine-induced hypersensitivity in guinea pigs, *Neurology (Minneap.)* (1979) **29**, 1054–1057.

176.   Weiss, G. & Hechtman, L. The hyperactive child syndrome, *Science* (1979) **205**, 1348–1354.

177.   Weissman, A., Koe, B.K. & Tenen, S.S. Antiamphetamine effects following inhibition of tyrosine hydroxylase, *J. Pharmacol. Exp. Ther.* (1966) **151**, 339–352.

178.   Willis, T. *The London Practise of Physick: or the Whole Practical Part of Physick*, London: Basset (1685) 397.

179.   Wyatt, R.J., Fram, D.H., Buchbinder, R. & Snyder, F. Treatment of intractable narcolepsy with a monoamine oxidase inhibitor. *New Engl. J. Med.* (1971) **285**, 987–991.

180.   Wyler, A.R., Wilkins, R.J. & Troupin, A.S. Methysergide in the treatment of narcolepsy, *Arch. Neurol.* (1975) **32**, 265–268.

181.   Yokel, R.A. & Pickens, R. Drug levels of d- and l-amphetamine during intravenous self-administration, *Psychopharmacologia* (1974) **34**, 255–264.

182.   Yoss, R.E. Treatment of narcolepsy. *Modern Treatment* (1969) **6**, 1263–1264.

183.   Yoss, R.E. & Daly, D.D. Treatment of narcolepsy with ritalin, *Neurology (Minneap.)* (1959) **9**, 171–173.

184.   Zarcone, V. Narcolepsy. A review of the syndrome, *New Engl. J. Med.* (1973) **288**, 1156–1165.

Index